toward a moral horizon

toward a moral horizon
Nursing Ethics for Leadership and Practice

EDITED BY

JANET L. STORCH, UNIVERSITY OF VICTORIA

PATRICIA RODNEY, UNIVERSITY OF VICTORIA

ROSALIE STARZOMSKI, UNIVERSITY OF VICTORIA

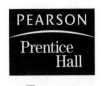

PEARSON
Prentice
Hall

Toronto

National Library of Canada Cataloguing in Publication Data

Toward a moral horizon : nursing ethics for leadership and practice / edited by Janet L. Storch, Patricia Rodney, Rosalie Starzomski. — 1st ed.

Includes bibliographical references and index.
ISBN 0-13-139716-8

1. Nursing ethics. I. Storch, Janet L., 1940- II. Rodney, Patricia Anne, 1955- III. Starzomski, Rosalie Catherine, 1956-

RT85.T68 2004   174'.2   C2003-904918-3

ISBN 0-13-139716-8

Vice President, Editorial Director: Michael J. Young
Executive Editor: Samantha Scully
Marketing Manager: Cas Shields
Developmental Editor: Angela Kurmey
Production Editor: Joel Gladstone
Production Coordinator: Andrea Falkenberg
Page Layout: Heidi Palfrey
Art Director: Mary Opper
Cover Image: Getty Images
Illustrations: Eileen Mosca, Graphic Artist, Vancouver, B.C.

1 2 3 4 5   08 07 06 05 04

Printed and bound in Canada.

Contents

Foreword

What you have before you is a unique, timely, scholarly book. Unique because it is the first nursing ethics book written for study at an advanced level. Timely because more and more nurses are seeking source materials that relate to the application of moral knowledge to ethical problems in everyday nursing practice, education, research, and management of nursing care. Nursing leadership for supporting the ethical practice of nurses and other health team members is desperately needed. Also, it is timely because of the increasing complexity of ethical problems, and because of the moral distress associated with nurses' working circumstances created by downsizing at all levels of health care.

It is a scholarly book because it is rooted in moral knowledge. To paraphrase Philip H. Phenix, it is rooted "in what a nurse *ought to voluntarily do.*" Part of the scholarliness of this book is the persistence of the authors and Editors in identifying the philosophical and historical cores of nursing ethical meanings, and in giving concrete nursing practice-based examples of issues and dilemmas, such as being faced with opposing ethical principles, the lack of nurses' autonomy to take action, and the complexity of trying to deal with interrelated individual, family, professional, and societal ethical problems. These practice-based narratives constitute powerful illustrations of how the *contexts* of ethical situations can profoundly affect the nature, occurrence, and complexity of nursing ethics.

The significance of this book extends far beyond nurses and nursing, for it is relevant—directly and indirectly—to all other health professionals and to those in other disciplines whose focus is on education, health, and social policy. Similarly, it is widely relevant to consumer groups and other NGOs, and to those in governments who "ought to voluntarily do" good in their practice.

In sum, this book is a nursing ethics moral integrity landmark.

Shirley M. Stinson, OC, AOE, RN, EdD, LLD (Hon), DSc (Hon)
Professor Emerita
Faculty of Nursing, and Department of Public Health Sciences
University of Alberta

Preface

We have talked about developing this book for a very long time. Initially we had intended it to be a text that we would author ourselves. An opportunity arose to begin the work (an opportunity motivated by approval of a new graduate course in advanced nursing ethics), and we seized the moment. At that juncture we considered the rich array of nursing ethics literature being developed by our nursing and other colleagues across Canada, and we decided to invite them into our project. One of the most enjoyable aspects of preparing this book was that our Canadian nursing colleagues said yes to our invitation to contribute, and that so many others were generous in reviewing chapters for us. The same has been true of our colleagues from other disciplines and other countries. Altogether, the support we have received has been energizing and inspiring.

Our original reasons for developing this book remain unchanged. To date, many wonderful nursing ethics texts have been developed for undergraduate students in nursing, including several in Canada. But what we found missing was a Canadian text in nursing ethics that both provided greater depth in nursing ethics and advanced the field of nursing ethics. We hope our book has achieved both of these goals. We envision this book being used in graduate nursing courses (and senior undergraduate courses), in clinical settings by senior nursing clinicians and advanced practice nurses, by nurse managers/administrators, in professional nursing associations and groups, in health policy units within provincial or federal governments, and by researchers conducting inquiry in health care or nursing ethics. We also hope that it will be of interest to other health professionals, both for what they can learn about nursing and what they might learn about health care ethics.

We three editors have enjoyed a long history in nursing ethics and health care ethics. Each of us has served on national committees related to nursing ethics, research ethics, or specific ethics areas; on provincial committees and with provincial nursing associations dealing with ethical issues; as "ethics consultants" to clinical agencies; and/or as members of clinical ethics committees; and all of us have studied, researched, written, and taught health ethics and nursing ethics. Based upon these experiences and particularly our nursing ethics research projects (completed and in progress), we are committed to the importance of addressing the issues of everyday ethics that nurses face, since these have too often been marginalized in health ethics. We have therefore endeavoured to create a text that is theoretically and practically relevant by including

- a wide range of moral concepts that undergird an approach to nursing ethics that focuses on the everyday as well as quandary (life-and-death) moral situations that nurses experience in their practice;
- a wider ethics vocabulary to describe the everyday as well as quandary situations that nurses experience;
- a range of topics to illustrate how these situations are experienced in practice—for example, in home care, in understanding care in situations of domestic violence, and in caring for children;
- "Ethics in Practice" narratives and cases in the chapters;

- "For Reflection" questions at the end of each chapter;
- extensive endnotes in many chapters to allow students, clinicians, teachers, and researchers to pursue related items of interest to them; and
- extensive references to support others to take up or continue work in nursing ethics.

Following the introductory chapter, we structure our book in three sections, which we have titled **Moral Landscape**, **Moral Climate**, and **Moral Horizons**. The first two chapters in Moral Landscape set the stage for the book by articulating the history of nursing ethics (Chapter 2) and the relationship to nursing philosophy (Chapter 3). We then move into a more detailed exploration of the interface of health care ethics with nursing ethics in the following four chapters (Chapters 4–7), after which we feature a chapter describing nurses' moral agency (Chapter 8). Thus, Moral Landscape provides an overview of the history and background within which nursing ethics needs to be understood.

The current sociopolitical and economic factors that affect nursing, and the ways in which these realities are being lived and described in practice, are explored in the second section of the book, Moral Climate. The first five chapters in this section provide a view of current funding challenges to health care delivery (Chapter 9), the challenges that nurses face in their workplaces (Chapters 10, 11, and 12), and the realities of end-of-life care (Chapter 13). We conclude this section with a chapter on narrative-based ethics, which offers both a description of the current climate and a means by which we can address that climate, as well as practical ideas for teachers of ethics (Chapter 14).

In the final section, Moral Horizons, the wider perspectives on health care, as well as social situations that inform nursing ethics, are explored in a number of issue-focused chapters (biotechnology, globalization, research, genetics, care of children, and violence against women are considered) (Chapters 15–20). While these chapters by no means cover the full scope of issues, we believe that the range we have selected is representative. In this section we then move to new ways to understand nursing ethics, including embodied knowing (Chapter 21), emotional sensitivity (Chapter 22), evolving spirituality (Chapter 23), and a deeply relational approach (Chapter 24). We conclude with a short chapter that attends to some issues foreshadowed but not addressed in the book, as well as questions for what are as yet largely unexplored horizons (Chapter 25).

The Appendices are meant to provide readers with supplemental resource materials. Appendix A provides a brief description of an Ethics in Practice study we have undertaken with other nursing faculty at the University of Victoria, and which we refer to at times in our own chapters; Appendix B includes three ethical decision-making frameworks; Appendix C contains the Canadian Code of Ethics for Registered Nurses; and Appendix D offers the Canadian Ethical Research Guidelines for Registered Nurses.

We acknowledge with deep appreciation the many people who helped make this book possible—they are and continue to be our network of support. We recognize with gratitude those who contributed chapters and those who served as reviewers: they are listed in the front section of our book. Here we want to thank them most sincerely for helping to create what we hope will be a memorable milestone publication in nursing ethics. Included in this company are numerous Canadians as well as colleagues from Australia, France, Norway, Sweden, and the United States. Our contributors and reviewers are primarily nurses, although we also benefitted from the expertise of colleagues in ethics, law, medicine, rehabilitation, sociology, and theology. We gratefully acknowledge permission granted by the

Canadian Association of Critical Care Nurses (CACCN) for the use of their members' poems in Chapter 14, "Narrative Ethics in Health Care." We also gratefully acknowledge Eileen Mosca, Graphic Artist, Vancouver, B.C., for permission to use her eagle illustrations to open each section of the book. We would like to extend our particular thanks to Lori d'Agincourt-Canning, who stood by to review manuscripts for us at a late date; Shirley Stinson who graciously agreed to write a foreword for this book; Kate Howe for her patient work on references; the staff of the Oak Bay Beach Hotel in Victoria for their hospitality; and all those in our lives who gave us concessions of time so we could complete this book. This includes Don Storch, John Thomasson, and the Starzomski family. It also includes our faculty colleagues on our research team: Colleen Varcoe and Gweneth Doane; the graduate students who have worked with us: Bernadette Pauly, Helen Brown, Gladys McPherson, and Karen Mahoney; and our able assistant, Jill Nichol. Included, as well, are the faculty and staff of the School of Nursing, University of Victoria who have kindly supported us in our work. The Canadian Nurses Association and the Canadian Bioethics Society have been fundamental to our continued networking opportunities. We offer both organizations our appreciation and praise.

Janet L. Storch, Patricia Rodney, and Rosalie Starzomski

About the Editors

Janet (Jan) Storch is a Professor at the University of Victoria School of Nursing. She has been a scholar in ethics since the mid-1970s and has served and continues to serve on numerous clinical and research ethics committees at local, regional, and national levels. She served as President of the Canadian Bioethics Society (1992–1993) and the National Council on Ethics in Human Research (1999–2001), Chair of the Canadian Nurses Ethics Advisory Committee (1997–2001), and she was Ethics Scholar in Residence at the Canadian Nurses Association (2001–2002). She is a Faculty Associate of the W. Maurice Young Centre for Applied Ethics at UBC, and Chair of the Human Research Ethics Committee at UVIC.

Patricia (Paddy) Rodney is an Associate Professor with the University of Victoria School of Nursing (located on the Lower Mainland Campus). Her clinical background in critical care nursing led to her long-standing interest in ethics. She has been a member of clinical ethics committees at St. Paul's Hospital and at BC Women's Hospital and Health Centre in Vancouver. Paddy is a Research Associate with Providence Health Care Ethics Services, a Faculty Associate with the W. Maurice Young Centre for Applied Ethics at UBC, and current Chair of the Canadian Nurses Association Ethics Committee.

Rosalie Starzomski is an Associate Professor with the University of Victoria School of Nursing (Lower Mainland Campus), an Ethics Consultant at the Vancouver Hospital and Health Sciences Centre, and a Faculty Associate of the W. Maurice Young Centre for Applied Ethics at UBC. Her clinical background includes many years as a nephrology/transplant advanced practice nurse. She is a member of the Canadian Council on Donation and Transplantation, Health Canada's Expert Advisory Committee for Xenograft Regulation, and the Board of Directors of the Canadian Organ Replacement Registry.

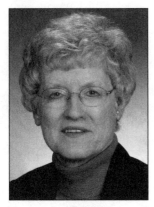 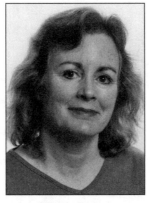 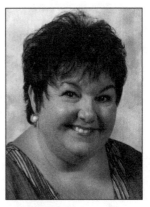

Janet Storch   Patricia Rodney   Rosalie Starzomski

Contributors

EDITORS

Janet (Jan) Storch, RN, MHSA, PhD
Professor, School of Nursing and Faculty Associate
W. Maurice Young Centre for Applied Ethics, UBC
University of Victoria, Victoria, BC

Patricia (Paddy) Rodney, RN, MSN, PhD
Associate Professor, School of Nursing and Faculty Associate
W. Maurice Young Centre for Applied Ethics, UBC
Lower Mainland Campus, University of Victoria
Vancouver, BC

Rosalie Starzomski, RN, MN, PhD
Associate Professor, School of Nursing and Faculty Associate
W. Maurice Young Centre for Applied Ethics, UBC
Lower Mainland Campus, University of Victoria
Vancouver, BC

OTHER CONTRIBUTORS

Wendy Austin, RN, MN, PhD
Associate Professor, Faculty of Nursing and
John Dossetor Health Ethics Center
Canada Research Chair (Relational Ethics in Health Care)
University of Alberta, Edmonton, AB

Vangie Bergum, RN, MEd, PhD
Professor, Faculty of Nursing and
John Dossetor Health Ethics Center
University of Alberta, Edmonton, AB

Helen Brown, RN, MSN, PhD (C)
Doctoral Candidate
School of Nursing, University of Victoria
Victoria, BC

Michael Burgess, PhD
Chair in Biomedical Ethics, The W. Maurice Young Centre for Applied Ethics
University of British Columbia, Vancouver, BC

Franco Carnevale, RN, MSc(A), MEd., MSc., PhD
Associate Professor, McGill University School of Nursing
Head Nurse, Montreal Children's Hospital
Montreal, PQ

Susan Cox, PhD
Assistant Professor and Michael Smith Foundation for Health Research Scholar
The W. Maurice Young Centre for Applied Ethics
University of British Columbia
Vancouver, BC

Gweneth Doane, RN, MA, PhD
Associate Professor, School of Nursing
University of Victoria, Victoria, BC

Joy Johnson, RN, MN, PhD
Professor, School of Nursing
University of British Columbia, Vancouver, BC

Marianne Lamb, RN, MN, PhD
Professor and Director, School of Nursing and
Associate Dean (Health Sciences)
Queen's University, Kingston, ON

Joan Liaschenko, RN, PhD
Associate Professor, School of Nursing and
Center for Bioethics, University of Minnesota
Minneapolis, Minnesota

Patricia Marck, RN, MN, PhD
Assistant Professor, Faculty of Nursing, University of Alberta
Adjunct Professor, John Dossetor Health Ethics Centre
Professional Practice Leader, Nursing, Royal Alexandra Hospital,
Edmonton, AB

Michael McDonald, PhD
Maurice Young Professor of Applied Ethics
The W. Maurice Young Centre for Applied Ethics
University of British Columbia, Vancouver, BC

Gladys McPherson, RN, MSN, PhD (C)
Doctoral Candidate
School of Nursing, University of British Columbia
Vancouver, BC

Jeffrey Nisker, MD, FRCS
Professor, Obstetric and Gynecology and Oncology
Faculty of Medicine and Dentistry
University of Western Ontario
London, ON

Per Nordvedt, RN, PhD
Associate Professor, Center for Medical Ethics
Medical Faculty, University of Oslo
Oslo, Norway

Kathleen Oberle, RN, MN, PhD
Associate Professor, Faculty of Nursing
University of Calgary, Calgary, AB

Bernadette Pauly, RN, MN, PhD (C)
Doctoral Candidate
School of Nursing, University of Victoria
Victoria, BC

Elizabeth Peter, RN, MScN, PhD
Assistant Professor, Faculty of Nursing
University of Toronto, Toronto, ON

Jane Simington, RN, MN, PhD
Adjunct Professor, Faculty of Nursing,
Adjunct Professor, St. Stephen's Theological College
Mental Health Consultant (Simington Consulting)
Edmonton, AB

Vicki Smye, RN, MHSc, PhD (C)
Visiting Lecturer, School of Nursing
Lower Mainland Campus, University of Victoria
Vancouver, BC

Annette F. Street, PhD
Professor, Cancer and Palliative Care Studies
Director, La Trobe/Health Clinical School of Nursing
Heidelberg West, Australia

Colleen Varcoe, RN, MEd, MSN, PhD
Associate Professor, School of Nursing,
Lower Mainland Campus, University of Victoria
Vancouver, BC

Reviewers

Susan Albersheim, BSc(Med), MD, FRCPC
Clinical Professor, Medicine, University of British Columbia
Staff Neonatologist, Children's and Women's Health Centre of BC

Wendy Amos, RN, MN
Clinical Nurse Specialist, Vancouver Island Health Authority
(South Island), Victoria, BC

Terry Anderson, BA, BD, STM, ThD
Professor Emeritus of Christian Social Ethics
Vancouver School of Theology, Vancouver, BC

Katherine Arnold, LLB
Co-Chair, BC Women's Hospital
and Health Centre Ethics Committee, Vancouver, BC

Anne-Marie Arseneault, RN, MSN
Professor, École de science infirmière, Université de Moncton
Moncton, NB

Elizabeth Banister, RN, PhD
Associate Professor, School of Nursing, University of Victoria
Victoria, BC

Danielle Blondeau, PhD
Professor, Faculté de sciences infirmières, Université Laval
Sainte-Foy, Quebec

Alister Browne, PhD
Chair, Dept. of Philosophy, Langara College and Ethics Consultant,
Vancouver Hospital & Health Sciences Centre, Vancouver, BC

Helen Brown, RN, MSN, PhD (c)
Doctoral Candidate
University of Victoria, School of Nursing
Victoria, BC

Laurel Brunke, RN, MSN
Executive Director, Registered Nurses Association of British Columbia
Vancouver, BC

Rabbi Dr. Reuven P. Bulka
Congregation Machzikei Hadas
Ottawa, Ontario

Mary C. Corley, RN, PhD
Associate Professor Emeritus, Virginia Commonwealth University
Richmond, Virginia

Lori d'Agincourt-Canning, MA, MSc, PhD
Post Doctoral Fellow, Department of Medical Genetics
University of British Columbia, Vancouver, BC

Anne Davis, RN, PhD, DSc (Hon.), FAAN
Professor Emerita, University of California, San Francisco
Professor, Part Time, Nagano College of Nursing, Japan

Raisa B. Deber, PhD
Professor, Department of Health Policy, Management and Evaluation,
University of Toronto
Director, From Medicare to Home and Community Research Unit, Toronto, ON

John B. Dossetor, OC, BM BCh, PhD
Professor Emeritus, Medicine/Bioethics, University of Alberta
Ottawa, ON

Mary Lou Ellerton, RN, MN*
Associate Professor, School of Nursing, Dalhousie University
Halifax, NS

Janet Ericksen, RN, MA (Nursing)
Assistant Professor Emeritus, School of Nursing, University of British Columbia
Vancouver, BC

Bethan Everett, PhD (c)
Doctoral Candidate, Interdisciplinary Studies, University of British Columbia
Vancouver, BC

Arthur W. Frank, PhD
Professor, Department of Sociology
Adjunct Professor, Faculty of Nursing
University of Calgary, Calgary, AB

Linda J. Frost, RN, MA
Education Practice Advisor, Vancouver Coastal Health Authority
Vancouver, BC

*We are sad to report that since serving as reviewer, our colleague Mary Lou Ellerton has died.

Sara T. Fry, RN, PhD, FAAN
Professor of Nursing Ethics, Boston College
Chestnut Hill, Massachusetts

Sally Gadow, RN, PhD
Professor of Nursing
University of Colorado Health Sciences Centre
and School of Nursing, Denver, Colorado

Angela Gillis, RN, PhD
Professor of Nursing, Saint Francis Xavier University
Antigonish, NS

Walter Glannon, PhD
Clinical Ethicist, BC Children's and Women's Health Centre of BC
Assistant Professor, The W. Maurice Young Centre for Applied Ethics,
University of British Columbia, Vancouver, BC

Lorraine (Laurie) Hardingham, RN, MA
Clinical Ethicist, St. Joseph's Hospital
London, ON

Christine Harrison, PhD
Director of Bioethics, The Hospital for Sick Children
Assistant Professor, University of Toronto
Toronto, ON

Virginia E. Hayes, RN, PhD
Associate Professor, School of Nursing, University of Victoria
Lower Mainland Campus, Vancouver, BC

Barry Hoffmaster, PhD
Professor, Departments of Philosophy and Family Medicine
University of Western Ontario, London, ON

Bashir Jiwani, MA
Former Special Projects Consultant, Provincial Health Ethics Network
Edmonton, AB

Megan-Jane Johnstone, RN, BA, PhD, FRCNA, FCN (NSW)
Professor of Nursing, Director of Research, Dept. of Nursing and Midwifery,
RMIT University, Melbourne, Australia

Bonnie Lantz, RN, MN
President, Registered Nurses Association of British Columbia
Director of Health Services, Fraser North, Fraser Health Authority
Burnaby, BC

Sandy Leadbeater, RN, PhD
Humber School of Health Sciences Program and
UNB Humber Collaborative Bachelor of Nursing Program, Toronto, ON

Kim Lutzen, RN, PhD
Professor and Director
Ersta-Skondal University College
Stockholm, Sweden

Abbyann Lynch, CM, PhD
Director, Ethics in Health Care Associates
Toronto, ON

Chris MacDonald, PhD
Assistant Professor, Department of Philosophy, Saint Mary's University
Halifax, NS

Marjorie McIntyre, RN, PhD
Associate Professor, University of Calgary
Calgary, AB

Gail Mitchell, RN, PhD
Assistant Professor, University of Toronto
Toronto, ON

W.J. Mussell, MEd
Chairman, Native Mental Health Association of Canada
Principal Educator, Sal'i'shan Institute Society
Chilliwack, BC

Astrid Norberg, RN, PhD
Professor, Department of Nursing, University of Umeå
Umeå, Sweden

Douglas P. Olsen, RN, PhD
Associate Director, Center for Health Policy and Ethics,
School of Nursing, Yale University, New Haven, Connecticut

Carole Orchard, RN, EdD
Associate Professor and Director
University of Western Ontario, London, ON

Eleanor Pask, RN, EdD
Sessional Assistant Professor
School of Nursing, York University, Toronto, ON

Mary Ellen Purkis, RN, PhD
Associate Professor and Director
School of Nursing, University of Victoria, Victoria, BC

Barbara K. Redman, RN, PhD, FAAN
Dean and Professor, College of Nursing, Wayne State University
Detroit, Michigan

Susan Sherwin, PhD, FRSC
University Research Professor, Department of Philosophy
Dalhousie University
Halifax, NS

Vicki Smye, RN, MHSc, PhD (C)
Visiting Lecturer, School of Nursing
Lower Mainland Campus, University of Victoria
Vancouver, BC

Morrie Steele, RPN, RN, MS
Instructor, University College of the Fraser Valley
Abbottsford, BC

Carol Taylor, CSFN, RN, MSN, PhD
Director, Center for Clinical Bioethics
Assistant Professor, Nursing, Georgetown University
Washington, District of Columbia

Theresa Thompson RN, BSN
Nurse Educator, Gerontology, Saint Paul's Hospital
Vancouver, BC

Jo Wearing, RN, MSN
Director, Policy Division, Registered Nurses Association of British Columbia
Vancouver, BC

George C. Webster, PhD
Clinical Ethicist, Health Care Ethics Service, Saint Boniface General Hospital
Winnipeg, MN

John Williams, PhD
Director of Ethics, World Medical Association
Ferney-Voltaire, France

Jenny M. Young, MSW
Patient Services Manager, Spinal Cord Program
GF Strong Rehabilitation Centre
Vancouver, BC

Lynne E. Young, RN, PhD
Associate Professor, School of Nursing, University of Victoria
Lower Mainland Campus, Vancouver, BC

Susan Young, RN, MN
Clinical Nurse Specialist, Nephrology
Providence Health Care/Saint Paul's Hospital
Vancouver, BC

chapter one

Nursing Ethics:

A Developing Moral Terrain

Janet L. Storch

... [N]ursing ethics is about being in relationship to persons in care. The enactment of nursing ethics is a constant readiness to engage our moral agency.

Nurses have always had to deal with a variety of ethical challenges. These challenges include determining how to ensure patients have the information they need prior to consenting to medical interventions, ensuring the safety of residents in long-term care without using physical restraints, or having to tube-feed patients who are actively resisting the procedure. It is only in the last three decades, however, that nurse scholars and senior nurse practitioners have identified nursing ethics as a unique area of inquiry (see, for example, Jameton 1984; Storch 1988; Fry 1989; Fry 1992; Benner, Tanner and Chesla 1996; Woods 1999; Tschudin 1999; Smith and Godfrey 2002; Storch et al. 2002; Rodney et al. 2002).

Since the mid-eighties, significant advances have been made in defining the academic and practice knowledge that comprise nursing ethics. The dominance of medical ethics, and bioethics as defined by medical ethics, has long seemed too limiting for nursing practice. Chambliss (1996), in his sociological study of caring, and Johnstone (1989, 1999), for example, draw attention to the fact that nurses have been bypassed and marginalized in the discipline of bioethics.[1] While bioethics and medical ethics have contributed to nursing ethics, nursing ethics is distinct from both (Fry 1989). Further, nurses' ethical concerns are not adequately addressed in either medical ethics or bioethics. Many nurses involved in the scholarship of ethics, as well as nurses providing direct care, have found the ethics of nursing practice to be separate and distinct. Nursing is a profession with a moral mandate that differs from the medical mandate in that nurses address the full diversity of need, with less emphasis on treatment and cure. Further, nurses occupy a unique moral in-between position in that they are answerable not only to patients or clients but also to organizations.

The editors of this text have recognized this reality for some time and, with the help of our colleagues, were determined to act on that knowledge. All three editors have been involved in providing direct nursing care, serving on ethics committees, providing ethics consultation, initiating dialogue about ethics with colleagues in nursing and other disciplines, and participating in scholarly inquiry. In 1999, along with several other nursing colleagues, we set out to explore what ethics means to nurses involved in direct practice, to nurses in advanced practice, and to student nurses.[2] The results of that research (see Appendix A for a synopsis), along with our background in nursing and in ethics, led to the development of this text. This book is designed to be a resource for nurses in graduate studies and in advanced practice. Fortunately, nurses in other parts of Canada and the Western world have also begun to research the unique features of nursing ethics (see, for example, Woods 1999; Smith and Godfrey 2002). Throughout this text, we draw upon our own research findings (Appendix A; Storch et al. 2002; Rodney et al. 2002) and those of other nurse scholars, as well as our own and other nurses' stories from practice.

Many nursing ethics texts and other ethics resources developed over the past decade offer a general overview of the issues involved in ethics, most intended for undergraduate students in nursing and other health professional disciplines. These resources have served us well because the level of ethical fitness amongst registered nurses and other direct care professions has been a developing field of inquiry.[3] Now that ethics is more fully recognized as an integral part of the nursing profession, we need to continue to explore and define the parameters of nursing ethics.

Nurses in every arena of practice face a myriad of challenges as they try to uphold the ethical standards of the profession in increasingly constrained practice environments. Our profession is in urgent need of nurse leaders who have had the opportunity to develop confidence in the language of ethics, and who can push inquiry forward in *nursing* ethics. This text is meant to provide support for such leadership. It is targeted at nurses who are ready for advanced studies in nursing ethics, whether they are students in undergraduate and graduate programs, nurses in direct practice, advanced practice nurses, administrators, researchers, educators, or nurses working in professional associations and unions. We need formal and informal leadership in ethics throughout every facet of our profession. And we need leadership that can support the ethical practice of our colleagues in other disciplines. We therefore hope that this text will also be relevant for members of other health care professions as well as for members of academic disciplines studying health care ethics. It is our hope not only that those in other health care professions and academia will be enabled to understand the ethics challenges facing nursing, but also that they will gain insights into the ethics involved in their own professional practices.

In the remainder of this chapter, we set the stage for what follows in the text. In particular, we lay out our understanding of the practical and theoretical challenges that our profession faces in articulating (and hence defending) the ethics of nursing practice.

DEFINING ETHICS

The classic textbook definition of **ethics** is "a generic term for various ways of understanding and examining the moral life" (see, for example, Beauchamp and Childress 2001, 1). **Practical ethics** then makes reference to "the use of ethical theory and methods of analysis to examine moral problems, practices, and policies in several areas, including the professions and public policy" (Beauchamp and Childress 1994, 4). **Professional ethics** emphasizes the primacy of relationships in ethics, often citing professional obligations to those served (Pellegrino and Thomasma 1988). **Bioethics** emerged as a field of inquiry in the mid-seventies and, in its most inclusive form, includes all ethics issues related to life, including animal rights and environmental concerns. **Medical ethics,** the moral ideals and virtues involved in the practice of medicine (including life and death decision-making), flourished within the field of bioethics. This was particularly so as newer technologies (such as respirators and dialysis machines) changed medical practice and caused a host of new ethical decisions to surface, including the need to change the criteria for determination of death. Since the inception of bioethics, medical ethicists and bioethicists have tended to assume that all other health professions neatly fit under the umbrella of bioethics and medical ethics. But as Fry (1989), Johnstone (1999), and others have noted, not all health providers can identify with the strong focus on the heroic issues of bioethics and medical ethics, and many disagree that medical ethics could or should subsume all health care providers. Thus, the language of **health care ethics,** as the field of inquiry involving individual provider-patient relationships as well as the organizational and societal ethics in health care and health policy, evolved as a broader approach to ethics in health care (Provincial Health Ethics Network 1995). Finally, nursing has focused on its own concerns in ethics and has identified **nursing ethics** as a unique field or discipline that deals with the moral dimension of nursing and its norms (Yeo and Moorhouse 1996). We believe that ethics is part of every nursing role and function because ethics is about relationships and about the moral commitments of nurses to those they serve.

Ethics versus Morality

Many basic ethics texts contain some initial discussion about the meaning of the words **ethics** and morals, or **morality.** Most writers agree that these two terms are quite interchangeable, since "ethics" is derived from ancient Greek (*ethikos* originally meaning "pertaining to custom and habit") and "morals" and "morality" are derived from Latin (*moralitas* originally meaning "custom or habit") (Johnstone 1999). Johnstone suggests that it is not incorrect to use these two terms interchangeably and that the choice is a matter of personal preference rather than of rigorous philosophical debate. Yet, until recently, use of the terms "morality" and "morals" has generally been avoided, with a preference for use of the words "ethics" and "ethical." One can only speculate on the reasons for this position. Perhaps "moral" contains too strong a religious connotation for some; for others it may be "too close to home," meaning that use of this vocabulary begins to involve them directly in that from which they have managed to distance themselves. Ethics can be held at an academic interest range; morality cannot. In this text, we choose to use the words interchangeably, although we will focus on the use of the word "moral" as an adjective to describe the range of circumstances experienced by individuals who try to be ethical.

Ethics in Practice

To provide tangible and steady links to nursing practice in this book, almost every chapter includes a practice story, a narrative, or a quote from a research transcript; these are called "Ethics in Practice." Through these stories we hope to stimulate moral imagination, foster meaningful engagement of our readers, and also provide practical tools for classroom teaching, unit discussion foci, and administrative consciousness-raising. We begin by using specific narratives from our own research as illustrations of the concepts that will be developed throughout this book. Following are four stories from practice as told by nurses in our research focus groups. (See Appendix A for details of the study in which these nurses participated.) These stories illustrate the meaning of ethics for nurses in practice and the important ethical leadership role of nurses in advanced practice. While each story provides a quick snapshot rather than a comprehensive account, we believe that together they start to capture some of the themes inherent in nurses' ethical practice. The story in Ethics in Practice 1-1 is told by a clinical nurse specialist.

Ethics in Practice 1-1	Moral Agency

One of the rewarding experiences I have had concerns ethical issues and advocacy for patients who are experiencing pain. When I first started in my role as clinical nurse specialist and pain management resource, there was a real move to better pain management and staff advocacy for patients in pain. This included standing up to physicians, families, and other care providers and focusing on what the patients need for appropriate pain management. I still remember one incident which was absolutely outstanding in my mind. One of the pain service physicians was arguing with a client and was actually verbally abusing this client. I got called about this and hurried to the Unit. As I entered the patient's room, there were two nurses who were actually physically taking the physician from the room and talking to him about pain management for that patient. They were attempting to get him out of the confrontation and were advocating for the person's pain management. Since the patient was an addict, for the staff to have come that far was mind-blowing!... That is the picture I have about advocacy.

In Ethics in Practice 1-1, the clinical nurse specialist (CNS) recognizes the way in which the staff nurses she has been working with have apparently accepted their **moral agency**—that is, their personal responsibility for advocating for care that best satisfies the patients' or clients' needs. The nurses have demonstrated their role as moral agents in their protection of the patient and in their protection of the physician as well. As the CNS noted, because the patient was an addict, the nurses' protective behaviour towards the patient, and their careful handling of a difficult situation to provide safety for each person involved, was ethically commendable. The concept of moral agency is a theme that will be developed further within this text.

Ethics in Practice 1-2	**Moral Sensitivity and Moral Dilemma**

I'm talking about a child dying at home. When the medical establishment, the treatment, failed, we lost credibility with the family. So the child went home on palliative care. Meanwhile the family brought in all these alternative therapies as a last ditch effort and (you can't blame them) they are desperate. But it meant that the child was not allowed to eat anything but green stuff, not allowed to watch TV because of radiation waves; and a lot of very odd and bizarre treatments were being tried. And the family was putting out mega bucks for this. And we knew it was not going to work, it wasn't going to change the outcome. But they don't believe us because we have lost credibility since our treatment did not work either. There is not a whole lot you can do about it because this is the family's choice, and if the child is old enough to know and knows that the parents are doing this out of love, then the child won't fight it. But for the nurses it is a real dilemma. Ethically, it's part of our Code to allow them to make their choice, but the other part is advocacy for the child. The question is, who is it right for? Best for who? And who gets to decide what is best? Do we really know what is best for the child? It's something the families live with the rest of their lives. We go out of their lives.

In Ethics in Practice 1-2, the nurse demonstrates a **moral sensitivity.** In other words, she is attuned to the physical, emotional, psychosocial, and spiritual needs of the persons for whom care is being provided. She is sensitive to the family's culture, including their faith in alternative therapy, that profoundly affects the dying child. Their right to hold these beliefs is not questioned by the nurse, who respects their autonomy in the situation. The nurse is also sensitive to the possibility that their behaviours may be motivated by desperation as they witness their child dying. But as the nurse observes, how does one acknowledge and respond to the needs of the child and the needs of the parents, knowing that the family is an integral unit? The nurse who strives to be ethical confronts this moral dilemma. A **moral dilemma** is a choice that involves opposing principles in support of mutually inconsistent courses of action. Moral dilemmas involving children and their parents will be discussed further in Chapter 19.

Ethics in Practice 1-3	**Moral Dilemma and Moral Distress**

I have come to a situation twice in my career, prior to working here, when I have ignored hospital policy because of my ethics. In both cases I found a person with terminal cancer, dead. And in both cases I didn't call a code. Because ethically I couldn't, I just simply couldn't. In both cases I was admonished by someone who said, "You have to call a code even if the person is dead." I'm sorry, I can't. End of story. The other time it was after the fact that I should have called a code because it is hospital policy. But just because the doctor forgot to write a "no code" on a terminal cancer patient, I can't continue the stupidity. But, I did contravene hospital policies twice and I will start doing it again and again. Because I cannot start jumping on somebody's chest just because the doctor forgot to write "no code." Ethically that is wrong in my gut, in my heart. I can't do it. And ethical is a feeling, it is honesty to me. Ethical is honest.

The situation described in Ethics in Practice 1-3 is one of the situations nurses most often identify as causing them the greatest feeling of **moral distress**—that is, the negative feelings resulting from a situation in which moral choices cannot be translated into moral action (Jameton 1984; Rodney and Starzomski 1993). In this story the nurse is caught between the official hospital regulation and the reality that, due to oversight, no order has been prepared to affect a person's "do not resuscitate" (DNR) status. In this case, others can certainly identify with the intensity of the nurse's moral distress and his or her feelings of anger, guilt, and frustration.

While some might suggest that the nurse is courageous in the stand she takes, this type of decision is not one any health professional should take alone. Communicating with others about the patient's distressing situation before the patient is in crisis is important for several reasons. The nurse may find that others can assist in changing the policy or in getting the DNR order prepared, or the nurse may find that others have information that assists in mitigating the distress she feels through new understanding about why no DNR order has been prepared. Difficult ethical situations require dialogue and reflection with others. Such interaction can be instrumental in preventing or alleviating moral distress. This situation also underscores the interface between ethical policy and practice. The nurse's ability to deal with the source of her moral distress would be greatly enhanced by supportive policy based on sound ethical principles—in this case a DNR policy that helps to address the patient, the family, and any potential interdisciplinary conflict may lead to a better outcome for all concerned. In Chapter 13, the dilemmas of DNR orders and other end-of-life decision-making are considered.

Ethics in Practice 1-4	Moral Distress and Moral Courage

I remember a situation where we had a family that needed to be supported in order to be able to remain together. That family was not able to provide enough resources to be able to care adequately for their mother who had become psychotic in the hospital. And, of course, English as a second language made it that much more difficult. What ended up happening, because resources weren't available, was that those children were apprehended at a time when the family needed to be supported in order to be able to remain together. We had an opportunity to sit down (all players). We looked at the sequence of events, why they happened, and how we could have made it a better outcome for the family. I

> think that ethically we really failed this family. It was not just a failure of community health but of the whole health care system, including the Ministry that holds the resources. We're saying people need resources, and then the fight begins in terms of trying to seek out those very few resources needed to keep that family together for the period of time it takes to get better. That doesn't happen in two days, three days, a week. It takes a longer period of time for some stability and for the crisis to ease, and to me that's very distressing.

In Ethics in Practice 1-4, the nurses could clearly see the possibility of the family overcoming the challenges they faced if they were provided with a modest amount of support from the health care system and from social welfare. They knew that keeping a family together can be health restoring for all of the family members; yet, they were unable to secure the resources needed to maintain the family unit. This situation was distressing to the nurses as they watched an all-too-common scenario unfold, in which resources were used to remove the children from the home: resources that might have been deployed to assist them to remain with their family. The nurses moved beyond their moral distress to demonstrate **moral courage**—the ability to overcome their fear of potential jeopardy as employees, the fear of increased interdepartmental conflict, and fear of job loss—to work with the health and social welfare team to review what had happened and what might have been done differently so that they might prevent future social injustices.

As these Ethics in Practice narratives illustrate, nursing ethics is about being in relationship to persons in care. The enactment of nursing ethics is a constant readiness to engage one's moral agency. Almost every nursing action and situation involves ethics. To raise questions about ethics is to ask about the good in our practice. Are we doing the right thing for this patient? Are we listening to this person's need for pain relief? Are we respecting a family's grief over their dying child as they struggle to squeeze out a few extra days or hours for the child through alternative therapies? Are we ready to stand up for what we know to be right when we face a situation requiring us to perform a procedure that we are confident is not appropriate and that violates the dignity of another human being? Are we willing to find time to debrief after complex situations to determine how we could have done better, with a commitment to doing everything in our power to prevent similar situations from occurring in the future?

Positive answers to these questions can lead to safe, competent, and ethical practice. But much more needs to be done. We need to educate student nurses, novice nurses, and often even experienced nurses, to imagine a different world—a world where ethical knowledge, skills, and attitudes are valued and rewarded. We also need to maintain a strong focus on and engagement in research in order to better understand ethics in practice and how it can be fostered. We hope that in the pages of this text nurses will see ways to understand and teach ethics differently, as well as recognize the need for further research in nursing ethics.

CONTEMPORARY ETHICAL CHALLENGES

One of the difficulties faced by those who would be ethical is that current practice environments are not the perfect places to ensure that nurses can engage in safe, competent, and ethical practice. Nurses face numerous challenges. The turbulence in the health care system, owing to cost restraints and serious lack of political foresight and action in Canada and virtually worldwide, is causing significant hardship for nurses and other staff members. The shortage of nurses, in particular, is one of the many manifestations of short-sighted thinking by governments at all levels. Nurses are working overtime, short-staffed, and under conditions that risk injury, illness, and low morale. Further, nurses are forced to accept casual and part-time employment because health care agencies are unable or unwilling to create full-time continuing positions (Varcoe and Rodney 2001; Duncan et al. 2001; Health Canada 2002; Storch 2003).[4]

Other ethical challenges exist as well, which both result from and are compounded by the problems we have cited above. First, nurses have difficulty in naming a situation as one that involves ethics. Second, the health care system has too few nursing leaders, and fewer yet who regard ethics as foundational to nursing practice. Third, we need to know more about ethics in practice, about strategies that help nurses become ethically fit, about how genuine teamwork can become a reality in all settings, and about better ways to address our ethical concerns. Within this text, we provide original work on ethics to augment the many ethics resources already available but with a specific focus on stimulating the development of a better **moral climate** for nurses (that is, an environment in which nurses are respected and enabled to provide safe, competent, and ethical care), as well as increased moral sensitivity to the ethics of the everyday in health care.

Ethical Awareness

Questioning whether various difficulties in health care and in nursing constitute an ethical issue, or an issue of another sort, is common in health care. Many nurses seem to be reticent to name situations as matters of ethics. Often this occurs because nurses' voices are silenced or, when nurses do name ethical issues, the response they receive suggests that ethics involves only one-to-one nurse-patient relationships, not organizational or political decisions that often lead to their ethical distress. It is only recently that nursing administration texts have begun to include chapters on ethics. Even then, many of these texts utilize business ethics or other non-nursing sources to discuss what is involved in being an ethical administrator. In doing so they ignore the unique responsibilities of nursing administrators in role modelling and teaching ethical behaviour, both in leadership with nursing staff as employees and as role models of ethical client care. Further, most texts have yet to show the everyday ethics of nursing administration.

The sidestepping of ethics occurs at all levels. Many documents that address the nursing shortage and the difficult conditions for nurses in practice (such as mandatory overtime, an overload in patient assignments, and interdisciplinary disputes) avoid naming these as matters of ethics. Why is this true? In national research reports, in federal policy discussions, and in the five-country study, naming concerns as ethical ones is not clearly evident (see, for example, Aiken et al. 2001; Baumann et al. 2001; O'Brien-Pallas, Baumann and Villeneuve 1994; Health Canada 2002; Havens and Aiken 1999; Scott, Sochalski and Aiken 1999). Some studies have shown that physicians and nurses have differing views on what constitutes an ethical problem (Prescott and Bowen 1985; Gramelspacher, Howell and Young 1986; Lindseth et al. 1994), but is it possible that there are widely different views about ethics and ethical problems amongst nurses as well? And if so, is that due to a lack of vocabulary to engage in ethical discourse? Is it because ethics seems too soft or sentimental? And if there are marked differences, what is at stake if we allow such divergent perspectives to continue to exist unchallenged?

We believe it is important that all nurses develop a greater ability to frame issues as matters of ethics. We believe that by naming issues appropriately, the search for solutions and the support for practitioners can be enhanced. This includes vocabulary that specifically focuses on ethical concerns at all levels of the health system, at the micro level (the level of client care), the meso level (the level of programs and organizations), and the macro level (the level of governments and other societal structures). In this text, we hope to be able to provide nurses with a language for ethics, greater sensitivity to ethics, and knowledge with which to enter into ethical discussion.

As important as it is to be able to identify situations as matters of ethics, it is more important to learn about how to use various ethics decision-making theories and models that can bring to nursing, and to health care teams overall, a meaningful way to address and resolve the issues nurses face in daily practice—in ways that result in positive patient/client outcomes. The past decade has seen significant development in the following theoretical perspectives in ethics: principle-based ethics, virtue ethics, contextual ethics (casuistry, feminist ethics), global ethics/ecological ethics, and political theory (see, for example, Botes 2000; Arras and Steinbock 1999). Attention has also been paid to resolving ethical differences amongst team members in a constructive manner in order to serve the needs of those in their care (see, for example, Canadian Healthcare Association et al. 1999; Miller et al. 2001).

Faculty and graduate students in nursing have adopted and developed newer theoretical perspectives and models more congruent with nursing's particular focus in care (Rodney 1991; Storch 1992; Alberta Association of Registered Nurses 1996; Bergum 1997; Starzomski 1998). In Chapters 4–7 of this text significant content is provided about the range of theoretical perspectives and about approaches to ethical decision-making. It is essential for nurses to know the theoretical origins of health ethics and nursing ethics, and their subsequent developments, to equip them to lead in practice, teaching, and research.

Ethical Leadership

Leaders in the nursing community who are committed to the development of nursing ethics have an opportunity to establish a **moral community**—a place in which the language of ethics is commonplace and in which the work environment promotes ethical discussion and action (Aroskar 1995; Storch 1999). Aroskar (1995) suggests that "nursing as a moral community initiates action to operationalize ethical principles and values in relationships among caregivers as a necessary co-requisite to compassionate care for clients."

During the past decade, the term "magnet hospitals" came to symbolize the best of practice, places where health professionals, and particularly nurses, flocked to work. These hospitals were known to allow nurses professional autonomy over their practice, as well as autonomy over their practice environments. They were also known for fostering effective communication amongst nurses, physicians, and administrators (Havens and Aiken 1999). These are all features of a workplace that makes safe, competent, and ethical practice possible. Although magnet hospitals did not give explicit attention to ethics, their practices accomplished the "good" and were found to make a significant difference to the persons in their care.

Nurses in the focus groups in our study (see Appendix A) spoke about the importance of nursing leadership in ethics and highlighted the challenges and opportunities in their work environment that allowed them to engage in ethical practice. For some nurses, the presence of structural resources such as ethics committees, ethics rounds, an ethics consultant, and ethics guidelines and protocols helped to create environments for them to grow and practice ethically. For others, the presence of similar resources had a limited effect on ethical nursing practice because, as one stated, "... what has not changed is the undercurrent of misunderstandings, miscommunications and not feeling heard."

In all but one of the 19 focus groups, nurses told us that the focus group session had allowed them to talk to other nurses—a luxury most said they did not have time for in their daily practice. The structures in nursing that formerly allowed nurses an opportunity to hear others discuss care of patients on the unit, and to gain a sense of the overall work of the unit for a given 12- to 24-hour period, have been lost on units where, for example, the "morning report," or any overall shift report for that matter, has been cancelled due to lack of time. Lost in such cancellations is the very substance of relationship building on a team, the time to deal with situations causing ethical distress, the opportunity to work together to problem solve in order to prevent bad care and bad outcomes, and the ability to take ownership for the work on the unit. All of these "goods" are lost in the rush of getting on with the work of caring for people who are intensely ill, dealing with greater numbers of admissions and discharges, and working with an insufficient number of staff to ensure safe, competent, and ethical individualized patient care.

In one focus group, the nurses reported that when they had expressed their need to talk to each other about their moral issues, organizational leaders had pointedly discouraged them from meeting as a group of professionals. Often the excuse was that nurses should be more inclusive of others. But as one nurse in our study said, "... other health professionals have not been criticized for wanting to meet together and be clear about their practice." Attempts to prevent nurses from sharing the burdens and joys of their work are a serious detriment to nursing morale, and lowered morale invariably proves to be detrimental to patient care.

Further, almost all continuing education opportunities, ranging from simple 15-minute sessions updating nurses on a new type of procedure, to more comprehensive sessions of an hour or a day or two, that allow nurses to keep current in their practice and to share their ethical concerns have vanished with cost cutting (Health Canada 2002; Storch et al. 2002). As a result, many nurses have cut themselves out of the system of caring, literally or figuratively. Continuing education cannot be regarded as a perk of the job: it is fundamental to competent practice and critical to nurses' sense of being valued for the emotional, mental, and physical work they do (Health Canada 2002).

Nursing leadership is desperately needed to demonstrate the value of nurses and nursing, both by leadership in practice and through political action to restore the losses and to retain nurses who are enabled to engage in ethical practice. Tschudin (1999) states her belief that "ethics is about power and how power is used." She suggests that nursing can use ethics as one way to reclaim its professional identity and move forward. Through this text we hope to better equip current and future nursing leaders to use ethical reflection, moral reasoning, and ethical theory as a way to move the system of care in the direction most effective for the well-being of persons of all ages who need good nursing care. Nurse leaders also need to know more to be able to do more. Research in nursing ethics and health ethics is critical to gain that knowledge and understanding.

Ethical Inquiry

Canada is fortunate to have a growing number of nurses engaged in research on ethics in nursing and in health care. Each year nurses have also presented refereed papers at the conference of the Canadian Bioethics Society (CBS). This national society (formed in 1988) has been instrumental in providing a forum for nurses—along with other health professionals and people from other academic disciplines—to explore ethics issues. Since the mid-nineties, lunch hour meetings during the conference have served as an occasion for nurses to get acquainted and reacquainted with each other and to share information and insights about developments in nursing ethics in Canada. Over the first 15 years of CBS conferences, more than a hundred presentations have been given by nurses, either individually, with nursing colleagues, or with other health professional colleagues, with increasingly sophisticated research presentations.[5] While no specific directory exists to catalogue the work of these nurses, an interim resource exists in the publication of the abstracts that is available at the annual conference of the CBS. Many nurses have been, and continue to be, involved in research that addresses specific ethical issues in health care, such as end-of-life decisions, advance directives, resource allocation, artificial nutrition and hydration, and new health care technologies. Recent nursing research has attended more thoughtfully to understanding nursing ethics, as noted earlier in this chapter. Pursuit of this inquiry is highly relevant to this text and to the continued development of nursing ethics. It is significant for nursing educators, nurses, and students. What seems clear to the editors is that the way we think about and teach nursing ethics must change to reflect current research and thus be more relevant in equipping nurses at all levels for practice.[6] We intend this text to be a rich resource for nursing educators in teaching nursing ethics.

We are fortunate to have several nursing journals inviting publications on nursing ethics, and two international journals in particular (*Nursing Ethics* and the *Journal of Advanced Nursing*, both based in Great Britain) that have helped foster dialogue and exchange of ideas amongst scholars in nursing ethics. Increasingly, the *Canadian Journal of Nursing Research* has featured nursing ethics research as well. The calibre of the research over the past few years has transcended the level of preliminary or exploratory studies to arrive at studies that carefully probe the ability of nurses to practise ethically under systems of serious fiscal constraint. The *Canadian Nurse Journal* and the Canadian Nurses Association have also fostered the ethics-mindedness of registered nurses across Canada, through policy papers, case and article publication, and the promotion of the network of nurses involved in ethics (in the form of networking breakfasts and lunches at both Canadian Bioethics Society conferences and Canadian Nurses Association conventions). These observations are in no way intended to dismiss the rich array of publications from our colleagues in the United States, Europe, Australia, and other places (nor the important international meetings featuring nursing ethics), but rather to spotlight our uniquely Canadian resources for the pursuit of nursing ethics scholarship.

INTERDISCIPLINARY CHALLENGES

The focus on nursing ethics must never become so narrow as to preclude attention to ethics concerns common to all health care providers. Nurses need to keep abreast of ethical issues impacting health care and to maintain a clear focus on the significance of those issues for nursing and safe, competent, and ethical nursing care. To that end, this text includes wide-ranging topics and discussions of matters impacting upon nursing practice.

Shared interdisciplinary ethics education can be important in assisting nurses to develop a firm footing in ethics and to be sensitized to new developments (such as xeno-transplantation and global ethics), as well as to areas marginalized or overlooked in ethics discourse (such as disability, and violence and women). Sociological studies often raise ethical questions about how we practise our professions and how we work in relationship to the other. These types of studies are also important for our understanding of everyday ethics (see Street 1992; Chamblais 1996).

A Common Code of Ethics?

Over the years, some ethics scholars largely outside of nursing, including philosophers, policy-makers, and administrators, have claimed that there should be a common code of ethics for all health professionals to reduce the likelihood of conflicting ethical positions. Pattison (2001) argues that basing all health professional and social welfare codes "within the context of clear, common, universal principles" would provide greater coherence in professional obligations and client expectations. At minimum, he suggests that

> A broad, inclusive framework of moral principles that was recognized as important and accept-able by a general audience of citizens may be a useful addition to most codes if they are actually to promote ethical behaviour in professionals in its widest and most proper sense. (10)

Clearly, each profession needs to know more about the values and ethical commitments of other health professionals, and some degree of common guidance could serve health teams well. But a common code might not be the best way to promote ethical practice because it is important to allow varying perspectives to be brought to bear on ethical prob-lems (Shannon 1997). When practitioners are willing to listen to each other's values and points of view, and to work together, they are often able to come up with ethical solutions that serve patients well and that are different and better than any one code or profession alone could contribute.

A Common Ethics Vocabulary

If an aggregated common code of ethics does not make sense, might there be good sense in developing and utilizing a common vocabulary to converse about ethics? Over a decade or more, nurses involved in ethics, as well as philosophers and others, have begun to shape a com-mon vocabulary to assist in naming the ethical situations in which we find ourselves. This allows parties engaged in ethics discussions to express their feelings about the situation and to be better understood. Contributors who stand out in the development of this vocabulary include Jameton (1984), credited with naming moral agency and moral distress, Rodney (1988) and Corley (1995) for further developing the concept of moral distress, and Webster and Baylis (2000) for articulating the concept of moral residue and clarifying other moral con-cepts as well. These concepts have been found helpful by bioethicists, nurses, and other health professionals in describing their ethics concerns by naming them, using terms such as "moral courage," "moral compromise," "moral uncertainty," "moral blindness," and "moral commu-nity." Such language assists in delineating the types of ethical concerns nurses and others expe-rience and contributes to interdisciplinary team communication through shared meanings.

Common Interdisciplinary Education

Common interdisciplinary ethics education is also of significant value because it can provide opportunities for nurses, physicians, and other health care professionals to understand each other's values and views. However, such education should not be seen as the only route to better working relationships. It seems increasingly clear that there is a need for a different kind of education, as well. There must be collaborative education that focuses on understanding what it means to be a team, on collaborating in practice, on learning to respect each other's professional knowledge and skills, and on seeking to understand each other (Miller, Freeman and Ross 2001). The richness of what each professional brings to practice can optimize patient benefit. Anything less than full team involvement cheats the patient of his or her right to the best possible care, and that, too, is a matter of ethics.

OUTLINE OF THE CONTENTS OF THIS TEXT

This text is organized into three sections: Moral Landscape, Moral Climate, and Moral Horizons. In the first section, we want to paint a picture of the moral landscape by providing this introduction and the subsequent thoughtful discussion and critique of historical perspectives in nursing ethics. Philosophical contributions to nursing ethics will then be highlighted as a prelude to four chapters that we consider a "theory quartet." The first provides a brief history of health care ethics and is followed by a chapter on diverse approaches to health care ethics. The third chapter in the quartet discusses applications in health care ethics, and the final chapter describes the landscape of nursing ethics today. Concluding the first section is a chapter on moral agency with a focus on relational connections and trust. Moral Climate, the second section, includes a range of health care system issues and practice setting–related challenges (privatization/profitization, home care and ethics, and end-of-life decision-making), as well as applications of theoretical approaches in practice (ecological theory, narrative ethics). The third and final section, Moral Horizons, includes an explosion of issues and ideas on the frontier of nursing ethics. Included in this section are chapters on biotechnology and ethics; global ethics challenges; research ethics; disability, genetics, and ethics; ethics in the care of children; and violence against women and ethics. The final chapters in the text focus on the ethical nursing practitioner's way of thinking and being in ethical practice. They include the embodiment of mind, emotion, and action; emotions and ethics; ethics and evolving spirituality; and relational ethics. We hope this final section will challenge readers to become involved in the creation and development of nursing ethics. The importance of this involvement was nicely summed up by one nurse in our study.

> Just speaking from personal experience, I think it's a developmental evolutionary kind of thing. When I was a baby nurse I probably felt the dissonance that there was something wrong but I probably couldn't name it. And over time as I experienced that feeling again and actually took a formal look at it through ethics education, I became aware of what the whole is about, what the literature informs us about, but also how that relates to professional practice.

FOR REFLECTION

1. In your nursing practice, have you considered yourself to be a "moral agent"?
2. Have you encountered situations that you might call "morally distressing"? At the time, did you consider those situations as having anything to do with ethics?

3. How might it help nurses to frame some of their concerns into the language of ethics?
4. What moral concepts might be particularly helpful to nursing leaders?

ENDNOTES

1. Johnstone (1989, 1999) provides a penetrating critique of how the medical profession, the media, interdisciplinary ethics seminars and conferences, the courts, government commissions and inquiries, and key publications in bioethics have marginalized nursing ethics.
2. Our research team was initiated with funding from Associated Medical Services, Incorporated (AMS) and continued with SSHRC (Social Sciences and Humanities Research Council) funding, as well as further research awards from AMS.
3. Ethical fitness is a concept developed by Kidder (1995). The term is used to draw a parallel between physical fitness and fitness for ethics encounters in practice. Both require good preparation, continual attention, and reflective performance.
4. Health Canada's release of the Canadian Nurses Advisory Committee Final Report occurred in August 2002. In it, some startling figures are revealed. The report contains estimates of Canadian registered nurses working a quarter million hours of overtime each week, which was judged to be the equivalent of 7,000 full-time jobs per year. Further, over a period of one year, in excess of 16 million hours are lost to registered nurse (RN) injury and illness. This was estimated to be the equivalent of almost 9,000 full-time nursing positions. Another finding addressed the issue of casual and part-time work for RNs. If involuntary part-time workers had been recruited to full-time work in 2001, it would have resulted in 4.7 million additional hours of nursing practice—the equivalent of 2,592 full-time nursing positions (Health Canada 2002, pp. 14–15).
5. This information is based upon a paper delivered by Storch at the ICN Conference in Copenhagen in 2001, titled "Nurses engaged in ethical research in Canada." This unpublished paper has been updated by Storch on a yearly basis.
6. A project currently underway with Gweneth Doane (Principal Investigator), and funded by Associated Medical Services, focuses on newer ways of teaching nursing ethics. Doane is a nursing faculty member at the University of Victoria, and she is joined on this project by Colleen Varcoe, Paddy Rodney, Bernie Pauly, Helen Brown, and Janet Storch, with an anticipated publication date of 2004.

REFERENCES

Alberta Association of Registered Nurses. 1996. *Ethical decision-making for registered nurses in Alberta: Guidelines and recommendations.* Edmonton: Alberta Association of Registered Nurses.

Aiken, L.H., Clarke, S.P., Sloane, D.M., Sochalski, J., Busse, R., Clarke, H., Giovannetti, P., Hunt, J., Rafferty, A.M. and Shamian, J. 2001. Nurses' report on hospital care in five countries. *Health Affairs, 20*(3), 43–53.

Aroskar, M.A. 1995. Envisioning nursing as a moral community. *Nursing Outlook, 43*(3), 134–138.

Arras, J.D., Steinbock, B. and London, A.J. 1999. Moral reasoning in the medical context. In J.D. Arras and B. Steinbock (Eds.), *Ethical issues in modern medicine,* 5th ed. (pp. 1–40). Toronto: Mayfield.

Baumann, A., O'Brien-Pallas, L., Armstrong-Stassen, M., Blythe, J., Bourbonnais, R., Cameron, S., Doran, D. I., Kerr, M., Hall, L.M., Vezina, M., Butt, M. and Ryan, L. 2001. *Commitment and caring: The benefits of a healthy workplace for nurses, their patients and the system.* Ottawa: Canadian Health Service Research Foundation.

Beauchamp, T.L. and Childress, J.F. 2001. *Principles of biomedical ethics.* 5th edition. New York: Oxford University Press.

Beauchamp, T.L. and Childress, J.F. 1994. *Principles of biomedical ethics.* 4th edition. New York: Oxford University Press.

Benner, P.A., Tanner, C.A. and Chesla, C.A. 1996. *Expertise in nursing practice: Caring, clinical judgment, and ethics.* New York: Springer.

Bergum, V. 1997. Knowledge for ethical care. *Nursing Ethics, 1*(2), 71–79.

Botes, A. 2000. An integrated approach to ethical decision-making in the health team. *Journal of Advanced Nursing, 32*(5), 1076–1082.

Canadian Healthcare Association, Canadian Medical Association, Canadian Nurses Association and Catholic Health Association of Canada. *Joint Statement on Preventing and Resolving Ethical Conflicts Involving Health Care Providers and Persons Receiving Care.* 1999. Ottawa: Canadian Healthcare Association, Canadian Medical Association, Canadian Nurses Association and Catholic Health Association of Canada.

Chambliss, D.F. 1996. *Beyond caring: Hospitals, nurses, and the social organization of ethics.* Chicago: University of Chicago Press.

Corley, M.C. 1995. Moral distress of critical care nurses. *American Journal of Critical Care, 4*(4), 280–285.

Duncan, S.M., Hyndman, K., Estabrooks, C.A., Hesketh, K., Humphrey, C.K., Wong, J. S., Acorn, S. and Giovanetti, P. 2001. Nurses' experience of violence in Alberta and British Columbia hospitals. *Canadian Journal of Nursing Research, 32*(4), 57–78.

Grammelspacher, G.P., Howell, J.D. and Young, M.J. 1986. Perceptions of ethical problems faced by nurses and doctors. *Archives of Internal Medicine, 146,* 577–578.

Fry, S.T. 1989. Towards a theory of nursing ethics. *Advances in Nursing Science, 11*(4), 9–22.

Havens, D.S. and Aiken, L.H. 1999. Shaping systems to promote desired outcomes: The Magnet hospital model. *Journal of Nursing Administration, 29*(2), 14–20.

Health Canada. 2002. *Our health, our future. Creating quality workplaces for Canadian nurses.* Final report of the Canadian Nursing Advisory Committee. Ottawa: Health Canada.

Jameton, A. 1984. *Nursing practice: The ethical issues.* Engelwood Cliffs, N.J.: Prentice Hall Inc.

Johnstone, M. 1999. *Bioethics: A nursing perspective.* 3rd edition. Toronto: Harcourt Saunders.

Johnstone, M.J. 1989. *Bioethics: A nursing perspective.* Toronto: W.B. Saunders.

Kidder, R.M. 1995. *How good people make tough choices: Resolving the dilemma of ethical living.* New York: Fireside.

Lindseth, A., Marhaug, V., Norberg, A. and Uden, G. 1994. Registered nurses and physicians' reflections on their narratives about ethically difficult care episodes. *Journal of Advanced Nursing, 20,* 245–250.

Miller, C., Freeman, M. and Ross, N. 2001. *Interprofessional practice in health and social care: Challenging the shared learning agenda.* London: Arnold.

O'Brien-Pallas, L.L., Baumann, A.O. and Villeneuve, M.J. 1994. The quality of nursing work life. In J.M. Hibberd and M.E. Kyle (Eds.), *Nursing management in Canada* (pp. 391–409). Toronto: W.B. Saunders.

Pattison, S. 2001. Are nursing codes of practice ethical? *Nursing Ethics, 8*(1), 5–18.

Pellegrino, E.D. and Thomasma, D.C. 1988. *For the patient's good: The restoration of beneficence in health care.* New York: Oxford University Press.

Prescott, P.A. and Bowen, S.A. 1985. Physician–nurse relationships. *Annals of Internal Medicine, 103,* 127–133.

Provincial Health Ethics Network. 1995. *Proposal for a Provincial Health Ethics Network in Alberta.* Developed and Submitted on Request of Alberta Health by the Steering Committee for Phase II Planning, J. Storch (Chair). Edmonton: Alberta Health.

Rodney, P.A. 1988. Moral distress in critical care nursing. *Canadian Critical Care Nursing Journal, 5*(2), 9–11.

Rodney, P.A. 1991. Dealing with ethical problems: An ethical decision-making model for critical care nursing. *Canadian Critical Care Nursing Journal, 1*(2), 8–10.

Rodney, P.A. 1997. *Towards connectedness and trust: nurses' enactment of their moral agency within an organizational context.* Unpublished doctoral dissertation. University of British Columbia, Vancouver, BC.

Rodney, P.A. and Starzomski, R. 1993. Constraints on moral agency of nurses. *Canadian Nurse, 89*(9), 23–26.

Rodney, P.A., Varcoe, C., Storch, J.L., McPherson, G., Mahoney, K., Brown, H., Pauly, B., Hartrick-Doane, G., and Starzomski, R. 2002. Navigating toward a moral horizon: A multi-site qualitative study of nurses' enactment of ethical practice. *Canadian Journal of Nursing Research, 34*(3), 75–102.

Scott, J.G., Sochalski, J. and Aiken, L. 1999. Review of Magnet hospital research: Findings and implications for professional nursing practice. *Journal of Nursing Administration, 29*(1), 9–19.

Shannon, S.E. 1997. The roots of interdisciplinary conflict around ethical issues. *Critical Care Nursing Clinics of North America, 9*(1), 13–27.

Smith, K.V. and Godfrey, N.S. 2002. Being a good nurse and doing the right thing: A qualitative study. *Nursing Ethics, 9*(3), 301–312.

Starzomski, R. 1997. *Resource allocation for solid organ transplantation: Towards public and health care provider dialogue.* Unpublished doctoral dissertation. University of British Columbia, Vancouver, BC.

Storch, J.L. 1988. Ethics in nursing practice. In A. Baumgart and J. Larsen (Eds.), *Canadian nursing faces the future: Development and change* (pp. 210–221). Toronto: Mosby.

Storch, J.L. 1992. Ethical issues. In A. Baumgart and J. Larsen (Eds.), *Canadian nursing faces the future,* 2nd ed. (pp. 259–270). Toronto: Mosby Year Book.

Storch, J.S. 1999. Ethical dimensions of leadership. In In J.M. Hibberd and M.E. Kyle (Eds.), *Nursing management in Canada* (pp. 351–467). Toronto: W.B. Saunders.

Storch, J. 2003. Nursing: Yesterday, today, forever. *Nursing Ethics, 10*(2), 120–121.

Storch, J.L., Rodney, P., Pauly, B., Brown, H. and Starzomski, R. 2002. Listening to nurses' moral voices: Building a quality health care environment. *Canadian Journal of Nursing Leadership, 15*(4), 7–16.

Street, A.F. 1992. *Inside nursing: A critical ethnography of clinical nursing practice.* Albany: State University of New York Press.

Tschudin, V. 1999. *Nurses matter: Reclaiming our professional identity.* London: Macmillan Press Ltd.

Varcoe, C., Hartrick, G., Pauly, B., Rodney, R., Storch, J., Mahoney, K., McPherson, G., Brown, H. and Starzomski, R. In press. Ethical practice in nursing: Working the in-betweens. *Journal of Advanced Nursing.*

Varcoe, C. and Rodney, P. 2001. Constrained agency: The social structure of nurses' work. In B.S. Singh and H.D. Dickinson (Eds.), *Health, illness and health care in Canada,* 3rd ed. (pp. 102–128). Scarborough, ON: Nelson Thomson Learning.

Webster, G.C. and Baylis, F.E. 2000. Moral residue. In S.B. Rubin and L. Zoloth (Eds.), *Margin of error: The ethics of mistakes in the practice of medicine* (pp. 217–230). Hagerstown, Maryland: University Publishing Press.

Woods, M. 1999. A nursing ethics: The moral voice of experienced nurses. *Nursing Ethics, 6*(5), 423–433.

Yeo, M. and Moorhouse, A. (Eds.) 1996. *Concepts and cases in nursing ethics.* 2nd edition. Peterborough, ON: Broadview Press.

section I

Moral Landscape

Patricia Rodney

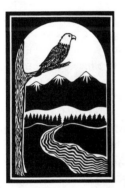

As nurses, we struggle to articulate the ethical concerns in our practice but find we are discounted or trivialized or sentimentalized. This has been damaging to individual nurses, the discipline of nursing, and patients. It is time for change. We need a moral language that will preserve a sense of the tragic, reminding us all that each of us is vulnerable to the contingencies of human life. We need a language that will enable us to sustain our patients and each other; that will serve as the vehicle for our ethical reflection; that will give voice to our ethical concerns (Liaschenko 1993, 9).

In her statement above, Liaschenko reminds us that, as nurses, we need to develop and embrace our own moral/ethical language. While a number of scholars in nursing and other disciplines have made (and continue to make) significant contributions to that language in the decade since Liaschenko wrote this piece, the work is far from finished. Thus, in this section we provide some theoretical foundations which other chapters in the text draw on—either directly or indirectly—and which we hope will be useful to anyone pursuing inquiry in nursing ethics as well as health care ethics. This section includes an orientation to the history of nursing ethics and to the contributions that philosophy has made to nursing ethics. We also explore the interface of health care ethics and nursing ethics, laying out some of the theoretical changes, challenges, and potential of each field. We conclude this section by reflecting on nurses' status as moral agents.

More specifically, in Chapter 2, Marianne Lamb provides a retrospective look at nursing ethics as it has developed over time. In examining the past, she reflects on what has changed and what has not changed about the ethical beliefs and values of nurses as they practised in varying time periods. Lamb argues that an historical perspective helps us to learn from the past and to connect our past to our future—it provides us with a context for current discussion and dialogue about nursing ethics and the thoughtful setting of directions for the future. Overall, she shows how scholarship in nursing ethics has grown over the decades and how this scholarship has been reflected in revised and expanded codes of ethics developed by nursing organizations.

In Chapter 3, Joy Johnson considers the ways in which philosophy can contribute to the evolution of nursing ethics. She begins by examining what we mean by nursing philosophy, the types of philosophical questions that are of concern to nurses, and the relationship of nursing theories to nursing philosophy. She then visits how the world of philosophy has contributed to the realm of nursing ethics. The chapter closes with an examination of some of the unresolved philosophical issues facing the field of nursing ethics. Johnson's thesis is that all nurses can benefit from becoming more strongly grounded in philosophy and from learning ways to use philosophical approaches to deepen their understanding of the nurse's world.

Following these two chapters, we launch into what we have come to think of as our "theory quartet," which elaborates on the interface of health care ethics and nursing ethics. The four chapters here have been developed as a set to be read in sequence but can also be read separately. In Chapter 4, Patricia Rodney, Michael Burgess, Gladys McPherson, and Helen Brown provide an orientation to the development of health care ethics, including an overview of its history and theoretical underpinnings, and some of the challenges we face in contemporary health care ethics. In this process, the authors endeavour to highlight the strengths and limitations of traditional approaches to health care ethics as guides to thinking in ethically troubling situations. They close by considering what it is that health care providers need from ethical theory. Then, in Chapter 5, Patricia Rodney, Bernadette Pauly, and Michael Burgess explore complementary approaches to ethics (especially cross-cultural and feminist). The authors show how such approaches can help us to understand and address the personal, social, and cultural aspects of health as well as the complex sociopolitical climates in which health care is delivered and in which resources for health are embedded. Chapter 6, by Gladys McPherson, Patricia Rodney, Michael McDonald, Janet Storch, Bernadette Pauly, and Michael Burgess, takes the insights from Chapter 4 and Chapter 5 and considers how they can be *applied* in health care ethics work. This includes an introduction of decision-making models for use with individuals and organizations. The quartet ends with Chapter 7, by Helen Brown, Patricia Rodney, Bernadette Pauly, Colleen Varcoe, and Vicki Smye. In it the authors provide an overview of the field of nursing ethics. They proceed first by positing nursing ethics as a distinct field of inquiry. This leads them to an examination of some of the major theoretical foundations of nursing ethics, including relationships between theory and practice and the various influences on and approaches to ethical theory. The authors pull together some conclusions in a case application, after which they anticipate the future heralded by postmodern shifts and postcolonial thinking.

Our *Moral Landscape* section ends with Chapter 8, by Patricia Rodney, Helen Brown, and Joan Liaschenko. The authors begin the chapter with a conceptualization of moral agency as inclusive of rational and self-expressive choice, notions of identity, social and historical relational influences, autonomous action, and embodied engagement. They contribute some details to this conceptualization for nursing, first by locating their analysis within the nature of nurses' knowledge and nurses' work. Following this, they comment on constraints to nurses' autonomous agency. They then posit that nurses and other individuals operate within a relational matrix as moral agents, and that matrix flourishes with authentic presence and trust. The authors conclude by articulating some of the implications of their analysis for collaborative practice.

As Editors, we hope that through the in-depth discussions of nursing ethics and health care ethics included in this section, readers can emerge with a sound comprehension of the moral landscape of nursing ethics. The section will prove useful for those wishing to pursue theoretical or empirical inquiry, as well as for those engaged in practice in nursing and health care ethics.

REFERENCE

Liaschenko, J. 1993. *Faithful to the good: Morality and philosophy in nursing practice.* Unpublished doctoral dissertation. University of California, San Francisco.

chapter two

An Historical Perspective on Nursing and Nursing Ethics

Marianne Lamb

It is clear that since the beginning of "modern" nursing in the 1800s, nurses have believed that their role in society brought with it specific moral obligations.

The intent of this chapter is to provide a retrospective look at nursing ethics as it has developed over time. In examining the past, we can reflect on what has changed and what has not changed about the ethical beliefs and values of nurses as they practised in varying time periods. Through such reflection, we can gain a deeper understanding of how our profession has influenced and been influenced by the social, political, and economic context of practice. An historical perspective helps us to learn from the past and to connect our past to our future—it provides us with a context for current discussion and dialogue about nursing ethics and the thoughtful setting of directions for the future.

   The starting point for this discussion of the historical aspects of nursing ethics is the late 1800s, when formal programs of education or training for nurses, many of them modelled on the one founded by Florence Nightingale, began to spread rapidly in North America and elsewhere. It was at this point that a body of literature began to develop that reflected the ideas and thoughts of those involved in the practice of nursing and the education of nursing students. This literature has grown and expanded to the present day; we now have many nursing journals that include articles on ethical aspects of nursing and an international journal, *Nursing Ethics*, devoted exclusively to the topic. The nursing literature serves as the major source of information about the evolution of nursing ethics over time, and although I have drawn on the international literature, most of the literature sources for this chapter are North American, with a focus on Canadian nursing.[1]

The ethical perspective of nurses at any point in history is inextricably linked to the context of nursing and such key factors as prevailing social thought on values and morality, how nursing work was organized, the economics of health care, the social role of women, and the pressing social issues of the day. All of these factors have shaped the ethical questions that nurses have raised, how nurses have thought about nursing ethics, and the issues that have been addressed by the organized profession. In this chapter, the evolution of nursing ethics is described in terms of three broad time periods: the late 1800s to the end of the 1920s, the 1930s to the late 1960s, and the 1970s to the present day. Given that changing thought on nursing ethics and practice can not be tied to any specific year, these time periods are somewhat artificial; however, they generally represent broad shifts in thinking about nursing ethics and nursing obligations.

THE EARLY YEARS: 1800s TO 1929

Following Florence Nightingale's founding of a training school for nurses in England in 1860, she was consulted by many hospitals in North America that wished to establish schools based on her model (Robb 1900; Woodham-Smith 1951).[2] Within several decades, nursing leaders emerged who began to organize the profession. The first professional association, the British Nurses' Association, was established in 1888; an American Society of Superintendents of Training Schools, composed of Canadian and American superintendents, was formed in 1893; and the International Council of Nurses (ICN) was formed in 1899 (Mussallem 1992). Nursing became firmly established as an occupation for women in North America, and although joint American and Canadian associations had to separate to develop national nursing associations, the initial link and exchange between nurses in the two countries continued and exists to the present day.[3] The initial ideas about ethics in nursing emerged in the writings of nurse leaders, who were generally superintendents of nursing schools and the authors of textbooks for nursing students. Over time, the voices of nurses who worked as graduates in private duty, in hospitals, or in public health were heard through articles in professional journals and books. The influence of French nursing sisters, which predated Florence Nightingale's influence in Canada, must be acknowledged for its significant contribution to the thinking and values of nurses through hospitals and schools of nursing founded in the Catholic tradition (Ross Kerr 1996).

Ethical Concepts: Character, Ideals, and Etiquette

In the early days of the development of nursing as a profession, the concept of "character" was central to nursing ethics. Character referred to the personal characteristics of the nurse that were required for nursing work, some of which were moral qualities and some of which were social qualities that led to success in nursing practice. Frequently mentioned characteristics included attentiveness to patients, vigilance, honesty, adaptability, patience, obedience and acceptance of authority, loyalty, unselfishness, tactfulness, devotion, and kindness (Broadhurst 1917; Crawford 1926; Dock 1893; Domville 1891; Robb 1900; Scovil 1917; Weeks-Shaw 1900). These qualities were considered to be those of the "good" nurse.

Moral conduct in nursing was considered to be largely dependent on character and the disposition to act in a certain manner. Within this view of morality, ideals were central concepts. The Christian ideal, the service ideal, and humanitarian ideals provided models that defined the sort of person whom the nurse should aspire to be (Potts 1921; Stewart 1918). Inspired by these ideals, the nurse would devote her abilities to the individual in her care.

Nursing Education: Character Formation

The focus on character was consistent with Victorian-era attitudes and the social role of women, but it was also due, in part, to the experimental nature of training young women for nursing. Training was a revolutionary idea at the time, and one not without opposition, particularly from physicians (Weeks-Shaw 1900; Woodham-Smith 1951). The confidence of the public was required if nursing was to be established as a reputable occupation because, in the early 1800s, hospitals and their "nurses" were places to be avoided. According to Robb (1900),

> The prevailing type of attendants upon the sick in the early years of the century had accustomed people to regard paid nurses as self-seeking menials, engaged in something far lower than domestic work, and whose only object was to benefit by others' misfortunes at the least expenditure of care and trouble on their own part (29).

Florence Nightingale recognized that if the "experiment" of a nursing school was to succeed, the behaviour of students of nursing must be above reproach. She emphasized the importance of character considerations in the selection of students, and each probationer was required to have a certificate of good character on admission. A monthly report on probationers included a "Moral Record" that addressed "punctuality, quietness, trustworthiness, personal neatness, cleanliness, ward management, and order" (Woodham-Smith 1951, 235). Training schools fulfilled their duty if they carefully selected candidates of good character; continued character formation through discipline and emphasis on obedience, loyalty, and respect for authority; and instilled the ideals of nursing as well as taught the etiquette required for successful practice.

Nightingale's emphasis on the qualities that denoted "character" and on the ongoing character training of nursing students was reflected in nursing education and nursing ethics for many decades (Crawford 1926; Broadhurst 1917; Parsons 1916; Cadmus 1916; AJN 1920). In the view of some, Nightingale's focus on forming character was interpreted by subsequent school superintendents in a way that led to indoctrination and an undue emphasis on discipline and etiquette (Brown 1966).

The Profession and Draft Codes of Ethics

As nursing developed as a profession, leaders began to write about the ethical nature of nursing. In an early book on nursing ethics, Isabel Hampton Robb (1900), a former Superintendent of Nurses and Principal of the Training School for Nurses at John Hopkins Hospital in Baltimore, wrote: "The rules of conduct adapted to the many diverse circumstances attending the nursing of the sick constitute *nursing ethics*" (14–15). She distinguished this from etiquette, which she viewed as important for nurses and as "the code of polite life," but she did not consider etiquette to have the same "moral weight" as ethics. Concerns of etiquette included appropriate dress and deportment, manners and expression, courtesy, and relationships with and respect for others ("A suggested code" 1926). Despite differing definitions, nursing ethics and nursing etiquette continued to be discussed together; the distinctions between the two were often unclear and they seemed to have equal importance. For example, in 1921, one nurse (Catton) proposed the development of the "Principles of Nursing Ethics and Etiquette of the CNATN" (Canadian National Association of Trained Nurses), citing lack of courtesy as a problem in nursing. Similarly, Aiken (1925), in a textbook titled *Studies in Ethics for Nurses*, identifies inappropriate behaviour that ranges from use of slang with doctors to leaving a private duty case without notice.

From the earliest days of the organized profession, calls were made for the development of a code of ethics, but leaders recognized that such an undertaking would take time and would require the building of a consensus among nurses. In 1898, Isabel Hampton Robb, who was active in the formation of a national association of nurses in the United States (the precursor to the American Nurses Association), wrote:

> Our work for the first few years must be constructive. A code of ethics is the first object mentioned in the constitution. But it cannot be among the first to be realized, for such a code should be the central point of thought of the association, reaching out in its influence and inspiration to our most remote branches.... Surely, it will be better to wait until we have taken sufficient and better form in the matter of numbers and closer organization, to learn the mind of the greater number on what shall constitute our national code of ethics (360).

The interest in developing a code of ethics to guide nursing conduct was evident in Canada and the United States during the 1920s (Catton 1921; "A suggested code" 1926). The Committee on Ethical Standards of the ANA (American Nurses Association) began work in 1924 and a suggested code was put forward (AJN 1926). This work showed some signs of a shift in the thinking about the ethical aspects of nursing, including the nurse-physician relationship and the obligations of the nurse. In this "suggested code," ideas of mutual respect, interdependence, and co-worker characterized the relationship. An editorial on the code noted that every nurse experienced "uneasiness when a rule and a principle came into conflict" (AJN 1926, 621). Similarly, there were some indications that "vaunted professional etiquette" was out of date (Fraser 1925), as was traditional respect for authority and discipline. At a discussion of professional ethics at the 1925 Congress of the International Council of Nurses (ICN), nursing leaders acknowledged that the younger generation would not submit to authority but would learn to use their judgment (Sidelights 1926). However, ideals, such as the "Golden Rule," loyalty, and respect for positions of authority continued to be highly valued in nursing ("A suggested code" 1926).

Private Duty Nursing Practice and Ethical Problems

The problems in nursing ethics of the early years were those related to private duty nursing, as this was the predominate form of nursing practice for graduates of nursing schools in Canada and the United States. An individual who was ill was usually cared for at home by a private physician and, if advised by the physician or requested by the family, by a private nurse. If hospitalization was necessary, the patient could hire a private nurse for "special" duty. Those who could not afford special nurses were cared for by student nurses. The major proportion of nursing services in Canadian hospitals was provided by students, even in small hospitals (Ellis 1927; Weir 1932).

To a great extent, the emphasis on nursing etiquette in these years is explained by the nature of private duty practice. First of all, the nurse had to work closely with the physician.

From her obligations to the patient stemmed those duties "owed" to the physician. Together, the nurse and physician formed a team in the battle against disease and death (Byers 1922). The physician was "captain of the team," and the nurse's role was to observe the patient, carry out the physician's orders, ensure that the patient was as comfortable and contented as possible, and to report her observations and concerns to the physician when he visited. Any discord in this team was viewed as not being in the best interests of the patient. The patient's recovery would be jeopardized by any lack of confidence in the nurse or physician (Scovil 1917).

A second reason why an emphasis on etiquette might be related to the predominance of private duty nursing is that the nurse was often on 24-hour duty in the home, and she had to be adaptable and tactful in fitting into family life while caring for her patient. Nurses were criticized for being "high-handed" (Perry 1929), and rather than being helpful, they needed "waiting on" (Humbly 1921). Laywomen told nurses that most of the complaints about private duty nurses involved the attitude, efficiency, and economy of the nurse in the private home. McWilliams (1921) reported that some nurses had a "too professional" air and lacked a tactful approach. If nurses could not "fit in" to a home, they were expected to resign from the case if they could arrange for a replacement (Kay 1926). The following description from a private duty nurse suggests how delicate the relationship between nurse and family might be:

> In her relation to the patient the nurse must shield her from all adverse influence and anxiety, standing between her and relatives, if necessary, and must see that all details are run smoothly for her advantage, at the same time studying her characteristics so as to determine when to yield and when to be firm in executing orders disagreeable to her (Clint 1914, 645–646).

Members of the CNATN (1922) discussed criticism of the private duty nurse, and the private duty section decided to establish a committee to investigate complaints. However, it would seem that most nurses did not consider unethical conduct to be a major problem and the matter was not pursued. Of greater concern than the behaviour of individual nurses was the concern about the costs of private duty nursing, the move to a shorter working day, and the access to private duty care by the middle income earner (Johns 1921).

By the 1920s, there was a growing concern that "materialism" was threatening traditional values, religion, and family life (Fairley 1923). Although nurses had long professed a belief in the need for self-sacrifice and altruism in nursing, during the early twenties, some implied that contemporary life was so characterized by a concern with money and goods that ethics and the altruistic ideal could become a thing of the past within the profession (Canadian Association of Nursing Education 1924). The movement by private duty nurses to shorten their hours of duty while maintaining their daily fee rate generated fears that nursing was becoming commercialized, although nursing was supposed to be above "mere money getting" (Field 1923). In Canada, private duty nurses organized a section within the national association in the hope that official nursing support would help their cause and deal with public criticism. In the United States, a famous American physician, Dr. Charles Mayo, accused the American nursing profession of "unionism" and selfishness for raising similar issues ("Nurses selfish" 1921). Over the decade of the twenties, increasing unemployment among private duty nurses gave rise to growing sympathy for the plight of graduate nurses, suggestions for government-sponsored plans for care of the sick, and a decrease in the call for self-sacrifice in nursing (Lamb 1981). Concerns about the costs of private duty nursing and accessibility to these services led to new systems of organizing nursing care: "group nursing," in which private duty nurses cared for two or more patients in hospital, and "hourly nursing," which involved home visits and charges for episodic, rather than continuous, care (Cameron 1927; Weir 1932).

In summary, the emphasis in the early years of nursing was on character, ideals, and etiquette as the basis for ethical conduct. The emphasis on etiquette served to prepare graduates to go into independent private duty, away from the influence of the military discipline of the training school, where they would have to succeed in practice, not only in terms of their professional knowledge and skill, but also in terms of their relationships with patients, family members, and physicians. Gradually, the traditional ideals of self-sacrifice and service were challenged as private duty nurses attempted to improve their income and working hours. Access to affordable nursing services became an issue, and solutions emerged to the dilemma of providing affordable nursing services while offering adequate income to nurses.

The organized profession was still in its infancy, focusing on such issues as building nursing organizations, achieving registration, developing public health nursing, improving nursing education, and instituting a shorter working day. Although organizations, such as the CNATN (later, the CNA) and the ANA, recognized the importance of nursing ethics, early calls for, or drafts of, a code of ethics did not result in definitive statements on ethics from the nursing profession during this early period.

THE MIDDLE YEARS: 1930s TO 1969

Between the thirties and the seventies, there was a major change in the location of nursing practice; most nursing care moved from the home to a hospital setting. While 60 percent of active nurses in Canada were engaged in self-employed private duty practice in 1930 (Weir 1932), more than 80 percent of nurses worked as employees in hospitals in 1970 (CNA 1971). The depression of the thirties had led to unemployment among private duty nurses and had exerted pressure on hospitals to hire graduate nurses and to rely less on student nurses for service, thus bringing about a decline in private duty nursing (Brown 1966). World War II brought about a severe shortage of nurses in the forties, generating subsequent efforts to increase enrolment in nursing schools (CNA 1947). The impact of these world events also led to developments in health and social policy in Canada: the growth of hospitals in the forties, publicly funded hospital insurance in the fifties, and medicare in the sixties, all of which had a profound effect on nursing. Following decades of continued effort by the profession to improve the education of nursing students, the practice of using nursing students to provide service ceased, and a major move of nursing education into systems of general education was underway by the late sixties and early seventies (Ross-Kerr 2003).

Ethical Concepts: Professional Obligation and Human Rights

The emphasis on the moral character of the individual nurse as a basis for nursing ethics gradually declined during the middle years, and the concept of the professional obligation of the nurse began to predominate. The changes in emphasis seemed to emerge from the experience of the growing profession and changes in society rather than from any formal ethical reflection and analysis.

One of the notable changes over the time period was thinking about the relationship of nurses to physicians. Around the world, nurses who subscribed to the instruction received by generations of nursing students that they must be obedient to the physician's orders were severely shaken by the 1929 "Somera case" involving a nurse in the Philippines who prepared an ordered drug that led to the death of a patient.[4] The nurse was sentenced to one year's imprisonment, despite testimony that this nurse "followed the rules which she had been taught" (Grennan 1930). Due to the intervention of the Philippine Nurses' Association, the International Council of Nurses, and women's groups, all of whom believed that the lower and higher court decisions were unjust, the nurse received a conditional pardon and was not imprisoned. This case was influential in changing the view of the nurse as "subservient" (Grennan 1930). Nurse educators, who later referred to the case, taught students that there must be nurse "judgement on each order so far as her action in carrying it out is concerned, in that she is held responsible for any act which she knows would be dangerous for the patient" (Dietz 1950, 148). The organized profession began, into the 1960s, to emphasize an obligation to carry out doctors' orders "intelligently and loyally" ("Code of ethics" 1965), and nurses were not expected to give "blind obedience" to physicians (Pelley 1964). By the end of the 1960s, nurses in Canada preferred to refer to their obligations to physicians in terms of co-operation and teamwork (Lindabury 1967).

A post-WWII focus on human rights led to the adoption of legislation related to discrimination and bills of rights in jurisdictions around the world, including the 1948 Universal Declaration of Human Rights by the United Nations (Storch 1977). This widespread focus on human rights led to a growing emphasis in nursing on non-discrimination in the provision of nursing care, respect for the religious beliefs of patients, and exhortations to "try and understand people of all sorts, irrespective of race, religion or color" (Spalding 1954, 102).

Education in Ethics: Professional Adjustments

The education of nursing students with respect to nursing ethics fell under the broad rubric of Professional Adjustments—courses designed to socialize students into professional life and to transmit ethical values, principles, and philosophies (Densford and Everett 1946). The degree to which these courses addressed ethical principles and ethical issues in nursing likely varied widely across nursing schools; much of the course material was devoted to career success, residence life, democratic ideals, and professional organizations. A 1958 CNA course guide on the teaching of Professional Adjustments in nursing programs, a course in which "professional nursing problems" were to be addressed, made reference to the 1953 ICN Code. The guide suggested the "discussion of professional, moral and personal responsibilities, according to [the] philosophy of individual schools" (CNA 1958, 16). However, this suggested discussion was a very small aspect of the overall course, which focused more on relationships with patients, hospital, physicians, and the profession. The reference in the guide to the philosophy of individual schools perhaps reflected differences between university and hospital schools of nursing and schools governed by secular and religious bodies, as representatives from all types participated in committee work.

Although not the norm in writings about nursing ethics, some schools did include attention to ethical theories and ethical principles. By the 1950s, Catholic hospitals in Canada had adopted the Moral Code. *Ethical and Religious Directives for Catholic Hospitals* and textbooks designed for nursing students in Catholic hospitals discussed moral philosophy, moral reasoning, and civil and ecclesiastical law, as well as specific ethical issues such as euthanasia and abortion (Godin and O'Hanley 1957; McAllister 1955).

In their textbook on ethics for nurses, Densford and Everett (1946), a nursing professor and a philosophy professor at an American university, discussed the "greatest-happiness principle" and principles of morality, as well as euthanasia and abortion. In a separate chapter, they also discussed issues of moral conflict in medicine and nursing. They noted that good rules can "go wrong" and that, despite the general obligation not to criticize a physician and to sustain confidence in him, the first rule was: "always do what is best for the patient" (157). They also stated that: "there are flagrant cases which justify breaking the rule of non-criticism" (160). Despite these indications that some nursing curricula addressed nursing ethics and that moral philosophy was influencing what was taught, references to "character formation" (Clermont 1953), "personal decorum," and "professional etiquette" (Pelley 1963) persisted in discussions of ethics.

The Profession and Adoption of Codes of Ethics

A Tentative Code (1940), drafted by a committee of ANA began with the statement that "Nursing is a profession" (977). This draft document contained a requirement to respect the religious beliefs of others, but for the most part was similar in tone to traditional views of nursing ethics in its references to "high ideals" and "honesty, understanding, gentleness, and patience" (978). Similarly, a draft Code of Ethics prepared by a committee of the Canadian Nurses Association in 1954 identified confidentiality, sympathy, understanding, and "the best in knowledge and skill" as obligations of the nurse to the patient. This draft code was not adopted, however, as the Canadian Nurses Association decided to adopt the ICN Code (CNA 1955).

During the 1950s, both the ANA ("What's in our code" 1952) and the ICN ("The ICN in Brazil" 1953) adopted codes of ethics that were almost identical and that departed considerably from earlier attempts to establish a code. First, these codes reflected the societal emphasis on human rights in that the preamble to these codes included a statement that nursing service was to be "unrestricted by consideration of nationality, race, creed, colour, politics or social status" (Tate 1977). Commentary on the Code in the *American Journal of Nursing* made explicit reference to the Universal Declaration of Human Rights and the "intrinsic dignity and value of each human being" ("What's in our code" 1952, 1248). The one significant change in the 1965 ICN Code of Ethics was the inclusion of the Red Cross Principles that stressed impartiality and universality ("Code of ethics" 1965).

For the most part, nursing codes and their revisions during the 1950s and 1960s did not expand on the rights of patients and continued to highlight relationships with physicians, including prohibitions not to treat (except in emergencies) to sustain confidence in the physician, and to "carry out the physician's orders intelligently and loyally, and to refuse to participate in unethical procedures" (CNA 1954; "Code of ethics" 1965). In these new codes, obligations of nurses were expanded more in terms of the profession and the larger community than in terms of the patient. Other new aspects of the Codes addressed the nurse's entitlement to "just remuneration," amounting to a prohibition against testimonials for commercial products and personal ethics that reflected well on the profession and citizenship responsibilities. Pellegrino (1964), in a review of codes of ethics for physicians and for nurses in the United States, identified that these codes still contained a number of statements of etiquette and noted that "their violation may impair the dignity of the some of the goals of professions, but they do not by their nature involve usurpation of the human rights of the patient," and that the "ethical core" of codes related to the "rights of the patient as a person" (41). This critique is consistent with Cianci's (1992) review of ANA draft and adopted codes, in which she notes that a focus on ethics in nursing education and the professional literature declined following adoption of the 1950 ANA code and did not re-emerge until the 1970s.

Hospital Nursing Practice and Ethical Problems

The major issues that arose during this period that challenged traditional ideals and values in nursing were those of "depersonalized care" and collective bargaining. By the late 1960s, health professionals were acutely aware of criticisms about Canadian health care services (Health Resources Directorate 1970; National Conference 1973). The demands for changes in the health care system were attributed not only to rising costs, but also to rising expectations about medical science, growth of the consumer movement, increasing public sophistication, and changing social values (Blishen 1970). One of the major criticisms was that patients were treated in an impersonal manner and given "assembly-line" treatment. Brown (1966) identified a "craving for individualized attention" and frustration among patients with the many different kinds of staff and fragmented care. As a personal service to human beings, nursing required a non-discriminating attitude, a patient-centred approach to care, and conduct respectful of the dignity and worth of the individual (Rogers and Ballantyne 1963). Many nurses, however, did not feel that these obligations were being met and expressed concern about the "dehumanizing" aspects of hospitalization towards the end of the sixties (McMurtry 1968). Hayter (1966), in an article on the meaning of "caring," emphasized the nurse-patient relationship and noted that "there is considerable guilt among nurses because they cannot give the kind of nursing care they would like to give" (31).

A second, but related, issue that raised ethical concerns for nurses over the years was how to improve their salaries and working conditions in a profession that had long emphasized service, personal sacrifice, and not abandoning patients who needed their care. As noted earlier, an increasing percentage of nurses became hospital employees during and after WWII, and nursing shortages were critical during the 1940s. In 1943, the CNA formed its first committee on labour relations following similar activities by several provincial associations (CNA 1968), and the national organization supported collective bargaining in nursing in 1944 (Lindabury 1968). However, in 1946, a CNA resolution affirmed that it was "opposed to any nurse going on strike at any time for any cause" (Lindabury 1968). Nevertheless, some provincial nursing associations who bargained collectively for nurses did not support such a "no-strike" policy, and services were withdrawn on a few occasions, albeit with great reluctance. By the mid-sixties, the salaries and working conditions of nurses were of widespread concern. MacLeod (1966) noted that nurses were becoming less reluctant to accept current salary levels:

> Prevalent in society today is a great concern for the welfare of the worker. Influenced by this trend, nurses feel strongly that they, too, have a right to better salaries, better hours, better conditions of work. But as a profession we have been inhibited by a guilty feeling that pressing for our rights somehow conflicts with the professional ethic of "putting the patient first" (20).

Although "many nurses still harboured reservations regarding the appropriateness of a profession participating in collective bargaining" (CNA 1968, 9–10), such sentiments gave way in both the United States and Canada, and nurses began to vote in support of strike action ("BC Nurses vote" 1968; Lindabury 1968).

In summary, between the thirties and the sixties, nursing organizations formalized nursing codes of ethics, reflecting a move away from a focus on the character of the nurse to a focus on the nurse's obligations and responsibilities as a professional. Gradually, the focus changed from who the nurse should *be* to what the nurse should *do*. Human rights and the dignity of the person began to receive emphasis, as well as a more frequent focus on the primacy of obligations to the patient. Although there was continued attention to relationships with physicians, obligations such as carrying out physicians' orders and not engaging in medical treatment were situational rather than blanket obligations. The early emphasis on etiquette, respect for authority, obedience to physicians' orders, and loyalty all but disappeared by the end of the 1960s, a decade that was marked by considerable distrust of public institutions and social protest. The gradually developing opinion within the profession was that nurses were independent professionals who were required to use their judgment. In addition to codes of ethics, the organized profession began to address the socio-economic welfare of nurses, collective bargaining, and strikes, a process that brought with it an end to discussions of the traditional notions of self-sacrifice and service.

THE LATER YEARS: 1970s TO THE PRESENT DAY

The human rights movement of the sixties led to a focus on patient rights in the seventies, which had a profound effect on nursing ethics and health care ethics in general. Storch (1977, 1982) traces the rise of a consumer rights movement in the late sixties and early seventies, the growing sense of health as a right, and the emergence of the Patient's Bills of Rights in the United States and Canada. This movement brought a focus to the meaning of patient rights in health care, articulated in the 1973 American Hospital Association's Statement on a Patient's Bill of Rights and by the Consumers' Association of Canada statement on Consumer Rights in Health Care ("Consumer rights" 1974). This latter statement identified the right of the individual to be informed, to be respected as the individual with the major responsibility for his or her own care, to participate in decision-making affecting his or her health, and to have equal access to health care. The assertion of these rights led to exploration of the rights of particular groups of patients in health care. In Canada, the rights of research subjects (Medical Research Council 1978), dying patients (Suzuki 1975), and the mentally handicapped (Greenland 1975) were studied and debated.

New developments in medical science and technology, from contraception to resuscitation techniques, raised a host of ethical questions surrounding their use in health care. Developments in the transplantation of human organs and genetic manipulation had increased interest in medical ethics in the late sixties and early seventies (Ramsey 1970; Siminovitch 1973), but by the mid-seventies, dramatic dilemmas, such as the Karen-Anne Quinlan case, focused public attention on the ethical complexities of life-prolonging intervention in health care delivery (Branson et al. 1976). Changing social attitudes towards death and dying and reproductive technology fuelled re-examination of abortion and euthanasia. A federal Law Reform Commission was appointed to investigate and recommend legislation on such issues as euthanasia and the definition of death (Baudouin 1977). (See Chapter 13.) The 1970s saw the rise of "bioethics," a term that emerged as individuals from a wide variety of academic disciplines and professions began to examine "ethical issues posed by developments in the biological sciences, and their application to medical practice" (Roy, Williams and Dickens 1994, 4).

Ethical Concepts: Patient Rights, Caring, and Nursing Ethics

The patient rights movement, concerns about dehumanizing care and the emergence of "life and death" issues with the development of new treatments, and moral pluralism in society challenged all health professionals to think about their moral obligations (Curtin and Flaherty 1982; Storch 1982). The early response to the patient rights movement in society generated bills of rights and an emphasis on the legal rights of patients to be informed about treatment or to refuse treatment. As consent to treatment and refusal of care by patients were major issues for nurses, there was early endorsement of such rights statements by the profession (Carnegie 1974). This legal focus was reflected in "contractual models of care" described by nurses (Curtin and Flaherty 1982; Ujhely 1973), and the notion that patients were to be full partners on the health team was consistent with several theories or conceptual models of nursing that had emerged in the United States during the late sixties and early seventies (Orem 1971). Tied to the notion of patient rights was the notion of patient advocacy, both reflecting the influence of legal concepts on nursing practice and nursing ethics (Jenny 1979). Adoption of the advocate role was viewed by some Canadian nurses as a natural extension of the traditional ethical obligation to protect patients from incompetent or unethical practice (Sklar 1979), while others believed that the role required a non-traditional and more active and assertive stance in view of the growth, rigidity, and complexity of health care bureaucracies ("Prepared to care" 1978). A number of nurses and others doubted that most nurses were in a position to advocate for patients, given their lack of power and employee status in health care settings (Sklar 1979; Storch 1977), and debate about the role continues to the present day (Hewitt 2002).

During the eighties and nineties, nurses moved beyond consideration of legal obligations to explore moral obligations in two parallel, but different, streams of study. The first stream fell within the realm of moral philosophy, biomedical ethics, and, subsequently, bioethics. Nurses, as part of the larger community of those interested in ethics in health care, examined nursing ethics in terms of moral philosophy and how ethical concepts, principles, and classical ethical theory could guide nurses in their practice (Davis and Aroskar 1978). Beauchamp and Childress's (1983) book, *Principles of Biomedical Ethics,* had a major influence on discussions of nursing ethics. Their analytic framework, which focused on four ethical principles—respect for autonomy, beneficence, nonmaleficence, and justice—was used by nurses to examine cases or situations that arose in daily nursing practice and the focus on principles was incorporated in ethical decision-making frameworks for nurses (Keatings and Smith 1995). The second way in which nurses examined nursing ethics had its roots in philosophic inquiry in nursing (Kikuchi 2003), nursing theory (Thorne 2003), and feminist ethics (Tong 1995). Nurses engaged in a fundamental exploration of nursing values, the nature of the nurse-patient relationship, and the social role of nursing in society to consider what these meant for ethical nursing practice. Central to this inquiry was the concept of "caring," which received increasing attention in the seventies, eighties, and nineties. Nurses had long considered themselves unique among health professionals in that their traditional focus was the "whole person" as an individual, rather than a limited interest in the disease condition or physical status (Murray 1970; Mussallem 1968). The word "care," as in nursing care, had always been used by nurses, but during the seventies, this word seemed to take on special meaning. Although not clearly defined by all who used the word, caring seemed to signify a humanistic philosophy of nursing, and the term conveyed a concern for the individual person, commitment to the welfare of the patient, empathy and sensitivity to the patient's emotional state, human compassion, and a respect for human worth and dignity. As expressed by various nurses, caring was a capacity (Poole 1973), an attitude (Christo 1979), a quality in nursing (Flaherty 1977), a natural human quality (Roach 1976), and a "basic way of being in the world" (Benner and Wrubel 1989, xi). Feminist scholarship from a variety of disciplines, such as Gilligan's (1982) work on women's moral development and Noddings' (1984) work on caring and the ethic of care, seemed to resonate with nurses (Crigger 2001; Fry 1989; Peter and Morgan 2001). Gilligan's empirical work found that women, when faced with a moral dilemma, tend to focus on relationships and the details of the situation and to seek solutions that maintain relationships. Noddings' ethic of care rejects the abstract rules of traditional ethics and requires an opening up to another person and acting on his or her behalf. In the past 20 years, scholarship in nursing ethics has grown. Nurses have continued to explore nursing ethics through theory development (Fry 1989; Peter and Morgan 2001) and empirical study (Crigger 2001; Crowley 1989; Ellenchild Pinch and Spielman 1996).

Education in Ethics: The Caring Curriculum and Bioethics

During the seventies, nurse educators emphasized the importance of nurturing caring attitudes in nursing students (DuGas 1973; Mesolella 1974) and caring as a moral ideal of nursing. In the view of Bevis (1989), this ideal should infuse the curriculum, and Watson (1989), citing the "transformative thinking" of feminist writers, advocated a nursing curriculum model based on human caring and values. Roy, Williams, and Dickens (1994) described bioethics as a "growth industry" and noted that courses that focus on ethics in health care are offered by departments and faculties of philosophy, religious studies, medicine, and nursing. As part of their nursing education, students may take courses from any one of these sources, but a required course in nursing ethics is probably not yet the norm in Canada. More likely, some nursing students take an elective course in nursing ethics, the majority learning about ethical aspects of nursing in core nursing courses that introduce students to the profession, in nursing theory courses, and in "issues" courses that address a wide variety of moral and non-moral issues and that represent the modern day version of the "professional adjustments" courses of the forties, fifties, and sixties.

A variety of textbooks are used that introduce students to nursing ethics and that provide guidance in terms of ethical ideals, theories, principles, and decision-making models (Blondeau 1986; Yeo and Moorhouse 1996; Davis, Aroskar, Liaschenko and Drought 1997). These books present cases and draw on nursing values, codes, and other resources to assist students in reflecting on the cases and their own practice. Professional associations also provide such guides designed to assist nursing students and practising nurses in their discussion and consideration of ethical challenges in everyday practice (CNA n.d.).

At the graduate level in particular, nursing education draws on a growing literature that addresses the relationship between theory development, research, and practice. This literature addresses such topics as the claim to a distinct nursing ethics (Twomey 1989), the integration of nursing theory and nursing ethics (Yeo 1989), the concepts of power and caring in nursing (Falk Rafael 1996), and the development of a theory of nursing ethics (Fry 1989).

The Profession: Revision of Codes of Ethics, Ethical Statements

Nursing organizations adopted or revised codes of ethics in the seventies, eighties, and nineties, and these revisions changed codes considerably from those of the sixties. The 1973 ICN code included an explicit statement on the primacy of the nurse's responsibility to the patient—the obligation to respect the "beliefs, values, and customs of the individual"—and deleted specific reference to physicians. To all health workers, the nurse owed co-operative effort. The one remaining reference to personal conduct now carried the modifier, "when acting in a professional capacity." According to Bergman (1973), nursing students were key in arguing for changes to the code and rejecting any statement that suggested the subservience of nursing to medicine or outdated customs.[5]

For many years, both the Canadian Nurses Association and many of the provincial nursing organizations responsible for nursing legislation in Canada had adopted the ICN Code of Ethics as their guide to ethical conduct, including the revision of 1973. In Quebec, new nursing legislation led to the adoption of a code of ethics for the Ordre des infirmières et infirmiers du Québec in 1976, and, in Ontario, the College of Nurses adopted the Guidelines for Ethical Behaviour in Nursing in 1980. In an era of standard-setting in nursing, these provincial codes and guidelines established expected standards of ethical conduct. The CNA adopted its own code in 1981, one that generated considerable controversy as it seemed to suggest to some nurses that participation in strikes was unethical. The subsequent CNA (1985) Code of Ethics for Nursing identified an obligation for nurses to take steps to protect patients in any job action (CNA 1985), an obligation that remained in subsequent revisions of the CNA Code (2002).

In addition to new and revised codes of ethics, the organized profession addressed specific ethical issues in policy statements and other publications. For example, the CNA, in a series of documents titled *Ethics in Practice*, addressed issues such as working with limited resources (CNA 2000), appropriate staff mixes (1998), and advance directives (CNA 1998). These guides acknowledged the reality of moral constraint, moral distress, and moral uncertainty for nurses who worked in a health care system that functioned at times with government cost constraints, scarce resources, and staff shortages.

New multidisciplinary organizations emerged in Canada that were devoted to the study of ethical issues in health care, and nurses participated actively in these. Philosophers, lawyers, nurses, and physicians began meeting at conferences to discuss bioethical issues (Davis, Hoffmaster and Shorten 1977), and, subsequently, a number of bioethics institutes were established in various parts of the country (Katz 1980). Two groups, the Canadian Society for Medical Bioethics and the Canadian Society of Bioethics, were created in 1986. The first organization was composed of physicians, and the latter was composed of individuals from a wide range of disciplines and professions, such as nursing, law, theology, and philosophy. These groups joined to form a single organization, the Canadian Bioethics Society, in 1988 (Roy, Williams and Dickens 1994).

Nursing Practice: Nursing Ethics and the Context of Practice

The patient rights movement of the 1970s brought with it continuing concerns about depersonalized care in a health care system that seemed increasingly fragmented, specialized, and subject to cost constraints (MacLellan 1976; Marcus 1975). Public complaints about impersonal care, especially in hospitals, alarmed many members of the profession. An ex-patient (Rose 1970) complained that "hospital nurses seem content to deal with patients as physical beings" (32), and, unlike public health nurses, they failed to provide patients with information and psychological support. One nurse (Guthrie 1973) related her unpleasant experience as a patient undergoing cardiac surgery. She attributed the problem of deper-sonalization, in part, to understaffing: "An overworked nurse is not blessed with the qual-ity of mercy, and her strain affects the patient" (33). In general, the seventies was a decade of protest by nurses about poor working conditions that affected their ability to provide the quality of care for which they felt accountable, an accountability emphasized in an era of standards development, quality assurance, and safety-to-practice programs in nursing ("Health Discipline Act" 1975; "Quality assurance" 1977). The introduction of federal government anti-inflation policies in 1975 not only set limits on wage levels, but also brought provincial cutbacks in health care spending, bed closures, and hiring freezes ("Belt-tightening hits" 1976).

Safe levels of staffing and quality of patient care were issues in a court case involving nurses in British Columbia (Hudson 1970), an arbitration board case in Sudbury ("Three Sudbury nurses" 1971), an arbitration board hearing in Toronto (Wahn 1979), and a year-long dispute at the Vancouver General Hospital during which several senior nursing administrators were fired. Nurses organized to demand, among other things, establishment of a Vice-President Nursing position. Inquiries were held into the firings, public protests by nurses were organized, the board of trustees was dismissed, and a public administrator was appointed, after which a new Vice-President of Nursing was also appointed ("Nurses fight" 1978; "Major changes" 1978). In a sociological analysis of the dispute, Lovell (1981) described the social organization of power in hospitals and how the "normative order" was challenged by nurses who believed that they were excluded from decision-mak-ing about nursing practice.

The Vancouver case could well have served as a Canadian example for Ashley's (1976) assessment of the situation in the United States. In her historical review of the development of nursing, she describes how nursing education and practice had been systematically con-trolled by hospital administration and the medical profession. She argues that sexism and paternalism oppressed nurses and hampered the reform of hospitals and health care in the United States and that nurses should "direct public pressure toward the formation of national health policies that will insure the full utilization of their abilities and talents" (Ashley 1976, 131). Nurses in Canada expressed similar opinions in the 1980s, as described in Growe's (1991) book titled *Who Cares? The Crisis in Canadian Nursing*. The book describes strikes by nurses, the treatment of nurses during the Royal Commission of Inquiry into the deaths at the Hospital for Sick Children, and the shortage of nurses by the end of the decade, highlighting stories of nurses that reinforce the picture of hospitals as paternal and rigid bureaucracies.

In the nineties, nurses identified organizational factors that constrained their actions as moral agents, sometimes with tragic consequences. Operating room nurses in a pediatric cardiac program in Winnipeg used "proper channels" to report problems in the program dur-ing 1994, but without results. In the subsequent Pediatric Cardiac Surgery Inquest Report (Sinclair n.d.; Sibbald 1997) following the deaths of 12 young patients, Judge Sinclair iden-tified how "serious and legitimate concerns" of nurses were dismissed and rejected and how this treatment delayed recognition of serious problems in the pediatric cardiac surgery program. The long-standing funding issues intensified in the nineties as governments sought to reduce debt. This focus led to cutbacks in health care and the layoff of nurses as hospitals closed large numbers of beds in Canada (Baumann et al. 2001). Reports of moral distress among nurses multiplied in all areas of health care but particularly in hospitals where the majority of nurses worked ("Managers must" 1997; CNA 2000). Varcoe and Rodney (2002) argue for the nursing profession to challenge resource allocation decisions at the societal level and blind acceptance of the emphasis on such corporate values as efficiency. Storch (1999) suggests that nurses should work collectively to establish a "moral community" that is supportive of the moral concerns of nurses in the workplace.

In summary, over the last three decades, the focus in nursing ethics has shifted from basic human rights to the rights of patients in health care to an exploration of the nature of the nurse-patient relationship as a basis for ethical conduct. Obligations to physicians, as an identified group, disappeared from codes, but increased interdisciplinary consideration of ethical questions and issues in health care emerged along with the development of bioethics. Increasingly, ethical issues that arose for nurses were tied to their ability to provide quality nursing care in the context of reduced funding and staffing and to their lack of authority in health care bureaucracies. Nursing scholarship in nursing ethics grew over the decades—in the areas of moral inquiry, theory development in nursing ethics, and descriptive ethics in nursing—and this scholarship has been reflected in revised and expanded codes of ethics developed by nursing organizations.

It is clear that since the beginning of "modern" nursing in the 1800s, nurses have believed that their role in society brought with it specific moral obligations. The emphasis shifted over time from the obligations of a nurse to physicians and those in authority to the nurse's obligations to the patient. The degree to which nursing, as a profession, has attended to ethical questions has varied from one time period to another. This level of attention has been influenced by developments in health care and by the broader concerns of society. What has been consistent over time is a sense of ethical distress related to the conditions under which nurses have worked, ranging from expectations of long hours for private duty nurses in the 1920s to the lack of an authoritative nursing voice in hospital bureaucracies and staff shortages in the 1990s. The last century and a half has culminated in a period of intense examination of ethics in nursing, a growing understanding of the moral dimension of nursing, and the beginnings of theory development in nursing ethics.

FOR REFLECTION

1. How did your nursing ethics education compare to that described in this chapter?
2. How has your perception of nursing ethics changed during your career?
3. Has your view of nursing obligations during your career been influenced by your work environment? By social issues and developments? By your professional organization?

ENDNOTES

1.   Much of the early twentieth century North American literature on nursing ethics, reviewed as a basis for this chapter, is comprised of books written by nurse educators and articles from the *American Journal of Nursing* and *The Canadian Nurse*. References from material in the former Archives of the Canadian Nurses Association are also included.

2.   Although Florence Nightingale has generally been identified as the founder of the first training school for nurses, non-secular training institutions, such as the St John's House Training Institution for Nurses, were established a few years prior to Nightingale's school (Summers 1997).

3.   Reverby (1987, 80) identifies Canadian women as the largest minority group in American training schools as Canadian hospitals schools were somewhat slower to develop.

4.   The "Somera Case," as it was known, was reported in the *International Nursing Review* in 1930 following the nurse's conditional pardon and was referred to in subsequent nursing texts to underscore that nurses were as equally responsible as doctors and were not subservient to them.

5.   According to Johnstone (1989), the nursing students who formally presented objections to "subservient" statements to both their national nursing association representatives and the ICN were Canadian, and, as a result, a clause in the code was deleted. There is continuing interest in ethics by nursing students—in the United States, the National Student Nurses' Association, Inc. (2001) has adopted a Code of Academic and Clinical Conduct.

REFERENCES

Aikens, C.A. 1925. *Studies in ethics for nurses.* 2nd edition. Philadelphia: Saunders.

American Journal of Nursing (AJN). 1920. The study of ethics in our schools of nursing. Paper presented at annual meeting of the CNA, 1919. *American Journal of Nursing, 20*(12), 988–989.

American Journal of Nursing. 1926. Editorial. *American Journal of Nursing, 26*(8), 621–625.

Ashley, J. 1976. *Hospitals, paternalism, and the role of the nurse.* New York: Teachers College Press.

Baumann, A., O'Brien-Pallas, L., Armstrong-Stassen, M., Blythe, J., Bourbonnais, R., Cameron, S., Irvine Doran, D., Kerr, M., McGillis Hall, L., Vezina, M., Butt, M. and Ryan, L. 2001. *Commitment and care: The benefits of a healthy workplace for nurses, their patients and the system.* Ottawa: Canadian Health Service Research Foundation.

Baudouin, J. 1977. Protection of life. *Canadian Nurse, 73*(6), 4.

Beauchamp, T.L. and Childress, J.F. 1983. *Principles of biomedical ethics.* New York: Oxford University Press.

BC Nurses vote to strike. 1968. News. *Canadian Nurse, 64*(7), 7.

Belt-tightening hits nurses, national outlook bleak. 1976. News. *Canadian Nurse, 72*(5), 10–11.

Benner, P. and Wrubel, J. 1989. *The primacy of caring. Stress and coping in health and illness.* Don Mills: Addison-Wesley.

Bergman, R. 1973. Ethics—concepts and practice. *International Nursing Review, 20*(5), 140–141, 152.

Bevis, E.O. 1989. The curriculum consequences: Aftermath of revolution. *Curriculum revolution: Reconceptualizing nursing education.* New York: National League for Nursing.

Blishen, B.R. 1969. Society's health expectations. In Health Resources Directorate, *Proceedings: National Health Manpower Conference*, October 7–10, 1969, Ottawa (pp. 31–41). Ottawa: Department of National Health and Welfare Canada.

Blondeau, D. 1986. *De l'éthique à la bioéthique: repères en soins infirmiers.* Chicoutimi, Québec: Gaëtan Morin.

Branson, R., Casebeer, K., Levine, M.D., Oden, T.C., Ramsey, P. and Capron, A.M. 1976. The Quinlan decision: Five commentaries. *Hastings Center Report, 6*(1), 8–19.

Broadhurst, J. 1917. Ethics of nursing. *American Journal of Nursing, 17*(9), 792–797.

Brown, E.L. 1966. Nursing and patient care. In F. Davis (Ed.), *The nursing profession: Five sociological essays* (pp. 176–203). New York: Wiley.

Byers, W.G.M. 1922. The ideals of nursing. *Canadian Nurse, 18*(2), 85–90.

Cadmus, N.E. 1916. Ethics. *American Journal of Nursing, 16*(5), 411–416.

Cameron, S. 1927. Nursing problems. *Canadian Nurse, 23*(10), 520–527.

Canadian Association of Nursing Education. 1924. *Proceedings of the convention*, June 26–28, Hamilton, ON.

Canadian Nurses Association. 1947. *Report of the Committee on nursing and nurse education. Bulletin No. 50.* Ottawa: Canadian Nurses Association.

Canadian Nurses Association. 1954. *Report—Committee to draft a code of ethics.* Ottawa: Canadian Nurses Association.

Canadian Nurses Association. 1955. *Minutes of the Executive Committee meeting,* February 17, 18, 19. Ottawa: Canadian Nurses Association.

Canadian Nurses Association. 1958. *Report of the special committee to study the teaching of professional adjustments in the basic programmes.* Ottawa: Canadian Nurses Association.

Canadian Nurses Association. 1968. *The leaf and the lamp.* Ottawa: Canadian Nurses Association.

Canadian Nurses Association. 1971. *Countdown. Canadian nursing statistics.* Ottawa: Canadian Nurses Association.

Canadian Nurses Association. 1985. *Code of ethics for nursing.* Ottawa: Canadian Nurses Association.

Canadian Nurses Association. 1998. *Advance directives: The nurse's role.* Ottawa: Canadian Nurses Association.

Canadian Nurses Association. 1998. *Ethical issues related to appropriate staff mixes.* Ottawa: Canadian Nurses Association.

Canadian Nurses Association. 2000. *Working with limited resources: Nurses' moral constraints.* Ottawa: Canadian Nurses Association.

Canadian Nurses Association. 2002. *Code of ethics for registered nurses.* Ottawa: Canadian Nurses Association.

Canadian Nurses Association. n.d.. *Everyday ethics.* Ottawa: Canadian Nurses Association.

Carnegie, M.E. 1974. The Patient's Bill of Rights and the nurse. *Nursing Clinics of North America, 9*(3), 557–562.

Catton, M.A. 1921. The question of a "Code of nursing ethics and etiquette" for Canadian nurses. *Canadian Nurse, 17*(9), 553–555.

Christo, S. 1979. Too tired to care? Input. *Canadian Nurse, 75*(11), 6–7.

Cianci, M. 1992. The code of ethics and the role of nurses: An historical perspective. *Nursing Connections, 5*(1), 37–42.

Clermont, D. 1953. Character formation of the nurse. *International Nursing Bulletin, 9*(4), 15–16.

Clint, M. 1914. Qualifications of a successful private nurse. *Canadian Nurse, 10*(10), 643–651.

Code of ethics as applied to nursing. 1965. *International Nursing Review, 12*(6), 38–39.

Consumer rights in health care. 1974. *Canadian Consumer, 4*(2), 1–3.

Crawford, B. 1926. How and what to teach in nursing ethics. *American Journal of Nursing, 26*(3), 211–215.

Crigger, N. 2001. Antecedents to engrossment in Noddings' theory of care. *Journal of Advanced Nursing, 35*(4), 616–623.

Crowley, M. 1989. Feminist pedagogy: Nurturing the ethical ideal. *Advances in Nursing Science, 11*(3), 53–61.

Curtin, L. and Flaherty, M.J. 1982. *Nursing ethics. Theories and pragmatics.* Bowie, Maryland: Prentice Hall.

Davis, A.J. and Aroskar, M.A. 1978. *Ethical dilemmas and nursing practice.* New York: Appleton-Century-Crofts.

Davis, A.J., Aroskar, M.A., Liaschenko, J. and Drought, T.S. 1997. *Ethical dilemmas and nursing practice.* 4th edition. Samford, Connecticut: Appleton & Lange.

Davis, J.W., Hoffmaster, B. and Shorten, S. (Eds.). 1977. *Contemporary issues in biomedical ethics.* Clifton, New Jersey: Humana Press.

Densford, K.J. and Everett, M.S. 1946. *Ethics for modern nurses. Professional adjustments I.* Philadelphia: Saunders.

Dietz, L.D. 1950. Professional adjustments II. 3rd edition. Philadelphia: Davis.

Dock, L.L. 1893. The relation of training schools to hospitals. In L. Petry (Ed.), *Nursing of the sick* (1949) (pp. 12–24). New York: McGraw-Hill.

Domville, E.J. 1891. *A manual for hospital nurses and others engaged in attending on the sick.* 7th edition. London: Churchill.

DuGas, B.W. 1973. Preparing tomorrow's practitioners. Innovations: A national view. In *National Conference on Nurses for Community Service,* November 13–16, 1973, Ottawa, (pp. 65–70). Ottawa: Canadian Nurses Association.

Ellenchild Pinch, W.J. and Spielman, M.L. 1996. Ethics in the neonatal intensive care unit: Parental perceptions at four years postdischarge. *Advances in Nursing Science, 19*(1), 72–85.

Ellis, B.L. 1927. Nursing education. *Canadian Nurse, 23*(9), 471–474.

Fairley, G.E. 1923. Report of the National Conference on Education and Citizenship. *Canadian Nurse, 19*(7), 414–421.

Falk Rafael, A.R. 1996. Power and caring: A dialectic in nursing. *Advances in Nursing Science, 19(*1), 3–17.

Field, C.C. 1923. Graduation address. Children's Hospital of Winnipeg, 1921. *Canadian Nurse, 19*(1), 14–17.

Flaherty, M.J. 1977. Accountability in health care practice: Ethical implications for nurses. In J.W. Davis, B. Hoffmaster and S. Shorten (Eds.), *Contemporary issues in biomedical ethics* (pp. 267–276). Clifton, New Jersey: Humana Press.

Fraser, E.M. 1925. Nursing service in hospital wards. *Canadian Nurse, 21*(12), 639–641.

Fry, S.T. 1989. Toward a theory of nursing ethics. *Advances in Nursing Science, 11*(4), 9–22.

Gardner, M.S. 1916. *Public health nursing.* New York: Macmillan.

Gilligan, C. 1982. *In a different voice. Psychological theory and women's development.* Cambridge, Massachusetts: Harvard University Press.

Grennan, E.M. 1930. The Somera case. *International Nursing Review, 5*(4), 325–333.

Growe, S.J. 1991. *Who cares? The crisis in Canadian nursing.* Toronto: McClelland & Stewart.

Godin, E. and O'Hanley, J. P. E. 1957. *Hospital ethics. A commentary on the Moral Code of Catholic Hospitals.* Bathurst, N.B.: Hotel Dieu Hospital.

Greenland, C. 1975. Consent to treatment—Problems of mental disability. In *Papers and Proceedings of the National Conference on Health and the Law,* September 23–25, 1975, Ottawa, (pp. 129–133). Ottawa: Canadian Hospital Association.

Guthrie, M. 1973. Cardiac surgery in the first person. *Canadian Nurse, 69*(9), 31–33.

Hayter, J. 1966. What does "caring" really mean? *Canadian Nurse, 62*(10), 29–32.

Health Disciplines Act proclaimed in Ontario. 1975. News. *Canadian Nurse, 71*(9), 12.

Health Resources Directorate. 1969. *Proceedings. National Health Manpower Conference,* October 7–10, Ottawa. Ottawa: Department of National Health and Welfare.

Hewitt, J. 2002. A critical review of the arguments debating the role of the nurse advocate. *Journal of Advanced Nursing, 37*(5), 439–445.

Hudson, B. 1970. Timely and revealing. Letters. *Canadian Nurse, 66*(10), 4.

Humbly, R.A. 1921. A new work of mercy. *Maclean's*, March 15, 64–66.

International Council of Nurses. 1977. *The nurse's dilemma. Ethical considerations in nursing practice.* Geneva: ICN.

Jenny, J. 1979. Patient advocacy—Another role for nursing? *International Nursing Review, 26*(6), 176–181.

Johns, E. 1921. The challenge of the future. *Canadian Nurse, 17*(1), 5–10.

Johnstone, M. 1989. *Bioethics. A nursing persepective.* Sydney: Saunders.

Katz, S. 1980. Life and death ethics. *Maclean's,* March 17, 45–47.

Kay, M.E. 1926. The private duty nurse. *Canadian Nurse, 22*(4), 192–193.

Keatings, M. and Smith, O. 1995. *Ethical and legal issues in Canadian nursing.* Toronto: Saunders.

Kikuchi, J.F. 2003. Thinking philosophically in nursing. In J.C. Kerr and M.J. Wood (Eds.), *Canadian nursing. Issues and perspectives* (pp. 103–115). Toronto: Mosby.

Lamb, M. 1981. Nursing ethics in Canada: Two decades. Unpublished Master of Nursing thesis. University of Alberta, Edmonton.

Lindabury, V.A. 1967. Editorial. *Canadian Nurse, 63*(9), 3.

Lindabury, V.A. 1968. Editorial. Withdrawal of service—A dilemma for nursing. *Canadian Nurse, 64*(7), 29.

Lovell, V. 1981. *"I care that VGH nurses care!" A case study and sociological analysis of nursing's influence on the health care system.* Vancouver: In Touch Publications.

MacLellan, B. 1976. Matthew my son: Prepared childbirth at the general. *Canadian Nurse, 72*(3), 38–39.

MacLeod, A.I. 1966. President's address. CNA 33rd general meeting. *Canadian Nurse, 63*(8), 19–22.

Major changes at Vancouver General Hospital. 1978. *RNABC News, 10*(7), 3–5.

Managers must help nurses beat moral distress. 1997. *Canadian Nursing Management, 115* (December), 3.

Marcus, C. 1975. Out of the mouths of patients. *Canadian Nurse, 62*(11), 16–17.

McAllister, J.B. 1955. *Ethics. With special application to the medical and nursing professions.* 2nd edition. Philadelphia: Saunders.

McMurtry, D. 1968. A life without dignity. *Canadian Nurse, 64*(8), 51–52.

McWilliams, M.S. 1921. A laywoman's view of the private duty nurse. *Canadian Nurse, 17*(1), 19–24.

Medical Research Council. 1978. *Ethical considerations in research involving human subjects. Report No. 6.* Ottawa: Supply & Services Canada.

Mesolella, D.W. 1974. Caring begins in the teacher–student relationship. *Canadian Nurse, 70*(12), 15–16.

Murray, V.V. 1970. *Nursing in Ontario. A study for the Committee on the Healing Arts.* Toronto: Queen's Printer.

Mussallem, H.K. 1968. The changing role of the nurse. *Canadian Nurse, 64*(11), 35–37.

Mussallem, H.K. 1992. Professional nurses' associations. In A.J. Baumgart and J. Larsen (Eds.), *Canadian nursing faces the future,* 2nd ed. (pp. 495–517). Toronto: Mosby.

National Conference on Nurses for Community Service. 1973. Ottawa: CNA.

National Student Nurses' Association, Inc. 2001. *Code of academic and clinical conduct.* Retrieved March 32, 2003, from http://www.nsna.org.

Noddings, N. 1984. *Caring: A feminine approach to ethics and moral education.* Los Angeles: University of California Press.

Nurses fight for better care. 1978. *RNABC News, 10*(4), 3–7.

Nurses selfish thinks Dr. Mayo. 1921. *The Toronto Star Weekly*, October 8, 14.

Orem, D. 1971. *Nursing: Concepts of practice.* Scarborough: McGraw-Hill.

Parsons, S.E. 1916. Ethics—the probationer. *American Journal of Nursing, 16*(10), 975–980.

Pellegrino, E.D. 1964. Ethical considerations in the practice of medicine and nursing. In American Nurses Association and American Medical Association (Eds.), *Medical and nursing practice in a changing world*, Proceedings of the First National Conference on Nurses and Physicians (pp. 39–48). Williamsburg, Virginia: American Medical Association.

Pelley, T. 1964. *Nursing. Its history, trends, philosophy, ethics and ethos*. Philadelphia: Saunders.

Perry, A.A. 1929. The high cost of sickness. *Chatelaine, 2*(2), 12–13, 44–47.

Peter, E. and Morgan, K.P. 2001. Explorations of a trust approach for nursing ethics. *Nursing Inquiry, 8*, 3–10.

Poole, P.E. 1973. Nurse, please show me that you care. *Canadian Nurse, 66*(2), 25–27.

Potts, F.J. 1921. Nursing ethics. *Canadian Nurse, 17*(4), 222–224.

"Prepared to care," Alberta nurses kick off province-wide campaign. 1978. News. *Canadian Nurse, 74*(7), 26.

Quality assurance off to a flying start. 1977. News. *Canadian Nurse, 73*(8), 12.

Ramsey, P. 1970. *The patient as person*. New Haven: Yale.

Reverby, S.M. 1987. *Ordered to care. The dilemma of American nursing, 1850–1945.* London: Cambridge University Press.

Roach, M.S. 1976. A framework for the nursing curriculum at St. Francis Xavier University. *Nursing Papers, 7*(4), 23–27.

Robb, I.H. 1898. The spirit of the associated alumnae. In L. Flanagan (Ed.) (1976), *One strong voice. The story of the ANA* (pp. 301–331). Kansas City: American Nurses Association.

Robb, I.H. 1900. *Nursing ethics. For hospitals and private use.* Cleveland: E.G. Koeckert.

Rogers, R. and Ballantyne, W. 1963. Basic qualities of a good nurse. *Canadian Nurse, 59*(10), 949–954.

Rose, S. 1970. A split in the family. *Canadian Nurse, 66*(4), 31–32.

Ross-Kerr, J.C. 1996. Nursing in Canada from 1760 to the present: The transition to modern nursing. In J.C. Ross-Kerr and J. MacPhail (Eds.), *Canadian nursing: Issues and perspectives,* 3rd ed. (pp. 11–22). Toronto: Mosby.

Ross-Kerr, J.C. 2003. The origins of nursing education in Canada: The emergence and growth of diploma programs. In J.C. Ross-Kerr and M.J. Wood (Eds.), *Canadian nursing. Issues and perspectives,* 4th ed. (pp. 330–348). Toronto: Mosby.

Roy, C. 1976. *Introduction to nursing: An adaptation model.* Englewood Cliffs, New Jersey: Prentice Hall.

Roy, D.J., Williams, J.R. and Dickens, B.M. 1994. *Bioethics in Canada.* Scarborough: Prentice Hall.

Scovil, E. R. 1917. The ethics of nursing. *Canadian Nurse, 13*(8), 462–472.

Sibbald, B. 1997. A right to be heard. *Canadian Nurse, 93*(10), 22–30.

Sidelights upon professional ethics with special reference to nursing. *The I.C.N., 1*(1), 7–28.

Siminovitch, L. 1973. Genetic manipulation: Now is the time to consider. *Canadian Nurse, 69*(11), 30–34.

Sinclair, C.M. n.d. *The report of the Manitoba Pediatric Cardiac Surgery Inquest: An inquiry into twelve deaths at the Winnipeg Health Sciences Centre in 1994.* Winnipeg: Provincial Court of Manitoba.

Sklar, C. 1979. Patient's advocate—a new role for the nurse? *Canadian Nurse, 75*(6), 39–41.

Spalding, E.K. 1954. *Professional nursing. Trends and relationships.* 5th edition. Philadelphia: Lippincott.

Stewart, I.M. 1918. How can we help to improve our teaching in nursing schools? *Canadian Nurse, 14*(11), 1393–1399.

Storch, J.L. 1977. *Consumer rights and nursing.* Edmonton: Masters in Nursing Research Trust Fund, University of Alberta.

Storch, J. 1982. *Patients' right: Ethical and legal issues in health care and nursing.* Toronto: McGraw-Hill Ryerson.

Storch, J. 1999. Ethical dimensions of leadership. In J.M. Hibberd and D.L. Smith (Eds.), *Nursing management in Canada,* 2nd ed. (pp. 351–367). Toronto: Saunders.

Suggested code, A. Code of ethics presented for the consideration of the American Nurses' Association. 1926. *American Journal of Nursing, 26*(8), 597–601.

A tentative code. For the nursing profession. 1940. *American Journal of Nursing, 40*(9), 977–980.

Summers, A. 1997. Nurses and ancillaries in the Christian Era. In I. Loudon (Ed.), *Western Medicine. An illustrated history* (pp. 236–244). Oxford: Oxford University Press.

Suzuki, D.T. 1975. The right to health, life and death—At what cost? In *Papers and proceedings of the National Conference on Health and the Lw,* September 23–25, 1975, Ottawa (pp. 236–244). Ottawa: Canadian Hospital Association.

Tate, B.L. 1977. *The nurse's dilemma. Ethical considerations in nursing practice.* Geneva: ICN.

The I.C.N. in Brazil. 1953. *Canadian Nurse, 49*(9), 687.

Thorne, S. 2003. Theoretical issues in nursing. In J.C. Kerr and M. J. Wood (Eds.), *Canadian nursing. Issues and perspectives* (pp. 116–134). Toronto: Mosby.

Three Sudbury nurses win hospital settlement after 13 months' fight. 1971. News. *Canadian Nurse, 67*(9), 14, 16.

Tong, R. 1995. What's distinctive about feminist bioethics? In F. Baylis, J. Downie, B. Freedman, B. Hoffmaster and S. Sherwin (Eds.), *Health care ethics in Canada* (pp. 22–30). Toronto: Harcourt Brace.

Twomey, J.G. 1989. Analysis of the claim to distinct nursing ethics: Normative and nonnormative approaches. *Advances in Nursing Science, 11*(3), 25–32.

Ujhely, G.B. 1973. The patient as equal partner. *Canadian Nurse, 69*(6), 21–23.

Varcoe, C. and Rodney, P. 2002. Constrained agency: The social structure of nurses' work. In B. S. Bolaria and H. Dickinson (Eds.), *Health, illness and health care in Canada*, 3rd ed. (pp. 102–128). Toronto: Harcourt Brace.

Wahn, E.V. 1979. The dilemma of the disobedient nurse. *Health Care in Canada, 21*(2), 43–44, 46.

Watson, J. 1989. Transformative thinking and a caring curriculum. In: E.O. Bevis and J. Watson (Eds.), *Toward a caring curriculum: A new pedagogy for nursing* (pp. 51–60). New York: National League for Nursing.

Webster, G.C. and Baylis, F.E. 2000. Moral residue. In S.B. Rubin and L. Zoloth (Eds.), *Margin of error. The ethics of mistakes in the practice of medicine* (pp. 217–230). Hagerstown, Maryland: University Publishing Group.

Weir, G.M. 1932. *Survey of nursing education in Canada.* Toronto: University of Toronto Press.

Weeks-Shaw, C.S. 1900. *Text-book of nursing. For the use of training schools, families, and private students.* 2nd edition. New York: Appleton and Company.

What's in our code? 1952. *American Journal of Nursing, 52*(10), 1246–1247.

Woodham-Smith, C. 1951. *Florence Nightingale.* Toronto: McGraw-Hill.

Yeo, M. 1989. Integration of nursing theory and nursing ethics. *Advances in Nursing Science, 11*(3), 33–42.

Yeo, M. and Moorhouse, A. 1996. *Concepts and cases in nursing ethics.* 2nd edition. Peterborough: Broadview Press.

chapter three

Philosophical Contributions to Nursing Ethics

Joy L. Johnson

Our leaders of tomorrow must be able to draw upon every tool available to them to support ethical nursing practice; one such tool is philosophy.

Philosophy has been described as "everybody's business." As humans, it is in our nature to try to make sense of our world and to ask questions about the meaning of life and our existence. When we wonder about what it means to be a good person, whether we have free will, or how language is possible, we are engaged in philosophical thinking. Such questions have generated wonder for thousands of years.

Unlike science and history, philosophy does not use investigative methods. To conduct a philosophic study we need not collect data; rather, we rely on our natural capacities to think and reason about the world in which we live. This capacity is captured in Plato's writings about Socrates, who philosophized by simply asking questions of the citizens of Athens. In answering Socrates' questions, the citizens did not need to collect or analyze data; rather, they were led to logical and justified conclusions by considering their own experiences in the world. The important point here is that philosophers do not conduct experiments; nor do they collect data to prove their theories. The practice of philosophizing involves exploring ideas and thinking through possible arguments for and against different positions. **Argumentation** is a key instrument of philosophy and involves providing logical reasons or evidence in support or denial of a particular position.

In drawing distinctions between philosophy and other realms of inquiry, Nagle (1987) maintains that the main concern of philosophy is to question and understand very common ideas that many of us take for granted. He illustrates the distinction between philosophy and other forms of inquiry by pointing out that while a historian might investigate past events, a philosopher would ask, What is time? Similarly, while anyone might ask a question, such as whether it is wrong to conceal the truth about a diagnosis from a patient, a philosopher would consider what makes an action right or wrong. The aim of this type of inquiry is to push our thinking and understanding of a matter and to deepen our insights.

Until recently, philosophy has not been embraced by nursing scholars as a legitimate form of inquiry. Accordingly, it represents an area of inquiry that is just beginning to receive the attention it deserves. Philosophy is also a frontier in that the questions that are considered by philosophers are seemingly limitless. The more we know, the more we are inspired to ponder what remains unknown.

In this chapter I consider the ways in which philosophy can contribute to the evolution of nursing ethics. I begin by examining what we mean by nursing philosophy, the types of philosophical questions that are of concern to nurses, and the relationship of nursing theories to nursing philosophy. I then briefly examine how the world of philosophy has contributed to the realm of nursing ethics. The chapter closes with an examination of some of the unresolved philosophical issues facing the field of nursing ethics. All nurses can benefit from becoming more strongly grounded in philosophy and learning ways to use philosophic approaches to deepen their understanding of the nurse's world. Our leaders of tomorrow must be able to draw upon every tool available to them to support ethical nursing practice; one such tool is philosophy.

WHAT IS NURSING PHILOSOPHY?

Many areas of nursing are taken for granted. Nurses can tend to go about their work without questioning why it is that they do the things they do. Nursing is a practice profession, and so it is appropriate that we focus on accomplishing tasks and completing nursing actions. While we would not accomplish our goals in nursing practice if we were forever questioning the very essence of nursing, it is highly appropriate that we, on occasion, step back and consider philosophic questions related to nursing. Just like the questions that philosophy addresses, nursing philosophy is directed toward considering "big" questions such as, What is the goal of nursing? What ought nurses to do when faced with difficult choices? and How can we distinguish nursing from other professional practices such as medicine? Practitioners in professions such as medicine and law similarly struggle to understand the nature of their work and the objectives toward which they should legitimately direct their efforts.

Nursing has an impressive philosophic legacy. Kikuchi and Simmons (1994) pointed out, "If the study of philosophical thought in nursing were to be undertaken, there would be no shortage of materials.... Nurses have reflected upon, and continue to reflect upon, the nature of their work and they continue to put their thoughts in writing, as a 'philosophy of nursing'" (1). Kikuchi and Simmons deliberately placed the term "philosophy of nursing" in quotations because, until lately, much of nursing scholarship, although philosophic in nature, was not recognized as philosophic writing. An excellent case in point can be found in the writings of Florence Nightingale, a well-known scholar of the 19th century. In writings such as *Notes on nursing: What it is and what it is not* and *Sick nursing and health nursing*, Nightingale applied logic and reasoning to consider the nature of nursing. She contrasted nursing to other forms of work and used her own experience to reason through possible solutions to problems such as determining "what nursing is, and what it is not."

Beginning in the 1970s several scholars, who became known as the "nursing theorists," developed conceptual frameworks for nursing practice. Numbered among these works are those by Dorothea Orem (1991), Martha Rogers (1970), and Rosemarie Parse (1981). The conceptualizations of nursing proposed in their works were developed to direct nursing practice and research by addressing questions such as, What is it good to do and seek in nursing? Although some might reject the idea of classifying these works as philosophic, they address questions that are philosophic in nature and appear to employ the methods of philosophy (that is, reason and logic). **Philosophies of nursing** are aimed at systematically articulating, through the methods of philosophy, the nature, scope, and object of nursing. In contrast, the term **philosophy in nursing** or **nursing philosophy** connotes the activity of philosophizing that focuses on questions relevant to nursing.

Since the 1990s nursing scholars have more fully embraced the role and contribution of philosophy. Conferences have been held and books and journal articles have been published that address nursing philosophic issues. Centres for the study of nursing philosophy have been established, and a journal titled *Nursing Philosophy* has been launched. These developments attest to the emergent field of nursing philosophy. With increasing frequency, nurses are recognizing that science is unable to answer many of the important questions facing nursing and have consequently turned to philosophy.

Nurses, whose work is grounded in Western philosophic traditions, have tended to focus their philosophic inquiries on three types of questions: ontological (concerning what is), epistemological (concerning how we know), and moral (concerning what we ought to do and seek). Examples of ontological questions are: What is the nature of nursing? What is the essence of the nurse-patient relationship? Examples of epistemological questions are: What is the nature of nursing knowledge? What is the type of evidence nurses need in their practice? and How can scientific findings be applied in particular situations? Finally, examples of moral questions that nurses have addressed include: What are nurses' obligations in relation to end-of-life decision-making? How should a nurse deal with matters of privacy and privilege? and How ought nurses ensure that their care is directed toward the needs of patients and not to the institutional system for which they work?

Ontological questions are the most fundamental in that assumptions about nursing must be presupposed if we are to begin to answer epistemological and moral questions. For example, to understand what *nursing knowledge* is, we must first understand what *nursing* is. Similarly, if we are to grapple with what a good action is for a nurse, we must understand the nature of nursing as well as the nature of goodness. As discussed earlier, philosophizing helps us to probe our common conceptions of nursing and to deepen our understanding of the problems facing nursing.

Much of the philosophical writing in nursing has been aimed at considering how the works of philosophers such as Kant, Merleau Ponty, and Foucault are relevant to nursing. These questions can be thought of as second order questions, and, while important, focusing solely on this type of question has its limitations. Knowledge of the first order is knowledge about reality; knowledge of the second order is knowledge about knowledge itself. It follows that in philosophy, first order questions are metaphysical or ontological in nature. These are questions about that which is or happens or about what we should do or seek. Examples of such questions include: What is the nature of nursing? What is the essence of the nurse-patient relationship? and What are the essential values that underlie nursing practice? In contrast, second order questions are about our first order knowledge. These are questions about how we know, think, or speak. Second order philosophic knowledge allows philosophy to be critical of its own concepts and language and to examine its own knowledge. Examples of second order questions include: What are the issues and controversies inherent in the ways that the art of nursing has been conceptualized by nursing scholars? and What are the limitations inherent in Parse's (1981) conception of nursing? In modern philosophy, we have seen an emphasis on second order questions. Thus, we see more philosophers concerning themselves with the limitations of our knowledge of the world than with knowledge of the world itself. We have spent considerable time accounting for the nature of nursing knowledge and relatively little effort considering the nature of nursing as nursing. This is cause for concern because an exclusive focus on questions about how or what we know is ultimately nihilistic in that it keeps a discipline from considering substantive questions necessary to push the frontiers of knowledge forward.

We need to philosophize about nursing. If we do not engage in this work, the nature of nursing work will be determined by whatever forces are the strongest, be they political, administrative, or the opinions of other health professionals. If we are unable to determine what nursing is, we will be unable to defend its borders or implement the interventions that we believe are required to achieve nursing goals. Philosophy also holds implications for our ethical actions as nurses. If nurses cannot articulate what it means to nurse well, they will be unable to make judgments about whether nurses have conducted themselves in ways that are consistent with an appropriate view of nursing. This type of work is difficult and will not easily yield clear answers; the aim of this work is to push our thinking and understanding about nursing and to deepen our insights.

A gradate student, in a moment of despair brought on by too much reading about philosophy of nursing, once asked me why we continue to ask and answer the "same old questions" such as, What is nursing? This type of inquiry seemed futile to the student, and she believed that it was senseless to continue asking questions that apparently could not be answered. My response to this student was that in the same way human beings continue to philosophize about the meaning of life, so too must nurses ask these questions about nursing. To do so is to tend to one's discipline, to carry the work forward, and to release oneself from simply assuming that nursing is what nurses do.

While there has been much debate among nurses about the nature of nursing and the type of knowledge required for nursing practice, there is wide agreement that nursing is a moral endeavour. Authors such as Carper (1978) have helped to articulate the essential elements of nursing knowledge and to secure the idea that an essential way of knowing in nursing is moral knowing. Nurses have vigorously pursued answers to questions regarding the moral realm of nursing. One approach used in this pursuit has involved drawing on knowledge from the realm of ethics and philosophy to help address nursing moral issues. Some of these philosophic influences are considered in the following section.

PHILOSOPHICAL INFLUENCES ON NURSING ETHICS

The discipline of philosophy has undergone numerous changes in the past two decades. Philosophers now consider topics that at one time might have been considered outside the proper domain of "academic philosophy." Among these topics is an enterprise commonly referred to as *applied ethics*. Here, general ethics theories are applied to social and professional problems that are fundamentally moral in nature. In the discipline of nursing we can observe nurses drawing upon various ethical theories to address moral problems. The notion that one can simply apply ethical theories to moral problems in nursing is somewhat of a misnomer. When working with these theories, one must analyze concepts and submit them to critical scrutiny, examine hidden presuppositions, and offer new accounts of the problem in question.

As demonstrated in the table of contents of this text, the branch of philosophic work known as "nursing ethics" covers a wide variety of topics and concerns. All of the papers in this text are influenced by philosophical assumptions related to what nursing is, what is knowable, and what is ethical. There is not agreement about what these assumptions are or should be, and so to examine any given conclusion one must consider the position on which the claim is based. A few examples can help to illustrate this point. In her paper on the ethics of care, Bowden (2000) draws on feminist philosophy to argue against considering "ethics in a vacuum." Feminist philosophy's concern with the subjectivity of experience and the ways that political and institutional structures shape experience inform her position. In contrast, in his paper on the ethics of care, Paley (2002) draws on a Kantian perspective (derived from the work of Emanuel Kant) and posits that Kant's work adequately accounts for the particularity of context and at the same time locates ethics in a fuller and universal account of moral conduct and moral character. While both of these papers address the ethics of care, each author is informed by different perspectives and draws different conclusions.

Nurses have drawn from a variety of philosophic works in their consideration of ethical questions. One need only scan the reference lists of papers related to ethical issues to see the variety of philosophic works that have been relied upon by nursing scholars in their consideration of moral issues in nursing. In general, nursing scholars have used these works to help position themselves and to provide context for the assumptions guiding an analysis, or they have applied key aspects of a philosopher's work to help shed light on problems or concerns. The philosophic works nurses have used can be roughly divided into a variety of schools or perspectives related to ontological positions such as **critical realism** (a position that emphasizes that our understanding of the world comes from an analysis of the world itself), **pragmatism** (a position that emphasizes that our understanding of the world should arise from an understanding of what works or is reasonable), **existentialism** (a position that emphasizes that our understanding of the world is subjective and emerges from a struggle with personal concerns and projects), and **postmodernism** (a position that emphasizes that our understanding of the world is constructed through social and political structures and that, accordingly, metatheories are to be rejected). There are of course numerous other perspectives that nurses draw on, and an attempt to classify them is beyond the scope of this chapter.

The majority of philosophers' works that nurses have drawn upon have emanated from the West. Eastern philosophy is a frontier that has been largely unexplored by nurses. There is an awakening interest among nurses in perspectives drawn from the East that challenge foundationalist approaches adhered to by Western philosophers. For example, Bruce (2002), in her dissertation, explores the notion of living with dying. She draws on a Buddhist perspective to deepen our understanding of notions of impermanence and to challenge our need for certainty and solidity. Rather than being consumed with "doing for" and "knowing that," she prompts us to consider how we might mindfully be with a person and acknowledge the impermanence of being. Her approach has profound ethical implications for how nurses might provide care in the midst of suffering. Rodgers and Yen (2002) also claim that the Eastern philosophic perspectives have a great deal to offer nursing and suggest that, given the growing globalization that surrounds us, nurses need to "empty their cups" and ponder different approaches to considering the discipline. The philosophic position one holds is based on assumptions about the nature of the world and the nature of knowledge and, therefore, has implications for the claims one makes about nursing and the conclusions one draws about what might be morally good or ethical. What this means is that rather than taking any position at face value, it is important to consider the assumptions upon which it rests and the implications that the position may hold for nursing thought and action.

THE CONTESTED BORDERS OF NURSING SCIENCE AND NURSING ETHICS

Nurses have become enamoured of science. I use the term "science" here to include a variety of methods, including quantitative, qualitative, descriptive, experimental, and interpretive. Science is a dominant branch of knowledge, and, in the current technological era, it is easy to believe that science will solve all of the problems facing modern society. Science, like philosophy, is a mode of inquiry concerned with phenomena in the world. Like philosophy, science is **empirical,** relying on sense experience. While philosophy is concerned with broad questions about the nature of the world, science is concerned with special experiences that are not accessible to us in our everyday worlds. Whereas scientific inquiry relies on the collection of data to answer questions, philosophical inquiry typically relies on reason and logic and "everyday" knowledge of the world. There are many questions that science cannot answer; Kikuchi (1992) pointed out that nurses have gotten themselves into a muddle by trying to answer philosophical questions with scientific methods. Science's investigative, interviewing, and measurement tools will not enable us to answer questions such as what nurses ought to do or what justice is. Similarly, Reed and Ground (1997) point out, "There are questions which scientists can and do ask themselves but which, purely as scientists, cannot be answered by them. Typically ethical questions are of this form" (65).

The sharp demarcation between science and philosophy that Kikuchi and Reed and Ground attempt to make is not shared by all, particularly in the field of ethics. It is widely recognized that the application of rationally based theory to moral problems in health care has not worked. A number of difficulties arise when we try to take philosophical theories and apply them to concrete practice problems. The theories lack specificity and cannot account for the variety of contextual issues that arise in the practice world.

Hoffmaster (1994) and others reject ethics' preoccupation with applying theory to practice in favour of **contextualism:** an approach that situates moral problems in institutional and organizational structures and in social and cultural backgrounds. Hoffmaster (1992) calls for the use of ethnographic studies of moral problems in health care to ensure that ethical theory is more responsive to the empirical dimensions of ethical problems. These studies are valuable in that they ground our understanding of ethical problems in the complex world in which they arise.

In nursing we have witnessed a burgeoning of studies that highlight the ethical dilemmas that nurses face. While these studies are not traditionally philosophical per se, they provide data about nurses' "everyday experiences" that provide rich ground for philosophizing. Often in the field of ethics a case is used to highlight salient points and to elucidate the complex nature of particular problems. Similarly, studies that collect data to highlight the dilemmas faced by nurses, and the approaches they use to resolve these dilemmas, provide grist for the philosophical mill. While ethnographic studies provide important information about the nature of the social world, strictly speaking, their methods stop short of transforming this knowledge into moral theory that can guide practice. Studies that apply solely the methods of science cannot answer questions about what nurses ought to do and seek. Deductions of what "ought to be" from "what is" have been referred to as **naturalistic fallacies.** This type of fallacy or mistake occurs when we try to derive ethical statements from non-ethical statements of fact. What is happening in a situation does not provide direction for what should be. To avoid this fallacy we must also employ the methods of philosophy and use principles and values to reason through an appropriate course of action. Science as a mode of inquiry can be helpful to ethics in that it can be used to describe phenomena, to study the conditions necessary to bring about a particular form of practice, or to highlight "taken for granted" aspects of nursing practice. Science alone, however, no matter how well executed, cannot provide answers to ethical matters. We must incorporate the tools of philosophy to develop theory about what nurses should do and seek. One of the challenges that lies ahead is to effectively blend the methods of social science and philosophy to ensure that relevant moral theory is developed.

While there are calls from many quarters for nursing practice to be based on scientific evidence, it is clear that solutions to problems cannot be simply achieved by using scientific findings to guide action. Evidence-based approaches to nursing care will not ensure that the practice of nursing is good or sound. This is true because while science is concerned with developing knowledge that can inform theory, ethical practice involves dealing with the particulars of a case (that is, many features which may be unique and require the practical judgment of the nurse). While science is an important tool for nursing, its potency must be circumscribed, a concern that is being increasingly acknowledged by nurses. For example, Winch, Creedy and Chaboyer (2002), drawing on a Foucauldian perspective, warn that evidence-based practice is a technique for governing nursing practice that ultimately might undermine the agency of the nurse. As we consider the frontiers of nursing ethics, it is clear that the borders between science and good practice will continue to be a topic that requires our attention.

UNRESOLVED ETHICAL NURSING ISSUES

Several unresolved philosophical issues remain in the field of nursing ethics that present significant challenges for the profession. In the following section, I highlight some of these issues and discuss why they are significant. These issues concern the role of ethical principles in nursing, the question of whether nursing has a unique ethical perspective, and issues related to what constitutes good, or artful, nursing practice.

The Role of Ethical Principles in Nursing

One issue concerns whether there are universal ethical principles—that is, principles about what constitutes good action that hold across time, place, and person. This is a central issue that has implications for nursing ethics as well as other forms of ethics. Do we believe that there can be a code of ethics that can be applied to all nurses in all situations, or do we acknowledge that there are always contingencies that must be taken into consideration? Can both positions be accommodated? Austin (2001) raised this issue when she asked, "Can we conceive of a macro-ethic that could guide our moral actions in a global community?" (11). Writers such as Gadow (2000), whose work is grounded in a postmodern perspective—a position that holds that knowledge is socially constructed and must be subjected to systematic deconstruction to reveal the ways in which it is partial—raise serious concerns about the very possibility of ethical principles. Others have suggested that rather than taking a principle-based approach to ensuring good practice, we should consider the virtues necessary to nurse well. If we are to endorse and use ethical guidelines and moral codes, we must come to a common understanding of what they are and how they should be used. If they are not possible, or useful, we need to acknowledge this and determine how we might ensure that nursing practice is moral.

If one holds that such principles are possible, how ought they to be derived? Possible responses are that principles ought to be derived from social consensus, from a notion of goodness that is grounded in an understanding of the nature of humans, or from some other approach. Depending on how one views the nature of the world and human beings, one would adopt different answers to this important question. This issue has been debated by moral philosophers for centuries. It is important to recognize that while it will likely remain unresolved, the perspective one takes has implications for the ways in which one might assess moral conduct in nursing practice.

Nursing's Unique Ethical Perspective

An important matter raised in a recent editorial by Carnevale (2002) concerns whether nursing has its own unique ethical perspective and is responsible for deriving ethical principles unique to nursing, or whether nursing's ethical perspectives should be drawn from the field of moral philosophy. Kikuchi (1992) suggested that while the field of moral philosophy addresses questions related to what is good to do and seek as humans, nurses are responsible for considering what it is we ought to do and seek as nurses.

Currently, there is considerable scholarly work being conducted to clarify nursing's unique ethical perspective. Scott (2000), for example, argued that any theory of ethics that denies the moral significance of the emotions would be problematic for nursing. Her approach brings us closer to understanding the essential elements of an ethics of nursing but does not fully address what else is required. Grace (2001), on the other hand, examines "advocacy" as an ideal ethic for nursing practice and concludes that a broad sense of advocacy that encompasses both individual and societal needs is appropriate for the practice of nursing. As the quest for an ethical perspective for nursing carries on, we can anticipate that philosophic work such as that conducted by Scott and Grace will continue. These types of analyses will help to push the frontiers of nursing ethics forward by broadening our understanding of moral conduct in nursing practice.

The Nature of Good Nursing Practice

Ethics is concerned with ensuring that our actions are morally good. When we think about good nursing practice, we often think about the required skills and values that are necessary.

The ability to nurse well is frequently referred to as the "art of nursing." An important question that has arisen in relation to nursing ethics is the relationship between nursing art and nursing ethics. While much disagreement exists about what it takes to be an artful nurse, the idea that nursing art is by nature a moral art is gaining acceptance.

Ethics in Practice 3-1	**The Artful Nurse**

A nurse is observed caring for a post-surgical patient. She assesses the client comprehensively and plans the care she will provide for the day. She anticipates all of the patient's post-surgical needs, providing pain medication when it is required, encouraging deep breathing and coughing, speaking with the patient and family and preparing him or her for discharge. The nurse appears to be very knowledgeable and has tremendous skill and efficiency. Toward the end of her shift, she strongly encourages the patient to sit in a chair, knowing this would be good for the patient. The patient is tired, scared, and unwilling to co-operate. The nurse persists and, eventually, with the help of another nurse, easily transfers the patient into a chair. The nurse is pleased that all the goals she set for the patient have been accomplished. The patient is clean, the dressing is changed, and the bedside is tidy. Is this an artful nurse?

At first glance, we might consider the nurse in Ethics in Practice 3-1 to be artful. But is skill in assessing and caring for a patient enough? The art of the nurse involves more than the skill and cunning required to make something occur. The nurse in this scenario selected a course of action that was scientifically sound and ignored the will of the patient. Unlike "artisans," who make things, nurses deal with human beings, and so, in addition to having specific skills, we expect nurses to comport themselves in particular ways. Not only must a nurse know what to do, she or he also must choose appropriately among means to decide the best course of action.

The question of the relationship between morality and art has long been a subject of debate among philosophers. Oscar Wilde summed up one position of this argument with the statement, "The fact of a man being a poisoner is nothing against his prose" (cited in Maritain 1959, 81). With this statement, Wilde implied that the world of art and morality are two entirely autonomous worlds. The fine artist (painter, poet, etc.) does not pursue a moral good, but rather the good of the work. A good writer need not be a good person, and good art is judged on its artistic merit alone, not on moral grounds. The same cannot be said for the art of nursing. A nurse may be technically competent and knowledgeable, yet if she or he does not make moral choices in the performance of nursing care, the nurse is not artful. According to this view, artful nursing is inextricably intertwined with human life and the achievement of particular human ends. Leah Curtin (1979), a pioneering nursing ethicist, summed up this notion:

The end or purpose of nursing is the welfare of other human beings. This end is not a scientific end, but rather a moral end. That is, it involves the seeking of good and it involves our relationship with other human beings. The science that we learn, the technological skills that we develop are shaped and designed by that moral end—much as an artist using a brush. Therefore, nursing is a moral art (2).

In even the smallest of actions, the nurse expresses the values to which she or he is personally committed. At almost every moment, a nurse is confronted with the need to choose between a greater and a lesser good (Lanara 1981). Accordingly, all nursing acts, to the extent that they are voluntary and affect human lives, are subject to moral judgment. Whereas the technician uses techniques that are evaluated by efficiency, "the professional makes decisions which are evaluated by the good" (Bishop and Scudder 1990, 69).

Although agreement is emerging that nursing art involves practising in such a way that a **moral good**—or an objective that is good for a person and is ethically defensible—is realized, there is little agreement about how this is best accomplished or what constitutes the good. Some authors, such as Beckstrand (1978), have suggested that moral practice can be achieved through the application of moral theory. Nurses need to simply apply ethical theory in their clinical reasoning processes. As discussed earlier, the problem with this approach is that it fails to accommodate the idiosyncrasies of a particular situation. In contrast, authors such as Gadow (1985) suggested that moral nursing practice can only be achieved when nurses enter into subjective caring relationships in which both the patient's and the nurse's values are considered. The moral good is thus achieved intersubjectively, between the nurse and the patient. In contrast, Benner (1991) took the position that nurses learn skilful ethical comportment over time as they participate in their practices and gain a sense of what it means to be "better" or "worse." An unresolved issue inherent in these positions is the question of whether a nurse's sense of what is morally good is **subjective**—arising from a personal sense of what is right—or whether there is some form of **objective** or external criterion with which to judge what is good. When a nurse chooses a course of action because she or he has a sense that it is a good course of action, or when a nurse and patient together choose a course of action, does this inherently make the action good? It would seem that neither the blind application of moral principles nor the nurse's personal sense of what is good is enough to ensure that an action is morally good. The answer to this issue may indeed lie in the melding of principles and perception so that the nurse carefully determines a correct course of action.

The notion of the good also applies to the realm of nursing leadership and administration. In these situations it is easy for nurses to lose sight of the good they are attempting to serve. What is "good" for the economic efficiency of a hospital is not necessarily "good" for patients; similarly, what is good for nurses is not always good for patients. Aristotle conceived of politics as a realm of philosophy related to ethics. While ethics is concerned with what is good for individuals, politics focuses on what is good for groups of humans, specifically the types of organizations that most benefit human beings. The moral art of nursing administration, or nursing leadership, is perhaps one of the least developed areas in nursing philosophy and is deserving of attention. What is the good that nursing administrators serve? What types of skills and virtues do artful nursing administrators require?

The Virtue of the Good Nurse

As has been discussed earlier in this chapter, nurses are coming to recognize that moral practice cannot simply be achieved by applying ethical principles to complex situations.

With the acknowledgment of the limitations of principle-driven approaches, attention has been increasingly focused on determining alternative approaches. Virtue-based approaches to moral practice are coming to be considered as alternatives. Sellman (2000), for example, applied MacIntyre's (1984) notion of virtue in considering the nature of nursing practice. This approach seeks to understand the **virtues,** or habits of good operation, that are required for moral practice. Instead of considering the principles that need to be applied for a moral practice, a virtue-based approach considers the virtues nurses require to be moral in their practice. The challenge this latter approach presents is for us to identify the virtues necessary to the practice of nursing.

Most would agree that the possession of skill and knowledge are necessary conditions for the moral conduct of nursing practice. It is hard to imagine a situation where incompetent nurses could morally conduct themselves in nursing practice; their lack of competency would not enable them to achieve desired goals. In identifying oneself as a professional, one is claiming a certain level of competence. The licence to practise nursing does not include permission to practise poorly. The moral responsibility of the nurse involves a commitment not only to nurse a patient competently, but also to "sustain excellent practice in the face of unreasonable demands and lack of appreciation on the part of patients" (Bishop and Scudder 1987, 37). The good nurse must not only be competent, but must consistently demonstrate competence in her or his practice no matter how arduous the circumstances. Pask (2001) emphasized this point, describing how nurses can feel challenged when "times get hard and they struggle to turn from their own suffering, to focus instead upon the needs of their patients" (45).

As suggested in Ethics in Practice 3-2, the other virtues that are required by nurses are moral virtues, or characteristics that ensure that a nurse makes good choices in her or his practice.

Ethics in Practice 3-2	**Nursing in Difficult Conditions**

It is three o'clock in the morning. The nursing unit is short staffed and all the nurses have been inordinately busy. There are several patients who are very ill and who require regular monitoring. The nursing staff are tired and have missed all their rest breaks. The patient in Room 200, not the sickest of the patients, has been "on the call bell all night." Every time one of the nurses makes the trek down the hall it is for some minor request or complaint. There is finally a lull and everyone has a chance to sit down, and the call bell goes on again. How will the character of the nurse who answers the call influence this situation?

Bishop and Scudder (1990) maintained that the possession of certain moral virtues enables a nurse to nurse artfully. Philosophers have long considered the nature of virtue: is it a natural propensity, or can it be cultivated? Most agree that it can be developed. Similarly, in nursing, while there is a sense that nurses must by nature be ethical, there is also a sense that the ability to comport oneself in difficult situations can be developed over time. Pask (2001), for example, suggested that it is "through the conscious training of their habitual responses, that a nurse comes disposed to respond, and to act with compassion" (51). What enables a nurse to act morally under difficult situations?

Since the time of Florence Nightingale nurses have discussed the virtues required to nurse artfully. Numbered among the primary virtues are charity, love, and compassion. In recent years caring has been upheld as the virtue that drives artful nursing. Benner and Wrubel (1989) suggested that the same act performed in a caring and uncaring way may have different effects, and only the nurse who cares will notice small differences in their patients' behaviours and create unique solutions to patients' needs. Jaegar (2001) suggested that moral sensitivity is the key capacity or virtue that must be fully developed by nurses. She maintains that being able to place oneself in another's position is not enough. One must be able to be open to the possibility that one does not share the same moral framework with the other person. Moral sensitivity is the capacity to be sensitive to these differences. Her concern is that, in today's environment, health care workers are in danger of losing their moral sensitivity and that moral theories describe too abstractly what it means to respect another person. Her claim is that the cultivation of moral sensitivity is an antidote to administrative policies that rely on the formulaic application of traditional moral theories.

Often, educators and administrators are focused on ensuring that nurses have skills and competencies. In addition to possessing these skills, nurses need to consistently use these competencies in an ethical manner. What virtues do nurses require? And how might nursing educators and administrators help to cultivate those virtues in the nurses they educate and supervise? Must a nurse possess these virtues innately, or can they be taught? What institutional factors need to be in place to support nurses to develop and use their virtues? These are important questions that require our urgent attention because answers to these questions have the potential to help us to assist nurses to develop the capacity to consistently respond in an ethical manner to the challenges they face.

In closing, philosophical contributions to nursing ethics are multifaceted. While the works of non-nursing philosophers provide valuable insights that can help to inform nursing ethics, these contributions cannot be simply applied to nursing situations and will not resolve nursing's fundamental ethical issues. Philosophical work focused specifically on nursing can help to answer questions related to the nature of nursing and the nurse-patient relationship and can provide valuable direction for the development of nursing ethics. The mandate to develop nursing philosophy cannot be relegated to nursing scholars; to do so is to condemn nursing philosophy to obscurity. If nursing philosophy is to be relevant, it must also be based on the contributions and insights of administrators, clinicians, and educators. This chapter has raised a number of philosophical questions related to nursing ethics that remain unanswered. In addition to considering the questions posed below, I encourage readers to consider the questions raised in the chapter and to attempt to formulate sound responses. Philosophy is, after all, every nurse's business.

FOR REFLECTION

1. Consider any one of the chapters in this text. What philosophical assumptions underlie the author's arguments? Are these assumptions implicit or explicit?

2. What do you contend is the nature, scope, and goal of nursing? What implications does your position have for ethical nursing practice?

3. Can a nursing leader be a good leader without a firm understanding of the nature of nursing?

4. Consider the practice of a nurse whom you consider to have demonstrated the finest attributes of nursing art. What are the virtues required by nursing, and how can they be cultivated?

5. What are the most important questions facing nursing ethics? How can these issues be resolved?

REFERENCES

Austin, W. 2001. Nursing ethics in an era of globalization. *Advances in Nursing Science, 24*(2), 1–18.

Barber, K. (Ed.). 1998. *The Canadian Oxford dictionary.* Toronto: Oxford University Press.

Beckstrand, J. 1978. The notion of a practice theory and the relationship of scientific and ethical knowledge to practice. *Research in Nursing and Health, 1*, 131–136.

Benner, P. 1991. The role of experience, narrative, and community in skilled ethical comportment. *Advances in Nursing Science, 14*(3), 13–28.

Benner, P. and Wrubel, J. 1989. *The primacy of caring: Stress and coping in health and illness.* Menlo Park, CA: Addison-Wesley.

Bishop, A.H. and Scudder, J.R. Jr. 1987. Nursing ethics in an age of controversy. *Advances in Nursing Science, 9*(3), 34–43.

Bishop, A.H. and Scudder, J.R. Jr. 1990. *The practical, moral, and personal sense of nursing: A phenomenological philosophy of practice.* Albany, NY: State University of New York Press.

Bowden, P. 2000. An 'ethic of care' in clinical settings: Encompassing "feminine" and "feminist" perspectives. *Nursing Philosophy, 1*, 36–49.

Bruce, W.A. 2002. *Abiding in liminal space(s): Inscribing mindful living/dying with(in) end-of-life care.* Unpublished doctoral dissertation. University of British Columbia, Vancouver, BC.

Carnevale, F. 2002. Betwixt and between: Searching for nursing's moral foundation. *Canadian Journal of Nursing Research, 34(2),* 5–8.

Carper, B.A. 1978. Fundamental patterns of knowing in nursing, *Advances in Nursing Science, 1,* 13–23.

Curtin, L.L. 1979. The nurse as advocate: A philosophical foundation for nursing. *Advances in Nursing Science, 1*(3), 1–10.

Gadow, S. 1985. Nurse and patient: The caring relationship. In A.H. Bishop and J.R. Scudder Jr. (Eds.), *Caring, curing, coping: Nurse physician, patient relationships* (pp. 31–43). Tuscaloosa, AL: University of Alabama Press.

Gadow, S. 2000. Philosophy as falling: Aiming for grace. *Nursing Philosophy, 1*, 89–97.

Grace, P.J. 2001. Professional advocacy: Widening the scope of accountability. *Nursing Philosophy, 2,* 151–162.

Hoffmaster, B. 1994. The forms and limits of medical ethics. *Social Science and Medicine, 39*, 1155–1164.

Hoffmaster, B. 1992. Can ethnography save the life of medical ethics? *Social Science and Medicine, 35*, 1421–1431.

Jaeger, S.M. 2001. Teaching health care ethics: The importance of moral sensitivity for moral reasoning. *Nursing Philosophy, 2,* 131–142.

Kikuchi, J. 1992. Nursing questions that science cannot answer. In J. Kikuchi and H. Simmons (Eds.), *Philosophic inquiry in nursing* (pp. 26–37). Thousand Oaks, CA: Sage.

Kikuchi, J. and Simmons, H. 1994. *Developing a philosophy of nursing*. Thousand Oaks, CA: Sage.

Lanara, V. 1981. *Heroism as a nursing value: A philosophical perspective*. Athens: Sisterhood Evniki.

MacIntyre, A. 1984. *After Virtue*. 2nd edition. Notre Dame, ID: University of Notre Dame Press.

Maritain, J. 1951. Art as a virtue of the practical intellect. In M. Weitz (Ed.), *Problems in aesthetics: An introductory book of readings* (pp. 76–92). New York: Macmillan.

Nagle, T. 1987. *What does it all mean? A very short introduction to philosophy*. Oxford: Oxford University Press.

Orem, D. 1991. *Nursing concepts of practice*. 4th edition. St. Louis, MO: Mosby Year Book.

Paley, J. 2002. Virtue of autonomy: The Kantian ethics of care. *Nursing Philosophy, 3,* 133–143.

Parse, R.R. 1981. *Man-living-health: A Theory of Nursing*. New York: Wiley.

Pask, E.J. 2001. Nursing responsibility and conditions of practice: Are we justified in holding nurses responsible for their behaviour in situations of patient care? *Nursing Philosophy, 2,* 45–52.

Reed, J. and Ground, I. 1997. *Philosophy for nursing*. London: Arnold.

Rodgers, B.L. and Yen, W. 2002. Re-thinking nursing science through the understanding of Buddhism. *Nursing Philosophy, 3,* 213–221.

Rogers, M.E. 1970. *An introduction to the theoretical basis of nursing*. Philadelphia: F.A. Davis.

Scott, P.A. 2000. Emotion, moral perception, and nursing practice. *Nursing Philosophy, 1,* 123–133.

Sellman, D. 2000. Alasdair MacIntyre and the professional practice of nursing. *Nursing Philosophy, 1,* 26–33.

Winch, S., Creedy, D. and Chaboyer, A.W. 2002. Governing nursing conduct: The rise of evidence-based practice. *Nursing Inquiry, 9,* 156–161.

chapter four

Our Theoretical Landscape: A Brief History of Health Care Ethics

Patricia Rodney,
Michael Burgess,
Gladys McPherson,
and Helen Brown

The Socratic injunction "know thyself" names the task at the entrance to the moral life. Through our upbringing and acculturation... we acquire numerous beliefs about right and wrong and good and bad. Beliefs thus acquired are deeply constitutive of who we are as adults, and may manifest themselves in our actions without our ever having reflected upon them.... The choice of the ethical life as expressed in the injunction "know thyself" commits one to bringing such unreflected beliefs to light and, having clarified them, to explicitly and responsibly embrace, reject, or modify them (Yeo 1996a, 11).

The challenge that Canadian philosopher Michael Yeo has articulated above applies to every one of us who practises in nursing and other health care professions. And it applies to ethical inquiry in each of our disciplines. Thus, a central tenet of this text is that **ethical practice** requires thoughtful scrutiny of the beliefs and values that underpin our adoption of ethical theories and our ethical theorizing. Ethical practice demands that we understand the sources of the theories that guide us, including the assumptions that are embedded in them, and how that theory is evolving. Most importantly, we must carefully consider how we might use—and shape—ethical theory to improve the practice of nurses and other health care professionals toward the goal of fostering the health and well-being of patients, families, and communities. In other words, our adoption and development of ethical theory should be thoughtful and conscious, and our theorizing (or application of theory) should involve processes of critical reflection.[1] In this chapter and the next three, we will address elements of both theory and theorizing.

More specifically, within this chapter it is our intent to provide an orientation to the development of **health care ethics,** including an overview of its history and theoretical underpinnings, and to describe some of the challenges we face in contemporary health care ethics. Theory and theorizing in health care ethics continue to evolve, and so it is important to have an historical sense of the field. As we lay out our understanding, we will be endeavouring to highlight the strengths and limitations of traditional approaches to health care ethics as guides to thinking in ethically troubling situations. We will close this chapter by considering what it is that health care providers need from ethical theory. In Chapter 5, we sketch out some of the newer theoretical possibilities opened up by cross-cultural, feminist, organizational, and political writings in health care ethics. We then explore the implications for applications in health care ethics in Chapter 6, and for the development of inquiry in nursing ethics in Chapter 7.

Although the overviews we provide in this chapter and the next three are not exhaustive, we believe that they set the stage for the subsequent chapters of this book. In these other chapters different authors will pick up various strands of ethical and related theory and weave them into their own arguments. Thus, the material presented in this chapter and the next three will be elaborated on throughout the text. We are not embarking on a process of delineating the best or correct approach to ethical theory or theorizing. Rather, our intent is to demonstrate some of the various forms and possibilities of ethical theories—for instance, cross-cultural theory (Chapter 5) and care-based theory (Chapter 7). And our intent is to demonstrate the various forms that ethical theorizing might take—for example, through consideration of the interests of children and elderly persons (Chapter 6) and through the use of narrative exploration (Chapter 14). Ultimately, the ethical theory we and other authors draw on will "look more like a tapestry composed of threads of many different hues than one woven in a single color" (Fraser and Nicholson 1990, 35).

Before we proceed, though, let us provide a few words about terminology. **Ethics** is a branch of philosophy.[2] In orienting to the field of ethics, it is important to note that, as generally understood, the major divisions of ethics as a discipline include descriptive ethics, normative ethics, and metaethics (Fowler 1987; Fry 1987; Yeo 1996a). *Descriptive ethics* focuses on factual descriptions of moral behaviour and belief systems or beliefs; *normative ethics* focuses on the formulation and defense of basic principles, values, virtues, and ideals governing moral behaviour[3], and *metaethics* focuses on an analysis of meaning, justification, and inferences of moral terms, concepts, and statements (Fowler 1987; Hoffmaster 2001). Whereas the term "ethics" usually refers to any of the above as a formal field of inquiry, "morality" usually refers to personal attributes and actions.

As distinguished from ethical theory, moral theory has recently been influenced by the field of developmental psychology—the study of at what point and under which circumstances individuals develop the capacities to act according to acceptable standards (see, for example, Damon 1988; Flanagan 1991; Kohlberg 1968). This is important because these origins colour prevailing beliefs about how persons act morally, a topic that we will elaborate on in later chapters (e.g., Chapters 7 and 19).

Unfortunately, the terms "bioethics," "biomedical ethics," "medical ethics," and "health care ethics" are often used interchangeably in common parlance. Our own preference is to use the term "health care ethics" (instead of "bioethics" or "biomedical ethics") to refer to ethical concerns that affect the health care system—concerns experienced by patients, families, health care professionals/providers, health care organizations, and society as a whole (Rodney 1997). Within health care ethics, there are concerns that are particular to the sciences of biomedicine (bioethics—for instance, debates about cloning), concerns that are particular to each of the professions (medical ethics, nursing ethics, pharmacy ethics, and so on, all of which are also related to professional ethics), and concerns that are particular to organizations (which are also related to business ethics).[4] When we use the term "bioethics" in this chapter, we will be referring to the more traditional (circumscribed) study of health care ethics that occurred early in the development of the discipline and continues to some extent today. Otherwise, our preferred term will be "health care ethics."

THE EVOLUTION OF HEALTH CARE ETHICS

Throughout the ages, philosophers have been engaged in dialogue about what has been described as the "ultimate task of morality"—that is, to find out "how best to live" (Hadot 1995) or how to lead the "good life" and enjoy well-being (Engelhardt 1986; Pojman 2001). Ethics has been popularly used as a generic term referring to "various ways of understanding and examining the moral life" (Beauchamp and Childress 1994, 4). Indeed, ethics has been the subject of rigorous philosophical debates in Western philosophy for almost 2500 years (Meilaender 1995; Pojman 2001). Despite the controversy about the task and methods of ethics, the works of the influential ancient Greek philosophers (namely Socrates, Plato, and Aristotle) firmly established ethics as a branch of philosophical inquiry which sought "dispassionate and rational clarification and justification of the basic assumptions and beliefs that people hold about what is to be considered morally acceptable and morally unacceptable behavior" (Johnstone 1999, 42). The application of ethics to health care has been greatly influenced by the historical evolution of philosophy and ethics.

Ethics: Recent Historical Trajectory

The recent history of ethics over the last few centuries has focused largely on metaethics (Winkler 1996). The objective of this theoretical enterprise is the working out of general theories that account for accepted moral judgments and assist in determining correct moral action in controversial circumstances. Most popular of these theories are versions of Immaneul Kant's *deontology* or duty-based ethics, John Stuart Mill's *utilitarianism* or consequentialist ethics, and John Rawl's *contractarian* approach.[5] (Arras, Steinbock and London 1999; Garner and Rosen 1967; Sher 1987; Tong 1997).

Philosophical writing has always used examples to illustrate the adequacy of ethical theory in elucidating right- or wrong-making characteristics. For example, one version of Kant's categorical imperative,[6] "Always act in a manner that in so doing you can will that your action become a universal principle," is typically used to explain why lying is immoral even when the consequences are better than that of telling the truth. This aspect of Kant's theory is often referred to as "universalizability." But the generalization can be limited by including very specific descriptions of the situation. For example, one might contemplate lying to an irreversibly ill person to allow her to fulfill her cherished plans for a long vacation. In this instance, if we hold truth-telling as a categorical imperative, ethical behaviour would not accommodate lying unless we can arrive at a more sophisticated categorical ethical principle. Universalizing the principle that lying in this example is defensible might yield a rule like, "Always lie to a patient who is dying if the truth will not provide any advantage and the lie may result in considerable benefit." Of course, such generalizations can lead to difficulties in practice.

In contrast to Kant's deontological perspective, utilitarianism assesses the morality of actions or policies based on their effects or consequences. The good and bad effects anticipated for each alternative action or policy must be compared. The morally required or "ethical" action or policy is that which produces the best outcomes. Some utilitarians use the standards of happiness and unhappiness to assess whether consequences are good or bad, while others judge consequences in terms of whether they produce pleasure or pain. It is also important to note that, in weighing consequences, most utilitarian theories demand that all persons affected by the action or policy are considered, whether taxpayers or bereaved relatives.

Contractarianism stands in opposition to utilitarianism, suggesting that the pursuit of happiness or pleasure is not the ultimate good and cannot be used as justification for means that impose unfair disadvantages on certain societal groups. This view is most often associated with the work of Rawls (1971) who articulated the notion of a *social contract*:

> [that] derives, from a strictly hypothetical and non-historical original position, the conclusion that, as a matter of (social) justice no one, or rather no group, has any business to be any better off than anyone else, or than any other group; save in so far as their being in this happier position is indirectly to the benefit of (not all those who are worse off but only) the least-advantaged group (Flew 1979, 299).[7]

In other words, while happiness or pleasure may be an unintended consequence of ethically justifiable action, it cannot be taken as the primary rationale for determining how we ought to act. Rawls' intent was to work towards a fair process for the distribution of societal goods such that the least well off in a society were protected. Many of our current health care systems reflect, at least to some extent, the results of this type of thinking.

While deontology, utilitarianism, and contractarianism were just three of the theoretical perspectives addressed by early modern ethical theory, they were some of the most influential on the development of bioethics. They remain important because of the significant influence they have had and continue to have on thinking about how health care services ought to be distributed and about the nature of professional-patient relationships. In other words, these theories have become entrenched in the more recently developed field of bioethics.

Other early influences on the development of bioethics came from theology and law (Arras, Steinbock and London 1999; Hoffmaster 1999; Roy, Williams and Dickens 1994). Theology had a particularly strong early influence. Thus, many early anthologies in bioethics included some version of natural law[8] or virtue ethics[9], typically based on some modification of Thomas Aquinas' work[10] as a sample of religious ethical theory. The law "provided a rich source of seminal cases, about matters such as refusal of treatment, the termination of life, and surrogate motherhood" (Hoffmaster 1999, 139–140). Although the law had an effect that was "overwhelmingly reactive in nature" (Hoffmaster 1999, 140), together with theology and liberal political ideology (Hoffmaster 1999, 140), it helped to entrench human rights[11] in early bioethics.

Thus, utilitarianism, deontology, contractarianism, natural law, virtue theory, and rights theory contributed a great deal to the development of early bioethics. Students in philosophy and early bioethics learnt the various theories and engaged in the critique of them from alternative perspectives. Although philosophers often argued for the superiority of a particular theory, more generally the field could reasonably be characterized as one of competition between incommensurable[12] moral theories. In other words, adherence to one perspective necessarily required that one held the position that other theories were, at best, misguided.[13]

Bioethics: Early Traditions

As the medical ethical historian Jonsen (1997) notes, "the work of healing, from time immemorial and in all cultures, has been wrapped in moral and religious meanings" (3). However, the biotechnological advances throughout the 1950s and 1960s, as well as post-World War II concerns about Holocaust medical experimentation, generated new problems that resulted in the birth of a new discipline—bioethics (Arras, Steinbock and London 1999; Evans 2000; Fox 1990; Jonsen 1995; 1997; Pellegrino 1993; Roy, Williams and Dickens 1994; Yeo 1996b). Bioethics emerged in response to grave and sometimes unanswerable questions that resulted from the use and institutionalization of new technologies of science—uses that could lead to immense good or unspeakable harm. The Nuremberg trials and related concerns about human experimentation (Trial of war criminals 1947), along with other discoveries, including publication of reports of blatant ethical misconduct in research involving human subjects (Beecher 1959; 1966), resulted in widespread fear about the clear dangers of unrestricted and unpoliced use of technology.[14] The resultant distrust of professionals and institutions was also manifested in the "anti-establishment" movement of the 1960s and was evident in the considerable attention given to iatrogenic effects of medical treatments. An early project of bioethics, one that soon became known as the doctrine of informed consent (discussed in more detail later), was initially intended to assure that human participants in medical research projects were truly voluntary. With the acceptance that informed consent was an essential element of medical treatment and participation in research, the cultural authority of physicians and medical institutions—although far from undermined—came under critical assessment.

Early bioethical issues, such as the problem of informed consent, were articulated as problems through the early modern discourse we described above. However, practitioners' intuitive responses about right actions or policies began to challenge the primacy of the philosophical theories. In this emerging world of biomedical technology and its associated ethical complexities, the offerings of philosophers seemed relatively humble. At the same time, theologically inclined theorists (who gained prominence in early bioethics work) were more concerned with practical problems individuals faced as they endeavoured to provide members of their faith with the means to reconcile their beliefs with ethical problems and to act in a manner consistent with their religious commitments. These changes in focus marked a shift from the use of health care examples in philosophical discourse to illustrate metatheoretical concepts to what we now know as bioethics—the topical discussion of health care issues from theoretical perspectives.

Initial efforts in bioethics proposed internally consistent, systematic approaches to ethical issues in health care. Although some philosophers maintained their commitment to particular ethical theories (for example, Singer 1986), many others seemed to abandon the search for unifying and justifying metaethical foundations. Instead, they focused on developing theories of bioethics that made sense of specific moral intuitions about health, health care, doctor-patient relationships, patient values, and social values. The result was a proliferation of bioethics texts (for example, Beauchamp and Childress 1989; Brody 1988; Engelhardt Jr. 1991; Gert 1988; Mappes and Zembaty 1991). The primary focus was on the theoretical support for agreement about what constituted the ethical elements of the problem. All of these texts shared a selective use of ethical theories to argue for the reasonableness of their claims that certain values were moral values and important (e.g., autonomy). Concepts developed to explain shared moral intuitions were used to provide guidance in the more controversial examples. While different positions were held on moral issues such as abortion, positions were not usually presented as strictly deduced from one specific moral theory. Many of the advances in bioethics were tied to cross-cutting conceptual analyses that clarified moral issues. Jane English's (1975) discussion of a self-defense argument for abortion and James Rachel's (1975) attack on the distinction between active and passive euthanasia stand as important examples of these conceptual advances.

Corresponding with the growth of bioethics was the growth of health professionals' interest in bioethics. Physicians, lawyers, nurses, chaplains, and a variety of other health-related professionals, as well as patients, administrators, and politicians, became interested in the concepts developed by those involved in bioethics. They were primarily interested in the concepts as tools to assist in the resolution of specific cases and policy issues. Collaboration between physicians and philosophers or theologians resulted in finer tuned presentations of clinical and personal details in specific ethical problems, clarifying the range and specific justification for practices and policies. Bioethics became a practice and academic discipline that was interdisciplinary in nature and was located in the institutions of health care, education, law, and policy.

The Principles of Bioethics

Introduction

As bioethics became established, practitioners and theorists sought an approach that would preserve the wisdom found in the ethical theories but would not demand the restrictions created by commitment to any one specific theory. They also sought an approach that would focus more strongly on particular situations. Ethical principles offered great promise here. An ethical principle was seen as "an essential norm in a system of thought or belief, forming a basis of moral reasoning in that system" (Beauchamp 1996, 81). "Principlism" was the belief that some set of principles could be arrived at from multiple ethical theories that would be useful in concrete applications. The search for and application of these principles consumed bioethicists throughout the last quarter of the 20th century. Moreover, there was a strong related interest on the part of government policy-makers. American groups such as the National Commission for the Protection of Human Subjects of Biomedical and Behavioral Research (in the 1970s) and the President's Commission for the Study of Ethical Problems in Medicine and Biomedical and Behavioral Science (in the 1980s) established principles that were used to justify policy positions and were applied in health care related decision-making (Evans 2000).

The most often cited work articulating ethical principles is Beauchamp and Childress's *Principles of Bioethics* (1994), a detailed explication of which was presented in the fourth edition of their book. Building on the work of the philosopher W.D. Ross, Beauchamp and Childress chose four *prima facie* principles especially appropriate for bioethics: autonomy, beneficence, nonmaleficence, and justice (Pellegrino 1993, 1160). As the medical ethicist Edmund Pellegrino (1993) explains, this "tetrad of principles had the advantage of being compatible with deontological and consequentialist theories and even with some aspects of virtue theory" (1160). Beauchamp and Childress's work was theoretically rich enough to be the object of philosophical study and adequately non-technical to encourage study by health care professionals interested in bioethics. Principle-oriented bioethics evolved into the rational, objective, and impartial application of the four ethical principles in bioethical theory and moral development theory (Arras, Steinbock and London 1999; Ackerman 1983; Cooper 1991; Mappes and Zembaty 1991; Omery 1989; Penticuff 1991; Tong 1997).

Autonomy

The principle of **autonomy** is central to the work of Beauchamp and Childress (1994), within the American commissions we cited above, and, subsequently, within bioethics in general (Arras, Steinbock and London 1999; Hoffmaster 1999; Tong 1997; Wolf 1994b). Autonomy can be understood as an observation about human nature and morality, with an ethical imperative drawn from it. The observation about human nature is that human beings *have the ability to act voluntarily based on information*. Evidence of human autonomy can be found in the moral experience of guilt, blame, or shame—emotions that are contingent on a belief that in a particular instance we could have acted otherwise. That we believe we would have behaved differently if we knew then what we know now is further evidence of our belief in autonomy. The observation about morality is that it makes sense to hold people morally responsible for their actions only if they actually could have chosen to act differently (that is, were autonomous). Coercion and incorrect belief are reasonable moral excuses because they qualify this sense of autonomy. It becomes evident that the doctrine of informed consent is rooted in the principle of autonomy (Arras, Steinbock and London 1999; Hoffmaster 1999; Tong 1997). The ethical imperative is that autonomy, as the element of human nature that makes morality possible, should be protected. Tristam Engelhardt Jr. (1986a) describes this form of argument as autonomy as a requirement of morality, per se, and therefore as a side-constraint on all theories.

   Some theorists have attempted to rebuild moral theory from the notion of autonomy as a central concept (for instance, Engelhardt 1989, 1991; Veatch 1981). Others have been content to illustrate how autonomy weighs relative to other moral concepts, such as doing good or avoiding harm to others (beneficence, nonmaleficence), fair distribution of goods (justice), control of information (confidentiality), veracity (truth-telling), and promise keeping (fidelity). Much of the early literature of bioethics was just such a weighing of these principles for specific issues, with various theorists proposing various approaches to determining the ranking of the principles in particular situations.

Beneficence and Nonmaleficence

The principles of **beneficence** and **nonmaleficence** are sometimes combined under the former term and, at other times, considered to be different from one another. In bioethics, these two principles may be used in either a Kantian or a utilitarian manner (Arras, Steinbock and London 1999; Tong 1997). In early bioethics, and in some more recent writings, there is a definite utilitarian flavour to the use of "beneficence" and "nonmaleficence" in that every act or option is subject to a harm-benefit analysis. This may be partially due to the nature of medical practice in which patient benefit is sought, but only by actions that are less harmful than beneficial. This has been characterized in ethics or philosophy of medicine as *primum non nocere*. On the other hand, a Kantian influence can be discerned when beneficence, or promoting benefit to other persons, is considered "weaker" than duties to avoid harm, such as nonmaleficence. Simply put, this means that, as a general rule, one should abstain from or justify any harm (maleficence) done to others, but one is obligated neither to perform every possible act of benefit to others nor to justify the omissions.

The implementation of the principles of autonomy, beneficence, and nonmaleficence can be illustrated by considering appropriate moral practice in delivering health care services. First, it is the duty of health care professionals to evaluate specific interventions to determine whether they are more beneficial than harmful when applied to the relevant population (that is, to those with a similar clinical condition). Similarly, the principles of beneficence and nonmaleficence are embodied in the clinical judgment of whether individual patients are at heightened risk or are likely to benefit (for example, contraindications). But even with the scrupulous application of beneficence and nonmaleficence, patients' autonomy must be respected. In more Kantian terms, patients are not to be treated simply as means to the end of their health, but as ends in themselves. This requires that persons who will be recipients of health care services themselves evaluate the options and possible harms and benefits and that they choose how to be treated. This additional requirement, labelled the "doctrine of **informed consent**," is an attempt to balance health care professionals' endeavours to benefit patients with patients' expression of informed choice. This is the challenge health care professionals face—negotiating between the tension created by competing perspectives on "the good" in general situations and applying these in particular moments of practice with particular persons.

Application: Informed Consent

This challenge is illustrated in the important discussions of the American commissions and Beauchamp and Childress' work where informed consent is emphasized. These works identify two important features of informed consent that a more static and legalistic notion might overlook. First, informed consent should be a reflection of continuing communication, collaboration, and commitment. Rather than being a one-time evaluation of information and a decision about how to proceed, the emphasis is on a *relationship* in which the health professional provides new information about effectiveness and risks and encourages patients to reflect on and express their interests. Patients are expected to attempt to understand the information as it is provided, to evaluate the information and their own concerns, and to consider continuing commitment or withdrawal of consent.

The second feature of informed consent emphasizes the role of the health care professional in the gatekeeping of information and services. Consent will often be only as informed as the health care professional allows since options may be omitted, risks or benefits may be emphasized or minimized, and professional opinions may carry considerable persuasive weight. Further, patient autonomy has never, in the complex version of principles of bioethics, been given full authority. For example, a request for service that a health professional considers harmful and without justified benefit does not establish an obligation to provide the service. Laetrile for cancer patients and heart surgery or organ transplants for patients who could not survive the surgery are typical examples. Decision-making is supposed to be done collaboratively between (hopefully) reflective and active patients and professionals who provide the information and expertise to assist in the interpretation of the choices the patient faces. But collaborative decision-making also recognizes that patient wishes do not always carry the authority to access the resources, often because the professional evaluates the service as unhelpful or too harmful. Individual patients are expected to make the right decisions for themselves if they are logical and if they are given the right information, and if they fail to do so, the professional (usually the physician) intervenes. If they are judged not competent, an individual proxy (substitute) decision-maker is appointed.[15]

The emphasis on continuing communication, collaboration, and commitment and the delineation of the professional-patient relationship (including boundaries) in the above conceptualization of informed consent are useful in clinical practice. *However, the emphasis is on the role of the health care professional in relation to individual, rational patients in this traditional view.* This leaves us with little insight into the role of emotion, conflict, or power imbalances in patient-professional relationships (Churchill 1997; Hoffmaster 1999; 2001; Rodney et al. 2002; Sherwin 1992; 1998; Tong 1997; Wolf 1994b). It also leaves us with little insight into the role of family or community in decision-making (Burgess et al. 1999; Nelson 1998; Nelson and Nelson, 1995).[16] We will say more about these limitations as we close this chapter and in Chapter 5.

Justice

The fourth principle, **justice,** is best known as a basis to argue for a right to health care (Arras, Steinbock, and London 1999; Buchanan 1989; Daniels 1985; McDonald 1999; Rawls 1971; 1993; Tong 1997). Over the history of bioethics, justice has been the least well operationalized ethical principle (Aroskar 1992; Daniels 1996), and, in our current sociopolitical era, it is under the most threat. As will be shown in Chapters 9 through 13 of this book, patients, families, communities, and health care providers currently face deep and disturbing questions about justice in health care delivery, so we will offer some elaboration here on this fourth principle. Indeed, it is more than a principle—it is also a theory and is closely tied to political philosophy. While we cannot elaborate on political philosophy here,[17] we can say more about the theory that underlies justice.

Justice, and in particular *distributive justice*, is an attempt to decide how to be fair in the distribution of resources. A right to health care is not so much based on some notion of what is essential to be respected as a person, but on what is fair treatment in a society with a particular set of medical and economic resources. Justice is also used to provide other reasons to limit patient demands for treatments. Some treatments are inadequately beneficial to justify resource dedication. On the other hand, beneficial treatments may be too expensive to meet the full demand without unacceptable loss of other important opportunities.

Philosophical discussions that enrich the use of justice in bioethics are broad and can be divided in two manners. One split is between *procedural* and *substantive* rules of justice. References to "due process" and lotteries or "first come–first served" maxims are examples of procedural rules of justice. John Rawls' (1971) mechanism of the "veil of ignorance" is an example of a procedural approach to determining justice in policy.[18] Substantive approaches to justice attempt to make a strong case for particular rules of distribution that are fair, such as "to each according to ability" or "to each according to need." Rawls' (1971) view of justice is based on a sophisticated form of a substantive rule that accepts as just rational self-interest arrived at through a process of reflective equilibrium.[19] Norman Daniels (1985) extends Rawls' work to health care, articulating a view of justice based on human needs and fair equality of opportunity.[20]

The second way of splitting the discussion of justice in bioethics is by *types of resources* being allocated. These discussions typically divide considerations of justice into three levels:

micro-, meso-, and macro-allocation (Kluge 1992; Yeo 1993; Yeo, Moorhouse, and Donner 1996). "Macro-allocation" is usually characterized as the division of societal resources into various types of services to benefit the population. The central question is how much to invest in each of the different ways to address the public's interests. The issue may be whether education and health care should receive similar or different levels of funding (or reductions). This decision-making is typically governmental. Proposals and commentaries for health care reform based on claims about citizens' rights to health or health care are also examples of macro-allocation. More recent efforts by health care economists and some ethicists emphasize that the goal of health care is to improve the population's health. They claim that determinants of health are more effective approaches to improving population health and to narrowing the gap of health between economic groups and between different countries. These efforts to determine a fair distribution of societal resources to health care are themselves embedded in claims about the role of health care in society. For example, Daniels (1985) claims that the moral goal of access to health care is to promote equality of opportunity and secondarily to compensate for irreversible loss of opportunity.

"Meso-allocation" is typically the division of a health care budget among various health care services. This decision-making can be governmental, regional, or institutional. Some meso-allocation policies come from professional bodies or from departments of health care professionals within institutions (e.g., whether to perform genetic testing for sex determination or cleft palate). The type of meso-allocation closest to macro-allocation is focused on determining what services to include in a publicly funded health care system. The Oregon Health Care Plan is now famous for its efforts, as well as for the criticism it has drawn (Blue et al. 1999; Hadorn 1991; 1992; Menzel 1992; Starzomski 1997). More specific policies regarding criteria for patients who are eligible for specific services such as transplants, other surgical techniques, and expensive diagnostic imaging are also meso-allocation decisions. Most of these policies operate implicitly on a material principle of justice of "to each according to need," whereby it is not unjust to deny access to a service from which one cannot benefit. This principle is inadequate to eliminate scarcity, because there are genuine shortages (for example, of organs), and because there is lack of will or ability to dedicate adequate resources at the macro level to cover all services that genuinely meet need.

Therefore, the material principle of meso-allocation is typically supplemented with some sort of procedural principle that allows persons of similar need (that is, those who stand a roughly equal chance of benefitting from the service if they receive it) to have an equal chance of getting the service. This may be first come–first served or a lottery. In Oregon's case, it was an attempt to construct a community-wide ranking of the importance of the services and a cutoff point on the list based on an estimate of what the state could afford to fund from a set budget. Neither approach is adequate. Better procedural principles for just meso-allocation decision-making are urgently needed in today's era of regionalization of health care services, and more comprehensive public participation in meso-allocation decision-making is crucial (see also Chapter 9 and Chapter 15). Recently, Daniels and a number of colleagues have been pursuing the operationalization of "accountability for reasonableness" in an attempt to work towards better procedural principles (Daniels and Sabin 1997; Martin, Abelson and Singer 2002). The conditions for accountability for reasonableness include relevance (based on sound evidence, reasons, and principles), publicity (public accessibility), appeals (a mechanism for challenges and dispute resolution), and enforcement (voluntary or public regulation) (Martin, Ableson and Singer

2002, 223; see also Chapter 6 of this text and McDonald's *An Ethical Framework for Making Allocation Decisions* in Appendix B).

"Micro-allocation" is the distribution of services to individual patients. The primary decision is professional determination of whether the individual would benefit from a service and whether the person wants the service. Individual health care professionals or health care teams typically make micro-allocation decisions. However, concerns about economic pressures sometimes motivate micro-allocation decisions that are more appropriately determined as meso-allocation issues. For instance, an expensive treatment might not be offered to a particular patient who, although she would benefit, does not have a supportive family or does not speak English. It is important to note that there is a danger that health care professionals will violate their ethical obligations if they try to save program costs (meso-allocation) through ad hoc rationing at the micro level (Council on Ethical and Judicial Affairs, American Medical Association 1999; Jennings, Callahan and Wolf 1987; Kjellstrand 1992; Pellegrino 1979; 1990; 1993; Sokolowski 1991; Starzomski and Rodney 1997). This is an especially real danger in today's era of escalating cost constraint (Caulfield 2002; Litman 2002; Mohr and Mahon 1996; Varcoe and Rodney 2002; Watson 1994; Wolf 1994a). The use of individual ethical decision-making models can help health care providers to work towards more just decision-making at the micro level (see also Chapter 6 of this text and McDonald's *An Ethical Decision Making Framework for Individuals* in Appendix B).

Transition

In summary, the principles of bioethics as described above have enabled a diverse set of professionals and academics, as well as some community members and advocacy groups, to find a language with which to discuss problematic health care situations. They provided some needed clarity in ethical debates, furnishing "an orderly way to 'work up' an ethical problem," leading to "fairly specific action guidelines," and avoiding "direct confrontation with the intractably divisive issues of abortion, euthanasia, and a host of other issues on which agreement seemed impossible" (Pellegrino 1993, 1160). Organizing the information about a case or information relevant to a policy around ethical principles has often encouraged discussion about the goals of treatment and the involvement of patients and family to assess goals, benefits, and harms from their particular perspectives. However, as we have indicated in our analysis so far (and will expand on in the section below and in Chapter 5), this traditional approach does not help us to understand and to deal with the personal, social, and cultural aspects of health as well as the complex sociopolitical climates in which health care is delivered and in which resources for health are embedded. In philosophical terms, we see the principles as necessary but not sufficient.

A CONFLICTED LANDSCAPE?

Critiques

Although the principle-oriented approach to health care ethics has been widely accepted, over the past two decades or so there have been serious concerns raised about its adequacy. It is important to note that some of the concerns may be related to how the principles have been used in practice rather than theoretical limitations in the principles themselves

(Churchill 1997; Levi 1996; Pellegrino 1993; Yeo 1994).[21] In the hands of busy clinicians, educators, and even ethicists, there has been a tendency to employ them in a non-contextual and reductionist manner. For instance, in applying the principle of autonomy to a dying patient's request not to have his family told of his prognosis, the discussion might quickly centre around whether he was competent, informed, and unconstrained, with little exploration of the meaning behind his request, his understanding of his own and his family's grief processes, the values he held about his family's well-being, and so on. The principle of autonomy, despite its rich theoretical traditions, can too easily be reduced to binary equations (competent/incompetent; informed/uninformed; constrained/unconstrained) if not handled with careful reflection and clinical insight.

Even given that many of the problems with bioethical principles may have to do with how they are used rather than with the underlying theory, there remain a number of problems with using principlism as the sole basis for work in health care ethics. It appears that there is a lack of consensus about the nature of fundamental ethical principles, and that ethical principles are not easily prioritized or applied to concrete moral situations (Ackerman 1983, 170–173). Principle-oriented ethics has been criticized for relying on ethical principles to the exclusion of other variables known to influence ethical practice, for not reflecting the breadth and diversity of concepts available in the general ethics literature, and for fostering a prescriptive formal approach by which principles are applied in a process-dominated manner (Penticuff 1991, 236–240). The sources of theory and the processes of theorizing are thus both being held up for scrutiny.

One area of critique comes (directly and indirectly) from **virtue**-based discourses. Beauchamp and Childress (1994) themselves acknowledge that "morality includes more than obligation" (452). They suggest that morality is a combination of the character traits of persons who make judgments as well as the obligations expressed in principles and rules. In this way, both virtue-based and principle-based approaches are required to describe the ethical obligations, ideals, "reliable character" and "moral good sense" in professional-patient relationships (Pellegrino 1985; 1993; 1995; 2001; Pellegrino, Veatch and Langan 1991; Smith and Godfrey 2002). Johnstone (1999) goes further, claiming that virtue ethics have been revitalized in response to dissatisfaction with dominant mainstream theories to provide an adequate account of the "moral life."

In our view, virtue-based accounts of morality are a useful supplement to principlism. They help to overcome the tendency for bioethical principles to place an undue emphasis on the moral minimum of obligations while largely ignoring characters and personal dispositions for their influence on moral deliberation and action. In other words, "we need to know what kind of person is involved, how the person thinks of other people, how he or she thinks of his or her own character, how the person feels about past actions and also how the person feels about actions not done" (Pence 1991, 256).

A second area of critique comes from discourses about **culture.** The principle-based approach has been criticized as "culturally specific and intellectually problematic" in terms of its "uncritical emphasis... on the individual and his or her rights (as opposed to the web of human relationships that engender mutual obligations and interdependence), the techniques of rational abstraction that uproot issues from their concrete human reality, and the assumption that these techniques and values have universal applicability" (Weisz 1990, 3).[22] What this means is that health care ethics has not, historically, attended very well to culture. And it has certainly not been terribly reflective about the cultural inheritance it has received from biomedicine, liberal individualism, and a variety of other sources. We will have more to say about this area of critique in Chapter 5.

Third, **feminist** theorists have made significant contributions to the critique—and reformulation—of theory and theorizing in health care ethics. Feminists have warned that health care ethics "has been strong on proclaiming individual autonomy to choose, but weak on insisting on access to health care and the creation of choices for those who have few" (Wolf 1994b, 402). Feminists have also warned that the rational, non-contextual application of ethical principles misses the subtle and pervasive power dynamics that infuse patient/family/provider relationships within hierarchical institutions.[23] Once again, we will have more to say about this area of critique in Chapter 5.

A Peace Proposal

Where do these critiques leave us in our pursuit of ethical theory and theorizing for practice in nursing and other health care disciplines? Put simply, we contend that no one theoretical schema—whether metaethical theories, ethical principles, virtues, or even cross-cultural or feminist theory—can furnish everything we need to inform the study and practice of health care ethics. As Arras, Steinbock, and London (1999) argue, we ought not to "view the various theoretical alternatives as mutually exclusive claims to moral truth. Instead, we should view them as important but partial contributions to a comprehensive, although necessarily fragmented, moral vision" (9).[24] This is a fairly recent development in the way that theory is developed and used in health care ethics. As we indicated at the outset of this chapter, the early history of work in ethics was such that adherence to one perspective necessarily required that one held the position that other theories were, at best, misguided. We believe that the growing call from theorists to work with more than one form of theory marks a significant shift and offers great promise. Indeed, the premise of this entire text is that we ought to consciously explore, develop, and apply the insights of theorists from various perspectives arising in philosophy, nursing, medicine, psychology, the social sciences, political sciences, cultural studies, and other related fields.

We are not arguing for the ad hoc and potentially sloppy development and application of theory. Rather, we are arguing for the use of a broad range of theory that best serves the ethical practice of nurses and other health care providers and best informs ethical health care policy work. This requires understanding the history, strengths, and challenges of whatever theory we work with, and it necessitates reconciling tensions between various forms of theory. As will be argued in the next chapter, for instance, we will want to hold onto the protection of individual rights that the ethical principle of autonomy offers but also to broaden autonomy to encompass relational and cross-cultural concerns (Burgess 1999; Sherwin 1998). *How* to manage a coherent and effective traverse of such a variety of perspectives is not yet entirely clear, but, fortunately, theorists such as Daniels are working on it.

In an insightful and entertaining chapter that tackles the current controversies in the use of theory in health care ethics, Daniels (1996) creates a Tolkien-esque metaphor of a war between three kingdoms (see Exhibit 4-1). He provides an historical exploration of the problems and interactions among three levels of theory (Kingdoms) and subsequently draws up a "peace proposal" for the three kingdoms. The first declaration in his peace proposal is "There is not one kind of ethical problem, but there are many kinds, and different problems require somewhat different approaches" (Daniels 1996, 112).

Exhibit 4-1	A War between Kingdoms (based on Daniels 1996)

The Uplanders: Theorists who subscribe to grand theories such as deontology

The Middle Kingdom: Principlists who subscribe to mid-range ethical principles

The Lowlanders: Contextualists (for instance, feminists and cross-cultural theorists) who prefer to rely on experiential knowledge

The application of Daniels' peace proposal relies on his adaptation of Rawls' (1971) concept of reflective equilibrium. Daniels articulates a notion of **"wide reflective equilibrium,"** which "seeks coherence among three divisions of moral thought" (Winkler 1996, 64)—that is, between the three kingdoms. More specifically,

> The method of wide reflective equilibrium... seeks coherence among three divisions of moral thought: our considered moral judgements, a set of principles designed to rationalize and order these judgements, and a set of relevant background theories or understandings about subjects such as human nature and psychology, the workings of the law and procedural justice, conditions for social stability and change, and the socio-economic structure of society (Winkler 1996, 64).

As we said at the outset of this chapter, our adoption and development of ethical theory should be thoughtful and conscious, and our theorizing should involve processes of critical reflection. In closing, we agree with Daniels and Winkler that we need to adopt and continue to refine theory from all three kingdoms. And we agree that our theorizing can benefit from processes such as wide reflective equilibrium. In Chapter 5 and Chapter 6 we will continue to explore both of these conclusions.

FOR REFLECTION

1. How might the values embedded in utilitarian theory differ from deontological theory?

2. One of the challenges in using principle-based ethics is that strategies to support one principle might threaten another. Can you think of clinical situations in which supporting autonomy might threaten beneficence?

3. Given that justice is the least understood and the least well operationalized principle, what are the implications for policy related to distribution of resources?

4. Think about Daniels' (1996) claim that "There is not one kind of ethical problem but there are many kinds, and different problems require somewhat different approaches" (112). Can you list some of the different kinds of ethical problems you encounter in your practice? You may find it helpful to distinguish between problems that you encounter at the micro, meso, and macro levels.

ENDNOTES

1. We would like to thank an anonymous reviewer of this chapter for emphasizing the importance of distinguishing between the adoption and development of ethical theory and the critical reflection involved in theorizing.

2. The other branches include epistemology (the nature of knowledge), metaphysics (the nature of reality), logic, and aesthetics.

3. In philosophy, "normative" has to do with questions of value. However, within the social sciences, the word holds a somewhat different meaning—normative implies what is standard, and hence normal.

4. This is by no means a well-standardized nomenclature, and many of the fields overlap (for instance, bioethical discussions about cloning also have relevance in the broader field of health care ethics when we consider access to reproductive technology and so forth). Many theorists see health care ethics (or bioethics), business ethics, and professional ethics as subsets of the larger field of applied ethics (for example, Beauchamp and Childress 1989; Fowler 1987; Mappes and Zembaty 1991; Singer 1986). It is worth noting that Roy, Williams, and Dickens (1994) warn that the concept of applied ethics itself is problematic, that by definition ethics is application—a guide to how humans ought to act in relation to one another.

5. In everyday language, utilitarianism can be thought of as "the end justifies the means," and deontology can be thought of as "do unto others as you would have them do unto you." Of course, various theorists have worked out a number of nuances of both forms of theory. Contractarianism focuses more on fair process.

6. Kant's (1949) categorical imperatives are essential moral rules that are rational and universal. These include such dictums as "the taking of life is wrong" or "always help those in need" (Bandman and Bandman 2002).

7. Rawls' social contractarianism has been described as Kantian because people are to be valued as ends in themselves in his theory—in other words, people are not to be used as the means to others' ends (Arras, Steinbock, and London 1999, 17–19). Rawls continued his work on contractarianism and his related theory of justice after the publication of his influential *A Theory of Justice* (1971), working towards an understanding of "justice as fairness as a form of political liberalism" (1993, xxix).

8. Natural law arises from theology, and consists of

   > A set of codes (rules, precepts) (a) intended by nature and grounded in some "higher" or "transcendent" reality, (b) which prescribes what should or should not be done, (c) which is universally binding upon all humans, and (d) which can be found by a rational examination of nature (Angeles 1981, 150).

9. Virtue theory has been strongly influenced by Aristotle and Aquinas. It is not a single moral theory, but, rather, a "family of moral theories that are specially concerned with or that give special priority to the role of virtues in the moral life" (Arras, Steinbock and London 1999, 30). Alisdair MacIntyre is a contemporary theorist on virtue ethics. He describes virtues as consistent dispositions manifested in varying kinds of situations, aimed at the pursuit of ethical goods and expressed in a consistent narrative of self (MacIntyre 1987). Interestingly, MacIntyre (1987; 1984) links virtues to the living traditions of institutions such as universities and hospitals, claiming that

   > Lack of justice, lack of truthfulness, lack of courage, lack of the relevant intellectual virtues—these corrupt traditions... [A]n adequate sense of tradition manifests itself in a grasp of those future possibilities which the past has made available to the present (587).

   The traditional virtues of health professionals have been proposed to derive from health care relationships (Johnstone 1999; Pellegrino 1985; 2001) and are frequently claimed to include compassion, discernment, trustworthiness, and integrity (although these virtues vary depending on the nature of the relationships) (Beauchamp and Childress 1994). Virtues are embedded in both professional roles and practices and embody social expectations as well as professional standards and internal ideals. See Kihlbom (2000) for an interesting analysis of a particularist version of virtue ethics.

10. St. Thomas Aquinas (c. 1225–1274) was an Italian Scholastic philosopher who, among his many contributions, made the works of Aristotle known and acceptable in the West (Flew 1979, 17–20).

11. A right is a justified claim or an entitlement (Sim 1995). Rights can be understood as constraining more powerful individuals from overriding certain interests of less powerful individuals. There are many views about what constitutes rights, how rights are claimed, and the power of rights (see, for example, Sumner 1987 and Thomson 1990 for comprehensive overviews of rights and Daniels 1985, 4–9, for a discussion of rights to health care). A perspective on rights as protected interests is a moderate view of rights. A stronger view of rights would be that rights are "trumps" (Freeman 1997).

12. Incommensurable means that they are so different from each other that they cannot be compared (Wehmeier 2000, 657).

13. For interesting and comprehensive overviews of the evolution of ethical theories, including the tensions between them, see Arras, Steinbock, and London (1999), Levi (1996), Pellegrino (1993), Tong (1997), and Wolf (1994b).

14. See also Chapter 17.

15. Chapter 6 provides a case discussion illustrating elements of substitute decision-making and advance directives.

16. See Chapter 6 for a discussion of family decision-making.

17. Political philosophy is an important field of study that can shed light on many of the justice problems we face in health care ethics. It covers theories such as utilitarianism, liberal equality, libertarianism, Marxism, communitarianism, and feminism (Jaggar 1988; Kymlicka 1990), as well as theories related to multicultural citizenship (Kymlicka 1995; Taylor 1992).

18. The veil of ignorance is a hypothetical procedure in which individuals make decisions about fair allocation of resources in a society. Their decisions are based on a general knowledge of human society, political affairs, economic theory, and so on, but *not* on knowledge of the particular circumstances of their own society or on what their particular position will be (Rawls 1971, 136–150). Because the individuals engaging in this procedure are rational and do not know how vulnerable their particular position might be, they will, Rawls (1971) argues, "prefer more primary social goods than less" (142).

19. Rawls' theory of justice (1971) is based on two components. One "proposes a criterion of justice that ranks feasible alternative basic structures by the minimum representative lifetime share of social primary goods each of them tends to generate" (Pogge 1989, 109). The second component "imposes two requirements upon the social and economic inequalities an institutional scheme may generate: the *opportunity principle* and the *difference principle* [emphases in original]" (Pogge 1989, 161). In the opportunity principle Rawls argues that there must be equality of opportunity, and in the difference principle he argues that the distribution of goods should benefit the least well off (Pogge, 161–165). In other words, both principles put limits on rational self-interest such that the worst off in society are advantaged. The process of reflective equilibrium—which we will say more about later in this chapter and in Chapter 5 and Chapter 6—is "the study of principles which govern actions shaped by self-examination.... A knowledge of these principles may suggest further reflections that lead us to revise our judgements" (Rawls 1971, 48–49). Thus, reflective equilibrium suggests that our moral judgments can be influenced by theory. We ought to be carefully reflective in our theorizing (that is, in the application of theory to our judgments).

20. Daniels' work on his theory of just health care—especially the application of it in policy—is ongoing (Daniels and Sabin 1997). See Daniels (1996) for an explanation of why, and Martin, Abelson, and Singer (2002) for an example of how.

21. In a chapter responding to various critiques of principlism, Beauchamp (1996) explains that he believes "that a misunderstanding of principles and a misleading account of the theories that are under attack appear in many of these criticisms" (80). He goes on to explain that he is using a *prima facie* rather than a robust conception of principles. This means that principles are "exceptionable and nonfoundational" (85) and we are therefore "free to view every moral conclusion supported by a principle and every principle itself as subject to rejoinder, refutation, and reformulation" (85).

22. See also Arras (1991); Churchill (1997); Evans (2000); Fox (1990); Fox and Swazey (1984); Hoffmaster (1990; 1991; 1993; 1999; 2001); Jennings (1990); Levi (1996); Rodney et al. (2002); Sherwin (1992; 1998); Tong (1997); Toulmin (1981); Winkler (1993; 1996); Watson (1994); Wolf (1994a; 1994b); and Yeo (1994).

23. See, for example, Anderson and Reimer Kirkham (1999); Liaschenko (1993); Rodney and Varcoe (2001); Sherwin (1992; 1998); Tong (1997), Warren (1992); Watson (1994); and Wolf (1994a; 1994b).

24. Susan Wolf (1994b) calls this approach the rise of a new pragmatism. See Rorty (1999) and Bernstein (1991) for thoughtful discussions of pragmatism and ethics.

REFERENCES

Ackerman, T.F. 1983. Experimentalism in bioethics research. *Journal of Medicine and Philosophy, 8*(3), 169–180.

Anderson, J. and Reimer Kirkham, S. 1999. Discourses on health: A critical perspective. In H. Coward and P. Ratanakul (Eds.), *A cross-cultural dialogue on health care ethics* (pp. 47–67). Waterloo, ON: Wilfrid Laurier University Press.

Angeles, P.A. 1981. *Dictionary of philosophy*. New York: Barnes & Noble.

Aroskar, M.A. 1992. Ethical foundations in nursing for broad health care access. *Scholarly Inquiry for Nursing Practice, 6*(3), 201–205.

Arras, J.D. 1991. Getting down to cases: The revival of casuistry in bioethics. *The Journal of Medicine and Philosophy, 16,* 29–51.

Arras, J.D., Steinbock, B. and London, A.J. 1999. Moral reasoning in the medical context. In J.D. Arras and B. Steinbock (Eds.), *Ethical issues in modern medicine,* 5th ed. (pp. 1–40). Mountain View, CA: Mayfield.

Bandman, E.L. and Bandman, B. 2002. *Nursing ethics though the life span.* 4th edition. Upper Saddle River, NJ: Prentice Hall.

Beauchamp, T.L. 1996. The role of principles in practical ethics. In L.W. Sumner and J. Boyle (Eds.), *Philosophical perspectives on bioethics* (pp. 79–95). Toronto: University of Toronto Press.

Beauchamp, T.L. and Childress, J.F. 1989. *Principles of biomedical ethics.* 3rd edition. New York: Oxford University Press.

Beauchamp, T.L. and Childress, J.F. 1994. *Principles of biomedical ethics.* 4th edition. New York: Oxford University Press.

Beecher, H.K. 1959. *Experimentation in man*. Illinois: Charles C. Thomas.

Beecher, H.K. 1966. Ethics and clinical research. *New England Journal of Medicine, 274,*1354–1360.

Bernstein, R.J. 1991. *The new constellation: The ethical–political horizons of modernity/postmodernity.* Cambridge, MA: MIT Press.

Blue, A., Keyserlingk, T., Rodney, P. and Starzomski, R. 1999. A critical view of North American health policy. In H. Coward and P. Ratanakul (Eds.), *A cross-cultural dialogue on health care ethics* (pp. 215–225). Waterloo, ON: Wilfrid Laurier Press.

Brody, B.A. 1988. *Moral theory and moral judgments in medical ethics*. Dorcrecht and Boston: Kluwer Academic.

Buchanan, A. 1989. Health-care delivery and resource allocation. In R.M. Veatch (Ed.), *Medical ethics* (pp. 291–327). Boston: Jones and Bartlett.

Burgess, M. 1999. Introduction: Part III: Ethical issues in the delivery of health care services. In H. Coward and P. Ratanakul (Eds.), *A cross-cultural dialogue on health care ethics* (pp.157–159). Waterloo, ON: Wilfrid Laurier University Press.

Burgess, M., Stephenson, P., Ratanakul, P. and Suwonnakote, K. 1999. End-of-life decisions: Clinical decisions about dying and perspectives on life and death. In H. Coward and P. Ratanakul (Eds.), *A cross-cultural dialogue on health care ethics* (pp. 190–206). Waterloo, ON: Wilfrid Laurier University Press.

Caulfield, T.A. 2002. Malpractice in the age of health care reform. In T.A. Caulfield and B. von Tigerstrom (Eds.), *Health care reform & the law in Canada: Meeting the challenge* (pp. 11–36). Edmonton: University of Alberta Press.

Churchill, L.R. 1997. Bioethics in social context. In R.A. Carson and C.R. Burns (Eds.), *Philosophy of medicine and bioethics: A twenty-year retrospective and critical appraisal* (pp. 137–151). Dordrecht, Netherlands: Kluwer Academic.

Cooper, M.C. 1991. Principle-oriented ethics and the ethic of care: A creative tension. *Advances in Nursing Science, 14*(2), 22–31.

Council on Ethical and Judicial Affairs, American Medical Association. 1999. *Medical futility in end-of-life care: Report of the Council on Ethical and Judicial Affairs. JAMA, 281*(10), 937–941.

Damon, W. 1988. *The moral child: Nurturing children's natural moral growth.* London: Collier Macmillan.

Daniels, N. 1985. *Just health care.* New York: Cambridge University Press.

Daniels, N. 1996. Wide reflective equilibrium in practice. In L.W. Sumner and J. Boyle (Eds.), *Philosophical perspectives on bioethics* (pp. 96–114). Toronto: University of Toronto Press.

Daniels, N. and Sabin, J.E. 1997. Limits to health care: Fair procedure, democratic deliberation and the legitimacy problem for insurers. *Philosophy and Public Affairs, 26,* 303–350.

Engelhardt, H.T,. Jr. 1986. *The foundations of bioethics.* 2nd edition. New York: Oxford University Press.

Engelhardt, H.T., Jr. 1989. Can ethics take pluralism?. *Hastings Center Report 19*(5), 33–34.

Engelhardt, H.T., Jr. 1991. *Bioethics and secular humanism: The search for a common morality.* Philadelphia: Trinity.

English, J. 1975. Abortion and the concept of a person. *Canadian Journal of Philosophy, 5*(2) 233–234.

Evans, J.H. 2000. A sociological account of the growth of principlism. *Hastings Center Report, 30*(5), 31–38.

Flanagan, O. 1991. *Varieties of moral personality: Ethics and psychological realism.* Cambridge, MA: Harvard University Press.

Flew, A. (Ed.). 1979. *A dictionary of philosophy.* 2nd edition. New York: St. Martin's.

Fowler, M.D.M. 1987. Piecing together the ethical puzzle: Operationalizing nursing's ethics in critical care. In M.D.M. Fowler and J. Levine-Ariff (Eds.), *Ethics at the bedside: A source book for the critical care nurse* (pp. 182–212). Philadelphia: J.B. Lippincott.

Fox, R.C. 1990. The evolution of American bioethics: A sociological perspective. In G. Weisz (Ed.), *Social science perspectives on medical ethics* (pp. 201–217). Philadelphia: University of Pennsylvania Press.

Fox, R.C. and Swazey, J.P. 1992. Leaving the field. *Hastings Center Report, 22*(5), 9–15.

Fraser, N. and Nicholson, L.J. 1990. Social criticism without philosophy: An encounter between feminism and postmodernism. In L.J. Nicholson (Ed.), *Feminism/postmodernism* (pp. 19–38). New York: Routledge.

Freeman, M. 1997. *The moral status of children: Essays on the rights of the child.* The Hague, ND: Kluwer Law.

Fry, S.T. 1987. Research on ethics in nursing: The state of the art. *Nursing Outlook, 35*(5), 246.

Garner, R.T. and Rosen, B. 1967. *Moral philosophy: A systematic introduction to normative ethics and meta-ethics.* New York: Macmillan.

Gert, B. 1988. *Morality: A new justification of the moral rules.* New York: Oxford University Press.

Hadorn, D. 1991. The Oregon priority-setting exercise: Quality of life and public policy. *Hastings Center Report, 21*(3), 11–16.

Hadorn, D. 1992. The problem of discrimination in health care priority setting. *JAMA, 268*(11), 1454–1459.

Hadot, P. 1995. *Philosophy as a way of life: Spiritual experience from Socrates to Foucault.* New York: Blackwell.

Hoffmaster, B. 1990. Morality and the social sciences. In G. Weisz (Ed.), *Social science perspectives on medical ethics* (pp. 241–260). Philadelphia: University of Pennsylvania Press.

Hoffmaster, B. 1991. The theory and practice of applied ethics. *Dialogue, 30,* 213–234.

Hoffmaster, B. 1993. Can ethnography save the life of medical ethics? In E.R. Winkler and J.R. Coombs (Eds.), *Applied ethics: A reader* (pp. 366–389). Oxford: Blackwell.

Hoffmaster, B. 1999. Secular health care ethics. In H. Coward and P. Ratanakul (Eds.), *A cross-cultural dialogue on health care ethics* (pp. 139–145). Waterloo, ON: Wilfrid Laurier University Press.

Hoffmaster, B. 2001. Introduction. In B. Hoffmaster (Ed.), *Bioethics in social context* (pp. 1–11). Philadelphia: Temple University Press.

Jaggar, A.M. 1988. *Feminist politics and human nature.* Totowa, New Jersey: Rowman and Littlefield.

Jennings, B. 1990. Ethics and ethnography in neonatal intensive care. In G. Weisz (Ed.), *Social science perspectives on medical ethics* (pp. 261–272). Philadelphia: University of Pennsylvania Press.

Jennings, B., Callahan, D. and Wolf, S.M. 1987. The professions: Public interest and common good. *Hastings Center Report, 17*(1), 3–10.

Johnstone, M.J. 1999. *Bioethics: A nursing perspective.* 3rd edition. Sydney, Australia: Harcourt.

Jonsen, A.R. 1995. Casuistry: An alternative or complement to principles? *Kennedy Institute of Ethics Journal, 5*(3), 237–251.

Jonsen, A.R. 1997. Introduction to the history of bioethics. In N.S. Jecker, A.R. Jonsen and R.A. Pearlman (Eds.), *Bioethics: An introduction to the history, methods, and practice* (pp. 3–11). Boston: Jones and Bartlett.

Kant, I. 1949. *Fundamental principles of the metaphysics of morals.* New York: Liberal Arts.

Kihlbom, U. 2000. Guidance and justification in particularistic ethics. *Bioethics, 14*(4), 287-309.

Kjellstrand, C.M. 1992. Disguising unjust rationing by calling it futile therapy. *The Bioethics Bulletin, 4*(2), 1–3.

Kluge, E.H.W. 1992. *Biomedical ethics in a Canadian context.* Scarborough, ON: Prentice Hall.

Kohlberg, L. 1968. Moral development. In D.L. Sills (Ed.), *International encyclopedia of the social sciences.* New York: Macmillan.

Kymlicka, W. 1990. *Contemporary political philosophy: An introduction.* Oxford: Clarendon.

Kymlicka, W. 1995. *Multicultural citizenship: A liberal theory of minority rights.* Oxford: Clarendon.

Levi, B.H. 1996. Four approaches to doing ethics. *The Journal of Medicine and Philosophy, 21*, 7–39.

Liaschenko, J. 1993. Feminist ethics and cultural ethos: Revisiting a nursing debate. *Advances in Nursing Science, 15*(4), 71–81.

Litman, M.M. 2002. Fiduciary law and for-profit and not-for-profit health care. In T.A. Caulfield and B. von Tigerstrom (Eds.), *Health care reform & the law in Canada: Meeting the challenge* (pp. 85–130). Edmonton: University of Alberta Press.

MacIntyre, A. 1987. The virtues, the unity of a human life, and the concept of a tradition. In G. Sher (Ed.), *Moral philosophy: Selected readings* (pp. 574–589). San Diego: Harcourt Brace Jovanovich.

Mappes, T.A. and Zembaty, J.S. 1991. *Biomedical ethics.* 3rd edition. New York: McGraw-Hill.

Martin, D., Abelson, J. and Singer, P. 2002. Participation in health care priority-setting: Through the eyes of the participants. *Journal of Health Services Research & Policy, 7*(4), 222–229.

McDonald, M. 1999. Health, health care, and culture: Diverse meanings, shared agendas. In H. Coward and P. Ratanakul (Eds.), *A cross-cultural dialogue on health care ethics* (pp. 92–112). Waterloo, ON: Wilfrid Laurier University Press.

Meilaender, G.C. 1995. *Body, soul, and bioethics.* Notre Dame: University of Notre Dame Press.

Menzel, P. 1992. Oregon's denial: Disabilities and quality of life. *Hastings Center Report, 22*(6), 21–25.

Mohr, W.K. and Mahon, M.M. 1996. Dirty hands: The underside of maketplace health care. *Advances in Nursing Science, 19*(1), 28–37.

Nelson, J.L. 1998. Death, medicine, and the moral significance of family decision making. In J.F. Monagle and D.C. Thomasma (Eds.), *Health care ethics: Critical issues for the 21st century* (pp. 288–294). Gaithersburg, Maryland: Aspen.

Nelson, H.L. and Nelson, J.L. 1995. *The patient in the family: An ethics of medicine and families.* New York: Routledge.

Omery, A. 1989. Values, moral reasoning, and ethics. *Nursing Clinics of North America, 24*(2), 499–508.

Pellegrino, E.D. 1979. Toward a reconstruction of medical morality: The primacy of the act of profession and the fact of illness. *Journal of Medicine and Philosophy, 4*(1), 32–56.

Pellegrino, E. 1985. The virtuous physician and the ethics of medicine. In E. Shelp (Ed.), *Virtue and medicine* (pp. 237–256). Dordrecht, Netherlands: Reidal.

Pellegrino, E.D. 1990. The medical profession as a moral community. *Bulletin of the New York Academy of Medicine, 66*(3), 221–232.

Pellegrino, E.D. 1993. The metamorphosis of medical ethics: A 30-year retrospective. *JAMA, 269*(9), 1158–1162.

Pellegrino, E.D. 1995. Is telling the truth a cultural artifact? In F. Baylis, J. Downie, B. Freedman, B. Hoffmaster and S. Sherwin (Eds.), *Health care ethics in Canada* (pp. 55–58). Toronto: Harcourt Brace.

Pellegrino, E.D. 2001. The internal morality of clinical medicine: A paradigm for the ethics of the helping and healing professions. *Journal of Medicine and Philosophy, 26* (6), 559–579.

Pellegrino, E.D., Veatch, R.M. and Langan, J.P. 1991. Preface. In E.D. Pellegrino, R.M. Veatch and J.P. Langan (Eds.), *Ethics, trust, and the professions: Philosophical and cultural aspects* (pp. vii–ix). Washington, DC: Georgetown University Press.

Penticuff, J.H. 1991. Conceptual issues in nursing ethics research. *Journal of Medicine and Philosophy, 16*(3), 235–258.

Pogge, T.W. 1989. *Realizing Rawls.* Ithaca: Cornell University Press.

Pojman, L.P. 2001. *Ethics: Discovering right and wrong.* Toronto: Wadsworth.

Rachels, J. 1975. Active and passive euthanasia. *New England Journal of Medicine, 292,* 78–80.

Rawls, J. 1971. *A theory of justice.* Cambridge, MA: Harvard University Press.

Rawls, J. 1993. *Political liberalism.* New York: Columbia University Press.

Rodney, P.A. 1997. *Towards connectedness and trust: Nurses' enactment of their moral agency within an organizational context.* Unpublished doctoral dissertation. University of British Columbia, Vancouver.

Rodney, P.A. and Varcoe, C. 2001. Toward ethical inquiry in the economic evaluation of nursing practice. *Canadian Journal of Nursing Research, 33*(1), 35–57.

Rodney, P., Varcoe, C., Storch, J. L., McPherson, G., Mahoney, K., Brown, H., Pauly, B., Hartrick Doane, G. and Starzomski, R. 2002. Navigating toward a moral horizon: A multi-site qualitative study of nurses' enactment of ethical practice. *Canadian Journal of Nursing Research, 34*(3), 75–102.

Rorty, R. 1999. *Philosophy and social hope.* London: Penguin.

Roy, D.J., Williams, J.R. and Dickens, B.M. 1994. *Bioethics in Canada.* Scarborough, ON: Prentice Hall.

Sher, G. 1987. Other voices, other rooms? Women's psychology and moral theory. In E.V. Kittay and D.T. Meyers (Eds.), *Women and moral theory* (pp. 178–189). Totonia, New Jersey: Rowman and Littlefield.

Sherwin, S. 1992. *No longer patient: Feminist ethics & health care.* Philadelphia: Temple University Press.

Sherwin, S. 1998. A relational approach to autonomy in health care. In S. Sherwin et al. (Eds.), *The politics of women's health* (pp. 19–47). Philadelphia: Temple University Press.

Sim, J. 1995. Moral rights and the ethics of nursing. *Nursing Ethics, 2*(1), 31–40.

Singer, P. 1986. *Applied ethics.* New York: Oxford University Press.

Smith, K.V. and Godfrey, N.S. 2002. Being a good nurse and doing the right thing: A qualitative study. *Nursing Ethics, 9*(3), 301–312.

Sokolowski, R. 1991. The fiduciary relationship and the nature of professions. In E.D. Pellegrino, R.M. Veatch and J.P. Langan (Eds.), *Ethics, trust, and the professions: Philosophical and cultural aspects* (pp. 23–43). Washington, DC: Georgetown University Press.

Starzomski, R.C. 1997. *Resource allocation for solid organ transplantation: Toward public and health care provider dialogue.* Unpublished doctoral dissertation. University of British Columbia, Vancouver.

Starzomski, R. and Rodney, P. 1997. Nursing inquiry for the common good. In S.E. Thorne and V.E. Hayes (Eds.), *Nursing praxis: Knowledge and action* (pp. 219–236). Thousand Oaks: Sage.

Sumner, L.W. 1987. *The moral foundation of rights.* New York: Oxford University Press.

Taylor, C. (with A. Gutmann, S.C. Rockefeller, M. Walzer and S. Wolf). 1992. *Multiculturalism and 'the politics of recognition'.* Princeton: Princeton University Press.

Thomson, J.J. 1990. *The realm of rights*. Cambridge: Harvard University Press.

Tong, R. 1997. *Feminist approaches to bioethics: Theoretical reflections and practical applications.* Boulder, CO: Westview.

Toulmin, S. 1981. The tyranny of principles. *Hastings Center Report, 11*, 31–39.

Trial of war criminals before the Nuremberg military tribunals under control council law 1947. (Military Tribunal I, Number 10). Washington, D.C.: U.S. Government Printing Office.

Varcoe, C. and Rodney, P. 2002. Constrained agency: The social structure of nurses' work. In B.S. Bolaria and H.D. Dickinson (Eds.), *Health, illness and health care in Canada,* 3rd ed. (pp. 102–128). Scarborough, ON: Nelson Thomson Learning.

Veatch, R. 1981. *A theory of medical ethics*. New York: Basic.

Warren, V.L. 1992. Feminist directions in medical ethics. *H.E.C. Forum, 4*(1), 19–35.

Watson, S.D. 1994. Minority access and health reform: A civil right to health care. *Journal of Law, Medicine & Ethics, 22,* 127–137.

Wehmeier, S. (Ed.) (with A.S. Hornby). 2000. *Oxford Advanced Learner's Dictionary.* 6th edition. Oxford: Oxford University Press

Weisz, G. 1990. Introduction. In G. Weisz (Ed.), *Social science perspectives on medical ethics* (pp. 3–15). Philadelphia: University of Pennsylvania Press.

Winkler, E.R. 1993. From Kantianism to contextualism: The rise and fall of the paradigm theory in bioethics. In E.R. Winkler and J.R. Coombs (Eds.), *Applied ethics: A reader* (pp. 343–365). Oxford: Blackwell.

Winkler, E. 1996. Moral philosophy and bioethics: Contextualism versus the paradigm theory. In L.W. Sumner and J. Boyle (Eds.), *Philosophical perspectives on bioethics* (pp. 50–78). Toronto: University of Toronto Press.

Wolf, S.M. 1994a. Health care reform and the future of physician ethics. *Hastings Center Report, 24*(2), 28–41.

Wolf, S.M. 1994b. Shifting paradigms in bioethics and health law: The rise of a new pragmatism. *American Journal of Law & Medicine, 20*(4), 395–415.

Yeo, M. 1993. *Ethics and economics in health care resource allocation*. Ottawa: Queen's-University of Ottawa Economic Projects.

Yeo, M. 1994. Interpretive bioethics. *Health and Canadian Society, 2*(1), 85–108.

Yeo, M.1996a. Introduction. In M. Yeo and A. Moorhouse (Eds.), *Concepts and cases in nursing ethics,* 2nd ed. (pp. 1–26). Peterborough, ON: Broadview.

Yeo, M.1996b. A primer in ethical theory. In M. Yeo and A. Moorhouse (Eds.), *Concepts and cases in nursing ethics,* 2nd ed. (pp. 27–55). Peterborough, ON: Broadview.

Yeo, M., Moorhouse, A. and Donner, G. 1996. Justice. In M. Yeo and A. Moorhouse (Eds.), *Concepts and cases in nursing ethics,* 2nd ed. (pp. 211–266). Peterborough, ON: Broadview.

chapter five

Our Theoretical Landscape: Complementary Approaches to Health Care Ethics

Patricia Rodney,
Bernadette Pauly, and
Michael Burgess

Most ethical problem solving cannot... be either top down or bottom up but must be multifaceted and responsive to the demands of both context and theory (Daniels 1996, 112).

While biomedicine has made great strides in understanding and treating a host of medical problems, and traditional bioethical theory has helped to promote respect for patients as self-determining persons, much more needs to be done. In particular, we need to better understand and address the personal, social, and cultural aspects of health as well as the complex sociopolitical climates in which health care is delivered and in which resources for health are embedded (Hoffmaster 1999; 2001; Sherwin 1992; 1998; Tong 1997; Wolf 1994a; 1994b). This entire text is constructed to help nurses as well as others involved in health care ethics to take up the challenge. This chapter is meant to point to some complementary sources of theory that can help.

CONTEXTUAL PERSPECTIVES

In Chapter 4 we argued that our adoption and development of ethical theory should be thoughtful and conscious, and that our theorizing should involve processes of critical reflection. We agreed with the ethicists Norman Daniels (1996) and Earl Winkler (1996) that we need to take up and continue to refine ethical theory/insights from three different levels: (1) general theories (such as utilitarianism, deontology, and contractarianism); (2) mid-range ethical principles (autonomy, beneficence, nonmaleficence, and justice); and (3) contextual (experiential or case) knowledge. And we agreed that our theorizing can benefit from processes such as wide reflective equilibrium.[1] The complementary approaches we explore in this chapter fall primarily in the third level, **contextualism.**

Winkler (1993) defines contextualism as

> the idea, roughly, that moral problems must be resolved within concrete circumstances, in all their interpretive complexity, by appeal to relevant historical and cultural traditions, with reference to critical institutional and professional norms and virtues, and by utilizing the primary method of comparative case analysis (344).[2]

We believe that it is most useful to think of contextualism as a lens through which we notice moral aspects that a different theoretical lens might tend to miss or distort. This does not mean that the distinction between context and theory is a "real" distinction—both intend to describe and appraise the moral components of life and often overlap. The essential feature to understand about contextualism is that it "moves from the bottom up" (Winkler 1996, 52). The various forms of contextualist ethics include (but are not limited to) a revival of casuistry, the call for an inductivism based on empirical information or ethnography, interest in narrative bioethics, the articulation of care-based ethics, and relational ethics (Wolf 1994b, 400).[3]

To start to illustrate how contextualism might work, let us consider how best to support a dying child and her grieving parents. We would want to understand her parents' unique circumstances and resources to deal with their grief (contextual features of the family as well as care theory), and we would also want to prevent the suffering of the child and engage her in decision-making as much as possible based on her unique wishes and capacities (beneficence, nonmaleficence, and autonomy as well as individual features of the child). In advocating contextualism, it is important to note that we are *not* subscribing to or promoting **ethical relativism.** As the anthropologist Clifford Geertz (2000) puts it, "the answers to our most general questions—why? how? what? whither?—to the degree they have answers, are to be found in the fine detail of lived life" (xi). Contextual ethical inquiry seeks to gather subjective as well as objective data about the real world in which ethical theory is to be implemented. In other words, contextualism draws our attention to particular people and particular relationships in particular contexts. While contextualism requires that specific ethical judgments are based on the relevant details of specific situations, it also benefits from and generates more general insight on what counts as ethically relevant details across situations. This situation-specific relevance of contextualism is distinct from the stronger claim of ethical relativism that all ethical judgments are only situation-specific expressions of approval or disapproval. This is why we believe that the ability to draw on all three levels of ethical thought is so important. Theories and principles propose general (at least provisional) standards, while contextual insights helps us to be more sensitive to nuance, personal meaning, and the influence of context as we move towards the implementation of such standards.[4]

In what follows in this chapter we will explore how cross-cultural and feminist ethics (which we treat as two large subsets of contextualist ethics) direct our attention to concerns about the particular. Both rely on an inductive approach and can include various forms of contextualist ethics. We will then move to a more explicit analysis of how concerns about the sociopolitical context lead to the insights offered by organizational and ecological ethics as well as by political theory.

The complementary approaches we explore in this chapter help us to identify and integrate contextual features into our ethical analysis and, subsequently, into our ethical practice. While the approaches we explore in this chapter (cross-cultural, feminist, organizational, and political) are fruitful, there are many others that are also capable of generating important insights for work in health care ethics. For instance, ethnography, critical social sciences, and economic analyses serve similar purposes. They can greatly enrich the approaches we discuss in this chapter.[5] Many of the various forms of contextualism will be elaborated on in more detail later in the text. For instance, Chapter 14 will explore the use of narrative-based ethics, Chapter 7 will explore care-based ethics, and Chapter 24 will explore relational ethics. *What these chapters share is the insight that moral problems ought to be addressed within real and concrete contexts and circumstances.*

Cross-Cultural Terrain

Critiques

Theorists and practitioners interested in **cross-cultural ethics** tell us that Western medicine is not neutral but, rather, "modern Western medicine is itself a culture alongside the other cultures" (Coward and Ratankul 1999, 3).[6] Traditional ethical theories such as utilitarianism, Kantian ethics, social contract theory, libertarianism, or other human rights–based theories reflect the cultural values and beliefs of the Western world and are dominated by European and American influences and infused with an inherent cultural ethnocentricity (Coward and Ratankul 1999; Fox 1990; Kleinman 1995). As one theorist has observed,

> In their analyses of complex situations, ethicists often appear grandly oblivious to the social and cultural context in which these occur, and indeed to empirical referents of any sort. Nor do they seem very conscious of the cultural specificity of many of the values and procedures they utilize when making ethical judgements (Weisz 1990, 3).

Although there has been significant progress since Weisz (1990) delivered his stinging critique, in Western health care and health care ethics we have tended to treat culture as being relevant only when we encounter people from "other" ethnic groups, forgetting that everyone, including those of us who have white skin and speak English, come from an ethnic background (Coward and Ratanakul 1999). **Culture** is much more than just ethnicity. It includes individualized as well as shared values and beliefs. A richer notion of culture is that of "shared meaning systems" (Shweder 1984, 1) that are fundamental to individuals' understandings of "what selfhood is" (Geertz 1984, 126; see also Coward and Ratanakul 1999). Culture is not static but is fluid and evolves over time. Furthermore, our conceptualization of culture ought to also be inclusive of notions of gender, race, and class.[7] It is important to note that "definitions and meanings of ethnicity and race are social constructions that shift constantly, reflecting the changing dynamics of gender, race/ethnic, and class relations over time" (Ng 1993, 227). Finally, culture permeates everything we do: "[C]ulture is a process occurring between people(s)... [T]he transmission and creation of both illness and health care are also cultural processes" (Stephenson 1999, 84). *This means that all of us involved in health care delivery and/or health care ethics come from our own disciplinary, specialty, and organizational cultures, as well as from our own background of personal, familial, and community values and beliefs.* Culture therefore operates in health care at all levels—from individual values, beliefs, and meanings, to group norms and practices, to organizational patterns and societal ideologies.

The understandings of culture we have articulated above have, historically, not been well operationalized in Western health care or Western health care ethics. There is evidence of a lack of sensitivity to social and cultural contexts and evidence of the effects of what happens when Western biomedicine dominates non-Western and traditional or Aboriginal cultures. Within the West, despite our liberal ideology, there are serious social inequities based on gender, race, and class.[8] When recent immigrants, people of Aboriginal ancestry, women, people who are impoverished, and the chronically ill, for instance, access the Western health care system, they frequently confront communication barriers and conflicts in ideology, if not outright discrimination.[9] In the case of Western health care in Canada for Aboriginal cultures,[10] there has been little opportunity for Aboriginal Canadians to engage in informed or participatory relationships with health care providers (Browne and Smye 2002; Kaufert and O'Neil 1990; Paulette 1993; Smye and Browne 2002; Stephenson 1999). In fact, Western health care delivery systems and other social systems (such as the residential schools that existed until a few decades ago) have disrupted the Aboriginal communities and systems of care that sustained people in more traditional times (Report of the Royal Commission on Aboriginal People 1996a; 1996b; 1996c).[11]

Western health care and health care ethics have been influenced by the evolution of a global corporate culture.[12] Thus, when Western health care is exported to other cultures, the results can be problematic. Education of health care professionals and the adoption of health care technology in other countries are often accompanied by implicit or explicit instruction in Western notions of health and health care ethics (Coward and Ratanakul 1999; Minami 1985). For example, in Thailand, where Buddhism is an important dimension of morality and ethics, high technology medicine "is increasingly supplanting traditional methods of treatment, reflecting the displacement of traditional models, with their holistic concept of health and health care. In its place, the Western model emphasizes technology, research, and specialized training" (Ratanakul 1990, 25). The Thai government has tended to fund high technology medicine at the expense of badly needed basic health care and services, thus threatening fundamental Buddhist notions of compassion and justice (Ratanakul 1990; 1999).

Overall, there is a certain ethnocentrism in Western health care ethics that devalues the contribution of other cultures to the process of ethical decision-making (Burgess 1999a; 1999b). While the concern in Western health care ethics to avoid ethical relativism is understandable, there has not been enough room left to negotiate between different meanings or to understand the influence of different contexts. Let us illustrate with an example. Ethics in Practice 5-1 comes from a focus group interview with nurses practising in an emergency department. The nurse we have quoted was participating in a study of nurses' ethical practice (see Appendix A). In this research transcript segment, she tells a story of an encounter that has left her troubled.

Our intent in citing the situation in Ethics in Practice 5-1 is not to judge whether the nurse's actions were right or wrong or to label the nurse as praiseworthy or blameworthy. Rather, in this chapter we want to use the emergency nurse's story to shed light on some of the practical challenges of health care ethics and to illustrate the promise of the insights that cross-cultural, feminist, organizational, and political perspectives can bring. We will therefore reflect on Ethics in Practice 5-1 at various points throughout the rest of the chapter.

Ethics in Practice 5-1	An Emergency Nurse's Story

There was a man not too long ago, his wife was miscarrying, and she didn't speak English—only he spoke English—so the surgeon explains [what is wrong with her and the proposed surgery] and the man is standing there supposedly translating to the woman. So I say to him, "She's going to sign the consent, ask her what she understands about it." He replied, "Doctor is going to fix it and make the baby okay." Because that's what he told her. So I say to the man,

"She doesn't understand." He replied, "Yes, that's what I want her to know." He wasn't too pleased with me because I got Interpreter Services to come and explain to her because she's signing a legal consent so that she understands what's going to happen to her. The man was so pissed off at me because he would tell her later in his own time that the baby was gone... or maybe not. (Adapted from Storch et al. 2001.)

For a start, on the face of it, the emergency nurse's story tells of her attempt to protect the patient's autonomy and uphold her right to informed consent.[13] These are important goals and, indeed, are enshrined in the code of ethics that directs the nurse's practice (Canadian Nurses Association 2002). However, the nurse has apparently focused on the patient in isolation from (in fact, in opposition to) her husband and possibly the rest of the patient's family.[14] As we indicated in Chapter 4, this kind of individualistic approach to autonomy has been part of the philosophical, legal, and political heritage of traditional bioethics. This does not make the nurse's worry about autonomy incorrect. It just means that there were other morally relevant features in the situation that she presumably overlooked.[15]

The patient and husband portrayed in Ethics in Practice 5-1 came from an ethnic background different from the nurse's and from the majority of other health care providers in the emergency department, and they were not fluent in English. Regardless of their ethnic background, it would have been important to find out more about how the husband was making sense of the situation and the personal meaning that he and his wife held about what she was going through. If he had a particular belief about protecting his family, it would have been important to find out more about that. *Such beliefs may or may not have been linked to his ethnic identity—it would have been crucial to avoid stereotyping him on the basis of language fluency, race, or any other characteristic.* Questions such as how he and his wife liked to make decisions in the family and what was important to him and his wife in this pregnancy would have been helpful. And more use of the hospital's interpreter services could have helped the nurse to better understand the wife's perspectives more directly. The nurse may have, in the end, made the same disclosure to the patient based on her concerns about autonomy, but she and the rest of the health care team would have *also* been better able to help the husband to understand and participate in the decision as much as possible. Instead, the husband was likely left feeling angry and betrayed, which would not help him to support his wife or help them both to deal with their grief.

The story recounted by the nurse in Ethics in Practice 5-1 also says something about the **culture of health care.** Health care delivery in general, and emergency departments in particular, are operating under a pervasive *ideology of scarcity* that rewards quick problem solving and efficient processing (Varcoe 1997; 2001; Varcoe and Rodney 2002; Varcoe, Rodney and McCormick in press). The nurse had a legitimate concern about the patient's informed consent but little time to more fully explore that concern. Indeed, she was almost certainly facing a backlog of other patients waiting for the patient's bed. The structure of work in the emergency department—including the expectations of her colleagues to clear the patient out to surgery quickly—mitigated against the nurse's ability to spend more time with the patient and the patient's husband even though she had access to (at least some) interpreter services. This is not to absolve the nurse of her responsibility to try to work more with the patient and the patient's husband and/or to bring in other resources. But it is to say that the culture of the emergency department she was operating in made it difficult. She was left with protecting the patient's right to informed consent as her default position.

As Ethics in Practice 5-1 indicates, the application of Western health care ethics to *all* cultures, and especially non-Western and traditional or Aboriginal cultures, needs critical examination. In the Western conception, a person has a bounded, unique, more or less integrated motivational and cognitive universe—a dynamic centre of awareness, emotion, judgment, and action supposedly organized into a distinctive whole. This whole is understood in isolation from other such wholes and in isolation from its social and natural background. Yet focusing on isolated individuals is a rather peculiar idea within the context of many of the world's cultures. Understanding others demands recognizing our individualistic orientation and seeing others' experiences within the framework of their own ideas of selfhood (Coward and Ratanakul 1999; Geertz 1984, 126).

An ethnographic and survey study of concealment and silence around cancer disclosure practices in Italy will help us to further explain what we mean. Researchers in Tuscany, Italy found that disclosure and informed consent as we know them in North America (which the researchers termed the "autonomy-control narrative") were enacted differently (Gordon and Paci 1997). Instead of a focus on the rights of the individual, there was a "social-embeddedness narrative" of social unity, protection, and hierarchy supporting non-disclosure (Gordon and Paci 1997). The researchers explain:

> Why is the question "to tell or not to tell" so dramatic for many in Italy? Because within this question is the much more essential question "to recognize or not to recognize the individual as separate and distinct from the family" (Gordon and Paci 1997, 1450).[16]

Gordon and Paci's study reminds us that we also ought to be open to the possibility that our North American valorization of autonomy may not be universally held.[17] At the same time, we ought not to stereotype any individual's values and beliefs according to ethnicity or any other attribute—including the values and beliefs of individuals from mainstream Western cultures. Reflecting back on Ethics in Practice 5-1, it may have been the case that the patient's husband, and quite possibly the patient herself, subscribed to something like a social-embeddedness narrative. As we have argued earlier, it would have helped if the nurse could have explored this further. Knowing more about what was important to the patient, her husband, and the rest of the family would have given the nurse a place from which to negotiate an ethical course of action—a course that, as much as possible, integrated the values of the patient and her family as well as the values of Western health care ethics (Burgess 1999a; 1999b; Gordon and Paci 1997; Jecker and Carrese 1995).

Possibilities

While the traditions of Western ethics have made considerable contributions, such as in the area of human rights, **cultural imperialism**[18] remains a serious challenge. The moral issue is that we have not recognized the worth of other cultures as resources for our ethical theory and theorizing (Jameton 1990; Taylor 1992). This occurs at least in part because we have failed to recognize the role of our own culture in our theories and judgments. Taylor (1992) suggests that we need to begin the study of any other culture with the presumption that "we owe equal respect to all cultures" (66). One major implication is that we ought to respect the contributions that the wisdom of various cultures can offer to Western health care ethics. If the culture of Western health care is to improve, we will need to have a richer composite of ethical approaches—as Daniels (1996) has articulated, theory and theorizing from general ethical theories, mid-range principles, and contextual approaches.

There is an opportunity here for us to draw on theories and traditions from various cultures for cross-cultural dialogue on the nature of ethics and the goals of health and health care. For example, Aboriginal belief systems in Canada are, in general, based on a notion of a balanced universe made up of energy fields, where the world, the environment, the community, the family, and the self are interwoven and move in harmony together. Thus, the four components of body, mind, emotion, and spirit are interwoven and are believed to be balanced in health and imbalanced in disease (Shestowsky 1993, 7).[19] Given the current critiques of the Western focus on isolated individuals, our development and use of ethical theory could be enriched by Aboriginal understandings of the need for balance and harmony between the self and the universe.[20]

Turning to another example, Western health care ethics could also be enriched by the Buddhist notion of compassion. Compassion is

> a central moral ideal in Buddhism.... [I]t is a universal and dispassionate love conjoined with knowledge. It radiates in the mind as a result of the recognition of human vulnerability to pain and suffering and the realization of the illusory nature of the Ego or the "I" that begets all form of self-seeking desires (Ratanakul 1999, 122).

The Buddhist definition of compassion could contribute substantially to current Western discussions of justice because of its acknowledgment of human vulnerability and its critique of self-interest.[21]

A second major implication is that we must find a way to negotiate between our own Western culture and the various cultural meanings that patients and their families hold (Jecker and Carrese 1995). Since morality is acted out in a cultural context, it is critical to try to engage in a dialogue with others about their cultural beliefs and practices before we pass judgment or implement decisions. We therefore need to acquire the knowledge and skills required to create the opportunity and space for enhanced intercultural exchange and understanding. In the situation in Ethics in Practice 5-1, for instance, we need to know more about *how* to approach the patient and her husband with questions about the patterns of decision-making in their family and about what was important to them in this pregnancy. Fortunately, there is a growing body of work by Western health care professionals and ethicists aiming at just this kind of knowledge and skill.[22] Moreover, there is an increasing array of theoretical, policy, and practice literature available that is written by individuals from a variety of ethnocultural groups.[23] Such literature can enhance cross-cultural understandings as well as the ongoing development of theory and theorizing in health care ethics.

Feminist Terrain

Some of the strongest challenges to the disciplinary history and the traditional theoretical focus of bioethics have been raised by feminist ethicists. **Feminist ethics** offers an alternate view of contemporary ethical issues and traditional ethical theory. Jagger (1991) notes, "The two parallel strands of feminist ethical work—the attention to contemporary ethical issues on the one hand and the criticism of traditional ethical theory on the other—together gave rise to the term 'feminist ethics,' which came into general use in the late 1970s and early 1980s" (81). Initially, feminist ethics brought the perspective of women's experience into the field of health care ethics and a belief that theory should be based on women's life experience (Warren 1989). While the early focus in feminist health care ethics was on reproductive issues, more recently, feminist ethics has taken on a wider range of issues, not just those that have to do with women's reproductive capacities (Wolf 1994b, 404–405).[24] The gender attentiveness of feminist ethics highlights the limitations of the first two levels of theory (general theories and principles) which are not sensitive enough to context and individual particularities (Wolf 1994b, 405).

A primary contribution of feminist ethics is the examination of a wider variety of ethical issues than in traditional bioethics, especially those issues related to sexism in health care delivery (Wolf 1994b). An important shift over the past two decades in feminist theory and feminist ethics has been the recognition that the experiences of all women are not the same and that factors such as race and resources have an important impact on experience.[25] That is, "The evaluation of medical practices must give primary attention to the impact of [medical] practices on women—not just individual women but on women as a group, including especially disadvantaged women such as poor women and women of color" (Lebacqz 1991, 12).

The Canadian ethicist Susan Sherwin is an important contemporary voice in feminist ethics. She further expands the scope of feminist ethics to address issues of **oppression** and **power inequities** more broadly. In her book, *No Longer Patient: Feminist Ethics and Health Care* (1992), she describes the intent of feminist approaches to health care ethics as follows:

> Feminism expands the scope of bioethics, for it proposes that additional considerations be raised in the ethical evaluation of specific practices: it demands that we consider the role of each action or practice with respect to the general structures of oppression in society. Thus medical and other health care practices should be reviewed not just with regard to their effects on the patients who are directly involved but also with respect to the patterns of discrimination, exploitation, and dominance that surround them.... In addition, feminism encourages us to explore the place of medicine itself in society (4–5).

Feminism explicitly raises issues such as the inequality and unequal treatment of women and others in health care (both patients and workers), discrimination on the basis of sexual orientation or (dis)ability or other personal attributes, sexist occupational roles in which gender roles of caring are assigned to female workers, job-related stress, and conflicts in relationships.[26] Embedded within these issues is the claim that ethical analysis requires attention to power in health care settings—"who has it, how it works, and how to fix the current inequities" (Wolf 1994b, 406). An additional claim made by feminist ethics is that "analysis of power and morality cannot proceed without careful attention to context and difference" (Wolf 1994b, 406). *Feminist theory draws attention to the quality of relationships—particularly the power in those relationships—at individual, organizational, and societal levels.*[27]

A number of applications of feminist ethics appear later in this text, particularly in Chapter 8 (on nurses' moral agency), Chapter 10 (on the moral climate for nursing practice), and Chapter 12 (on ethical issues in home care). For now, let us return to our consideration of Ethics in Practice 5-1. As a theoretical lens, feminist ethics raises somewhat different issues than those we have discussed so far in relation to cross-cultural ethics.

First, feminist ethics reminds us to consider the power relations that might be at play in the situation in Ethics in Practice 5-1. We ought to inquire about the quality of the relationship between the patient, her husband, and the rest of the family, and we ought to be sensitive to the fact that she (or any other patient) may be living in an abusive situation. This is one further reason why it was important for the nurse to ensure that the woman had some time alone with herself or another health care provider and a translator who was not a member of her family. It takes strong clinical and communication skills to make this kind of assessment without jeopardizing the relationships between the health care providers, the patient, and the family. We ought *not* to proceed with the inaccurate (but widely held) stereotype that only women who come from immigrant, Aboriginal, or impoverished families experience violence (Varcoe 1997; 2001; see also Chapter 20). As we have said earlier, the husband's preference for non-disclosure may have come from a sincere desire to protect his wife.

Other power relations we ought to consider include how, in Ethics in Practice 5-1, the staffing and rapid pace in the emergency department made it difficult for the nurse to sit down and listen to the patient. Feminist theory will help us to understand why nurses in that emergency department—and in almost every other arena of health care delivery—are so excessively stretched.[28]

Second, feminist ethics will help us to further explore the ethical principle of **justice** in situations such as Ethics in Practice 5-1. As was identified earlier, justice is probably the least understood and the least well operationalized principle in health care ethics. At the heart of feminist ethics is the ideal of achieving social justice. Feminist ethics therefore brings greater understanding to the concept of justice.

One feminist theorist, Young (1990), argues that contemporary theories of justice are dominated by a distributive paradigm and that it is a mistake to reduce social justice to distribution, claiming that the distributive paradigm "tends to ignore the social structures and institutional context that often help determine distributive patterns" (15). She argues that notions of distributive justice cannot illuminate class relations or provide critical analysis of such relations: "The concepts of domination and oppression, rather than the concept of distribution, should be the starting point for a conception of social justice" (16). Domination and oppression are not always overt. They can be manifested in policies and structures that create covert barriers to health care access (Henry, Tator, Mattis and Rees 2000). Reflecting on Ethics in Practice 5-1, this means we ought to consider questions such as how the patient's lack of fluency in English affected her access to prenatal care, whether she and her family were able to afford transportation to health care services, whether they were able to afford adequate nutrition, and so forth. As was identified at the beginning of this chapter, the challenge before us in health care ethics is to better understand and address the personal, social, and cultural aspect of health as well as the sociopolitical climate of health care delivery. What our analysis has suggested is that feminist ethics, through new understanding and insights into justice, has much to offer in addressing this challenge.

Third, feminist theory contributes to the study and debate of ethical questions by introducing diversity in how health care ethics is pursued and by encouraging the exploration of ethics from many different perspectives (DeRenzo and Strauss 1997; Tong 1997; Warren 1989; Wolf 1994b). In feminist theory, attention is paid to how people relate in ethics discussions. As one feminist observer notes,

> In academia, the Ethics Game is sometimes played to one-up the opposition. The goals include proving oneself right (about what is morally right) and proving the "opposition" wrong. Moral theories and arguments are used as weapons (Warren 1989, 83).

Discussions in health care ethics have too often been demeaning—focused on someone "winning" rather than on finding meaning or truth (Warren 1989). In other words, feminist ethics asks us to consider how we treat each other and our patients and their family members as well as the power dynamics in the organizational and societal structures in which we operate. It also asks us to consider the ways in which we conduct ourselves as we practise, study, teach, and/or do research and policy work in health care ethics.

In summary, feminist ethics draws our attention to important contextual features of peoples' lives and social circumstances. It especially draws our attention to particulars involving gender, power, and justice. Returning to Daniels' (1996) proposal for the use of diverse sources of theory in ethics, we note that his second premise is "Because there are many types of problems and a division of moral labor is reasonable, many people from many different disciplines and training backgrounds can expect to make important contributions in bioethics" (112). Thus, we would like to suggest that *both* cross-cultural and feminist insights can help us to engage more effectively in health care ethics. We need insights from anthropologists, sociologists, religious scholars, and feminist theorists, as well as from philosophers/ethicists and health care providers.[29] In Chapter 6 we will start to say more about *how* we might draw from these diverse insights.

A WIDER TERRAIN

In concluding this chapter, we wish to reflect on a wider terrain foreshadowed in both cross-cultural and feminist ethics. In thinking of culture, we are reminded to think of the culture of health care institutions, and in thinking of feminism, we are reminded to consider relationships and power dynamics in organizations. Furthermore, cross-cultural analyses point us to global considerations, and feminist analyses point us to societal values and expectations. *This means that the theoretical diversity in health care ethics that Daniels (1996) calls for (and that we support) ought to include more organizational, ecological, and political contributions.*[30] This is necessary if those of us engaged in health care ethics are to better understand and deal with the complex sociopolitical climates in which health care is delivered and in which resources for health are embedded.

Organizational

For a start, we need to understand the ways in which the social processes of health care institutions affect health care practices and outcomes (Mishler 1981, 79). As Anderson, Blue and Lau (1991) have stated, "the vocabularies of the larger social organization are reproduced in micro level interactions between [patients/families] and health professionals through a set of ideologies that structure health care delivery" (102).[31] Thinking of **ethics at the organizational level** can help us to both unpack and strategize around these kinds of issues.

Organizations such as hospitals, long-term care facilities, community centres, and research institutes are characterized by hierarchy, a complex division of labour, administrative positions based on technical expertise and/or knowledge, collective outputs, reliance upon rules and policies, and multiple institutional/staff relationships (Buchanan 1996, 419–420). Health care agencies are therefore entities that have responsibility and accountability that transcend the responsibility and accountability of individual health care providers. This means that health care agencies have a role in the resolution *and* the creation of ethical problems in health care (Storch, Rodney and Starzomski 2002). For instance, in Ethics in Practice 5-1, the way that the staffing and services were organized in the emergency department made it difficult for the nurse to better attend to the patient and her husband.

Attention to the ethics of organizations is a relatively new phenomenon but is gaining increasing attention in a number of fields of applied ethics, including health care.[32] We have learned—often through painful experience—that organizations do not always operate in the best interests of the people they serve and/or the people they employ. In the aerospace industry, for example, the 1986 *Challenger* disaster (when the space shuttle exploded immediately after take off) raised questions about the willingness of management to listen to the advice of its engineers (Boisjoly, Curtis and Mellican 1991). In health care, the unexpected deaths of 12 infants who had undergone cardiac surgery in Winnipeg between March and December 1994 raised questions about the willingness of management to listen to the concerns of nurses practising in the operating room (Sinclair 2000; see also Chapter 2). The nurses (and some physicians) had repeatedly expressed concern about the unexpected complications that the infants were experiencing but were left feeling not listened to, and even threatened. Associate Chief Judge Murray Sinclair's *Pediatric Cardiac Surgery Inquest Report* (2000) determined that the pediatric cardiac surgery program at the involved Winnipeg hospital was under-resourced, the competence of the sole pediatric cardiac surgeon was questionable, and the nurses and physicians had been justified in taking their concerns to hospital management. Tragically, their concerns were not acknowledged until after many preventable deaths had occurred.

High profile incidents such as the *Challenger* disaster and the infant cardiac surgery deaths in Winnipeg—and multiple everyday problems such as short staffing—make it clear that we need to pay attention to the ethics of organizations, not just those of professionals/providers. The scope and character of organizational ethics include (but are not limited to)

- theories of organizational ethics (e.g., the organization as moral agent);
- issues that are particularly relevant for organizations (e.g., conflict of interest, allocation of resources);
- the use of professional guidelines or explicit statements of responsibilities for individuals at all levels the organization (e.g., codes of ethics and job descriptions);
- virtues that contribute to organizational ethics (e.g., promise keeping, prudence, and trustworthiness); and
- structures and processes which contribute to organizational ethics (e.g., mission and value statements, policies and procedures, and ethics committees). (Adapted from Boyle et al. 2001, 17–18.[33])

In a sense, what we aim to do in organizational ethics is to change the *cultural ethos* (Jameton 1990; Liaschenko 1993) of the organization so that it better serves the diverse but legitimate interests of the people it serves as well as the people it employs. Within health care, we have much more work to do to figure out *how* to achieve this change. As we will explain in Chapter 6, organizational ethics committees can play a role. And, as the authors of many of the chapters in Section II: Moral Climate will argue, we ought to listen to nurses and other health care providers and involve them—as well as the people they serve—in making decisions about their conditions of work.[34]

Action at the organizational level is important, but it is not enough. Liaschenko (1993) reminds us that cultural ethos is "a complex term that includes both explicit and implicit ideals of conduct, ideology, and social and political structure and organization" (71). In other words, the push to launch the *Challenger* on schedule and the push to have an active pediatric cardiac surgery program in Winnipeg were embedded in influences that went beyond organizational walls.

Ecological and Political

Organizations exist within a nexus of complex structural, geographic, biological, social, and political environments. For this reason, an organization "can be considered an ecosystem, and its study an ecology" (Boyle et al. 2001, 7). As Marck will explore in Chapter 11, we need to better understand some of these relationships in order to foster the ethical practice of nurses and other health care providers. For instance, the relative geographical isolation of Winnipeg in the middle of the Prairies meant that there were not as many specialized medical resources for the pediatric cardiac surgery program as there might have been in a city like Toronto.[35] And the unique specialization and geographic isolation of the operating room meant that it was not easy for the nurses and physicians to have their concerns about standards of practice heard.

We ought to be concerned about how complex structural, geographic, biological, social, and political environments affect the ethical dimensions of health care delivery. This wider view is especially important in reflecting on the concept of justice. Writing from the field of ethics and geography, David Smith (2000) warns of "a fundamental and deeply geographical distinction in morality: between sympathy for close and familiar persons and concern for distant and different others" (9). Our discussion earlier in this chapter of cross-cultural and feminist ethics would suggest that our concern for the latter group is not well developed, or at least not well acted upon.[36] This means that the individualistic orientation of much of health care shapes the ethical focus to be those about identifiable individuals and not populations—about familiar case or management problems and not the political-social-economic context that shapes them. It is therefore our conviction that ethicists, policy-makers, and health care providers need to better explore the interface of ethics and **politics.**[37]

On the basis of his experiences in national policy work, Daniels (1996) notes "the gap between principle and guidance in institutional design is quite wide and... we do not yet know how to fill it" (108). His conclusion is that "we must pay much more attention to problems of fair process and to refinements of democratic theory" (112). We could not agree more. We would add that paying attention to problems of fair process and democratic theory means engaging all individuals so that they can have meaningful participation in decisions that will affect the communities that they live and/or work in (Mann 1994; McGowan 1998). This requires promoting a constructive dialogue that embraces diverse viewpoints—

processes that are at the heart of democracy (Chinn 1995; Mouffe 1993).[38] This is past/future terrain. Almost three thousand years ago, Aristotle (350 BCE/1985) is reported to have spoken on politics immediately after he spoke on ethics. He saw these two disciplines as continuous and interdependent. We have lost this insight in our "modern" era, and it is time to retrieve it. The contemporary political philosopher Mark Kingwell (2000) claims that we need to re-think citizenship for ethics to be actualized through politics:

> What we don't have, but desperately need, is a global politics to balance and give meaning to these troubling universal realities.... At its best, a best we have yet to realize, citizenship functions as a complex structure for realizing our deeply social nature, even as it acknowledges and copes with the terrible vulnerability of humans, the myriad fragilities and risks of our existence on the mortal plane (3–5).

We are, indeed, diverse people experiencing diverse realities but sharing existential vulnerabilities. Throughout this chapter, we have made the case that health care ethics, therefore, needs to draw on diverse sources of wisdom—sources that we hope will continue to evolve and flourish.

FOR REFLECTION

1. Culture is more than ethnicity. Identify cultural characteristics (shared values and beliefs) of a health care specialty you are familiar with. What are some of the consequences of those characteristics?

2. What do you think a feminist analysis of the under-reporting and under-treatment of cardiac disease in women might include?

3. Whistleblowers—individuals who call external attention to organizational problems—are often ostracized, if not punished. How can organizations be proactive instead of reactive with whistleblowers?

4. How can we obtain more diverse input into public discussions about health care resource allocation? Project some examples.

ENDNOTES

1. As it was defined in Chapter 4, the method of wide reflective equilibrium

    seeks coherence among three divisions of moral thought: our considered moral judgements, a set of principles designed to rationalize and order these judgements, and a set of relevant background theories or understandings about subjects such as human nature and psychology, the workings of the law and procedural justice, conditions for social stability and change, and the socio-economic structure of society (Winkler 1996, 64).

2. Winkler's (1993) definition may be somewhat narrow since contextualism does not always proceed by comparative case analysis and may, in fact, also use ethical standards in addition to specification of institutional and professional norms and virtues. Nonetheless, Winkler's definition is helpful in starting to delineate the field of contextual ethics.

3. Casuistry is an inductive approach to ethics that proceeds through case analyses (Arras 1991; Jonsen 1995; Jonsen and Toulmin 1988; Levi 1996; Toulmin 1981). Inductivism is a more general term referring to the use of qualitative and quantitative data to inform ethical theorizing (Hoffmaster 1991; 1993; Jameton and Fowler 1989). Narrative bioethics has emerged as a means to use story to inform ethical practice (Brody 2002; Frank 1998). Care-based ethics entails a primary focus on relationships and care (Bergum 1993; Flanagan 1991; Gilligan 1982), while relational ethics entails a primary focus on human meaning and connectedness (Bergum 1993; Sherwin 1998a; see also Chapter 8 and Chapter 24). For other sources describing contextual approaches, see Bergum (1993); Churchill (1997); Gadow (1999); Hoffmaster (1999; 2001); Kaufman (2001); Levi (1996); and Yeo (1994).

4. See also Susan Sherwin's (1992) chapter on "Feminism and Moral Relativism" (58–75). For an interesting critique of debates about relativism in philosophy and anthropology, see Clifford Geertz's (2000) chapter on "Anti-Anti Relativism" (42–67).

5. See, for example, Churchill (1997); Donath (2000); Harding (1995); Hoffmaster (1990; 1993; 2001); Jennings (1990); Kaufman (2001); Kleinman (1995); Rodney et al. (2002); and Varcoe, Rodney and McCormick (In press).

6. See also Burgess (1999a; 1999b); Burgess and Brunger (2000); Fox (1990); Kleinman (1995); Stephenson (1999); and Weisz (1990).

7. Anderson and Reimer Kirkham (1998; 1999); Bannerji 1993; hooks 1990; Ng 1993; see also Chapter 7.

8. Bannerji (1993); Blue et al. (1999); Cassidy, Lord and Mandell (1995); hooks (1990); Kaufert and O'Neil (1990); Li 1988; Ng (1993).

9. Anderson and Reimer Kirkham (1998; 1999); Browne and Smye (2002); Bunting (1992); Henry, Tator, Mattis and Rees (2000); Institute of Medicine (2002); Lynam et al. (2003); Smye and Browne (2001); Speck (1987); Stevens (1992); Thorne (1993; 2002).

10. There are three Aboriginal (indigenous) populations of people in Canada: First Nations, Inuit, and Métis. There is a rich diversity of history, traditions, and beliefs among these peoples. All three groups do, however, share an unfortunate history of dominance and colonization by Anglo-European settlers.

11. We would like to thank an anonymous reviewer for emphasizing the importance of this history.

12. See, for instance, Anderson and Rodney (1999); Hui et al. (1999); Laxer (1998); McQuaig (2001); Shiva (1997); and Williams (1993). See also Chapter 16 for a discussion of globalization and ethics.

13. See Chapter 4 for a discussion of rights and informed consent.

14. In an actual case review we would, of course, need much more information. We are extrapolating on the basis of our knowledge of the rest of the focus group interview, related research, and our own experiences in ethics consultations and policy work.

15. In Chapter 6, we talk about the use of ethical decision-making models that can assist in the fuller exploration of morally relevant features in ethical situations. Two such models (McDonald's *Ethical Decision Making Framework for Individuals* and Storch's *Model for Ethical Decision-Making for Policy and Practice*) are available in Appendix B.

16. See also Dalla-Vorgia et al. (1992) and Diego Gracia (1993) for discussions of differences between Italian/Mediterranean and other European and North American ethical traditions.

17. See also Hoffmaster (1999) and Keyserlingk (1999).

18. Said (1993) has been an insightful commentator on cultural imperialism, linking culture to narration. He explains:

    The main battle in imperialism is over land, of course; but when it came to who owned the land, who had the right to settle and work on it, who kept it going, who won it back, and who now plans for its future—these issues were reflected, contested, and even for a time decided in narrative (xii–xiii).

    We believe that a similar claim can be made about health care ethics. That is, we see similar contested questions about who owns the "correct" ethical theory, who has the right to use their theory, and where, and how that theory should evolve. Such questions involve issues of Western dominance over non-Western, traditional, and Aboriginal cultures and are at least in part reflected by how we narrate our approaches to health care ethics.

19. See also Burgess et al. (1999); Kaufert and O'Neill (1990); Paulette (1993); and Willms et al. (1992).

20. This is not an argument for cultural appropriation of Aboriginal philosophy or ethics. Instead, we are suggesting that an egalitarian and ongoing dialogue between theorists and practitioners in Western, non-Western, traditional, and Aboriginal cultures could help to move theory and theorizing ahead in health care ethics.

21. See Chapter 4 for a discussion of the challenges we currently face to our conceptualization and operationalization of justice in health care ethics.

22. See, for example, Bowman (2000); Jecker and Carrese (1995); Kaufert and Putsch (1997); and Thompson (1991).

23. For example, Advisory Group on Suicide Prevention (2003); Bannerji (1993); hooks (1990); and Tuhiwai Smith (1999).

24. Feminist theory is by no means a homogenous whole. See Jaggar (1991); Olesen (1994); and Tong (1997) for interesting descriptions of some of the various forms of feminist theory.

25. Anderson and Reimer Kirkham (1998; 1999); Bannerji (1993); Collins (1990); Lebaczq (1991); Lugones (1991); Ng (1993); Olesen (1994); Sherwin (1992); Williams (1993); Wolf (1994a; 1994b).

26. Card (1991); Chinn (2001); Holmes and Purdy (1992); Sherwin (1992; 1998); Shogan (1992); Tong (1997); Warren (1989); Wolf (1994b).

27. Baier (1994); Mann (1994); Sherwin (1992; 1998); see also Chapter 7 and Chapter 8.

28. Rodney and Varcoe (2001); Varcoe and Rodney (2002); see also Chapters 10–12.

29. Note that all these categories overlap. Many feminist scholars theorize about cross-cultural considerations (e.g., Anderson and Reimer Kirkham 1999; Sherwin 1992). This is becoming linked to a rich and evolving post-colonial literature (Anderson 2002; Bhaba 1994; Browne and Smye 2002; see also Chapter 7).

30. We are claiming this in the future tense because, as we write, these forms of theory are only beginning to flourish in health care ethics.

31. See also Kleinman (1995) and Waitzkin (1983).

32. See, for example, Boyle et al. (2001); Buchanan (1996); Goold (2001); Pentz (1999); and Reiser (1994).

33. Note that in Canada addressing the ethics of health care organizations also requires addressing the ethics of the health care regions they are usually clustered in. See Yeo, Williams and Hooper (1998).

34. See also Jameton (1990); Liaschenko (1993); Raines (2000); Rodney and Varcoe (2001); Varcoe and Rodney (2002); and Chapter 10.

35. This is *not* to say that specialized medical resources ought not to be located in cities such as Winnipeg, which serve a number of isolated communities. Across Canada, there are serious regional (especially rural) inequities in access to health care (Blue et al. 1999; Commission on the Future of Health Care in Canada 2002).

36. See also Chapter 16. And for an interesting application of moral geography, see Valentine (2003).

37. One ethicist puts it this way:

    Bioethics will need to provide leadership in the hardest moral tasks of our time, what is at stake is the way we think about health and citizenship, about the nature and the duty of the state, the regulation of the power of scientific knowledge (Zoloth 2001, 39).

38. See also Chapter 10 and Chapter 15.

REFERENCES

Advisory Group on Suicide Prevention. 2003. *Acting on what we know: Preventing youth suicide in First Nations.* Report of the Advisory Group on Suicide Prevention. Ottawa: Advisory Group on Suicide Prevention.

Anderson, J. 2002. Toward a postcolonial feminist methodology in nursing research: Exploring the convergence of postcolonial and black feminist scholarship. *Nurse Researcher, 9*(3), 7–27.

Anderson, J.M., Blue, C. and Lau, A. 1991. Women's perspectives on chronic illness: Ethnicity, ideology and restructuring life. *Social Science and Medicine, 33*(2),101–113.

Anderson, J. and Reimer Kirkham, S. 1998. Constructing nation: The gendering and racializing of the Canadian health care system. In V. Strong-Boag, S. Grace, A. Eisenberg and J. Anderson (Eds.), *Painting the maple: Essays on race, gender, and the construction of Canada* (pp. 242–261). Vancouver: UBC Press.

Anderson, J. and Reimer Kirkham, S. 1999. Discourses on health: A critical perspective. In H. Coward and P. Ratanakul (Eds.), *A cross-cultural dialogue on health care ethics* (pp. 47–67). Waterloo, ON: Wilfrid Laurier University Press.

Anderson, J.M. and Rodney, P. 1999. Part IV: Conclusion: Health policy: A cross-cultural dialogue. In H. Coward and P. Ratanakul (Eds.), *A cross-cultural dialogue on health care ethics* (pp. 257–261). Waterloo, ON: Wilfrid Laurier University Press.

Aristotle. 350 BCE/1985. *Nicomachean ethics.* Translator: T. Irwin. Indianapolis, IN: Hackett.

Arras, J.D. 1991. Getting down to cases: The revival of casuistry in bioethics. *The Journal of Medicine and Philosophy, 16*, 29–51.

Baier, A.C. 1994. *Moral prejudices: Essays on ethics.* Cambridge, MA: Harvard University Press.

Bannerji, H. 1993. *Returning the gaze: An introduction.* In H. Bannerji (Ed.), *Returning the gaze: Essays on racism, feminism, and politics* (pp. ix–xxix). Toronto: Sister Vision Press.

Bergum, V. 1993. Participatory knowledge for ethical care. *The Bioethics Bulletin, 5*(2), 4–6.

Bhabha, H. 1994. *The location of culture.* London: Routledge.

Blue, A., Keyserlingk, T., Rodney, P. and Starzomski, R. 1999. A critical view of North American health policy. In H. Coward and P. Ratanakul (Eds.), *A cross-cultural dialogue on health care ethics* (pp. 215–225). Waterloo, ON: Wilfrid Laurier Press.

Boisjoly, R.P., Curtis, E.F. and Mellican, E. 1991. Roger Boisjoly and the Challenger disaster: Ethical dimensions. In D.C. Poff and W.J. Waluchow (Eds.), *Business ethics in Canada,* 2nd ed. (pp. 178–192). Scarborough, ON: Prentice Hall.

Bowman, K.W. 2000. Communication, negotiation, and mediation: Dealing with conflict in end-of-life decisions. *Journal of Palliative Care, 16*, S17–S23.

Boyle, P.J., DuBose, E.R., Ellingson, S.J., Guinn, D.E. and McCurdy, D.B. 2001. *Organizational ethics in health care: Principles, cases, and practical solutions.* San Francisco: Jossey-Bass.

Brody, H. 2002. Narrative ethics and institutional impact. In R. Charon and M. Montello (Eds.), *Stories matter—The role of narrative in medical ethics* (pp. 149–153). New York: Routledge.

Browne, A.J. and Smye, V. 2002. A postcolonial analysis of health care discourses addressing Aboriginal women. *Nurse Researcher, 9*(3), 28–41.

Buchanan, A. 1996. Toward a theory of the ethics of bureaucratic organizations. *Business Ethics Quarterly, 6*(4), 419–440.

Bunting, S.M. 1992. Eve's legacy: An analysis of family caregiving from a feminist perspective. In J.L. Thompson, D.G. Allen and L. Rodrigues-Fisher (Eds.), *Critique, resistance, and action: Working papers in the politics of nursing* (pp. 53–68). New York: National League for Nursing Press.

Burgess, M. 1999a. Part III: Introduction: Ethical issues in the delivery of health care services. In H. Coward and P. Ratanakul (Eds.), *A cross-cultural dialogue on health care ethics* (pp.157–159). Waterloo, ON: Wilfrid Laurier University Press.

Burgess, M. 1999b. Part III: Conclusion: Ethical issues in the delivery of health care services. In H. Coward and P. Ratanakul (Eds.), *A cross-cultural dialogue on health care ethics* (pp. 207–209). Waterloo, ON: Wilfrid Laurier University Press.

Burgess, M. and Brunger, F. 2000. Collective effects of medical research. In M. McDonald et al. (Eds.), *The Governance of health research involving human subjects.* Ottawa: The Law Commission of Canada. Available online: www.lcc.gc.ca/en/themes; www.ethics.ubc.ca/people/burgess/lccburgess.pdf

Burgess, M., Rodney, P., Coward, H., Ratanakul, P. and Suwonnakote, K. 1999a. Pediatric care: Judgments about best interests at the outset of life. In H. Coward and P. Ratanakul (Eds.), *A cross-cultural dialogue on health care ethics* (pp. 160–175). Waterloo, ON: Wilfrid Laurier University Press.

Canadian Nurses Association. 2002. *Code of Ethics for Registered Nurses.* Ottawa: Canadian Nurses Association.

Card, C. (Ed.). 1991. *Feminist ethics.* Lawrence, KS: University of Kansas Press.

Cassidy, B., Lord, R. and Mandell, N. 1995. Silenced and forgotten women: Race, poverty, and disability. In N. Mandell (Ed.), *Feminist issues: Race, class and sexuality* (pp. 32–66). Scarborough, ON: Prentice Hall.

Chinn, P.L. 1995. *Peace & power: Building communities for the future.* 4th edition. New York: NLN Press.

Chinn, P.L. 2001. *Peace & power: Building communities for the future.* 5th edition. Sudbury, MA: Jones and Bartlett.

Churchill, L.R. 1997. Bioethics in social context. In R.A. Carson and C.R. Burns (Eds.), *Philosophy of medicine and bioethics: A twenty-year retrospective and critical appraisal* (pp. 137–151). Dordrecht, Netherlands: Kluwer Academic.

Collins, P.H. 1990. *Black feminist thought: Knowledge, consciousness, and the politics of empower-ment.* Boston: Unwin Hyman.

Commission on the Future of Health Care in Canada. 2002. *Building on values: The future of health care in Canada.* ("The Romanow Report.") Ottawa: Commission on the Future of Health Care in Canada.

Coward, H. and Ratanakul, P. 1999. Introduction. In H. Coward and P. Ratanakul (Eds.), *A cross-cultural dialogue on health care ethics* (pp. 1–11). Waterloo, ON: Wilfrid Laurier University Press.

Dalla-Vorgia, P., Katsouyanni, K., Garanis, T., Drogari, G. and Koutselinis, A. 1992. Attitudes of a Mediterranean population to the truthtelling issue. *Journal of Medical Ethics, 18,* 67–74.

Daniels, N. 1996. Wide reflective equilibrium in practice. In L.W. Sumner and J. Boyle (Eds.), *Philosophical perspectives on bioethics* (pp. 96–114). Toronto: University of Toronto Press.

DeRenzo, E.G. and Strauss, M. 1997. A feminist model for clinical ethics consultation: Increasing attention to context and narrative. *HEC Forum, 9*(3), 212–227.

Donath, S. 2000. The other economy: A suggestion for distinctively feminist economics. *Feminist Economics, 6*(1), 115–123.

Flanagan, O. 1991. *Varieties of moral personality: Ethics and psychological realism.* Cambridge, MA: Harvard University Press.

Fox, R.C. 1990. The evolution of American bioethics: A sociological perspective. In G. Weisz (Ed.), *Social science perspectives on medical ethics* (pp. 201–217). Philadelphia: University of Pennsylvania Press.

Frank, A.W. 1998. First-person microethics: Deriving principles from below. *Hastings Center Report,* (July–August), 37–42.

Gadow, S. 1999. Relational narrative: The postmodern turn in nursing ethics. *Scholarly Inquiry for Nursing Practice, 13*(1), 57–69.

Geertz, C. 1984. "From the native's point of view": On the nature of anthropological understanding. In R.A. Shweder and R.A. Levine (Eds.), *Culture theory: Essays on mind, self, and emotion* (pp. 123–136). Cambridge: Cambridge University Press.

Geertz, C. 2000. *Available light: Anthropological reflections on philosophical topics.* Princeton: Princeton University Press.

Gordon, D.R. and Paci, E. 1997. Disclosure practices and cultural narratives: Understanding conceal-ment and silence around cancer in Tuscany, Italy. *Social Science and Medicine, 44*(10), 1433–1452.

Gilligan, C. 1982. *In a different voice: Psychological theory and women's development.* Cambridge, MA: Harvard University Press.

Goold, S.D. 2001. Trust and the ethics of health care institutions. *Hastings Center Report, 31*(6), 26–33.

Gracia, D. 1993. The intellectual basis of bioethics in southern European countries. *Bioethics 7,* 97–107.

Harding, S. 1995. Can feminist thought make economics more objective? *Feminist Economics, 1*(1), 7–32.

Henry, F., Tator, C., Mattis, W. and Rees, T. 2000. *The colour of democracy: Racism in Canadian society.* 2nd edition. Toronto: Harcourt.

Hoffmaster, B. 1990. Morality and the social sciences. In G. Weisz (Ed.), *Social science perspectives on medical ethics* (pp. 241–260). Philadelphia: University of Pennsylvania Press.

Hoffmaster, B. 1991. The theory and practice of applied ethics. *Dialogue, 30,* 213–234.

Hoffmaster, B. 1993. Can ethnography save the life of medical ethics? In E.R. Winkler and J.R. Coombs (Eds.), *Applied ethics: A reader* (pp. 366–389). Oxford: Blackwell.

Hoffmaster, B. 1999. Secular health care ethics. In H. Coward and P. Ratanakul (Eds.), *A cross-cultural dialogue on health care ethics* (pp. 139–145). Waterloo: Wilfrid Laurier University Press.

Hoffmaster, B. 2001. Introduction. In B. Hoffmaster (Ed.), *Bioethics in social context* (pp. 1–11). Philadelphia: Temple University Press.

Holmes, H.B. and Purdy, L.M. (Eds.). 1992. *Feminist perspectives in medical ethics.* Bloomington, IN: Indiana University Press.

hooks, b. 1990. *Yearning: Race, gender, and cultural politics.* Boston: South End Press.

Hui, E., Tangkanasingh, S. and Coward, H. 1999.Threats from the Western biomedical paradigm: Implications for Chinese herbology and traditional Thai medicine. In H. Coward and P. Ratanakul (Eds.), *A cross-cultural dialogue on health care ethics* (pp. 226–235). Waterloo, ON: Wilfrid Laurier University Press.

Institute of Medicine. 2002. *Unequal treatment: Confronting racial and ethnic disparities in health care.* Available online: www.nap.edu/openbook/030908265X/html

Jaggar, A.M. 1991. Feminist ethics: Projects, problems, prospects. In C. Card (Ed.), *Feminist ethics* (pp. 78–104). Lawrence, KS: University of Kansas Press.

Jameton, A. 1990. Culture, morality, and ethics: Twirling the spindle. *Critical Care Nursing Clinics of North America, 2*(3), 443–451.

Jameton, A. and Fowler, M.D.M. 1989. Ethical inquiry and the concept of research. *Advances in Nursing Science, 11*(3), 11–24.

Jecker, N.S. and Carrese, J.A. 1995. Caring for patients in cross-cultural settings. *Hastings Center Report 25*(1), 6–14.

Jennings, B. 1990. Ethics and ethnography in neonatal intensive care. In G. Weisz (Ed.), *Social science perspectives on medical ethics* (pp. 261–272). Philadelphia: University of Pennsylvania Press.

Jonsen, A.R. 1995. Casuistry: An alternative or complement to principles? *Kennedy Institute of Ethics Journal, 5*(3), 237–251.

Jonsen, A.R. and Toulmin, S. 1988. *The abuse of casuistry: A history of moral reasoning.* Berkeley, CA: University of California Press.

Kaufert, J.M. and O'Neil, J.D. 1990. Biomedical rituals and informed consent: Native Canadians and the negotiation of clinical trust. In G. Weisz (Ed.), *Social science perspectives on medical ethics* (pp. 41–63). Philadelphia: University of Pennsylvania Press.

Kaufert, J.M. and Putsch, R.W. 1997. Communication through interpreters in healthcare: Ethical dilemmas arising from differences in class, culture, language, and power. *The Journal of Clinical Ethics, 8*(1), 71–86.

Kaufman, S.R. 2001. Clinical narratives and ethical dilemmas in geriatrics. In B. Hoffmaster (Ed.), *Bioethics in social context* (pp. 12–38). Philadelphia: Temple University Press.

Keyserlingk, E. 1999. Comparing the participation of Native North American and Euro North American patients in health care decisions. In H. Coward and P. Ratanakul (Eds.), *A cross-cultural dialogue on health care ethics* (pp. 176–189). Waterloo, ON: Wilfrid Laurier University Press.

Kingwell, M. 2000. *The world we want: Virtue, vice, and the good citizen.* Toronto: Penguin.

Kleinman, A. 1995. *Writing at the margin: Discourse between anthropology and medicine.* Berkley: University of California Press.

Laxer, J. 1998. *The undeclared war: Class conflict in the age of cyber capitalism.* Toronto: Penguin.

Lebacqz, K. 1991. Feminism and bioethics: An overview. *Second Opinion, 17*(2), 10–25.

Levi, B.H. 1996. Four approaches to doing ethics. *The Journal of Medicine and Philosophy, 21*, 7–39.

Li, P.S. 1988. *Ethnic inequality in a class society*. Toronto: Wall and Thompson.

Liaschenko, J. 1993. Feminist ethics and cultural ethos: Revisiting a nursing debate. *Advances in Nursing Science, 15*(4), 71–81.

Lugones, M.C. 1991. On the logic of pluralist feminism. In C. Card (Ed.), *Feminist ethics* (pp. 35–44). Lawrence, KS: University of Kansas Press.

Lynam, M.J., Henderson, A., Browne, A., Smye, V., Semeniuk, P. and Blue, C. 2003. Healthcare restructuring with a view to equity and efficiency: Reflections on unintended consequences. *Canadian Journal of Nursing Leadership, 16*(1), 112–140.

Mann, P.S. 1994. *Micro-politics: Agency in a postfeminist era*. Minneapolis: University of Minnesota Press.

McGowan, J. 1998. *Hannah Arendt: An introduction*. Minneapolis: University of Minnesota Press.

McQuaig, L. 2001. *All you can eat: Greed, lust, and the new capitalism*. Toronto: Penguin.

Minami, H. 1985. East meets west: Some ethical considerations. *International Journal of Nursing Studies, 22*(4), 311–318.

Mishler, E.G. 1981. Social contexts of health care. In E.G. Mishler, L. Amara Singham, S.T. Hauser, R. Liem, S.D. Osherson and N.E. Waxler (Eds.), *Social contexts of health, illness and patient care*. Cambridge, U.K.: Cambridge University Press.

Mouffe, C. 1993. *The return of the political*. London: Verso.

Ng, R. 1993. Sexism, racism, Canadian nationalism. In H. Bannerji (Ed.), *Returning the gaze: Essays on racism, feminism, and politics* (pp. 223–241). Toronto: Sister Vision Press.

Olesen, V. 1994. Feminisms and models of qualitative research. In N.K. Denzin and Y.S. Lincoln (Eds.), *Handbook of qualitative research* (pp. 158–174). Thousand Oaks, CA: Sage.

Paulette, L. 1993. A choice for K'aila. *Humane Medicine, 9*(1), 13–17.

Pentz, R.D. 1999. Beyond case consultation: An expanded model for organizational ethics. *The Journal of Clinical Ethics, 10*(1), 34–41.

Ratanakul, P. 1990. Thailand: Refining cultural values. *Hastings Center Report, 20*(2), 25–27.

Ratanakul, P. 1999. Buddhism, health, disease, and Thai culture. In H. Coward and P. Ratanakul (Eds.), *A cross-cultural dialogue on health care ethics* (pp.17–33). Waterloo, ON: Wilfrid Laurier University Press.

Reiser, S.J. 1994. The ethical life of health care organizations. *Hastings Center Report, 24*(6), 28–35.

Report of the Royal Commission on Aboriginal People. 1996a. *Volume 1, Looking forward, looking back*. Ottawa: Report of the Royal Commission on Aboriginal People.

Report of the Royal Commission on Aboriginal People. 1996b. *Volume 3, Gathering strength*. Ottawa: Report of the Royal Commission on Aboriginal People.

Report of the Royal Commission on Aboriginal People 1996c. *Volume 4, Perspectives and realities*. Ottawa: Report of the Royal Commission on Aboriginal People.

Rodney, P.A. 1997. *Towards connectedness and trust: Nurses' enactment of their moral agency within an organizational context*. Unpublished doctoral dissertation. University of British Columbia, Vancouver, BC.

Rodney, P.A. and Varcoe, C. 2001. Toward ethical inquiry in the economic evaluation of nursing practice. *Canadian Journal of Nursing Research, 33*(1), 35–57.

Rodney, P., Varcoe, C., Storch, J. L., McPherson, G., Mahoney, K., Brown, H., Pauly, B., Hartrick Doane, G. and Starzomski, R. 2002. Navigating toward a moral horizon: A multi-site qualitative study of nurses' enactment of ethical practice. *Canadian Journal of Nursing Research, 34*(3), 75–102.

Said, E.W. 1993. *Culture and imperialism*. New York: Vintage.

Sherwin, S. 1992. *No longer patient: Feminist ethics & health care.* Philadelphia: Temple University Press.

Sherwin, S. 1998. A relational approach to autonomy in health care. In S. Sherwin and the Feminist Health Care Ethics Research Network (Eds.), *The politics of women's health* (pp. 19–47). Philadelphia: Temple University Press.

Shestowsky, B. 1993. *Traditional medicine and primary health care among Canadian Aboriginal people: A discussion paper with annotated bibliography.* Ottawa: Aboriginal Nurses Association of Canada.

Shiva, V. 1997. *Biopiracy: The plunder of nature and knowledge.* Toronto: Between the Lines.

Shogan, D. 1992. Conceptualizing agency: Implications for feminist ethics. In D. Shogan (Ed.), *A reader in feminist ethics* (pp. 333–355). Toronto: Canadian Scholars' Press.

Shweder, R.A. 1984. Preview: A colloquy of culture theorists. In R.A. Shweder and R.A. Levine (Eds.), *Culture theory: Essays on mind, self, and emotion* (pp. 1–24). Cambridge, U.K.: Cambridge University Press.

Sinclair, M. 2000. *Pediatric cardiac surgery inquest report.* Winnipeg, Manitoba: Manitoba Chief Medical Examiner.

Smith, D.M. 2000. *Moral geographies: Ethics in a world of difference.* Edinburgh: Edinburgh University Press.

Smye, V. and Browne, A. 2002. "Cultural safety" and the analysis of health policy affecting aboriginal people. *Nurse Researcher, 9*(3), 42–56.

Speck, D.C. 1987. *An error in judgement: The politics of medical care in an Indian/White community.* Vancouver: Talonbooks.

Stephenson, P. 1999. Expanding notions of culture for cross-cultural ethics in health and medicine. In H. Coward and P. Ratanakul (Eds.), *A cross-cultural dialogue on health care ethics* (pp. 68–91). Waterloo, ON: Wilfrid Laurier University Press.

Stevens, P.E. 1992. Who gets care? Access to health care as an arena for nursing action. *Scholarly Inquiry for Nursing Practice, 6*(3), 185–200.

Storch, J., Hartrick, G., Rodney, P., Starzomski, R. and Varcoe, C. 2001. *The ethics of practice: Context and curricular implications for nursing.* Research study. University of Victoria School of Nursing, Victoria, BC.

Storch, J., Rodney, P. and Starzomski, S. 2002. Ethics in health care in Canada. In B.S. Bolaria and H. Dickinson (Eds.), *Health, illness, and health care in Canada,* 3rd ed. (pp. 409–444). Toronto: Harcourt Brace.

Taylor, C. 1992. *Multiculturalism and "The politics of recognition."* Princeton: Princeton University Press.

Thompson, J.L. 1991. Exploring gender and culture with Kymer refugee women: Reflections on participatory feminist research. *Advances in Nursing Science, 13*(3), 30–48.

Thorne, S.E. 1993. *Negotiating health care: The social context of chronic illness.* Newbury Park, CA: Sage.

Thorne, S.E. 2002. Health promoting interactions: Insights from the chronic illness experience. In L.E. Young and V. Hayes (Eds.), *Transforming health promotion practice: Concepts, issues, and applications* (pp. 59–70). Philadelphia: F.A. Davis.

Tong, R. 1997. *Feminist approaches to bioethics: Theoretical reflections and practical applications.* Boulder, CO: Westview.

Toulmin, S. 1981. The tyranny of principles. *Hastings Center Report, 11,* 31–39.

Tuhiwai Smith, L. 1999. *Decolonizing methodologies: Research and indigenous peoples.* London: Zed Books.

Valentine, G. 2003. Geography and ethics: In pursuit of social justice—Ethics and emotions in geographies of health and disability research. *Progress in Human Geography, 27*(3), 375–380.

Varcoe, C. 1997. *Untying our hands: The social context of nursing in relation to violence against women.* Unpublished doctoral dissertation. University of British Columbia, Vancouver, BC.

Varcoe, C. 2001. Abuse obscured: An ethnographic account of Emergency Unit nursing in relation to violence against women. *Canadian Journal of Nursing Research, 32*(4), 95–115.

Varcoe, C. and Rodney, P. 2002. Constrained agency: The social structure of nurses' work. In B.S. Bolaria and H. Dickinson (Eds.), *Health, illness, and health care in Canada,* 3rd ed. (pp. 102–128). Toronto: Harcourt Brace.

Varcoe, C., Rodney, P. and McCormick, J. In press. Health care relationships in context: An analysis of three ethnographies. Manuscript accepted for publication with *Qualitative Health Research.*

Waitzkin, H. 1983. *The second sickness: Contradictions of capitalist health care.* New York: Free Press.

Warren, V.L. 1989. Feminist directions in medical ethics. *Hypatia, 4*(2), 73–87.

Weisz, G. 1990. Introduction. In G. Weisz (Ed.), *Social science perspectives on medical ethics* (pp. 3–15). Philadelphia: University of Pennsylvania Press.

Williams, P.J. 1993. Disorder in the house: The new world order and the socioeconomic status of women. In S.M. James and A.P.A. Busia (Eds.), *Theorizing black feminisms: The visionary pragmatism of black women* (pp. 118–123). London: Routledge.

Willms, D.G., Lange, P., Bayfield, D., Beardy, M., Lindsay, E.A., Cole, D.C. and Johnson, N.A. 1992. A lament by women for "The People, The Land" [Nishnawbi-Aski Nation]: An experience of loss. *Canadian Journal of Public Health, 83*(5), 331–334.

Winkler, E.R. 1993. From Kantianism to contextualism: The rise and fall of the paradigm theory in bioethics. In E.R. Winkler and J.R. Coombs (Eds.), *Applied ethics: A reader* (pp. 343–365). Oxford: Blackwell.

Winkler, E. 1996. Moral philosophy and bioethics: Contextualism versus the paradigm theory. In L.W. Sumner and J. Boyle (Eds.), *Philosophical perspectives on bioethics* (pp. 50–78). Toronto: University of Toronto Press.

Wolf, S.M. 1994a. Health care reform and the future of physician ethics. *Hastings Center Report, 24*(2), 28–41.

Wolf, S.M. 1994b. Shifting paradigms in bioethics and health law: The rise of a new pragmatism. *American Journal of Law & Medicine, 20*(4), 395–415.

Yeo, M. 1994. Interpretive bioethics. *Health and Canadian Society, 2*(1), 85–108.

Yeo, M., Williams, J.R. and Hooper, W. 1998. Ethics and regional health boards. In L. Groarke (Ed.), *The ethics of the new economy* (pp. 125–141). Waterloo, ON: Wilfrid Laurier University Press.

Young, I.M. 1990. *Justice and the politics of difference.* Princeton: Princeton University Press.

Zoloth, L. 2001. Heroic measures: Just bioethics in an unjust world. *Hastings Center Report, 31*(6), 34–40.

chapter six

Working within the Landscape: Applications in Health Care Ethics

Gladys McPherson,
Patricia Rodney,
Michael McDonald,
Janet Storch,
Bernadette Pauly, and
Michael Burgess

The purpose of inquiry is to achieve agreement among human beings about what to do, to bring about consensus on the ends to be achieved and the means to be used to achieve those ends (Rorty 1999, xxv).

The ends we want to achieve in ethics include the right, the good, and the fitting action.[1] In Chapter 4 we provided an overview of the history, theoretical underpinnings, and challenges we face in contemporary health care ethics. In Chapter 5, building on Daniels' (1996) argument for theoretical diversity in health care ethics, we sketched out some of the newer theoretical possibilities opened up by cross-cultural, feminist, organizational, and political writings in health care ethics. In this chapter we want to say more about how we might *apply* the theory in health care ethics we have visited thus far. While Chapter 7 and subsequent chapters in the text will explore the implications of ethical theory for nursing in particular, there are a number of practical insights from health care ethics more generally that we wish to highlight here.

Conceptually, we have been taking direction from Daniels' notion of **wide reflective equilibrium.** Daniels explains that "'Doing ethics' involves trying to solve very different kinds of problems answering to rather different interests we may have, some quite practical, others more theoretical" (1996, 102). Thus, we have suggested that the ethical theory we adopt, develop, and apply ought to draw on general ethical theories and mid-range ethical principles as well as contextual insights (particularly from cross-cultural and feminist approaches) (Daniels 1996; Winkler 1996). This means we have been promoting the use of a variety of sources of moral wisdom to solve problems[2] in the real world of practice—in Rorty's (1999) words, above, to figure out "what to do" as well as *how* to do it. *In this chapter we will therefore consider how conceptual thinking can be brought to bear in practical ethical problems.*

We commence with some reflections on the autonomy and interests of persons, especially those who are vulnerable. We illustrate our reflections on interests first by focusing on children. This leads us to consider practical dimensions of ethical decision-making with and for individuals in health care settings, at which point we focus on elderly persons' interests through a case illustration. In following through on our discussion of interests, we also address the interests of families in the case illustration. Because health care ethics often engages with problems at an organizational level, we conclude this chapter with some reflections on ethical action for organizations.

REFLECTIONS ON AUTONOMY AND INTERESTS

Relational Autonomy

When we think about moral obligations to others, and especially when ethical decision-making takes place in relation to persons whose capacities for autonomous decision-making may be limited, we are challenged to find ways of thinking that take into account an array of (sometimes competing) views. In any ethically challenging situation, we may be informed by mid-range theoretical perspectives. As we discussed in Chapter 4, the four mid-range bioethical principles—beneficence, nonmaleficence, autonomy, and justice—have had a great influence in health care ethics. But, as we have also noted in Chapter 4 and Chapter 5, while these approaches raise important considerations in ethically troubling situations, taken alone they can be limited in assisting us to decide what principle should predominate in any particular situation.

Consider, for example, the principle of **autonomy** and the complexities of incorporating this principle in ethically troubling situations. Conventional views of autonomy hold that an autonomous individual has the capacity to (1) be "sufficiently competent" to make a decision; (2) choose reasonably from the available options; (3) obtain adequate information and demonstrate understanding of the information related to the options available; and (4) not be coerced by others (Sherwin 1998). When we think of this principle in light of a contextual approach to ethics, the application of autonomy as a guide to ethical decision-making becomes far more complex. An important challenge we face is that, in Western societies, the value of respect for autonomy as a principle of ethical practice has tended to be accepted as a universal truth (Burgess et al. 1999a; see also Chapter 5). Furthermore, as we explained in Chapters 4 and 5, conventional perspectives on autonomy have been challenged by feminist theorists in reaction to notions of Kantian individualism and claims related to invariant developmental sequencing of moral orientations (Gilligan 1993; Sherwin 1998).

Sherwin (1998) draws our attention to what a broader and more contextualized understanding of what autonomy might mean in health care decision-making.[3] She posits an alternative view that she labels **relational autonomy.** Sherwin defines relational autonomy as "a capacity or skill that is developed (and constrained) by social circumstances. It is exercised within relationships and social structures that jointly help to shape the individual while also affecting others' responses to her efforts at autonomy" (36).

Conventional views of autonomy have also been disputed by post-structural theorists, who suggest that the very idea of autonomy is a sort of illusion of the Enlightenment conception of person (Foucault 1981; Mackenzie 2000). Whereas feminist theorists tend to support a more relationally composed understanding of autonomy, post-structural theorists insist that understandings of self and identity, and consequently of autonomy, are mere products of language and power.[4] Post-structuralist and feminist theorists therefore remind us to think about the power dynamics of the sociopolitical contexts we operate in as moral agents. And feminist theorists (especially Sherwin) remind us to consider the complex network of relationships that the persons we serve—and we ourselves—are embedded in. The models of ethical decision-making we articulate later in this chapter are designed to help to assess both power and relationships.

The Interests of Persons

The moral challenge of assessing the level of capacity of persons to participate in health care decisions and the responsibility of nurses and other health care providers to do so are ethical challenges that play out in many ways and in many places in contemporary Western health care. Not all humans are able to act autonomously. Some are, for example, partially or totally incompetent, unable to rationally assess options, or unable to act freely. However, some who could exercise autonomy are indirectly constrained from doing so by health care providers and/or the health care system. As we stated in Chapter 5, in Western health care we are sometimes not very reflective about who does or does not have the opportunity to have meaningful input into their treatment and care—that is, to have their autonomy respected. We are not very reflective about how attributes such as income level, religion, language fluency, gender, sexual orientation, substance use, mental and physical abilities, and age influence health care providers' assumptions about people's competence to participate in heath care decisions. It is the authors' belief that a better understanding of the **interests**[5] of all persons—especially those who are unable to act autonomously or who are at risk of having their autonomy overlooked or overridden—can move us towards better ethical practice.

For the purposes of illustration in this chapter, we first discuss ethical decisions with and for children (which will be expanded on in Chapter 19). We argue that addressing the interests of children, as well as other persons' requires that we understand their rights, needs, and relationships.[6] Let us start with a story about a patient in pediatric intensive care.

Ethics in Practice 6-1	**Clarence**

Clarence was a twelve-year-old boy who suffered serious and rare complications of a bacterial respiratory infection. Within days of the onset of the illness Clarence's lungs began to fail and he required artificial ventilation. In addition, he developed bilateral pneumotho-races and pneumomediastinum.[7] In spite of two weeks of aggressive treatment in intensive care, Clarence's condition continued to deteriorate.

A decision was made by the physicians and his parents to start ECMO[8] therapy. From that point on, Clarence endured a multitude of complications, including persistent bleeding in various sites (including his lungs), periods of low blood pressure, and infection. Many invasive procedures were performed in an effort to save his life. In spite of these aggressive efforts, Clarence died approximately 30 days after the onset of his illness.

Clarence was very sick from early in the course of his treatment. Although Clarence was sedated and received large doses of analgesia, he was conscious some of the time during his hospitalization. Because of the tubes in his airway, he was unable to speak. He could only communicate through gestures and facial expressions. For periods of days, he was pharmacologically paralyzed[9] and consequently unable to communicate in any way. Clarence was never asked if he wanted to proceed with treatment and no one is sure he ever knew the severity of his illness. When not paralyzed, there were times when Clarence was obviously dreadfully frightened and tried to pull at tubes or tried to get up. At those times, he needed to be physically restrained and required additional sedation.

Clarence's parents were at his bedside constantly. Throughout his illness, they spoke on his behalf, seeking to make the Clarence whom they knew visible to the nurses, physicians, and technicians involved in his care. Their wish was that everything possible be done for Clarence, and they provided their consent for every procedure that might offer any hope. When it became evident that Clarence could not survive, his parents found comfort in their religious faith that led them to believe that this illness was the will of God and that, when Clarence died, he would be going to a better place.

Caring for Clarence was troubling for many nurses. The aggressive nature of the illness, the age of this child, and the experimental nature of the treatment created a tense climate. Staff voiced concerns about the extent to which Clarence could or should be involved in decisions about his care and questioned the extent to which his parents' interests could reasonably be assumed to truly represent Clarence's interests. These concerns compounded an already perplexing situation. One of the main questions that nurses struggled with was, did they, as nurses, have an obligation to foster Clarence's participation in decisions made about his health care?[10]

Honouring Rights

Claims that children and other persons have certain **rights** reflect particular beliefs about their moral status (see also Chapter 4 and Chapter 19). Children's rights are generally considered to be of three types: the right to resources, including knowledge; the right to protection from harm or abuse; and the right to autonomy or freedom.[11]

Some have suggested that appeals to children's rights (and rights in general) have been made too often, resulting in the dilution of the power of these claims. Others see rights claims as particularly powerful instruments that bring considerations of children's moral status to the forefront, reminding us of what interests our society has committed to protect. Seen this way, rights constrain more powerful individuals (such as health care providers and other adults) from overriding certain interests of less powerful individuals (such as children and the elderly). Rights promote a consensus about the moral status of children and other persons. Thus, in any given interaction with children or other persons, considerations of rights may be particularly useful in sorting out what interests we deem most important to protect.

In regard to children's participation in decisions about their health care, claims to rights help us to hold in mind the positioning of children within our health care system and heighten our awareness of power differentials between children and adults, as well as between children as health care recipients and nurses as health care providers. Thus, the situation in Ethics in Practice 6-1 may cause us to wonder if the (well-intended) power differentials between Clarence, his parents, and the health care providers interfered with Clarence's right to participate in decisions about his treatment. But these claims to rights to participate cannot stand alone. Somehow, participation must be appropriate to the patient's capabilities, contextually structured to enhance the particular individual's participation, and considerate with regard to stimulating the patient's growth as a moral agent.[12] While Clarence's active participation in decisions about his treatment might have been appropriate to his age, and might have engaged him as an active agent, the contextual features of the suddenness and cascading severity of his illness made active participation difficult, though not impossible.

It becomes evident that while thinking about the rights of children and other persons causes us to ask important questions, rights are limited in the degree to which they can help us discern correct action in specific situations. For example, it can be argued that children have the right to participate as much as they are able in matters that concern them. Simultaneously, adults have responsibility to protect children and act in children's best interests. Between participation and protection, nurses and other health care providers are sometimes left to negotiate difficult territory—ensuring that children have opportunity to participate as fully as possible in decisions about their care, while at the same time ensuring that children's best interests are protected. The challenge is to look more closely at this issue of children's interests to find a reasonable way to make judgments about "best interests." We need a more nuanced way to think about how to weigh different interests—how to consider the relationship of one person's interests to the interests of others. Rights are a necessary component of our understanding of children's and other persons' interests but are not sufficient to provide guidance in complex situations where rights compete with one another and where other needs and relationships come into play.

Considering Needs

Thinking about rights may alert us to the critical features that must always be accounted for in the way we treat children and other vulnerable persons. Arguing against rights as the foundation for making decisions about how health care ought to be organized and delivered, Daniels (1985) writes, "appeals to rights do not take us past our disagreements and uncertainties about the scope and limits of such right claims" (5).[13] Daniels suggests that in considerations of health care, theories about **needs** provide a more intricate means by which to sort out what is fair and just. When we look in this direction, another important body of theory and research informs our thinking. Like rights thinking, a needs perspective has little to do with the specifics of particular moments of practice and more to do with our understanding of who persons are and what they are capable of.

For instance, a child's basic needs can be understood as what he or she requires to live the normal life, to flourish rather than merely survive (Honderick 1995). In this view, if a child's needs are unmet, that child experiences harm. Thinking about needs assists us to prioritize the meeting of most basic requirements but also leads us to ask other questions, the answers to which may enhance our understanding of children's interests in particular situations. Our understanding of children's needs is supported by substantial theory in the field of child development. Reflecting back on Ethics in Practice 6-1, this should cause us to ask not only whether Clarence's right to respect was being protected, but also whether his needs were being attended to. Developmental theories would help us to understand his need for privacy, connection to his family, and so forth. These are not unique needs of the individual child; nor are they respect for his autonomy or unique individuality. These are needs based on seeing beyond the technical aspects of health care services to recognize the requirements of children and other persons as human beings.

What children need will vary depending on the child's health condition, experience, and unique characteristics.[14] In each of these areas, research and theory inform us about potential ways in which these factors shape children's interests. For example, experience with illness and the health care system has been shown to be often as important as age and stage in shaping a child's capacity to participate in decision-making (Alderson 1993; Bluebond-Langner 1978). Considering this knowledge, health care providers would do well to take children's previous experience into account in making determinations of their interests and in making judgments about their participation in health care decision-making. For this reason, it would have been relevant to know more about Clarence's previous experiences with health care. This kind of experiential background is also relevant for other persons. For example, research has shown that experience with illness and (especially) the health care system profoundly affects the quality of life of adults and older adults with a chronic illness (Rogers et al. 2000; Thorne 1993; 2002).

Respecting Relationships

Consideration of the rights and needs of children and other vulnerable persons enables us to better appreciate individual characteristics that are important in judgments of their interests. While generally not included in discussions about interests, **relationships**—who individuals are as members of families and communities—can be seen as important elements in judgments made about benefits for persons, and hence in making ethically sound decisions. In Ethics in Practice 6-1, for example, respecting Clarence's relationships leads us to consider the role of his parents in interpreting his interests and to think about the preservation of his relationships with his parents and others as an important dimension of addressing his best interests.

In an interesting analysis of judgments about best interests of infants, Burgess et al. (1999b) explore the case of K'aila, an Aboriginal infant with liver disease for whom a liver transplant offered the only hope of long-term survival. K'aila's parents resisted the transplant on the basis of their cultural and spiritual values.[15] Legal efforts to apprehend K'aila in order that the transplant could be performed failed, and K'aila died of liver failure at 11 months of age. Burgess et al. (1999b) make the point that spiritual and cultural beliefs— the kind of beliefs that define relationships to family, community, and the cosmos—are not always taken into account in determinations of children's best interests. We argue that in order to attend to the interests of children and other persons, they ought to be.

In summary, responding to the interests of children and other persons requires that we attend to their rights as well as their needs. Responding to the interests of children and other persons also requires that we understand and promote the family, community, and team relationships that can support and nurture each person. Further, we have argued that responding to the interests of those who are vulnerable because of attributes such as income level, religion, language fluency, gender, sexual orientation, substance use, mental and physical abilities, and age makes it *especially* important that we attend to their rights, needs, and relationships.[16] Within health care we require approaches to ethical action that can foster this kind of responsiveness.

ETHICAL ACTION FOR INDIVIDUALS

Ethical Decision-Making

Ethical decisions are necessary at those times when value-based questions give rise to difficulties in selecting among health care options or determining respectful care in the course of health care interactions, especially in situations of uncertainty. Whether the product of deliberate and considered thinking or not, the decisions made in such moments are ethical in nature because they have an inherent value component. Ethical decisions may have to do with issues such as the type or extent of medical or nursing care, the disclosure of information to patients, the maintenance of patient privacy and confidentiality, interdisciplinary team and family conflict, access to health and social resources, and so on—an infinite range of quandary[17] and everyday issues (Rodney et al. 2002). It is important to note that awareness of the moral dimensions of a particular situation and attentiveness to the possibility of alternate courses of action are prerequisites for ethical deliberation.[18]

Ethical decision-making can be thought of as a more formal process—a structured form of moral deliberation that occurs when an individual confronts an ethical situation (Beyerstein 1993, 422; Rodney and Howlett in press). Over the past two decades a number of models of ethical decision-making have evolved for clinical practice. Most early models followed a process of rational analysis and drew on a principle-based approach to ethical theory. Ethical principles were applied and weighed, which included explaining the ranking of the principles in each case and providing reasons for preferring one principle over another when they conflicted (Beyerstein 1993, 419). Recently, a more nuanced approach to ethical decision-making that is sensitive to context has had increased influence (Rodney et al. 2002).[19] Contextual approaches to ethical decision-making encourage us to undertake a careful assessment of the patient's physiological status, personal wishes, cultural and spiritual beliefs, and overall quality of life (Hoffmaster 2001; Rodney and Howlett in press; Winkler 1993; 1996). They also encourage us to consider the patient in the context of his or her family and social environment. *Such models can therefore help us to better understand each person's unique interests.*

The fundamental concepts we have available for ethical decision-making include the traditional principles of autonomy, beneficence/nonmaleficence, and justice as well as more contextual concepts such as fidelity and care (Arras, Steinbock and London 1999).[20] Moreover, incorporating Sherwin's notion of relational autonomy (1998) can strengthen our use of decision-making models. Approaches to ethical decision-making, such as McDonald's, are therefore consistent with Daniels' (1996) notion of wide reflective equilibrium. A composite approach to theory is taken such that general theories (e.g., deontology, virtue theory), mid-range ethical principles (e.g., autonomy, beneficence/nonmaleficence, and justice), and more experiential/relational concepts (e.g., fidelity, care, and relational autonomy) are implicit in various portions of the model (Rodney and Howlett in press). Furthermore, some of the models also provide guidance for interpersonal and group processes that can foster consensus.[21]

Turning to Ethics in Practice 6-2, we will now look at how we might sort through a particular situation involving an elderly patient (whom we will call Mr. Johansen), his daughter (whom we will call Stephanie), and the health care team using McDonald's *Ethical Decision Making Framework for Individuals*. The story in Ethics in Practice 6-2 is based on an advanced practice nurse's account of a practice situation in which a number of morally challenging factors converged. In what follows, we highlight some of the special interests of elderly patients and families. We then put those insights into action through the application of McDonald's framework.

Ethics in Practice 6-2	**Mr. Johansen**

In my role as clinical nurse specialist, with a focus on gerontology, I was asked to see an elderly man who had been living with his daughter, had had a stroke, and had been in hospital on a busy general medical unit for a while. This is very typical for me. The nurses are having difficulty, so they call me saying, "He's just not getting any better, the confusion is getting worse, come and see." He had delirium after he came in following his stroke and that seemed to resolve somewhat, but that label of confusion that was placed on him at admission remained firmly attached to him. The nurses told me that he was now worse than he had been originally. Apparently, his daughter is there every single day. She is very knowledgeable, having read up on stroke, dementia, and delirium. And, by asking many questions, she has driven the physicians away—they tend to avoid her like the plague. I go through his chart and see that there are a variety of issues at play here.

The nurses mentioned that their earlier efforts to draw this patient's increasing confusion and delirium to the attention of the attending physician resulted in a sarcastic response. But the attending physician was away and there was an on-call physician taking over for him. I phoned the on-call doc. She was willing to talk to me, so she and I went over some of the facts, including the patient's increasing dehydration, his elevated WBC [white blood cell count], and the nurses' suspicion that he had a urinary tract infection (UTI). Because the on-call physician didn't know the patient, she came in right away. When she saw him, he was lying in bed, with his legs over the side rails, picking things out of the air. His daughter was at his bedside, clearly distressed. As it turns out, this man did have a UTI. When the UTI was treated, the delirium disappeared. Although he was still somewhat confused, the hallucinations and delirium were gone. The daughter was really relieved. However, when the attending physician returned, he told me that he wouldn't have bothered to treat the patient's UTI if I had called him, saying, "He's just going to die anyway."

But the question I ask is, "What about the daughter's health?" She felt so much better having her father back to somebody she could relate to, even though she knew he would never recover from his stroke. She had been so distressed because in the middle of his delirium he said something like, "I think it's time for the move." To her that meant that he wanted to die. The daughter had tried to say this to the [attending] physician.... She would pick out all these threads from his confusion, what he was trying to convey about how he was feeling.... She was becoming a thorn in their [the attending physician's and the specialist's] sides.

I had a sense that the daughter felt relieved to have her father back again to somewhat of the person she knew before, even though he'd had this stroke. But to see him and... to hear his terror as he verbalized his hallucinations and his delusions... that kernel of what was going on inside him, she knew him so well that she could figure it out... it was so distressing for her. (Adapted from Rodney 1997.)

Interests of the Elderly

Clearly, Ethics in Practice 6-2 raises important issues about the interests of the elderly gentleman, Mr. Johansen, and his daughter, Stephanie. We claimed earlier that responding to the interests of all persons requires that we attend to their rights, needs, and relationships. It will be important to start to understand more about all three categories for Mr. Johansen, Stephanie, and the rest of their family as a prerequisite to engaging in an effective ethical decision-making process. We explored all three categories for children in some detail. While it will not be possible to do a full analysis of the elderly or their family members (or other vulnerable persons), we can make at least a few observations here. Let us start with Mr. Johansen.

First, the *right* of Mr. Johansen to be respected as a unique, self-determining being (founded in the ethical principle of autonomy) was under threat. Whether or not he was dying, he deserved to have some relief of what were treatable symptoms.[22] He did not deserve to have treatment and care withheld because of an assumption that "he was just going to die anyway." Further, he deserved to have his **dignity** protected and to have some choices in his treatment and care. At the time of the story in Ethics in Practice 6-2, Mr. Johansen was no longer competent to enact this right, but his daughter apparently was competent as his proxy (substitute) decision-maker. Threats to patient autonomy are, unfortunately, all too common for the elderly when they experience health challenges. Whether they are in their homes, in long-term care facilities, or in acute care hospitals, they may experience a lack of respect from care providers, particularly if their level of consciousness is impaired (Agich 1998; 1999; Randers and Mattiasson 2000). Further, despite significant progress in **advance directives** over the past few years[23], the elderly continue to have little control over how treatment and care decisions unfold throughout their illness trajectories, especially as they approach death.[24]

Second, the unique *needs* of elderly persons are often not well attended to in health care delivery. For instance, it took expertise in gerontology to understand that Mr. Johansen's confusion was worsened by his UTI. And it took expertise to understand how much rehabilitation potential he still had post-stroke (he may not, in fact, have been close to death). Although gerontology and geriatric medicine have become important new specialties, mainstream health care has a long way to go in understanding and, hence, addressing the needs of the elderly—how they experience pain, social isolation, financial barriers, and a host of other challenges.[25] As a society, we have even further to go in understanding capabilities of the elderly as well as their needs.

Third, the story in Ethics in Practice 6-2 raises some important questions about Mr. Johansen's *relationships* with the health care delivery system and with his family. As Sherwin (1998) reminds us, relational autonomy should call our attention to organizational as well as interpersonal relationships.[26] Behind the scenes of this account were troubling questions about the allocation of resources for the elderly. The acute medical unit where this patient was placed had many other elderly patients, many of whom were not receiving adequate nursing resources (Rodney 1997). This is by no means atypical. Current gerontological and ethical literature resounds with warnings that the elderly are bearing the brunt of fiscal policy changes.[27] That is, they are experiencing a progressive erosion of access to appropriate resources for treatment and care in acute and long-term care facilities and in home care situations.[28] Elderly women, and women who must stay home as caregivers, are especially vulnerable. This should cause us to wonder, for instance, what kind of home supports Mr. Johansen and Stephanie had available to them.

Interests of Families[29]

One of the most important challenges in contemporary health care ethics is to understand and attend to our ethical obligations to families—as individual **family** members, as family units, and as both connected to and distinct from patients (Blustein 1993; 1998; Nelson 1998; Nelson and Nelson 1995). Attending to families requires that we understand and work with the community within which families and patients are located (which will be explored further in Chapter 12). In Ethics in Practice 6-1, for instance, the family was very present and was interpreting Clarence's intentions and desires. In Ethics in Practice 6-2, on the other hand, we saw a family member, Stephanie, who was also very much present yet was not acknowledged. Furthermore, we lacked information about the roles, relationships, and stories from the rest of Mr. Johansen's family. It appeared that Stephanie was more vulnerable because she was alone.

Although we are given limited information, it is likely that Stephanie was having her rights as a proxy decision-maker ignored. Unfortunately, this is not uncommon, especially in end-of-life situations. Research tells us that families have a difficult time having their voices heard on behalf of their family members at the end of life.[30] The sources of this difficulty are multi-faceted and include lack of information or advanced discussion about the patient's illness, lack of understanding of advance directives per se, conflict between family members, and, perhaps most commonly, communication breakdown between the family, the patient, and the health care team (Rodney and Howlett in press). This is not to say that the rights of the family ought to outweigh the rights of the patient. But it is to say that we need to re-think how we involve families in decisions that unfold over time and that have an impact on family members as well as on patients.[31] As one leading theorist in the field explains,

> The notion that patients need to be empowered in [health care institutions] is exactly right; the mistake is in thinking this is likely to happen if patients are allowed to be alienated from their own sources of personal affirmation and authority in the name of giving such authority formal protection (Nelson 1998, 293).

There has been substantial research done on the needs of families in **critical care** settings. This research tells us that one of the foremost needs of family members, such as Clarence's parents in Ethics in Practice 6-1 and Stephanie in Ethics in Practice 6-2, is access to health care team members—especially physicians—for comprehensible and up-to-date information about the patient.[32] Research from **palliative and chronic care** contexts reminds us that family needs include access to adequate resources for treatment and care in the home and/or health care facility (including respite care), as well as access to financial, social, and psychological support.[33] Throughout all of the research, there is an implicit or explicit focus on the importance of supportive relationships between patients, family members, community members, and health care team members.

In summary, we can say that attending to family interests requires, at the least,

- respect for family members as individuals and for the family as a unit that has evolved (and will evolve) over time;
- regular communication between the family, the patient, and the health care team;
- anticipatory guidance to prepare for expected and unexpected health challenges; and
- careful attention to the resources the family will need to support the well-being of the patient, family members, and the family as a unit.[34, 35]

It appears that Stephanie would have benefitted from all of the above. In her case anticipatory guidance would include grief work and making the most of the time she has remaining with her father. In the words of an ethicist who is worried about how the elderly are viewed in our society, "Soon enough, we will no longer be able to walk hand in hand, but it matters deeply that we treasure the companionship while we can" (Lachs 1999, 203).

McDonald's Ethical Decision-Making Framework for Individuals

Thus far we have unpacked some of the important interests in Ethics in Practice 6-2. Let us now put those insights into action through the application of **McDonald's *Ethical Decision-Making Framework for Individuals*** (the full text of which can be found in Appendix B).[36] While it is not possible to fully illustrate all the components of the framework, we hope to say enough to promote the application of this framework (or other models or frameworks) to practice.

The details of the story in Ethics in Practice 6-2 bring what might be understood as a typical ethical issue in the care of elderly persons into a particular context, where the problem—to treat or not to treat—becomes much more complex. The problem depicted in this story could be described as a case of "the futility of treating terminally ill elderly persons" or "the problem of power dynamics in nurse-physician relationships." The nurse clearly moves beyond an understanding of this issue as an example of a "generic" ethical case. Within her account of the problem is an array of knowledge that has ethical relevance. Knowledge about the clinical problem, the daughter's experience, and the staff nurses' concerns all entered into her inquiry about this issue.

Effective ethical decision-making models can support description and analysis of the problem in a complex and contextualized way and promote movement toward a negotiated consensus. *Perhaps the greatest asset that models and frameworks such as McDonald's offer us is that they prompt us to ask particular questions of ethically troubling situations and to take the knowledge gleaned from these questions into our analyses.* McDonald's *Ethical*

Decision-Making Framework for Individuals consists of five iterative steps: (1) collect information and identify the problem; (2) specify feasible alternatives; (3) use your ethical resources to identify morally significant factors in each alternative; (4) propose and test possible resolutions; and (5) make your choice—live with it and learn from it. It is important to note that this framework is not a linear problem-solving guide or algorithm.[37] As the process unfolds, new information may generate new alternatives for treatment and care. [38]

Furthermore, no model or framework stands alone. What becomes evident is that, in addition to the structures for thinking that a model or framework supplies, education in critical thinking, ethical theory, the application of ethical decision-making models, and related ethical issues is also required. In Ethics in Practice 6-2, related ethical issues include contemporary thinking about withholding and withdrawing treatment, controversies about the concept of futility, and the use of advance directives. They also include, as we have argued above, an appreciation of the interests of the patients and family members involved. Similarly, substantive knowledge in the practice area is beneficial. In Ethics in Practice 6-2, this included, for instance, knowledge of neurology, gerontology, rehabilitation, grief theory, family theory, and conflict resolution theory.

Application of McDonald's Framework to Ethics in Practice 6-2

1. COLLECT INFORMATION AND IDENTIFY THE PROBLEM.

This step is foundational to the success of the entire decision-making process. In identifying and describing the problem, McDonald suggests that we ought to take into account multiple perspectives. This requires that we seek input from the patient, family, friends, and other health care team members and involve these individuals as much as possible through every step of the process. For Mr. Johansen in Ethics in Practice 6-2, the individuals we needed input from included himself (that is, his prior expressed values and wishes), his daughter Stephanie, other family members and friends, the nurses on the medical unit, his home care nurses and care aides, his family physician, the medical specialists involved in his care, his attending physicians on the medical unit, his social worker(s), and his rehabilitation therapist(s). It takes time and communication skill to identify and then gather information from such diverse parties.[39] Indeed, information gathering should be continuous throughout the ethical decision-making process.

As we proceed, we ought to ask questions about the patient's physical, psychological, social, cultural, and spiritual status, including changes over time. For instance, more information about Mr. Johansen's symptoms of stroke, and how those progressed, was important. What were his explicit and implicit **values** in the way he lived his life before the stroke? Did religious faith play an important role in his life? and so on. We also ought to investigate the patient's assessment of his or her own **quality of life** and his or her wishes about the treatment/care decision(s) at hand. This includes determining the patient's **competency** and determining who is available to speak for him or her. In Ethics in Practice 6-2, this meant finding out if Mr. Johansen had an advance directive and trying to determine what he had told others about his beliefs about life-sustaining treatment and who he wanted making decisions for him. A **family assessment** is crucial, including roles, relationships, and relevant "stories." We have already raised questions about the apparent isolation of Stephanie. What other family members or friends were available locally? At a distance? How had the decision for her to become her father's caregiver been arrived at? Further, we ought to identify the health care team members involved and the circumstances affecting them. In this situation, for instance, it appears that the staff nurses had been disempowered, that their voices had not been heard (or that they had not raised them effectively) in previous efforts to address this issue. Why was that? What were the **power dynamics** in the organization? And why were the attending physicians apparently so reluctant to treat the patient? Were they under pressure to admit other patients to his acute care bed? Conversely, were they afraid that the daughter was going to launch legal action if they discharged the patient?

As we start to put the information together, we ought to summarize the situation briefly but with all the relevant facts and circumstances, trying to get a sense of the patient's overall illness trajectory. It is also important that we determine what decisions have to be made and by whom. Thus, a detailed and specific description of the ethical problem—a description that captures the multiple points of view—is helpful for the contextual component of ethical decision-making. **Thin descriptions** of the problem fail to provide a contextual understanding (see also Chapter 14). The stronger our contextual understanding of the problem, the more effective and relevant the following steps in the process and the more likely that the resolution will attend to the interests of all involved and be ethically defensible.

Consider the difference between these two descriptions of the problem in the story in Ethics in Practice 6-2:

1. Mr. Johansen, an elderly man who had suffered a stroke, is experiencing increasing confusion. His daughter and the nurses involved in his care believe that he should be assessed and treated. His attending physician feels this is a waste of scarce resources. Should he be assessed and treated, or not?

2. Mr. Johansen, an elderly man who recently suffered a stroke, is experiencing increased confusion and is having periods of delirium. His daughter and the nurses who are caring for him have noticed this change and suspect that this increased confusion may be the result of a treatable problem. The attending physicians indicate that because of Mr. Johansen's pre-existing confusion, his age, and his impending death, he should not receive additional medical treatment. This ethical problem has at least four tracks: (1) What authority should the voices of the daughter and the nurses have in this decision-making process? How are they reflecting Mr. Johansen's interests? (2) Should Mr. Johansen be offered medical assessment and treatment that may well improve the quality of his life even though it will not likely change its duration? What symptom management can be achieved? (3) How can the well-being of Mr. Johansen's family be attended to as they face his uncertain prognosis and possible death? And (4) how can we deal with the interdisciplinary team conflict that has exacerbated this situation?

Notice that the two descriptions of the problem, while related, will lead in quite different directions. The first is much more one dimensional. It reduces complex issues to two "win-lose" questions: Which patients benefit most when resources are scarce? and Who has the final authority here? The second description is more deeply embedded in the context of the particular situation and is, we would argue, more likely to promote ethical practice. It moves significantly beyond simple black-and-white or win-lose choices.

2. SPECIFY FEASIBLE ALTERNATIVES FOR TREATMENT AND CARE.

In this second step of the ethical decision-making process, we consider what possibilities exist for action. Although in Ethics in Practice 6-2 we do not have an account of the nurse's reasoning process as she decided on her course of action, important questions about how to treat and care for Mr. Johansen and Stephanie arise for us as we work through the case we are provided. At a juncture such as this, creative and critical thinking are essential and must be informed by sound **clinical judgment**. **Moral imagination** and ongoing **self-reflection** are also immensely helpful (see also Chapters 14, 21, and 22). We should lay out sets of options ("tracks") in accordance with how we have identified the problems.

For Mr. Johansen, this means that we need carefully tailored options to address each of the four tracks. *First,* we need to make a decision about who is best able to speak for Mr. Johansen in accordance with his prior wishes and any advance documentation we are able to find. In doing this, it is important for us also to carefully attend to Mr. Johansen's (albeit somewhat confused) expression of his feelings and concerns. *Second,* in this and in most challenging ethical situations, there are more fine-grained alternatives than "treat" or "not treat"—or worse, "heroics" and "no heroics." For example, antibiotics may be appropriate for a **palliative** patient if they help relieve symptoms of confusion and agitation in an elderly patient. Furthermore, palliative care ought to be integrated in to all levels of care (Quill 2000; Rocker 2002; Rodney and Howlett in press; Roy 2000). In other words, even if Mr. Johansen were to be treated with a full range of medical therapy, he and Stephanie should still have the opportunity to benefit from the pain and symptom management and the personal and social **support** that palliative care provides.[40] *Third,* we need options for the personal and social support Mr. Johansen and his daughter will require whether he is discharged home or whether he stays in hospital, and regardless of when he dies. This includes, for instance, home care services, grief counselling, and pastoral care involvement. *Fourth,* we need to identify means by which we can better understand and deal with the intra- and inter-disciplinary **team conflict** that the various team members are reacting to.[41]

3. USE ETHICAL RESOURCES TO IDENTIFY MORALLY SIGNIFICANT FACTORS IN EACH ALTERNATIVE.

Once we have identified sets of alternatives organized around the tracks in the situation, we need to sort out which alternatives are most ethically defensible. Informed by our understanding of the interests of the patient and family, and also attentive to the interests of the health care team, we should evaluate the alternatives according to ethical principles/concepts, professional standards, and personal judgments and experiences. There may also be a need for a formal ethics case conference, ethics committee meeting, or case consultation in situations that are especially complex and/or conflicted (Rodney and Howlett in press).

To illustrate, for Mr. Johansen in Ethics in Practice 6-2, we might consider a set of alternatives (drawn from each track) that involve (1) formally designating Stephanie as proxy decision-maker; (2) medical treatment for his UTI, with a period of more intense physiotherapy and nursing care in hospital and involvement of social work and the family physician to commence planning for his eventual discharge from hospital; (3) referral of Stephanie to the clinical nurse specialist and a pastoral care liaison for ongoing support and **grief** work; and (4) calling a meeting between medical and nursing staff to discuss the communication challenges they are facing and to help them generate some solutions, including continuing **education** on end-of-life issues. We would reflect on each of these in terms of ethical principles/concepts, professional standards, and personal judgments and experiences. For example, our understanding of justice and relational autonomy would help us to identify the importance of mobilizing (arguing for) better acute care and eventual home care resources. Our professional standards around palliative care and rehabilitation would help us to come up with a care plan while Mr. Johansen is in hospital and a care plan for his transition home. Our personal judgments and experiences would help us to work out how best to approach Stephanie and recover her trust before helping her with her grief. And our personal judgments and experiences would help us to know how to proceed with getting the health care team together to start to face their own conflict.

4. PROPOSE AND TEST POSSIBLE RESOLUTIONS.

Here we move to select the best alternatives, all things considered—in other words, realizing that we may not achieve either certainty or perfection. The individuals closest to Mr. Johansen, including, for instance, Stephanie, other family members, his family physician, and his church minister, will be crucial players here. Proposing and testing possible resolutions includes performing a sensitivity analysis and considering our choices critically: Which factors would have to change to get us to alter our decisions? In Ethics in Practice 6-2, for example, our alternatives would shift if we learned that Mr. Johansen's death was imminent. We also need to think about the effects of our choices upon others' choices: Are we making it easier for others (health care providers, patients and their families) to act ethically? The fourth set of strategies for Mr. Johansen are targeted explicitly in this direction as we are hoping to help the members of the team learn from the situation and from each other.

We also need to ask if this is what a compassionate health care professional would do in a caring environment. Here it is helpful to formulate our choices as general maxims for all similar situations. This includes thinking of situations where they do *not* apply as well as where they do. For example, if Mr. Johansen's daughter was estranged from her father, we might be looking elsewhere for a proxy decision-maker. Finally, we need to ask if, as decision-makers, we are still comfortable with our choices. If there is not reasonable consensus, we need to revisit the process.

5. MAKE THE CHOICE—LIVE WITH IT AND LEARN FROM IT.

This is, perhaps, the most difficult step—to take action on what has been decided. Making the choice ought to include delineating *how* to implement what has been decided. In Mr. Johansen's situation, for instance, this would include: (1) following the agency policy to designate Stephanie as proxy decision-maker; (2) communicating with the hospital physicians, physiotherapists, nurses, social workers, and family physician(s) who would be involved in Mr. Johansen's treatment and care; (3) arranging for Stephanie to meet with the clinical nurse specialist and a pastoral care liaison; and (4) getting a commitment from medical and nursing staff to discuss the communication challenges they are facing.

Living with the decision means accepting the **responsibility** to monitor the **outcomes.** Most importantly, this includes getting feedback from the patient (if possible), from the family, and from health care team members. Given that ethical decision-making is a nonlinear process, this may also mean triggering further review or further action.

Learning from the decision should be both informal and formal. Informally, we should talk with colleagues who were involved in the situation, share experiences, and reflect on our feelings. Formally, we ought to have periodic **case reviews** of situations such as Mr. Johansen's—not to allocate blame, but to be more prepared for the next situation like his that arises and to recognize when we have made improvements in our ethical practice. Furthermore, our reviews may raise the need for proactive **policy** work to prevent what will otherwise be recurring problems. In Mr. Johansen's situation, for instance, a review of policies (and education around policies) for end-of-life care would seem warranted. Finally, there is a role for **research** here to more formally evaluate the outcomes of ethical decision-making processes. For example, a carefully designed qualitative study to explore the experiences of family members such as Stephanie could be beneficial.

In concluding our discussion of Mr. Johansen's story, we can see how the use of an ethical decision-making model helped us to move towards a plan of action that was more ethical than what was occurring prior to the clinical nurse specialist's intervention.[42] What might otherwise be seen as a case of an elderly person experiencing the normal course of deterioration toward death was instead understood as an event in which treatment and care improved the quality of this man's remaining life and the life of his daughter.

Towards Consensus

In closing this section of the chapter, we want to elaborate on the notion of **consensus** that appears at the end of McDonald's *Ethical Decision-Making Framework for Individuals*. The theoretical landscape of health care ethics has progressed to the point at which we are better able to appreciate the unique interests of individuals, including how those interests change with time and experience. However, it takes **negotiation** to support individuals and their varied interests within complex and often conflicted family, community, and health care organizational contexts. We therefore wish to advocate for an inclusive and ongoing process of negotiating consensus as a goal of ethical work. This is not a prescription for an imperialist view of health care ethics; nor is it a descent into ethical relativism (see Chapter 5). Rather, it is meant to be a thoughtful and dialectical process consistent with the concept of wide reflective equilibrium. We are advocating an approach to reasoning that draws on both deductive and inductive modes of thinking—a contextual approach that does not neglect the wisdom offered by philosophical positions and theoretical perspectives. We believe that McDonald's *Ethical Decision-Making Framework for Individuals* offers one means of engaging in both deductive and inductive thinking (see Chapter 4 and Chapter 5).

A crucial focal point in a conversation about the application of ethical theory/insights with individuals is to think about who these individual human beings (the persons we refer to as patients) are within their relationships with their family and community, with health care professionals, with the health care system, and with society. It takes **interpersonal skill** to come to this understanding and to hear the voices of all those affected by the situation at hand—not just the loudest voices or the voices representing official organizational roles. *Hence, ethical action is as much about process as it is about theory.* What we envision is ethical practice as a dynamic process of building consensus (in contrast to a static group decision)—that is, a "healthy community of open, inclusive moral discovery and growth" (Jennings 1991, 461–462).[43] While this dynamic process is not easy to achieve, it is not impossible to move towards, especially with guidance from effective decision-making models and frameworks and with adequate organizational support.

ETHICAL ACTION FOR ORGANIZATIONS

Preamble

Ethical action for individuals is, to a significant extent, dependent on the **moral climate** of the organizational context of health care delivery (see also Chapter 10). For example, the alternatives we posited for Mr. Johansen will be difficult to achieve if there are inadequate policies on end-of-life decision-making and advance directives, if palliative care and home care expertise is not available, if the clinical nurses specialist and pastoral care liaison are not able to allocate time to spend with Mr. Johansen's daughter, and if the nursing staff on the medical ward have such excessive workloads that they cannot attend staff meetings. *While the individuals involved each have responsibility for their own actions, there is also a level of responsibility that transcends individual action.*

As we stated in Chapter 5, attention to the **ethics of organizations** is a relatively new phenomenon but is gaining increasing attention in a number of fields of applied ethics, including health care.[44] The call for organizational attention to ethics and ethical behaviour is not unique to health care organizations. Recent breaches of trust by companies once considered highly trustworthy have alerted organizational leaders and the public to the importance of ethics. However, the centrality of ethics to health care and to health care organizations creates a moral imperative to respond by placing ethics and ethical practices as a high priority in health care organizations (see Exhibit 6-1).

Exhibit 6-1   Characteristics of an Ethically Healthy Organization

Developed by the Vancouver Island Authority (South Island) Regional Ethics Committee[45]

1. A philosophy of ethics permeates the organization.
2. A clear statement of the vision/mission/values of the organization is available.
3. Ways and means are in place by which all decision-making is made through an "ethics lens" (including financial, policy and procedural, and clinical decisions).
4. The budget reflects ethical commitments.
5. An organizational body is charged with championing ethics, and it has an organization-wide profile as well as a community profile.
6. There is a common framework and language for ethical discussion, as well as an organizational code of ethics.
7. It is evident to newcomers and clients that procedures include ethical considerations in everything the organization does.
8. Staff feel supported in their practice and respected in their work.
9. Ethics is part of recruitment, selection, orientation, and continuing education, and there is safety for all who identify ethical concerns or moral distress.
10. Organizational ethics committees and ethics consultants are two vehicles that can help to move health care agencies towards placing ethics and ethical practices as a high priority.

Health Policy

Health care organizations are imbued with policy. The integration of ethics into **health care policy** development and decision-making is becoming increasingly important in the current health care environment. Relative to the attention paid to the resolution of individual cases, bioethics has, until recently, tended to underplay issues related to development of health policy and health care delivery (Fox 1990; see also Chapter 5). We are only now coming to realize that all levels of health policy have a significant moral dimension (Blue et al. 1999; Malone 1999; Mitchell 2001). Thus, the interface of ethics and health policy is important—both in terms of generating policies to address ethical issues and in critiquing existing policies in term of their ethical implications (Sherwin 2001; Storch, Rodney and Starzomski 2002).

Resource Allocation

Ethics in Practice 6-2 raises some significant policy questions around end-of-life care and resource allocation. While Chapter 13 will further explore policy around end-of-life care, we would like to pick up some of the **resource allocation** questions arising at the meso (organizational) level here.[46] Interestingly, while the initial focus of **ethics committees,** from their inception in the late 1970s, was on difficult decision-making at the micro level, a number of ethics committees are also beginning to grapple with meso-level decisions about the allocation of resources (Storch, Rodney and Starzomski 2002).

As we noted earlier, if palliative care and home care expertise are not available, if the clinical nurses specialist and pastoral care liaison are not able to allocate time to spend with Mr. Johansen's daughter, and if the nursing staff on the medical ward have such excessive workloads that they cannot attend staff meetings, it will be difficult to implement ethical care for Mr. Johansen. How can decisions about the allocation of these kinds of resources be made ethically? This poses a huge challenge for health care agencies and health care regions—a challenge that is gaining more explicit ethical reflection. Health care organizations face diverse economic, social, political, and legal pressures from different publics (e.g., patients versus taxpayers). The public expects careful stewardship, with fair and efficient use of resources, while patients (such as Mr. Johansen) expect that their interests will be served (Commission on the Future of Health Care in Canada 2002). At this time, health care administrators and regional health authorities wield significant power as intermediate and mediating figures (Yeo, Williams and Hooper 1998).

From an ethical stance, meso-level resource allocation decisions should proceed with fair processes as well as fair outcomes. Thus, ethical decision-making frameworks are beneficial for resource allocation decisions as well as patient-focused decisions. More work needs to be done to provide ethical direction for health care providers and administrators involved in resource allocation at the meso level. In the meanwhile, in Appendix B we have made available McDonald's *Ethical Framework for Making Allocation Decisions*, which is a promising resource.[47]

Organizational Ethics Resources

The creation of structures and mechanisms to foster ethical decision-making in organizations has included (but is not limited to) the growth of **ethics committees** and the use of clinical **ethics consultants** (Storch, Rodney and Starzomski 2002). Ethics committees are an important resource for health care agencies in the areas of ethics education, case consultation, and policy formulation (Storch et al. 1990; Storch and Griener 1992). An ethics consultant is

someone who has the knowledge, abilities, and attributes of character to facilitate... ethical discourse in case consultation on ethical issues in clinical care or clinical research, and in ethics
consultation to ethics committees, to research ethics boards (institutional review boards), and to
policy formulation committees (Baylis 1994, 28).

Thus, consultants—who may come from a variety of disciplinary backgrounds—serve
as an important adjunct to committees. Overall, ethics committees and ethics consultants
can help to improve the moral climate of health care agencies (Storch, Rodney and
Starzomski 2002). Reflecting back on Ethics in Practice 6-1, for example, an ethics committee and/or an ethics consultant could help Clarence's parents and the members of the
health care team to decide how best to involve Clarence in decisions about his treatment
and care. Similarly, in Ethics in Practice 6-2, an ethics committee and/or an ethics consultant could help to lead Mr. Johansen's daughter Stephanie and the health care team through
a structured ethical decision-making process and/or help them to resolve an impasse they
may have reached in their decision-making. An ethics committee and/or ethics consultant
could also help to develop or update policies on end-of-life decision-making and advance
directives. And they could help with the debriefing and education of members of the health
care team for Ethics in Practice 6-1 and Ethics in Practice 6-2. Each situation will have
taken an emotional toll on team members as well as the patients' families.

It is important to note that a substantial evaluative literature has evolved around ethics
committees and ethics consultants. While attempting to redress some of the cultural problems that are inherent in health care delivery, both resources are also subject to some of
those cultural problems themselves. For instance, they may not be visible, they may function in an autocratic manner, they may be under-resourced, and they may be morally constrained by administration.[48] On the other hand, effective ethics consultants and/or ethics
committees have the following attributes (Rodney and Howlett in press):[49]

- a clear focus on the well-being of patients and families;
- a commitment to maintaining the moral integrity of health care team members;
- visibility and accessibility for health care team members, patients, and families;
- strong skills in interpersonal communication, group process, and conflict resolution;
- knowledge of and support from the employing health care organization;
- sensitivity to organizational and professional power dynamics;
- a commitment to an egalitarian approach that fosters trust;
- transparency in decision-making and subsequent recommendations; and
- a commitment to education, policy development, and ongoing evaluation of their own
  effectiveness.

TOWARD ETHICAL PRACTICE

Achieving wide reflective equilibrium in ethically challenging situations can be a daunting
process. Whether it takes place in the context of interaction with an individual or group of
individuals or transpires in activities of policy development, ethical decision-making is a
complex and nuanced process. Our goal in this chapter has not been to simplify the complex and contextual nature of ethical decision-making, but rather to provide some tools to
assist nurses and others in navigating through the maze of theories, principles, contextual

features, and interests. Decision-making frameworks such as those introduced in this chapter are intended for this purpose: they are maps to assist in sorting out the terrain when ethical questions arise. As authors, our experiences in ethics consultations, policy work, and education have convinced us that such maps *can* make a difference in the turbulent and challenging world of practice.

This chapter sets the stage for the remainder of the book, where we and other authors consider specific aspects of ethics in nursing practice. As we and other authors look at a variety of issues in the chapters that follow, we endeavour to cast light on theoretical and contextual considerations that must be taken into account if the equilibrium we seek to achieve is indeed "wide."

FOR REFLECTION

1. How does Sherwin's (1998) notion of relational autonomy strengthen the traditional ethical principle of autonomy?

2. We have argued that understanding the interests of persons requires understanding their rights, needs, and relationships. Sketch out what you would consider necessary to understand the rights, needs, and relationships of persons with disabilities.

3. Compare the McDonald (individual) and Storch models of decision-making (Appendix B). What are their similarities? Their differences?

4. What impact might a model such as McDonald's *Model for Allocation Decisions* (Appendix B) have for health policy work at the organizational level?

ENDNOTES

1. We wish to thank an anonymous reviewer for this phrasing.

2. We are using the term "ethical problems" quite broadly. We consider ethical problems to involve questions about what is right or good at individual, interpersonal, organizational, and even societal levels.

3. See also Burgess and Brunger (2000) for a relational approach to autonomy that extends to family and community.

4. These comments about feminism and post-structuralism do not, of course, do justice to the range of perspectives within these fields or the overlap between them.

5. We are using the term *interests* to reflect what persons as unique individuals situated in multi-faceted relational contexts require for their well-being. This is in contrast to an objective reasonable person standard where we make assumptions about what an "average prudent person" would want. See Kluge (1992, 111–140) for a related discussion of objective and subjective standards for informed consent.

6. This conceptual approach to interests has been developed by the first author of this chapter (McPherson).

7. Pneumothoraces and pneumomediastinum are both types of air leakage from the lungs into the chest cavity. They are the result of severe injury to the lung tissue and cause further deterioration in lung function.

8. ECMO is an acronym for Extra-Corporeal Membrane Oxygenation. This is a highly technical procedure in which a heart-lung machine takes over the work of the child's heart and lungs for a period of days in order, in Clarence's case, to give his lungs time to heal. The use of this technology is controversial. It is a relatively new and very invasive technology that is also highly expensive and resource intensive.

9. Pharmacological paralysis makes a child or any other person unable to move or breathe but has little effect on sensory experiences and cognition.

10. Ethics in Practice 6-1 is adapted (and fictionalized) by McPherson from her clinical experiences and experiences of her colleagues. See also McPherson (1999).

11. Alderson (2000); Alderson and Montgomery (1996); Bandman (1999); de Winter, Caerveldt and Koolstra (1999); Franklin (1986); Lowes (1996).

12. See Chapter 8 and Chapter 19 for related discussions of moral agency.

13. This argument reflects one version of rights-based discussions ("rights as trumps"—e.g., right to choice versus right to life), but not of notions of rights as *prima facie* starting points for nuanced discussion.

14. Unique characteristics are often addressed through terms such as "personality" and "temperament."

15. K'aila's parents' beliefs about human beings and spiritual life were grounded in their Aboriginal culture. In his mother's words, "As Native American people, whose cultural and spiritual traditions are steeped in a reverence for the wisdom inherent in the Creator's natural order, we felt we might be committing a grave error if we tried to recreate our son's body... [W]hile trying to play God, we would run the risk of violating K'aila's spiritual as well as physical identity" (Paulette 1993, 14).

16. See also Anderson and Reimer Kirkham (1999); Cassidy, Lord, and Mandell (1995); Daniels (1985); Sherwin (1992; 1998); Smith (2000); Stephenson (1999); Taylor (1992); and Warren (1992).

17. By quandary we mean high profile life or death decisions, such as treatment withdrawal, euthanasia, abortion, and cloning.

18. This has implications for basic and continuing ethics education. As people who engage in ethics education and ethics consultation, we authors find it useful to start by asking people to notice "when their gut is in a knot." (See also Chapters 21 and 22 about the role of emotion in ethics, and Hartrick Doane [2002a; 2002b] about moral identity and ethics education.)

19. See, for instance, Kuhl and Wilensky (1999) and Jonsen, Sieglar, and Winslade (1986) as well as Appendix B (McDonald's *Ethical Decision-Making Framework for Individuals* and Storch's *Model for Ethical Decision-Making for Policy & Practice*).

20. See also Chapter 5. Fidelity is a concept that directs our attention to trust (including, but not limited to, truth-telling), while care directs our attention to enhancing patent/family/team relationships (in the present and over time).

21. For example, DeRenzo and Strauss (1997), Kuhl and Wilensky (1999), and McDonald's *Ethical Decision-Making Framework for Individuals* (Appendix B).

22. Jennings, Ryndes, D'Onofrio and Baily (2003); Roy (1994); Smith (2002); Subcommittee to Update "Of Life and Death" of the Standing Senate Committee on Social Affairs (2000); see also Chapter 13.

23. An advance directive is "a written document containing a person's wishes about life-sustaining treatment" that "extend[s] the autonomy of competent patients to future situations in which the patient is incompetent" (Singer 1994, 111; see also Gordon, 2000; Storch, Rodney and Starzomski 2002). One form of an advanced directive is an *instructional directive*, in which the individual articulates "what or how healthcare decisions are to be made in the event that he or she becomes incompetent" (Health Canada Secretariat on Palliative and End-of-Life Care 2002, 84). The second form is a *proxy directive* (also known as a durable power of attorney for health care decisions), in which the individual articulates "who is to make healthcare decisions in the event that he or she becomes incompetent" (Health Canada Secretariat on Palliative and End-of-Life Care 2002, 84). Advance directives are best when they include both types of articulation (Dossetor and Cain 1997; Singer 1994). The appointment of a proxy decision-maker who knows the patient and can represent his or her best interest is an important means of ensuring that someone speaks on behalf of the individual's prior decisions (Rodney and Howlett in press; see also Sullivan 2001 and Chapter 13).

24. Fried et al. (1999); Kaufman (2001); Gallagher et al. (2002); Gallagher and Hodge (1999); Rodney and Howlett (in press); Sawchuk and Ross-Kerr (2000); and Sheehan (1998).

25. Bernabei et al. (1998); Gallagher et al. (2002); Gallagher and Hodge (1999); National Advisory Committee (2000); Penning (2002); Post (1998); Volbrecht (2002).

26. See also Chapter 5 and Chapter 8.

27. See also Chapter 9 and Chapter 10.

28. Bell (1992); Binstock (1998); Commission on the Future of Health Care in Canada (2002); Gallagher et al. (2002); Gallagher and Hodge (1999); Lachs (1999); Penning (2002).

29. Within this chapter, we are using the term "family" quite broadly (Rodney 1997). We agree with family theorists that "it is quite possible for people to have a family experience (including the feelings of intimacy, connectedness, commitment, and so forth) with people who are not in one's actual family" (Hartrick and Lindsey 1995, 154). Therefore, we take it that the "most useful definition of family [is] "Who the family says it is." Furthermore, who "counts" as family may vary depending on the health concern" (Robinson 1995, 119).

30. Chamber-Evans (2002); Hiltunen et al. (1999); Nelson (1998); Stajduhar (2003); Tilden et al. (1999).

31. Of course, some family members will not be acting in the patient's best interest—see, for instance, Chapter 19 for a discussion of serious family conflicts jeopardizing the well-being of children and Chapter 20 for a discussion of violence against women.

32. Abbott et al. (2001); Curtis et al. (2001); Hiltunen et al. (1999); Tilden et al. (1999); Vandall-Walker (2002); see also Chapter 13.

33. Hayes and McElheran (2002); Mårtensson, Dracup and Fridlund (2001); Rodney and Howlett (in press); Stajduhar (2003); Tapp (2001); Wilson (2000).

34. Abbott et al. (2001); Chamber-Evans (2002); Curtis et al. (200)1; Hayes and McElheran (2002); Hiltunen et al. (1999); Mårtensson, Dracup, and Fridlund (2001); Nelson (1998); Nelson and Nelson (1995); Rodney and Howlett (in press); Stajduhar (2003); Tapp (2001); Tilden et al. (1999); Vandall-Walker (2002); Wilson (2000).

35. An anonymous reviewer of this chapter has quite correctly pointed out that this level of family involvement presupposes that the (capable) patient has chosen to have his or her family engaged in his or her treatment and care. Some patients may want to circumscribe the level of their family's involvement. Other patients are estranged and/or isolated from their next of kin and may choose to define their friends or neighbours as family.

36. There are, of course, a variety of effective ethical decision-making models or frameworks available to choose from. We have made an alternate model available in Appendix B, Storch's *Model for Ethical Decision-Making for Policy and Practice*.

37. Storch's *Model for Ethical Decision-Making for Policy and Practice* (Appendix B) is for this reason constructed as a circle.

38. In our experience, linear approaches or algorithms do not work well in the real world of practice where we are often dealing with uncertainty and where new information generates new alternatives. We usually have to cycle back and forth between information, reflection, and alternatives. Furthermore, one of the challenges we face with most models or frameworks (including McDonald's) is to try to capture a process that changes over time as the patient's illness trajectory unfolds (see also Rodney et al. 2002).

39. For patients and family members for whom English (or French in francophone communities) is not the first language, the availability of trained interpreters throughout the process is crucial (Kaufert and Putsch 1997).

40. In fact, there are a growing number of research studies and practice guidelines promoting the integration of palliative care interventions within critical care (Nelson and Danis 2001; Nelson-Marten, Braaten and English 2001; Quill 2000; Rocker, Shemie and Lacroix 2000).

41. See also Chapter 8 and Chapter 10.

42. In the story recounted by the clinical nurse specialist in Ethics in Practice 6-2, the clinical nurse specialist, the physician on call, and the nursing staff implemented an ethical decision-making process, although not necessarily with the use of a formal model or framework. They were able to work out and implement a number of ethically sound alternatives. In other words, a formal model/framework and consultation process were not required. In many complex or conflicted situations, though, the use of a formal model or framework is beneficial. Calling for an interdisciplinary team meeting and possibly a formal ethics consultation *as early as possible* can prevent deteriorations in patient/family care and escalations in family/team conflict.

    It is important to note that a follow-up case review with staff involved in Ethics in Practice 6-2 would have been beneficial. Such follow-up is usually helpful in any situation where there has been conflict and uncertainty.

43. For more information about egalitarian and practical approaches to group process that foster consensus, see Bowman (2000), Chinn (2001), and DeRenzo and Strauss (1997). It is important to note that in using the word "consensus" we are talking about processes that work towards an equalization of power, respect a diversity of perspectives, and generate a range of carefully crafted options. We are *not* talking about processes in which the majority rules, where there is "groupthink," or where dissent is silenced. The latter three processes are too often (incorrectly, we believe) attributed to consensus.

44. Boyle et al. (2001); Buchanan (1996); Goold (2001); Pentz (1999); Reiser (1994).

45. The development of these characteristics was based on the outcomes of a regional retreat, January 20th, 2003. The authors would like to thank the Vancouver Island Authority (South Island) Regional Ethics Committee for permission to use Exhibit 6-1.

46. Macro (societal) levels of resource allocation will be addressed in Chapter 9. See also Chapter 4 for a discussion of the principle of justice and meso-allocation.

47. As we write this chapter, the Alberta Provincial Health Ethics Network and a Canadian/American group of philosophers are embarking on a research project to develop and test more meso-level resource allocation models. See also Daniels and Sabin (1997), Martin, Ableson and Singer (2002), Sherwin (2001), and Chapter 4. Moreover, a recent article by Galarneau (2002) emphasizes the importance of *community* in justice-based deliberations. Galarneau (2002) explains:

    Because conflicts of meaning and value within and between communities are inevitable, we will need political processes that ensure effective community voice, deliberation, and decision making (38).

48. Howe (1999); Jurchak (1998); Storch and Griener (1992); Thomasma and Monagle (1998).

49. See also Baylis (1994); Brodeur (1998); DeRenzo and Strauss (1997); Dowdy, Robertson and Bander (1998); Jurchak (1998); Pellegrino (1999); Redman (1996); Rubin and Zoloth (2000); and Storch and Griener (1992).

REFERENCES

Abbott, K.H., Sago, J.G., Breen, C.M., Abernethy, A.P. and Tulsky, J.A. 2001. Families looking back: One year after discussion of treatment withdrawal or withholding of life-sustaining support. *Critical Care Medicine, 29*(1), 197–201.

Agich, G.J. 1998. Respecting the autonomy of elders in nursing homes. In J.F. Monagle and D.C. Thomasma (Eds.), *Health care ethics: Critical issues for the 21st century* (pp. 200–211). Maryland: Aspen.

Agich, G.J. 1999. Ethical problems in caring for demented patients. In S. Govoni, C.L. Bolis and M. Trabucchi (Eds.), *Dementia: Biological bases and clinical approach to treatment* (pp. 297–308). Milano: Springer-Verlag Italia.

Alderson, P. 1993. *Children's consent to surgery*. Buckingham: Open University Press.

Alderson, P. 2000. *Young children's rights: Exploring beliefs, principles and practice*. London: Jessica Kingsley Publishers.

Alderson, P. and Montgomery, J. 1996. *Health care choices: Making decisions with children*. London: Institute for Public Policy Research.

Anderson, J. and Reimer Kirkham, S. 1999. Discourses on health: A critical perspective. In H. Coward and P. Ratanakul (Eds.), *A cross-cultural dialogue on health care ethics* (pp. 47–67). Waterloo, ON: Wilfrid Laurier University Press.

Arras, J.D., Steinbock, B. and London, A.J. 1999. Moral reasoning in the medical context. In J.D. Arras and B. Steinbock (Eds.), *Ethical issues in modern medicine*. 5th edition. (pp. 1–40). Mountain View, CA: Mayfield.

Bandman, B. 1999. *Children's right to freedom, care and enlightenment*. New York: Garland.

Baylis, F.E. (Ed.). 1994. *The health care ethics consultant*. Totowa, NJ: Humana Press.

Bell, N.K. 1992. If age becomes a standard for rationing health care…. In H.B. Holmes and L. Purdy (Eds.), *Feminist perspectives in medical ethics* (pp. 82–90). Bloomington: Indiana University Press.

Bernabei, R., Gambassi, G., Lapane, K., Landi, F., Gatsonis, C., Dunlop, R., Lipsitz, L., Steel, K. and Mor, V. 1998. Management of pain in elderly patients with cancer. *JAMA, 279*(23), 1877–1882.

Beyerstein, D. 1993. The functions and limitations of professional codes of ethics. In E.R. Winkler and J.R. Coombs (Eds.), *Applied ethics: A reader* (pp. 416–425). Oxford: Blackwell.

Binstock, R.H. 1998. Older people and long-term care: Issues of access. In J.F. Monagle and D.C. Thomasma (Eds.), *Health care ethics: Critical issues for the 21st century* (pp. 177–188). Maryland: Aspen.

Blue, A.W., Keyserlingk, E.W., Rodney, P. and Starzomski, R. 1999. A critical view of North American health policy. In H. Coward and P. Ratanakul (Eds.), *A cross-cultural dialogue on health care ethics* (pp. 215–225). Waterloo, ON: Wilfrid Laurier University Press.

Bluebond-Langner, M. 1978. *The private worlds of dying children*. Princeton: Princeton University Press.

Blustein, J. 1998. The family in medical decision making. In J.F. Monagle and D.C. Thomasma (Eds.), *Health care ethics: Critical issues for the 21st century* (pp. 81–91). Maryland: Aspen.

Bowman, K.W. 2000. Communication, negotiation, and mediation: Dealing with conflict in end-of-life decisions. *Journal of Palliative Care, 16*, S17–S23.

Boyle, P.J., DuBose, E.R., Ellingson, S.J., Guinn, D.E. and McCurdy, D.B. 2001. *Organizational ethics in health care: Principles, cases, and practical solutions.* San Francisco: Jossey-Bass.

Brodeur, D. 1998. Health care institutional ethics: Broader than clinical ethics. In J.F. Monagle and D.C. Thomasma (Eds.), *Health care ethics: Critical issues for the 21st century* (pp. 497–504). Maryland: Aspen.

Buchanan, A. 1996. Toward a theory of the ethics of bureaucratic organizations. *Business Ethics Quarterly, 6*(4), 419–440.

Burgess, M. and Brunger, F. 2000. Collective effects of medical research. In M. McDonald et al. (Eds.), *The governance of health research involving human subjects.* Ottawa: Law Commission of Canada. Available online: www.lcc.gc.ca/en/themes; www.ethics.ubc.ca/people/burgess/lccburgess.pdf

Burgess, M., Stephenson, P., Ratanakul, P. and Suwonnakote, K. 1999a. End-of-life decisions: Clinical decisions about dying and perspectives on life and death. In H. Coward and P. Ratanakul (Eds.), *A cross-cultural dialogue on health care ethics* (pp. 190–206). Waterloo, ON: Wilfrid Laurier University Press.

Burgess, M., Rodney, P., Coward, H., Ratanakul, P. and Suwonnakote, K. 1999b. Pediatric care: Judgments about best interests at the onset of life. In H. Coward and P. Ratanakul (Eds.), *A cross-cultural dialogue on health care ethics (*pp. 160–175). Waterloo, ON: Wilfred Laurier University Press.

Cassidy, B., Lord, R. and Mandell, N. 1995. Silenced and forgotten women: Race, poverty, and disability. In N. Mandell (Ed.), *Feminist issues: Race, class and sexuality* (pp. 32–66). Scarborough, ON: Prentice Hall.

Chambers-Evans, J. 2002. The family as window onto the world of the patient: Revising our approach to involving patients and families in the decision-making process. *Canadian Journal of Nursing Research, 34*(3), 15–32.

Chinn, P.L. 2001. *Peace and power: Building communities for the future.* 5th edition. Boston: Jones and Bartlett.

Commission on the Future of Health Care in Canada. 2002. *Building on Values: The Future of Health Care in Canada.* ["The Romanow Report"] Ottawa: Commission on the Future of Health Care in Canada.

Curtis, J.R., Patrick, D.L., Shannon, S.E., Treece, P.D., Engelberg, R.A. and Rubenfeld, G.D. 2001. The family conference as a focus to improve communication about end-of-life care in the intensive care unit: Opportunities for improvement. *Critical Care Meicined, 29*(2, supplement), N26–N33.

Daniels, N. 1985. *Just health care.* Cambridge: Cambridge University Press.

Daniels, N. 1996. Wide reflective equilibrium in practice. In L.W. Sumner and J. Boyle (Eds.), *Philosophical perspectives on bioethics* (pp. 96–114). Toronto: University of Toronto Press.

Daniels, N. and Sabin, J. 1997. Limits to health care: Fair procedures, democratic deliberation, and the legitimacy problem for insurers. *Philosophy and Public Affairs, 26*(4), 303–350.

DeRenzo, E.G. and Strauss, M. 1997. A feminist model for clinical ethics consultation: Increasing attention to context and narrative. *HEC Forum, 9*(3), 212–227.

de Winter, M., Caerveldt, C. and Koolstra, J. 1999. Enabling children: Participation as a new perspective on child-health promotion. *Child: Care, Health and Development, 25*(1), 15–23.

Dossetor, J.B. and Cain, D.J. (Eds.). 1997. *A handbook of health ethics.* Alberta: Bioethics Centre, University of Alberta.

Dowdy, M.D., Robertson, C. and Bander, J.A. 1998. A study of proactive ethics consultation for critically ill and terminally ill patients with extended lengths of stay. *Critical Care Medicine, 26*(2), 252–259.

Foucault, M. 1981. The order of discourse. In R. Young (Ed.), *Untying the text: A poststructuralist reader* (pp. 48–78). Boston: Routledge and Kegan Paul.

Fox, R.C. 1990. The evolution of American bioethics: A sociological perspective. In G. Weisz (Ed.), *Social science perspectives on medical ethics* (pp. 201–217). Philadelphia: University of Pennsylvania Press.

Franklin, R. 1986. *The rights of children*. London: Blackwell.

Fried, T., van Doorn, C., O'Leary, J., Tinetti, M. and Drickamer, M. 1999. Older persons' preferences for site of terminal care. *Ann Intern Med, 131*, 109–112.

Galarneau, C.A. 2002. Health care as a community good: Many dimensions, many communities, many views of justice. *Hastings Center Report, 32*(5), 33–40.

Gallagher, E., Alcock, D., Diem, E., Angus, D. and Medves, J. 2002. Ethical dilemmas in home care case management. *Journal of Healthcare Management, 47*(2), 85–96.

Gallagher, E.M. and Hodge, G. 1999. The forgotten stakeholders: Seniors' values concerning their health care. *International Journal of Health Care Quality Assurance, 12*(3), 79–86.

Gilligan, C. 1993. *In a different voice: Psychological theory and women's development*. Cambridge, MA: Harvard University Press.

Goold, S.D. 2001. Trust and the ethics of health care institutions. *Hastings Center Report, 31*(6), 26–33.

Gordon, R.M. 2000. The emergence of assisted (supported) decision-making in the Canadian law of adult guardianship and substitute decision-making. *International Journal of Law and Psychiatry, 23*(1), 61–77.

Hartrick, G.A. and Lindsey, A.E. 1995. The lived experience of family: A contextual approach to family nursing practice. *Journal of Family Nursing, 1*(2), 148–170.

Hartrick Doane, G.A. 2002a. In the spirit of creativity: The learning and teaching of ethics in nursing. *Journal of Advanced Nursing, 39*(96), 521–528.

Hartrick Doane, G.A. 2002b. Am I still ethical? The socially-mediated process of nurses' moral identity. *Nursing Ethics, 9*(6), 623–635.

Hayes, V.A. and McElheran, P.J. 2002. Family health promotion within the demands of pediatric home care and nursing respite. In L.E. Young and V. Hayes (Eds.), *Transforming health promotion practice: Concepts, issues, and applications* (pp. 265–283). Philadelphia: F.A. Davis.

Health Canada Secretariat on Palliative and End-of-Life Care. 2002. *Discussion paper: National Action Planning Workshop on End-of-Life Care*. Ottawa: Health Canada.

Hiltunen, E.F., Medich, C., Chase, S., Peterson, L. and Forrow, L. 1999. Family decision making for end-of-life treatment: The SUPPORT nurse narratives. *The Journal of Clinical Ethics, 10*(2), 126–134.

Hoffmaster, B. 2001. Introduction. In B. Hoffmaster (Ed.), *Bioethics in social context* (pp. 1–11). Philadelphia: Temple University Press.

Honderick, T. (Ed.). 1995. *The Oxford companion to philosophy*. New York: Oxford University Press.

Howe, E.G. 1999. Ethics consultants: Could they do better? *The Journal of Clinical Ethics, 10*(1), 13–25.

Jennings, B. 1991. Possibilities of consensus: Toward democratic moral discourse. *The Journal of Medicine and Philosophy, 16*, 447–463.

Jennings, B., Ryndes, T., D'Onofrio, C. and Baily, M.A. 2003. Access to hospice care: Expanding boundaries, overcoming barriers. *Hastings Center Report (Special Supplement), 33*(2), S3–S59.

Jonsen, A.R., Sieglar, M. and Winslade, W.J. 1986. *Clinical ethics: A practical approach to ethical decisions in clinical medicine*. 2nd edition. New York: Macmillan.

Jurchak, M. 1998. Clinical ethics consultants: Survey and practice. In J.F. Monagle and D.C. Thomasma (Eds.), *Health care ethics: Critical issues for the 21st century* (pp. 471–483). Maryland: Aspen.

Kaufert, J.M. and Putsch, R.W. 1997. Communication through interpreters in healthcare: Ethical dilemmas arising from differences in class, culture, language, and power. *The Journal of Clinical Ethics, 8*(1), 71–86.

Kaufman, S.R. 2001. Clinical narratives and ethical dilemmas in geriatrics. In B. Hoffmaster (Ed.), *Bioethics in social context* (pp. 12–38). Philadelphia: Temple University Press.

Kluge, E.-H.W. 1992. *Biomedical ethics in a Canadian context.* Scarborough, ON: Prentice Hall.

Kuhl, D.R. and Wilensky, P. 1999. Decision making at the end of life: A model using an ethical grid and principles of group process. *Journal of Palliative Medicine, 2*(1), 75–86.

Lachs, J. 1999. Dying old as a social problem. In G. McGee (Ed.), *Pragmatic bioethics* (pp. 194–203). Nashville: Vanderbilt University Press.

Lowes, L. 1996. Paediatric nursing and children's autonomy. *Journal of Clinical Nursing, 5*, 367–372.

MacDonald, M. 2003. *McDonald's Ethical Decision-Making Framework for Individuals.* Vancouver: Centre for Applied Ethics, University of British Columbia. Available online: www.ethics.ubc.ca/mcdonald/decisions.html

Mackenzie, C., and Stoljar, N. 2000. Autonomy refigured. In C. Mackenzie and N. Stoljar (Eds.). *Relational autonomy: Feminist perspectives on autonomy, agency, and the social self* (pp. 130–141). New York: Oxford University Press.

Malone, R.E. 1999. Policy as product: Morality and metaphor in health policy discourse. *Hastings Centre Report,* (May–June), 16–22.

Mårtensson, J., Dracup, K. and Fridlund, B. 2001. Decisive situations influencing spouses' support of patients with heart failure: A critical incident technique analysis. *Heart and Lung, 30*(5), 341–350.

Martin, D., Abelson, J. and Singer, P. 2002. Participation in health care priority-setting through the eyes of the participants. *Journal of Health Services Research & Policy, 7*(4), 222–229.

McPherson, G. 1999. Treating children as people: Exploring nurses' practice to preserve children's personal integrity. Unpublished masters thesis, University of British Columbia, Vancouver, B.C.

Mitchell, G.J. 2001. Policy, procedure and routine: Matters of moral influence. *Nursing Science Quarterly, 14*(2), 109–114.

National Advisory Committee. 2000. *A guide to end-of-life care for seniors.* Ottawa: Health Canada.

Nelson, J.L. 1998. Death, medicine, and the moral significance of family decision making. In J.F. Monagle and D.C. Thomasma (Eds.), *Health care ethics: Critical issues for the 21st century* (pp. 288–294). Maryland: Aspen.

Nelson, J.E. and Danis M. 2001. End-of-life care in the intensive care unit: Where are we now? *Critical Care Medicine, 29*(supplement 2), N2–N9.

Nelson, H.L. and Nelson, J.L. 1995. *The patient in the family: An ethics of medicine and families.* New York: Routledge.

Nelson-Marten, P., Braaten, J. and English, N.K. 2001. Promoting good end-of-life care in the intensive care unit. *Critical Care Nursing Clinics of North America, 13*(4), 577–585.

Paulette, L. 1993. A choice for K'aila. *Humane Medicine, 9*(1), 13–14.

Pellegrino, E.D. 1999. Clinical ethics consultations: Some reflections on the report of the SHHV-SBC. *The Journal of Clinical Ethics 1999, 10*(1), 5–12.

Penning, M.J. 2002. The health of the elderly: From institutional care to home and community care. In B.S. Bolaria and H. Dickinson (Eds.), *Health, illness, and health care in Canada,* 3rd ed. (pp. 292–308). Toronto: Harcourt Brace.

Pentz, R.D. 1999. Beyond case consultation: An expanded model for organizational ethics. *The Journal of Clinical Ethics, 10*(1), 34–41.

Post, S.G. 1998. Treating senility and dementia: Ethical challenges and quality-of-life judgements. In J.F. Monagle and D.C. Thomasma (Eds.), *Health care ethics: Critical issues for the 21st century* (pp. 189–199). Maryland: Aspen.

Quill, T.E. 2000. Perspectives on care at the close of life. Initiating end-of-life discussions with seriously ill patients: Addressing the "elephant in the room." *Journal of the American Medical Association, 284*(19), 2502–2507.

Randers, I. and Mattiasson, A.C. 2000. The experiences of elderly people in geriatric care with special reference to integrity. *Nursing Ethics, 7*(6), 503–519.

Redman, B.K. 1996. Responsibility of healthcare ethics committees towards nurses. *HEC Forum, 8*(1), 52–60.

Reiser, S.J. 1994. The ethical life of health care organizations. *Hastings Center Report, 24*(6), 28–35.

Robinson, C.A. 1995. Beyond dichotomies in the nursing of persons and families. *Image, 27*(2), 116–120.

Rocker, G. 2002. End-of-life care: An update. *Critical Care Rounds, 3*(5). Available online: www.criticalcarerounds.ca

Rocker, G.M., Shemie, S.D. and Lacroix, J. 2000. End-of-life issues in the ICU: A need for acute palliative care? *Journal of Palliative Care, 16*(supplement), S5–S6.

Rodney, P.A. 1997. *Towards connectedness and trust: Nurses' enactment of their moral agency within an organizational context.* Unpublished doctoral dissertation. University of British Columbia, Vancouver, BC.

Rodney, P. and Howlett, J. (In press). Elderly patients with cardiac disease: Quality of life, end of life, and ethics. In D. Fitchett (Ed.), *Canadian Cardiovascular Society Consensus Document on Care of the Elderly with Cardiac Disease.*

Rodney, P., Varcoe, C., Storch, J. L., McPherson, G., Mahoney, K., Brown, H., Pauly, B., Hartrick Doane, G. and Starzomski, R. 2002. Navigating toward a moral horizon: A multi-site qualitative study of ethical practice in nursing. *Canadian Journal of Nursing Research, 34*(2), 75–102.

Rogers, A.E., Addington-Hall, J.M., Abery, A.J., McCoy, A.S.M., Bulpitt, C., Coats, A.J.S. and Gibbs, J.S.R. 2000. Knowledge and communication difficulties for patients with chronic heart failure: Qualitative study. *BMJ, 321*, 605–607.

Rorty, R. 1999. *Philosophy and social hope.* London: Penguin.

Roy, D. 1994. Those days are long gone now. *Journal of Palliative Care, 10*(2), 4–6.

Roy, D.J. 2000. The times and places of palliative care. *Journal of Palliative Care, 16*(supplement), S3–S4.

Rubin, S.B. and Zoloth, L. (Eds.). 2000. *Margin of error: The ethics of mistakes in the practice of medicine.* Hagerstown, MA: University Publishing Group.

Sawchuk, P.J. and Ross-Kerr, J. 2000. Choices, decisions and control: Older adults and advance care directives. *Canadian Nurse, 96*(7), 16–20.

Sheehan, M.N. 1998. Technology, older persons, and the doctor–patient relationship. In J.F. Monagle and D.C. Thomasma (Eds.), *Health care ethics: Critical issues for the 21st century* (pp. 432–441). Maryland: Aspen.

Sherwin, S. 1992. *No longer patient: Feminist ethics and health care.* Philadelphia: Temple University Press.

Sherwin, S. 1998. A relational approach to autonomy in health care. In S. Sherwin and The Feminist Health Care Ethics Research Network (Eds.), *The politics of women's health: Exploring agency and autonomy* (pp. 19–47). Philadelphia: Temple University Press.

Sherwin, S. 2001. *Towards an adequate ethical framework for setting biotechnology policy.* Paper prepared for the Canadian Biotechnology Advisory Committee Stewardship Standing Committee: 17. Ottawa: Canadian Biotechnology Advisory Committee. Available online: http://cbac-cccb.ca

Singer, P.A. 1994. Advance directives in palliative care. *Journal of Palliative Care, 10*(3), 111–116.

Smith, D.M. 2000. *Moral geographies: Ethics in a world of difference.* Edinburgh: Edinburgh University Press.

Smith, R. 2002. A good death: An important aim for health services and for us all. *BMJ, 320*(7228), 129–130.

Stajduhar, K.I. 2003. Examining the perspectives of family members involved in the delivery of palliative care at home. *Journal of Palliative Care, 19*(1), 27–35.

Stephenson, P. 1999. Expanding notions of culture for cross-cultural ethics in health and medicine. In H. Coward and P. Ratanakul (Eds.), *A cross-cultural dialogue on health care ethics* (pp. 68–91). Waterloo, ON: Wilfrid Laurier University Press.

Storch, J., Rodney, P. and Starzomski, S. 2002. Ethics in health care in Canada. In B.S. Bolaria and H. Dickinson (Eds.), *Health, illness, and health care in Canada,* 3rd ed. (pp. 409–444). Toronto: Harcourt Brace.

Storch, J.L. and Griener, G.G. 1992. Ethics committees in Canadian hospitals: Report of the 1990 pilot study. *Healthcare Management Forum, 5*(Spring), 19–26.

Storch, J.L., Griener, G.G., Marshall, D.A. and Olinek, B.A. 1990. Ethics committees in Canadian hospitals: Report of a 1989 survey. *Healthcare Management Forum, 3,* 3–8.

Subcommittee to Update "Of life and death" of the Standing Senate Committee on Social Affairs. 2000. *Quality end-of-life care: The right of every Canadian.* Ottawa.

Sullivan, W.J. 2001. Autonomy and the terminally ill patient. *BC Medical Journal, 43*(6), 342–345.

Tapp, D.M. 2001. Conserving the vitality of suffering: Addressing family constraints to illness conversations. *Nursing Inquiry, 8*(4), 254–263.

Taylor, C. 1992. *Multiculturalism and "The politics of recognition."* Princeton: Princeton University Press.

Thomasma, D.C. and Monagle, J.F. 1998. Hospital ethics committees: Roles, memberships, structure, and difficulties. In J.F. Monagle and D.C. Thomasma (Eds.), *Health care ethics: Critical issues for the 21st century* (pp. 460–470). Maryland: Aspen.

Thorne, S.E. 1993. *Negotiating health care: The social context of chronic illness.* Newbury Park, CA: Sage.

Thorne, S.E. 2002. Health promoting interactions: Insights from the chronic illness experience. In L.E. Young and V. Hayes (Eds.), *Transforming health promotion practice: Concepts, issues, and applications* (pp. 59–70). Philadelphia: F.A. Davis.

Tilden, V.P., Tolle, S.W., Nelson, C.A., Thompson, M. and Eggman, S.C. 1999. Family decision making in foregoing life-extending treatments. *Journal of Family Nursing, 5*(4), 426–442.

Vandall-Walker, V.A. 2002. Nursing support with family members of the critically ill: A framework to guide practice. In L.E. Young and V. Hayes (Eds.), *Transforming health promotion practice: Concepts, issues, and applications* (pp. 174–189). Philadelphia: F.A. Davis.

Volbrecht, R.M. 2002. *Nursing ethics: Communities in dialogue.* New Jersey: Prentice Hall.

Warren, M.A. 1997. *Moral status: Obligations to persons and other living things.* Oxford: Clarendon Press.

Wilson, D.M. 2000. End-of-life care preferences of Canadian senior citizens with caregiving experience. *Journal of Advanced Nursing, 31*(6), 1416–1421.

Winkler, E.R. 1993. From Kantianism to contextualism: The rise and fall of the paradigm theory in bioethics. In E.R. Winkler and J.R. Coombs (Eds.), *Applied ethics: A reader* (pp. 343–365). Oxford: Blackwell.

Winkler, E. 1996. Moral philosophy and bioethics: Contextualism versus the paradigm theory. In L.W. Sumner and J. Boyle (Eds.), *Philosophical perspectives on bioethics* (pp. 50–78). Toronto: University of Toronto Press.

Yeo, M., Williams, J.R. and Hooper, W. 1998. Ethics and regional health boards. In L. Groarke (Ed.), *The ethics of the new economy* (pp. 125–141). Waterloo, ON: Wilfrid Laurier University Press.

chapter seven

Working within the Landscape: Nursing Ethics

Helen Brown,
Patricia Rodney,
Bernadette Pauly,
Colleen Varcoe,
and Vicki Smye

Ethical behavior is not the display of one's moral rectitude in times of crises. It is the day-by-day expression of one's commitment to other persons and the ways in which human beings relate to one another in their daily interactions (Levine 1977, 846).

In the previous three chapters we have attempted to orient the reader to the theoretical landscape that we have found most useful in understanding health care ethics from the vantage point of nurses and other health care providers. We have argued for theoretical diversity in our use of theory, carefully choosing from a variety of (evolving) traditions as we work towards the health and well-being of the patients, families, and communities we serve. We have further argued that our theoretical approaches must also help us to attend to the moral integrity of health care providers and of health care organizations within their diverse and often conflicted sociopolitical-cultural contexts. Throughout, we have been in agreement with the ethicist Norman Daniels' (1996) claim that "Most ethical problem solving cannot... be either top down or bottom up but must be multifaceted and responsive to the demands of both context and theory" (112; see also Chapters 4–6).

This chapter is our final "snapshot" of the landscape. In it we provide an orientation to the field of nursing ethics. This particular terrain is evolving even more quickly than the other fields we have surveyed, and so we are by no means claiming the final word on the state of nursing ethics. Rather, we are offering our own understandings, knowing that the rest of the chapters in this text will take the exploration further and confident that readers of this text will themselves continue to push inquiry in nursing ethics forward.

We will proceed first by positing nursing ethics as a distinct field of inquiry. This will lead us to an examination of some of the major theoretical foundations of nursing ethics, including relationships between theory and practice and the various influences on and approaches to ethical theory. We will pull together some conclusions in a case application, after which we will look towards the future heralded by postmodern shifts and post-colonial thinking.

A DISTINCT FIELD OF INQUIRY

For a start, it is important to note that for nursing to claim **nursing ethics** as a distinct field of inquiry (and hence practice) has taken some time. As nursing ethics literature and research began to flourish in the 1970s and 1980s, the tendency was for nurses to borrow heavily from medicine and adopt theory and principles from traditional biomedical ethics.[1] In this approach, nursing ethics was treated as a subcategory of medical ethics.[2] For instance, one prominent ethicist argued that "there is very little that is morally unique to nursing" (Veatch 1981, 17). According to this view, both nursing and physician ethics were subcategories of the larger field of biomedical ethics. Nursing ethics was seen as the analysis of ethical decisions by nurses and physician ethics was seen as the analysis of ethical decisions by physicians.

Principlism and its dominance created a *medicocentric* focus throughout bioethics (see also Chapter 4). A medicocentric focus placed emphasis on the legal and ethical dimensions of "exotic" issues arising from medical science and technology such as euthanasia, transplantation, abortion, reproductive technologies, and genetic engineering, among others (Fox 1990; Johnstone 1999). The dominance of principlism and the ensuing medicocentric focus of health care ethics heavily influenced the evolution of nursing ethics.[3] As the Australian nurse ethicist Johnstone (1999) explained, "not only has mainstream bioethics come to refer to and represent these issues, but, rightly or wrongly, [it] has given legitimacy to them—through the power of naming—as *the* most pressing bioethical concerns of contemporary health care in the Western world" (44, italics in original). This meant that everyday (and widespread) ethical problems nurses faced, such as excessive workloads, did not make it onto the list of "valid" ethical issues in traditional bioethics.[4]

The medicocentric focus of bioethics did not serve nursing well.[5] The exotic issues of medical science are relevant to nursing but do not constitute the bulk of nurses' moral concerns of everyday practice of caring for patients and families. Also, in our view, the dominance of principlism, despite the value of having a common theoretical language to share with other health care disciplines, has created a gulf between theory and practice as nurses struggle to use the relatively abstract language of principlism to make ethical decisions in everyday practice.

Fortunately, the historical dominance of medicine and principlism over nursing ethics has not been taken as a given. As our lead-in quotation for this chapter indicates, as early as 1977, a nurse theorist (Levine) argued that there were ethical challenges to be found in everyday activities of professional practice that have been overlooked in favour of an emphasis on life-and-death issues. An American ethicist, Andrew Jameton (1984), argued that nursing ethics was unique as a form of ethical inquiry that contributes to developments in philosophical ethics. A leading American nurse ethicist, Sara Fry, agreed that nursing ethics was unique, but saw it as a subset of bioethics, just as she saw medical ethics as a subset of bioethics (1987; 1989). In both views of nursing ethics as unique, the tools of philosophical analysis were brought to bear to describe the moral phenomena of nursing practice (Fry 1989). In other words, nursing ethics came to be seen as a distinct field of inquiry in its own right, within the discipline of philosophy. Fry emphasized the importance of distinguishing nursing ethics from medical ethics:

> Present theories of medical ethics… do not fit in with the practical realities of nurses' decision making in patient care and…, as a result, tend to deplete the moral agency of nursing practice rather than enhance it. Any theory of nursing ethics should consider the nature of the nurse–patient relationship within health care contexts and should adopt a moral point of view that focuses directly on this relationship (Fry 1989, 20).

At the same time, an increasing number of nurse theorists and nurse ethicists in the United States and a number of other countries were working to articulate the **philosophical foundations** as well as the moral uniqueness of nursing.[6] While different theorists offered different definitions of nursing ethics, Johnstone (1999) characterized it as *"the examination of all kinds of ethical and bioethical issues* from the perspective of nursing theory and practice *which, in turn, rest on the agreed core concepts of nursing"* (46, italics in original).[7]

In our view, nursing ethics is both similar to and distinct from medical ethics. For example, issues arising from genetic engineering enter the professional domains of *both* nurses and physicians, yet, how these issues present to nurses and what their associated concerns are may differ substantially from those of physicians. Despite the fact that ethical issues present themselves differently to nurses and physicians, these practitioners often share concerns about what constitutes ethical care in relationships with patients and families. For example, both nurses and physicians are concerned about ethical relationships with patients and with one another as members of multidisciplinary teams. Mutual respect, **trust,** and **fidelity** are ethical dimensions of relationships between nurses, physicians, patients, families, and other health care providers. Nursing and medicine, therefore, both have important contributions to make that can reshape mainstream health care ethics in a way that is beneficial to patients, families, and communities. For these reasons, theoretical inquiry in nursing ethics is both a distinct endeavour and one that is ultimately related to the ethical means and ends of medicine, social work, administration, research, physiotherapy, and other disciplines in health care.

FOUNDATIONS

In the above passage from Fry (1989), she claimed that nursing needs to articulate a unique moral point of view. In a later discussion of future directions in nursing philosophy, Fry (1999) articulated the need for further exploration of two related questions: "What are the moral concepts that guide nursing practice and what are their foundations?" and "What is the relevance, nature and type of ethical theory needed for nursing practice?" (11). The answers to these questions are far from clear. There has been, and continues to be, significant disagreement about the moral phenomena of nursing and the appropriate theoretical bases from which to understand nursing's moral phenomena. Nonetheless, we believe that it is still useful to lay out our pathway of understanding.

Early Stages

As inquiry in nursing ethics progressed in the 1980s, a number of theorists claimed that the development of nursing ethics was essential to enhancing professionalism within nursing and improving the **practice** of nursing for the benefit of society. Canadian ethicist Michael Yeo (1989) explained:

> A more radical questioning has occurred about the nurses' role and responsibility in relation to patients, other health care professionals, and society in general. Both nursing theory and nursing ethics attempt to come to terms with such issues and define a distinct professional identify for nursing (33–34).

Yeo argued that both nursing ethics and nursing theory are important to the development of nursing as a profession in that a profession requires both a set of ethical standards and a unique knowledge base. Similarly, Pamela Reed (1989) argued that ethical inquiry is essential to the development of nursing theory. She articulated the importance of recognizing that theorizing about nursing is essentially an ethical activity and that ethics should be an *a priori* consideration in nursing research and theory development: "Nursing theorizing, whether it occurs at the outset or emerges during the process of inquiry, is inescapably linked to the theorist's value choices and beliefs about human beings, the environment and health" (Reed 1989, 2). Thus, she reminded us that theorists are morally obligated to examine the value foundations in the development of nursing theory and research to ensure they are true to the aims and values of nursing: "An ethical framework in nursing reflects not only a basic concern for human welfare, but also a moral commitment to the discipline." (Reed 1989, 7; see also Mitchell 2001 and Noureddine 2001).

Another American nursing ethics theorist, Anna Omery (1989), advocated for the development of nursing ethics that adequately addressed issues in practice, research, and education. She warned that if nursing did not identify its ethics, "nursing itself and society will continue to confuse and/or equate medical ethics with all of bioethics" (Omery 1989, 506). She also warned that "nursing will stand to lose practitioners as they try but fail to articulate their professional nursing oughts and shoulds for themselves and their patients" (Omery 1989, 506; see also Nagle 1999). While the development of nursing ethics will benefit nurse researchers and educators, she pointed out, "the greatest benefit will be, however, to the practicing nurse as she/he struggles with giving excellent nursing care consistent with a positive nursing ethic" (Omery 1989, 507).

In summary, in its early stages, the development of nursing ethics came to be seen as essential to the development of nursing theory, research, and, most importantly, professional nursing practice. More recently, we have begun to realize that progress in nursing ethics has the potential to contribute to ethical theory and examination of ethical issues for other disciplines and in health care overall (Rodney et al. 2002). For instance, long-standing problems of consent to treatment withdrawal are confounded by fragmented communication, interdisciplinary team conflict, and family grief. Nursing ethics inquiry can help to more fully explore, and hence move towards resolving, many such problems.[8]

Development

Ultimately, the development of nursing ethics is important for the purpose of promoting the health and well-being of the public. In order to achieve these goals, thoughtful consideration of the development of the **theoretical foundations** of nursing ethics is needed. These foundations are diverse and "are laden with different theoretical presuppositions and the potential for influencing the way that the nurse recognizes ethical conflict, and names and addresses it as part of the clinical judgment process" (Fry 1999, 11). In what follows, we will explore the diverse foundations of nursing ethics in terms of (1) application of traditional biomedical ethical theory; (2) nursing theory and practice as the foundation for the development of nursing ethics; (3) perspectives on relationships; and (4) perspectives on care. Of course, some of these categories overlap—for instance, perspectives on relationships share some theoretical foundations with perspectives on care. Yet there are significant differences between the categories, especially as they have evolved over time.

Application of Traditional Biomedical Ethical Theory

In Chapter 4 we explored the strengths as well as the limitations of traditional **biomedical ethical theory.** We concluded that health care ethics needs to be able to draw on traditional metatheory and mid-range principles as well as on newer contextual approaches such as those entailed in feminist and cross-cultural ethics (see also Daniels 1996). This is true for nursing ethics as well as health care ethics. In his early article on nursing ethics, for instance, Yeo (1989) described the pitfalls of reductionist approaches to traditional biomedical ethics in which specific theories were applied to particular situations to provide direction for action. He argued that such "formula" ethics is misguided because it simplifies ethical positions, "reduces ethical practice to correct technique, and promotes an overly mechanical (and therefore insensitive) comportment to ethical problems" (39). According to Yeo, the implications of this approach for nursing are that the moral situation of nursing is squeezed into imported categories that are applied in a top-down fashion. The danger is that the experience of nursing is "distorted or otherwise denied" (Yeo 1989, 39).

In the early 1990s, Benner (1991) argued that rights and principles cannot stand alone because they do not provide statements of good but "are dependent on an everyday practical knowledge of the good to sustain them" (2). She claimed that disengaged reasoning may allow for thoughtful reflection on the principles and reveal some issues, but it does not reveal the good being threatened in situations and misses the wisdom of those engaged in the situation: "It is in disembodied and conceptual distance that normative ethics fails to grasp essential embodied human distinctions of worth, such as honor, courage, and dignity" (4). Additionally, she claimed that a focus on disengaged principles obstructs accurate understanding and action in a particular situation and should therefore not be given a privileged status over "engaged knowledge of the particular situation" (Benner 1991, 4). Benner (1991) therefore proposed that there is room for more than one source of ethical knowledge. She suggested that dialogue between ethical theory and skilful moral comportment is needed and that one shapes the other. She further argued that **narrative** has a promising role to play in addressing relational and contextual issues (Benner 1991; see also Chapter 14). Nelson (1992) made a similar argument in the same time period as Benner. She claimed, "Nursing is intimate, but it is an intimacy directed at strangers, so it is a social rather than a familial or friendly intimacy. It requires, then, an ethics that is sensitive to the particulars of a given personal relationship yet still leaves room for action in the wider society" (Nelson 1992, 12).

Taken together, the authors we have cited above argued for nursing ethics to embrace a moral foundation that includes attention to particular relationships as well as a call to action on issues in the broader health care context. The application of traditional biomedical ethics to nursing came to be seen as insufficient (though not irrelevant) as a moral foundation for nursing.

Nursing Theory and Practice as the Foundation for the Development of Nursing Ethics

Some authors have suggested that the moral foundation for a system of nursing ethics is embedded in **nursing theory** and/or **nursing practice.** Such approaches are attempts to articulate a system of nursing ethics that is unique and reflective of nursing values. Additionally, these approaches would be consistent with a view that nursing ethics is a unique branch of philosophical ethics related to but not subsumed by health care ethics.[9]

For instance, Yeo (1989) advocated that nursing ethics should arise "from nursing itself" and asked nurses to consider nursing theory in their exploration of a foundation for the development of nursing ethics (39). As Yeo (1989) observed, nursing ethics and nursing theory attempt to address the same issues, such as "the nurses' role and responsibility in relation to patients, other health care professionals, and society in general," and have the shared goal of defining a professional identity for nurses. Yet there has been little communication between the two (33). Yeo also observed that nursing ethics and nursing theory have historically been developed independently of the other, separated by the ideal of science. Legitimacy in nursing theory was initially based on scientific criteria. *In nursing ethics there is more recognition of the limitations of science in sorting out questions of value.* "Nursing ethics is above all concerned with values and value conflicts arising out of nursing practice and research" (Yeo 1989, 34). Its development has therefore been influenced more by moral philosophy and developmental psychology than by science. It is important to note that Yeo (1989) advocated for a reexamination of nursing theory in the development of nursing rather than uncritically adopting from moral philosophy or developmental psychology.

Other theorists and researchers emphasized the importance of nursing practice more than nursing theory as a foundation for the development of nursing ethics. The essence of this approach is that the meaning of what is good is found in nursing practice and that the notion of ethics is embedded in practice (Benner 1991; 1994; 2000; Bishop and Scudder 1987; 1991; 2001). Nursing is viewed as an inherently ethical activity and ethics is integral to the practice of the nurse: "To examine notions of the good life, what is worth being and preserving, one must study everyday ethical expertise and narrative embedded in the practices of communities" (Benner 1991, 1).

Let us turn to an example. In a grounded theory (qualitative) study of the everyday moral decision-making of eight experienced nurses in New Zealand, one researcher found that: "In essence,... the ethic that served as the central guide or driving force behind every moral decision and action of morally competent nurses had its origins, development and usefulness in everyday nursing practice, rather than in formal ethics education" (Woods 1999, 426). The researcher told of a situation in which a young child dying from cancer wished to defy his parents' wishes and refuse life-prolonging treatment—in this case, blood transfusions (Woods, 423–424). In his description, the researcher foregrounded how the nurse negotiated between her own values and those of the seven-year-old boy to whom she was providing care. The boy was adamant that he did not want further treatment, even in the face of a shortened life span. The nurse listened to the boy and helped to organize a meeting between the boy, his physicians, and his father so that the boy's decision could be heard.

Here, the quandary was not reduced only "to continue or not continue treatment," which would tend to be the primary focus with the application of traditional biomedical ethical principles. Instead, the relational and contextual complexity of the situation was shown. In this case, the nurse was apparently trying to negotiate the conflict by aligning herself with her patient and mediating the other relationships in the situation (Varcoe and Rodney 2003).

Perspectives on Relationships

As Woods' (1999) study indicates, much of what is unique in nursing ethics is focused on relationships and care. Here we will discuss developments in the literature on **relationships,** and in the next section, we will further explore perspectives on care. The two fields are related but have somewhat different theoretical foundations and therefore somewhat different implications for nursing ethics.[10]

Since nurses' primary ethical and professional commitments are to patients, the nurse-patient relationship is often viewed as constituting the moral foundation of nursing practice (Peter and Morgan 2001) and, hence, represents a central site of nursing work.[11] A primary commitment to relationships with patients means that nursing by its very nature is seen as a moral endeavour.[12] Since nursing places considerable importance on nurse-patient relationships, there is an abundance of theoretical literature focused on nursing practice as defined by the primacy and ethical nature of these relationships. Historically, nurse-patient relationships have most often been described as based on *contracts, advocacy,* and *care.*[13] While we will further explore care in the section that follows, here we would like to note that ethical obligations in nurses' relationships with patients have been primarily explored through the concept of **advocacy,**[14] which is premised on an individual's right to autonomy. Advocacy, then, underlies a nurse's actions to help a client exercise his or her self-determination. From this perspective, advocacy became the "middle ground" as nurses sought to reconcile paternalistic practices and consumer movement in health care. Gadow's (1990) work on existential advocacy as a philosophy of care, among other work in this area (e.g., Curtin 1979), effectively forges a connection between nurses' primary commitment to patients and the moral dimensions of nursing practice.

Various critiques have been raised about the limitations of these approaches. For one, it is next to impossible to view health care relationships as **contractual**[15] since there are usually unequal power relations between care providers and patients, even if providers attempt to lessen the inequality (May 1989). Furthermore, the concept of advocacy in nursing has been critiqued for lacking empirical support, for placing the patient in a passive stance, for ignoring nursing's relative powerlessness within the health care system, for ignoring the advocacy performed by other health care providers, and for working against an interdisciplinary team approach (Hewitt 2002; Storch 1999; Wurzbach 1999). Returning to reflect on the story from Woods' (1999) study, for instance, neither the seven-year-old boy nor his father were in a position to negotiate as equals with the highly specialized health care providers. Accounting for the relationships in terms of contract would therefore not be accurate. In fact, a notion of **covenant**—whereby we acknowledge asymmetrical power relationships and work to uphold trust despite this asymmetry—would be more useful.[16] Furthermore, while the nurse stepped forward to advocate for the boy by helping him to have his voice heard, she did more than act as an advocate for him. She had to be knowledgeable about the family and team relationships, and she had to be in a position of sufficient personal power herself to have *her* voice heard in an emotionally charged and conflicted situation. As the nurse recounts, "I mean it was very traumatic... to be really strong and stand up not only to the father, but the consultant [physician] as well, and to say this is what is needed" (Woods, 424). Although we do not have further information about the story, we can conjecture that the nurse's ethical actions would have been even more effective if she could also work to help the father and the rest of the family with their grief and negotiate an interdisciplinary palliative care plan with the other health care providers. In other words, understanding the nurse's actions only in terms of advocacy for the boy would miss some other morally relevant relationships and considerations.[17]

All this is not to say that notions of contract and advocacy have not been useful. They have helped us to reflect on and better understand the ethical nature of nursing relationships. However, in order to account for ethical relationships more fully we need a wider repertoire of theory about relationships to draw on. Fortunately, there is a growing body of such work available.

Other theoretical work in nursing describes the **everyday** relational context of nursing practice as essential to ethical deliberations.[18] For instance, there is writing that emphasizes the relational nature of interdisciplinary teamwork (Taylor 1997), professional autonomy (MacDonald 2002), the importance of connectedness and trust for enacting moral agency (Peter and Morgan 2001; Rodney 1997; see also Chapters 8 and 12), the development of moral identity (Hartrick Doane 2002a; 2002b; see also Chapter 21), and philosophical questions about the nature of nurse-patient relationships (Gadow 1999). Furthermore, there is emerging theoretical attention to the notion that nursing knowledge and practice within nurse-patient relationships are situated productions whose meanings are both relational and contextual (Campbell 2001; McMahah, Hoffman and McGee 1994; Purkis 1994). In other words, these latter works emphasize that we cannot fully understand the nature of nurse/provider/patient/family/organizational relationships without also accounting for the often taken-for-granted discourses and ideologies in the larger sociopolitical contexts. For instance, the physicians, nurses, and family of the boy dying from cancer (Woods 1999) were all influenced by an ideology of cure in cancer treatment, by the taken-for-granted status of children in health care decision-making (see also Chapter 19), and by societal norms of physician and male authority.

Nursing scholars working in ethics are increasingly calling into question contextual constraints on ethical practice in nurse–patient relationships. In particular, Varcoe et al. (in press) point to how nurses perceive that they must ration their care in ways that interfere with their moral obligations in relationships with patients. Nurses describe how the lack of time means that they have few, if any, meaningful conversations with patients. They cite the reason for not asking patients relevant questions as having no time to listen to their answers. It has been argued that an **"ideology of scarcity"** structures much of nursing practice (Varcoe 1997; 2001; Varcoe, Rodney and McCormick in press); basic conditions for ethical relationships with patients are not met due to what nurses experience as a scarcity of resources and the increased needs of the patients and families they serve.[19] The impact of the **sociopolitical context** on nurses' relationships is thus getting more attention in the literature on nursing ethics. In fact, Nortvedt (2001), questioning whether or not patient advocacy ought to be assumed as "the" way to respect autonomy within nurse-patient relationships, claims that what is central to nursing practice now in terms of relationships with patients is "not how to give the best care for one's patients, but instead how to minimize potential harm to patients created by socio-economic circumstances" (112).

Perspectives on Care

Care is a construct that is often employed in descriptions of the moral foundations of nurse-patient relationships. For a start, we would like to point out that the emphasis on caring in the development of nursing ethics has arisen out of criticisms of justice-based biomedical ethics as an appropriate foundation for nursing ethics. Nursing's affinity for caring theory in ethics has been based on the need to accommodate the relational bases of nursing, the need to recognize the context of ethical decision-making, and the need to recognize persons, not just acts, as important to ethics (Salsberry 1992).

The development of care-based discourses can be traced primarily to women's studies and to psychological studies of moral development. These traditions distinguished between how women display an ethic of care and men predominantly exhibit a justice-oriented ethic of rights and obligations. Both Carol Gilligan (1982; 1988), as a psychologist, and Annette Baier (1994), as a feminist philosopher, have played prominent roles in the development of care-based approaches. These authors, among others, criticize the liberalist underpinnings of Western moral theory, thereby challenging the notion of blind impartiality as necessary for moral life. In particular, proponents of an ethics of care argue that the primacy of the autonomous self and rational individualism in modern ethical theory excludes the moral relevance of our relatedness as human beings. Such a moral stance has been argued to leave us blind to the special needs of and relationships with others.[20] In addition, care-based approaches challenge the notion that good and mature moral judgment occurs only with moral distance.

Moreover, care-based discourses have expressed a disdain for abstract principles supposedly applied with impartiality, finding them irrelevant, ineffectual, and constricting. A rejection of principle-based accounts of ethics means that care-based approaches have turned towards two important themes: the responsibility of attending to mutual interdependence in relationships and the important moral role of emotions in choosing a path of ethical action (Heckman 1995). Noddings (1984) claims that ethical caring is rooted in natural caring, defined as "that relationship in which we respond as one caring out of love or natural inclination" (50). In ethical caring, one acts out of natural caring, the remembrance of natural caring, or the desire to be virtuous. In taking up these kinds of perspectives on care, nursing authors have emphasized caring as a feminine ethic using work from developmental psychology (for example, Cooper 1989; Huggins and Scalzi 1988). They have also conceived of caring as both a value (e.g., Watson 1988; Gadow 1985; 1990; Fry 1989) and a virtue (e.g., Salsberry 1992).

However, care-based approaches are not without criticism from outside and within nursing. They have been seen to include an inherent gender- and sexual-orientation bias, reinforcement of negative stereotypes of servile women, promotion of dependency of the one cared for, and over-involvement and burnout by the caregiver. More specifically, Gilligan's work has been accused of creating a dualism between care and cure, nursing and medicine, women and men. And Nodding's work has been criticized for being a feminine rather than feminist ethic since it does little to acknowledge its inherent gender bias. Finally, care theory has been criticized for being inattentive to culture, race, and class, and for lacking theoretical clarity and empirical support.[21] In other words, care-based approaches help us to understand and promote human connection in certain relationships, but they do not necessarily help us to understand caring by and for persons of different genders and sexual orientations, they do not necessarily help us to understand the goals in caring relationships, and they do not necessarily help us to understand how power operates in relationships between individuals, groups, organizations, and society.

Thus, despite the important focus on relationships as morally relevant in care-based perspectives, we argue that care-based perspectives are necessary but not sufficient as a theoretical basis for determining what makes a relationship ethical in health care.[22] Contributing to the insufficiency of care-based perspectives as a theoretical basis for nursing ethics has been the lack of clarity about caring as a virtue, a value, or a quality of relationships. For example, the locating of caring solely as a feminine virtue in relationships has been criticized for failing to attend to the sociopolitical context in which those relationships take place and in which nursing is often constrained.[23] Furthermore, some feminist theorists argue that an "ethic of care,"[24] while being valuable for its challenge to dominant conventions of justice-oriented moral theory, fails to confront the "morality of gender inequality itself and, in fact, perpetuates the reign of the dominant by encouraging self-sacrifice and servility in the guise of care" (Bowden 2000, 8).

Such dialogue about the sufficiency of care-based perspectives is critical to the development of theoretical works that thoughtfully examine the implications of both dichotomizing justice from care (such as constructing morality as gendered) and combining justice and care perspectives in moral theory as a basis for nursing ethics. We believe that dialogue about the ethical significance of "caring" relations ought to involve philosophical analysis that reflects the enormous diversity and complexity of moral experience—both within the context of gender and beyond. It seems particularly problematic to equate nursing ethics primarily with care-based ethics that do not account for gendered, social inequalities. Despite the potential of care-based perspectives to provide a gender sensitive corrective to conventional moral theories, nursing ethics ought to account for feminist criticisms arguing that "celebrations of caring reduce and simplify the range of women's moral possibilities to those displayed in practices of care" (Bowden 2000, 8). Fortunately, theoretical work in **feminist ethics** accounts for these criticisms.

Caring from a *feminist* (rather than a *feminine*) perspective holds more potential for nursing ethics since it not only evokes a responsibility to develop a capacity to experience another person and be receptive to his or her needs, but also accepts the responsibility to improve the welfare of all human beings. As Sherwin (1992a; 1998) and others[25] remind us, caring is about more than relationships among individuals; it also reflects a social conscience that moves beyond individuals to families, groups, communities, and societies. Sherwin argues that for caring to reflect such a social conscience, it must also entail notions of **justice**.[26] She explains that

> Because feminism arises from moral objections to oppression, it must maintain a commitment to the pursuit of social justice; that commitment is not always compatible with preferences derived from existing relationships and attitudes. Hence we must recognize that feminist ethics involves a commitment to considerations of justice, as well as to those of caring (Sherwin, 1992b, 52).

A number of nursing theorists and researchers echo Sherwin's position. Studies of nurses' moral reasoning have shown that nurses (and physicians) employ care as well as justice and other ethical constructs when they confront ethical situations.[27] For instance, in one study where 31 staff nurses were interviewed about preselected ethical dilemmas, they showed a moral "richness" in their ethical decision-making (Sherblom, Shipps and Sherblom 1993). As the investigators of the study explain,

In addition to clear justice and care concerns raised for each dilemma, nurses express integrated concerns connecting deceit, truthfulness, trust, and the role that trust plays in a caregiving relationship; a conception of advocacy as an overall commitment to patients' well-being; and patients' right and need to know the seriousness of a terminal illness to prepare for their death (Sherblom, Shipps and Sherblom 460).

Nursing and other theorists are thus calling for nurses to purposefully embrace feminist constructions of justice as well as care so as to recognize the complexity and diversity of nurses' moral experience.[28] Moreover, researchers and theorists are calling for an even broader integration of morally relevant constructs. In Sherblom, Shipps, and Sherblom's (1993) study, for instance, deceit, truthfulness, and trust were also important. Other studies have also profiled the importance of trust (Peter and Morgan 2001; Rodney 1997). Hope (Simpson 2002), compassion (Armstrong, Parsons and Barker 2000; Gaul 1995), and empathy (Reynolds, Scott and Austin 2000) are among the other constructs flagged as important in nurses' ethical relationships. In the meantime, there remain a number of interesting questions to pursue—for example, whether such constructs are virtues, emotions, or duties and the relationship of the constructs to justice-based theories (Armstrong, Parsons and Barker; Liaschenko 1999; Reynolds, Scott and Austin 2000).

As will become clear later in this chapter, the dialogue about care-based perspectives and their ethical relevance intersects with postmodern understandings of diversity of human experience in light of the "totalizing" effects of modernism. In other words, any work in nursing ethics arising from care-based perspectives ought to reject universalizing attempts to theorize the meaning of "ethical caring." Such an approach denies the local and contextual relevance of "caring" practices and relations.

In summary, when caring is viewed as being a diverse and multidimensional concept that has ethical relevance in relationships, it may then hold more potential for nursing ethics. Caring can be seen as being about a professional commitment to the diversity and complexity of nurses' moral experience. Moreover, when care-based perspectives are informed by feminist concerns about social justice, nursing ethics may then begin to pay critical attention to ethical concerns such as the political structures that shape ethical practice. The task of liberating caring from a notion reducible to women's work towards a postmodern recognition of the complexity and diversity of moral experience and feminist conceptions of social justice holds much promise for nursing ethics.

Application of the Foundations of Nursing Ethics

Thus far, we have provided an orientation to (our understanding) of the diverse and rapidly evolving field of nursing ethics. In order to bring more colour to that orientation, we wish to explicate another story to add to the one we have drawn on from Woods (1999). This second story, in Ethics in Practice 7-1, comes from a feminist ethnographic study of nurses' ethical practice on an acute medical ward in a community hospital (Rodney 1997). In it, a nurse research participant is recounting her concerns about a recent night shift that she worked when she had a student with her. The interviewer (Rodney) spent a number of shifts as a participant observer with the nurse participant and so has some understanding of the context described by the nurse. In what follows, we will synthesize the conclusions drawn in this chapter so far and link these conclusions to the story for purposes of illustration.

| Ethics in Practice 7-1 | **"A Patient Who Was Really, Really Ill..."** |

[W]ell last week, we had a patient who was really, really ill. Actually, she should have been in ICU [the Intensive Care Unit] but... in the hospital at the time we had two other codes [arrests] plus we had a few people from emergency and... everything, it seems to happen all in one night.... And so, the supervisor was saying, "We don't have any beds in ICU, can you hang onto this person?" So they [the ICU medical staff] came up and took a look at this lady and they said, "Well, as long as you can keep her 0₂ sats [oxygen saturation] above 90." Well, she kept deteriorating through the night and... she had absolutely no urine output at all, like not even a drop, and so we were sitting there trying everything. We gave her 240 mg of IV [intravenous] Lasix.... It was really nice that I was the extra because I basically just looked after this patient.... It was L.'s [another nurse's] patient and I ended up looking after her, and S. [the student the nurse participant was working with] looked after our group, came to me when she needed help, and I popped in and made sure S. was all right....

[A]t the end of the night we were all tired; we were all late getting off. I got off at, um, I think it was nearly, well, eight, quarter after eight and... so I got off late and L... got off late and it was actually kind of irritating because some of the [nurses] on days [didn't help us].... like this lady [the critically ill patient], all of a sudden her blood pressure just bottomed out, and they [the physicians] wanted the monitor put on her and you know, so that they could keep a close eye on her blood pressure and we don't have a monitor on our floor so we had to go to another building to get a monitor. On days nobody was going, nobody wanted to go and L. kept saying, "Can anybody go and get this, is anybody not busy?" and there were a few sitting at the desk and talking and I wanted to go and kick them. Finally I said, "Forget it, you don't understand how sick she is."... And of course they wouldn't because they weren't there at night and they were on a different group and they weren't directly involved so they didn't see the urgency. So anyway I went and got it [the monitor]... but the patient ended up coding [having a cardiopulmonary arrest] at ten and... ended up in ICU and she ended up in [another hospital] on dialysis is what I heard, but... I kept thinking thank goodness I was extra.... Because if I wasn't extra... she would have been on her own.... And... she was really distressed... her breathing was really, really distressed and it was scary, she was terrified, she thought she was going to die and she almost did (Rodney 1997, 157–158).

Conclusion 1:

For nursing to claim "nursing ethics" as a distinct field of inquiry (and hence practice) has taken some time.

Until fairly recently, it would have been difficult to engage in a full ethical analysis of the problem described by the nurse in Ethics in Practice 7-1. Traditional biomedical ethical approaches would have focused on the patient's consent to treatment and access to acute care resources. While these are important elements of the story, the traditional approach would have missed the ethically relevant problems of excessive workload and intra- and interdisciplinary **team conflict**. Both of the latter were values-based problems that interfered with "the good" in the nurses' and other health care providers' practice.

Conclusion 2:

The development of nursing ethics came to be seen as essential to the development of nursing theory, research, and, most importantly, professional nursing practice.

Nursing theory helps us to conceptualize the person we are interacting with, the nature of nursing and our interventions, the **health** or **well-being** we are aiming for, and the effects of the environment. In Ethics in Practice 7-1, the nurse was worried about the patient as a person ("she was terrified") and had a notion of health in mind that her patient was clearly not achieving ("her breathing was really, really distressed"). Her interventions were aimed at some level of restoration of the patient's health and protection from further harm—particularly from the cardiopulmonary arrest she later suffered. The nurse also recognized that specialized equipment and care were required, and she was worried about deficiencies in her current environment. While we do not have the full story (for instance, how the nurse might have supported the patient's family), it is apparent that her practice was informed by her theorizing about nursing whether or not she was using a particular nursing model. Her practice was directed towards fulfilling what she saw as her ethical obligations. In the language of today's version of the Canadian Nurses Association Code of Ethics for Registered Nurses (2002), for example, those obligations would relate to "safe, competent, and ethical care," "health and well-being," "justice," and "accountability."

Conclusion 3:

Progress in nursing ethics has the potential to contribute to ethical theory and examination of ethical issues for other disciplines and in health care overall.

Conclusion 4:

The application of traditional biomedical ethics to nursing came to be seen as insufficient (though not irrelevant) as a moral foundation for nursing.

Violation of **informed consent** is a persistent and widespread problem in health care ethics. This story shows some of the complexity of involving the patient and her family in autonomous decisions about instituting life-saving treatment. The relative isolation of the acute medical unit from the specialized providers and resources in the intensive care unit meant that the patient was constrained in her real choice of treatment options. Indeed, in ethics consultations, the authors of this chapter have seen similar situations result in the patient's and the family's loss of trust in the team. This loss of trust can proceed to the extent that when (even appropriate) treatment withdrawal is later suggested, the patient and family do not believe that the health care providers have the patient's best interest at heart. Nursing ethics inquiry, with its attention to particular relationships and particular contexts, can help to unpack and hence move towards resolving such problems. For instance, an earlier assessment by the Intensive Care Unit providers and an earlier meeting with the patient, her family, and the nurses looking after her (with or without an earlier transfer to the Intensive Care Unit) could have helped the patient and her family to be more informed and to have more trust in the health care team.

Conclusion 5:
Much of what is unique in nursing ethics is focused on relationships and care.

Conclusion 6:
The impact of the sociopolitical context on nurses' relationships is getting more attention in nursing ethics.

The nurse in this story expressed a great deal of concern about the care she was trying to provide for the patient—to keep the patient safe and help her to feel less short of breath and less afraid. The nurse's concerns about relationships also extended to the nursing colleague she was assisting and the student nurse she was working with. However, constraints in the **sociopolitical environment** of the hospital meant that she did not get the support from relationships with health care providers in the intensive care unit or physicians on the medical ward. And, perhaps most troubling to her, she could not get the nurses who arrived on the day shift on her ward to pitch in to help her care for the patient in a timely fashion ("because they weren't there at night and they were on a different group and they weren't directly involved"). While it is difficult to account for this lack of support on the basis of the story we are provided with, a persistent finding in the study overall was the intense time pressures nurses had to work under because of the excessive workloads they had to manage (Rodney 1997). The day-shift nurses did not likely welcome an interruption to their "beat-the-clock" morning routine. This nurse expressed a commitment to relationships and care, but the context in which she was working did not make it easy for her to fulfill her commitment.

Conclusion 7:
Caring and feminism—when united through concerns about social justice—can reflect a commitment to dignity, humanity, and equality, and draw critical attention to the political structures that shape such possibilities.

There were a number of **power** issues inherent in the situation the nurse encountered. For one, the structure of the hospital meant that the "general" practice of acute medicine did not have nearly as many structural and human resources as the Intensive Care Unit, even for patients who were sick enough to require intensive care[29] (Rodney 1997). The fact that it was a nurse and a woman, rather than a physician and/or a male, trying to get more assistance for the (female) patient did not help matters. Finally, we are left to wonder if the day-shift nursing staff's behaviour was a form of passive aggression towards the night nurse, the colleague she was helping, and her student. In other words, the day staff's reluctance to help their colleagues may have been related to more than just time pressures. They may have felt that it was the night shift nurses' fault that they were behind because they had not been efficient. Unfortunately, nursing has a long history of similar kinds of horizontal violence, or unsupportive behaviour among nursing colleagues.[30] We will say more about these kinds of power issues in the next section of this chapter.

TOWARDS THE FUTURE

The landscape of theory and practice we have described thus far is diverse and changing. In closing this chapter we wish to reflect on two emerging theoretical trends for further work in nursing ethics—postmodern shifts and post-colonial thinking.[31] Both offer us the means to expand our thinking in relation to Conclusion 7 above. Postmodern shifts in the philosophy of science help us to question taken-for-granted power dynamics in relationships between individuals, organizations, and sociopolitical structures. And post-colonial thinking can help us to re-think our relationships with some of those who have been most marginalized in Western health care. While both postmodern and post-colonial theory have already had an influence on nursing and many other disciplines in academia as well as health care, we believe that they could be particularly beneficial in shaping the future of nursing ethics.

Postmodern Shifts

We are using the term **postmodern** to describe the current philosophical, social, political, cultural, economic, and global context in which old and new questions are related to phenomena such as nursing ethics. Postmodern thinking has generally been characterized by a loss of belief in an objective world and incredulity towards the meta-narratives of legitimation (Kvale 1995).[32] Critiques are forwarded about the grand narratives of modernism, such as science, where totalizing theories are advanced as universally applicable (Bernstein 1991; Heckman 1995; Lyotard 1984). Within postmodern thinking there has been an expansion of rationality to go beyond the cognitive and scientific domain to include also the ethical and aesthetic domains of life in reason (Bernstein 1991). Challenging the dominance of a technical means-ends rationality creates space for going beyond the Kantian split of science, morality, and art and involves a "rehabilitation of the ethical and aesthetic domains" (Nussbaum 2001).

Thus, postmodern critiques have opened up space for questioning the previously unquestioned, which invariably leads to new possibilities for considering the meaning of ethical relationships. Questions about the value of *either* normative (see Chapter 4) *or* local knowledge about ethical relationships become less of an *either/or* and more of a *both/and,* particularly as, for instance, nurses work back and forth in practice between a professional code of ethics and their obligation to be responsive to the particular needs, experiences, and contexts of patients' lives. When grand narratives, such as the narrative of ethics and science, are no longer seen as monolithic "truths" and are revealed for their taken-for-grantedness in the everyday world, possibilities arise for seeing knowledge, relationships, culture, and "truth" as situated, unstable, and fluid. Such a way of thinking presumes that, when asking the question about ethical relationships, one ultimate answer is neither possible nor desirable. However, postmodern thinking does not mean that any answer is adequate or that there are no right answers or no better answers (Varcoe and Rodney 2003). In other words, postmodern thinking does not necessarily mean that we have to commit to a stance of ethical relativism in which "anything goes" (Squires 1993; see also Chapter 5). To the contrary, while postmodern thinking increases the challenge by making it clear that there are no *easy* answers, we still agree with philosophical pragmatists such as Rorty (1999) that the purpose of inquiry is to "achieve agreement among human beings about what to do, to bring about consensus on the ends to be achieved and the means to be used to achieve those ends" (xxv)—to solve real problems in the real world of practice. There is a value-based direction from which we proceed and towards which we are moving, though the specifics of individual paths will vary.

We find the metaphor of **"moral horizons"** useful in understanding this value-based direction (Rodney et al. 2002). While the metaphor has been described by various theorists in different ways, we believe that it tells us something about the values we are operating from as well as the value-based plurality of landscapes we may move towards (Bernstein 1991; Taylor 1992). Furthermore, these horizons are political as well as ethical. As another philosophical pragmatist, Bernstein, explains:

> Although we can distinguish ethics and politics, they are inseparable. For we cannot understand ethics without thinking through our political commitments and responsibilities. And there is no understanding of politics that does not bring us back to ethics. Ethics and politics as disciplines concerned with *praxis* are aspects of a unified practical philosophy (9, italics original).

A postmodern frame therefore influences how we view human relationships generally and in health care specifically. Whereas modern thinking tends to divorce individuals from their social context, postmodern thinking (re)centres the idea that human relations are rooted in both social and historical contexts.[33] Liberal theories that privilege a view of persons as "rugged individuals" and moral theories that posit a dualistic perspective of the autonomous self and subject-object relations have tended to obscure the important notion that social relations shape and are shaped by individuals within them, and that relationships exist within a broader discursive context (see also Chapters 5 and 8).

A fruitful example of where nursing ethics can draw from postmodern insights comes from Canadian feminist ethicist Sherwin's (1998) formulation of the concept of **"relational autonomy"** in health care. As was noted in Chapter 6, Sherwin proposes a relational concept of autonomy that can be termed socially situated or contextualized: "Under a relational view, autonomy is best understood to be a capacity or skill that is developed (and constrained) by social circumstances. It is exercised within relationships and social structures that jointly help to shape the individual while also affecting others' responses to her efforts at autonomy" (36). An important dimension of relational autonomy is that it takes account of social and political structures and their impact on the lives of individuals. Relational autonomy thus draws our attention to barriers and constraints that might interfere with individuals' abilities to *enact* their autonomy.

Conclusion 8:
Postmodern thinking (re)centers the idea that human relations are rooted in both social and historical contexts.

In situations where some patients and families are less articulate than others and have access to fewer resources, Sherwin's notion of relational autonomy is most useful. For example, we might ask, "Were there adequate opportunities for respectful encounters with health care providers in which patients were able to reflect on the values informing their decisions and choices?" This kind of question was certainly relevant, for instance, to the boy and his family in Woods' (1999) study. And it was relevant for the critically ill woman in Ethics in Practice 7-1 (Rodney 1997). In both situations, there were significant barriers for patients and families as well as nurses and other health care providers.

Post-Colonial Thinking

As we said in Chapter 5, theorists, researchers, and practitioners in health care ethics have recently become more aware of the complex and intersecting **cultural contexts** of their work. The same is true for theorists, researchers, and practitioners in nursing ethics. For example, Lützén (1997) and Lützén and Nordin (1993) have begun to explore moral concepts and principles in relation to culture in the development of nursing ethics (see also Cortis and Kendrick 2003; Zoucha and Husted 2000). Others have attempted to adapt traditional ethical theory and ethical decision-making frameworks to include a cultural component (e.g., Griepp 1995). **Post-colonial** theory can be a good adjunct to cross-cultural theory for nursing ethics because it can help us to re-think our relationships with some of those who have been most marginalized in Western health care.

In the last decade, post-colonialism has taken its place with other theories as a major critical discourse in the humanities (Gandhi 1998). This discourse provides a special point of scrutiny regarding knowledge development, taking us from the experiences of those "who have suffered from the sentence of history—subjugation, domination, diaspora, [and] displacement" (Bhabha 1994, 172) to examine the social and historical location from which dominant discourses have been produced (Anderson 2002). The "post" in post-colonial does not connote the notion of "after" colonialism but, rather, refers to a studied reflexive process attuned to colonialism as it existed *and exists* both locally and globally. Post-colonialism takes us back and forth between ideas of the past to the solutions in the present and the structures that create them (Bhabha 1994; McConaghy 1997; Quayson 2000). This reflexive process that characterizes the post-colonial

> is a sign that we are now more aware of our historical locatedness, less sure of the rightness of our policy decisions, more alert to the possibility that our decisions may be colonizing rather than decolonizing in their consequences, more able to be responsive to new situations of disadvantage and more able to correctly analyze and redress the specifics of local oppressions (McConaghy 1997, 86; see also Smye and Browne 2002).

It is important to note that "post-colonial" does not mean the end of colonialism. For example, the socio-cultural, economic, and political positioning of Aboriginal people in Canadian history has meant, and continues to mean, that Aboriginal people have significantly poorer health status on almost every measure than do non-Aboriginal people (Stephenson 1999). The jurisdictional debate between federal and provincial governments related to who is responsible for Aboriginal health continues to wreak havoc in the lives of Aboriginal people. In other words, Aboriginal peoples in Canada and other countries continue to experience colonialism in their everyday lives (see also Chapter 5).

An understanding of post-colonialism assists us in recognizing the voices at the margins of mainstream Western society. Furthermore, it offers a dialogue to reframe dominant discourses and to create a perspective on knowledge development that reflects multiple social locations (Anderson 2002). Today, as we engage in debates about health and social policy issues in the context of health reform, we need to understand that, in a sense, "we are making decisions about what constitutes colonialism" and "what we have determined to be the essential aspects of anti-colonial work" (McConaghy 1997, 82). Our challenge is to determine when and under what circumstances an initiative (practice, policy, or research) might be "oppressive" and "limiting" and when it might be "emancipatory" (McConaghy 1997, 82; see also Smye and Browne 2002). It is significant to note, for instance, that the boy and his father in Woods' (1999) study were Aboriginal individuals from New Zealand. This ought to cause us to wonder how the conflict had been influenced by the family's possible isolation from large Westernized treatment centres, their previous experiences with non-Aboriginal care providers, the physicians' and nurses' awareness of how their own values and beliefs were similar to and different from the boy's and his father's, and so on. Furthermore, we ought to wonder what the Aboriginal community members' experiences of Western-based research were. There is growing evidence that indigenous peoples often feel disempowered and even stigmatized by biomedical research (Stephenson 1999; Tuhiwai Smith 1999). For example, did the father believe that the possible benefits of science were truly exhausted for his son, or did he feel that the treatment his son had received was being limited because of his Aboriginal status? As this (brief) illustration shows, a post-colonial interpretation locates health and social conditions in the domains of the structural disadvantages that shape them (Browne and Smye 2002). This kind of interpretation is important for future work in nursing ethics, especially for ethical practice with Aboriginal and immigrant peoples.[34]

Conclusion 9:

Post-colonial theory can be a good adjunct to cross-cultural theory for nursing ethics because it can help us to re-think our relationships with some of those who have been most marginalized in Western health care.

In summary, then, post-colonial perspectives can help nurses to think about colonizing experiences and knowledge that not only constrain ethical practice but also serve to perpetuate the unproblematized discourses that currently pervade Western health care culture. More explicit attention to post-colonial, postmodern, and feminist theory can infuse nursing ethics with concerns about social justice—for *all* those involved in the provision and receipt of health care. Nursing ethics ought to be responsive to the contextual, relational, and power-laden nature of nurses' experiences and actions as they engage in the everyday work of caring. This responsiveness can lead to better ethical practice for individuals such as the Aboriginal boy in Woods' (1999) study and the critically ill woman in Ethics in Practice 7-1, for their families, and for the communities they live in.

This brings to a close our orientation to the field of nursing ethics. We have offered our own understandings of a swiftly evolving terrain, organizing our insights into nine statements of conclusion. We commenced by positing nursing ethics as a distinct field of inquiry which led us to an examination of some of the major theoretical foundations of nursing ethics, including relationships between theory and practice and the various influences on and approaches to ethical theory. We used two case situations (Woods 1999 and Ethics in Practice 7-1) to illustrate our orientation, after which we looked towards the future heralded by postmodern shifts and post-colonial thinking. It will be an interesting and productive future, as the subsequent chapters in this text attest.

FOR REFLECTION

1. What historical influences likely made it difficult for nursing to articulate a distinct field of nursing ethics two decades ago?

2. How do you think nursing ethics ought to influence nursing theory, and vice versa, in the future?

3. Comment on how a postmodern understanding of relational autonomy (Sherwin 1998) might affect the ongoing development of nursing ethics.

4. What impact do you imagine that post-colonial thinking might have on the development of codes of ethics and ethical policies for nurses in the future?

ENDNOTES

1. Fry (1989); Johnstone (1999); Omery (1989); Rodney and Varcoe (2003); Yeo (1989).

2. Fry (1989a); Fry and Veatch (1987); Melia (1994); Veatch (1981).

3. Johnstone (1999); Liaschenko (1993a; 1993b); Yeo (1989); Woods (1999).

4. Chambliss (1996); Liaschenko (1993); Rodney (1997); Rodney and Varcoe (2003); Storch et al. (2002); Varcoe et al. (in press)

5. The medicocentric focus in traditional bioethics did not necessarily serve medicine or other disciplines all that well either. For instance, some physician ethicists have emphasized the importance of understanding the virtues inherent in clinical practice rather than just the duties inherent in the application of autonomy, beneficence, and justice (Gillett 1995; Pellegrino and Thomasma 1993; Pellegrino, Veatch and Langan 1991).

6. See also Benner, Tanner, and Chesla (1996); Edwards (2001); Fry (1999); Gadow (1999); Johnstone (1999); Kikuchi and Simmons (1992; 1994); Omery, Kasper, and Page (1995); Nordvedt (1998); and Chapters 3 and 22 in this text.

7. It is worth noting that Johnstone also characterized nursing ethics as *descriptive* (describing nurses' values, beliefs, and practices), *normative* (establishing standards and rules of conduct), and *meta* (undertaking a critical examination of the nature, logical form, and language of nursing ethics) (1998, 39–69; 1999, 47). This delineation parallels the structure of ethics as a discipline (see also Chapter 4).

8. See, for example, Chamber-Evans (2002); Godkin (2002); Hiltunen et al. (1999); Jezewski (1994); Sawchuk and Ross-Kerr (2000); Taylor (1995); Tilden et al. (1999); and Chapter 13 in this text.

9. As we explained in Chapter 4, within health care ethics, there are concerns that are particular to the sciences of biomedicine (bioethics—for instance, debates about cloning), concerns that are particular to each of the professions (medical ethics, nursing ethics, pharmacy ethics, and so on, all of which are also related to professional ethics), and concerns that are particular to organizations (which are also related to business ethics). When we use the term "bioethics," we are referring to the more traditional (circumscribed) study of health care ethics that occurred early in the development of the discipline and continues today, to some extent.

10. There is an emerging literature on relational ethics. See, for example, Sherwin (1998) and Chapter 24 in this text.

11. Bishop and Scudder (1990; 2001); Gadow (1990; 1999); Yarling and McElmurry (1986).

12. Bishop and Scudder (1990; 2001); Georges and Grypdonack (2002); Johnstone (1999); Paterson and Zderad (1988); Smith and Godfrey (2002); Yarling and McElmurray (1986).

13. Bandman and Bandman (2002); Benner and Wrubel (1989); Curtin (1982); Flaherty (1982); Fry (1987); Fry and Johnstone (2002); Gadow (1990); Kohnke (1990); Peter and Morgan (2001); Storch (1992; 1999); Thompson, Melia, and Boyd (1994); Yeo (1989); Winslow (1990).

14. One definition of "advocacy" is

    the active assistance to patients in their self-determination concerning health alternatives. Advocacy not only safe-guards but contributes positively to the exercise of self-determination. It is the effort to help patients become clear about what they want in a situation, to assist them in discerning and clarifying their values and examining available options in light of those values (Gadow 1990, 53).

15. The notion of a contract implies two autonomous and unconstrained individuals freely entering into negotiations on a level playing field (May 1989).

16. Cooper (1988); May (1983); Rodney (1997); Stenberg (1979).

17. In his article, Woods (1999) does an excellent job of exploring a variety of morally relevant relationships and considerations.

18. Bergum (1998); Gadow (1999); Hartrick (2002a; 2002b); MacDonald (2002); Rodney (1997); Rodney et al. (2002); Taylor (1997); Chapter 24 in this text.

19. Corley and Goren (1998); Gaudine and Beaton (2002); Johnstone (2002); Rodney and Varcoe (2001); Varcoe and Rodney (2002); Weiss et al. (2002); Chapter 10 in this text.

20. Baier (1994); Bowden (2000); Gilligan (1982); Noddings (1984).

21. Baier (1994); Blum (1994); Bowden (2000); Curzer (1993); Flanagan (1991); Flanagan and Jackson (1993); Fry (1991); Houston (1989); Kottow (2001); Kuhse (1997); Levi (1996); Liaschenko (1993); Morse et al. (1992); Nelson (1992); Olsen (1992); Pellegrino (1993); Puka (1989); Seigfried (1989); Sher (1987); Sherwin (1992a; 1992b); Shogan (1992); Tronto (1993); Wolf (1994).

22. Kuhse (1997) makes a similar point:

    While those approaching ethics from a perspective of care have done much to highlight the importance of dispositional [health-related] care, the importance of context and the uniqueness of persons, "care" in this sense can always constitute only a necessary, not a sufficient component of ethics. It does not and cannot constitute the whole of ethics (157).

23. Baier (1994); Bowden (2000); Kuhse (1997); Sherwin (1992a; 1992b; 1998); Tronto (1993).

24. An ethic of care primarily arose from Gilligan's (1982) work that challenged the dominant conventions of moral theory—primarily justice-oriented perspectives. Despite the critique of the adequacy of evidence for Gilligan's claims for gender-related difference in ethical thought, the acknowledgment of a significant (but overlooked) female voice of women's moral experience became the basis from which some feminist philosophers and theorists have looked towards the implications of care as an ethical concept (Bowden 2000).

25. For example, Baier (1994); Bowden (2000); Heckman (1995); Kuhse (1997); Mann (1994); Nussbaum (2001); Shogan (1992); Tong (1997); Tronto (1993).

26. It is worth noting that Nelson (1992) cautions that one cannot just "add justice and stir," as the concepts arise from quite different philosophical approaches.

27. For example, Botes (2000a; 2000b); Chally (1992); Cooper (1991); Lipp (1998); Omery (1991); Sherblom, Shipps, and Sherblom (1993); Starzomski (1997).

28. Bowden (2000); Cameron (1991); Frost (2003); Liaschenko (1993); Kuhse (1997); Rodney (1997); Volbrecht (2002); see also Chapters 8, 10–12, and 20 in this text.

29. This is not to say that intensive care ought to have fewer resources. It is to say that the lack of resources for non-specialty areas can be unjust (Rodney 1991; 1997).

30. Corley and Goren (1998); David (2000); Roberts (1983); Varcoe and Rodney (2002); Varcoe, Rodney, and McCormick (in press).

31. A third is ecological thinking in ethics. This will be examined in Chapter 11.

32. In using the term, we have some reservations about its distinctiveness. Specifically, we are cautious about the ambiguous and diverse meanings of modernity/postmodernity within and across cultural groups and academic disciplines (Bernstein 1991) and how this intellectual tradition has become a discursive practice "dominated primarily by the voices of white male intellectuals and/or academics elites who speak to and about one another with coded familiarity" (hooks 1995, 118). In the last decade, the term "postmodern" has become an increasingly popular label for the intellectual period at the end of the 20th century. Despite the assumption that the term "postmodern" represents a cohesive response to conditions of modernity, philosophical opinion about postmodernism is deeply divided. Cahoone (1996) claims that

    > for some, postmodernism connotes the final escape from the stultifying legacy of modern European theology, metaphysics, authoritarianism, colonialism, racism and domination. To others it represents the attempt by disgruntled left-wing intellectuals to destroy Western civilization. To yet others it labels a goofy collection of hermeneutically obscure writers who are really talking about nothing at all (1).

33. Hartrick (2002a); MacKenzie and Stoljar (2000); Sherwin (1992a; 1992b; 1998); Strum (1998).

34. An interesting related concept here is that of **cultural safety.** Cultural safety is the opposite of cultural risk, which occurs when people from one culture believe they are "demeaned, diminished or disempowered by the actions and the delivery systems of people from another culture" (Wood and Schwass 1993, 2). From a cultural safety perspective people feel their indigenous worth is reflected in health care provision (Reimer Kirkham et al. in review). The central themes of cultural safety include: (1) recognition of all health care interactions as bicultural; (2) the need to examine our own cultural realities as bearers of culture; (3) the ongoing interrogation of unequal power relations; and (4) a commitment to change the policies and structures that institutionalize inequitable treatment and sometimes outright racism (Polaschek 1998; Ramsden 1993; Ramsden and Spoonley 1993). See Kanitsaki, Giger and Davidhizar (2000) for a review and a critique of cultural safety.

REFERENCES

Anderson, J. 2002. Toward a postcolonial feminist methodology in nursing research: Exploring the convergence of postcolonial and black feminist scholarship. *Nurse Researcher, 9*(3), 7–27.

Armstrong, A.E., Parsons, S. and Barker, P.J. 2000. An inquiry into moral virtues, especially compassion, in psychiatric nurses: Findings from a Delphi study. *Journal of Psychiatric and Mental Health Nursing, 7*, 297–306.

Baier, A. 1994. *Moral prejudices: Essays on ethics.* Cambridge: Harvard University Press.

Bandman, E.L. and Bandman, B. 2002. *Nursing ethics through the life span.* 4th edition. Upper Saddle River, NJ: Prentice Hall.

Benner, P. 1991. The role of experience, narrative and community in skilled ethical comportment. *Advances in Nursing Science, 14*(2), 1–21.

Benner, P.A. 1994. Caring as a way of knowing and not knowing. In S. Philips and P.A. Benner (Eds.), *The crisis of care: Affirming and restoring caring practices in the helping professions* (pp. 42–62). Washington, D.C.: Georgetown University Press.

Benner, P. 2000. The roles of embodiment, emotion and lifeworld for rationality and agency in nursing practice. *Nursing Philosophy, 1*, 1–14.

Benner, P., Tanner, C.A. and Chesla, C.A. 1996. *Expertise in nursing practice.* New York: Springer.

Benner, P. and Wrubel, J. 1989. *The primacy of caring: Stress and coping in health and illness.* Menlo Park, CA: Addison-Wesley.

Bergum, V. 1998. Relational ethics. What is it? *In touch: The Provincial Health Ethics Network, 1*(2), 1–2.

Bernstein, R.J. 1991. *The new constellation: The ethical–political horizons of modernity/postmodernity.* Cambridge, MA: MIT Press.

Bhabha, H. 1994. *The location of culture.* London: Routledge.

Bishop, A.H. and Scudder, J.R. 1987. Nursing ethics in an age of controversy. *Advances in Nursing Science, 9*(3), 34–43.

Bishop, A.H. and Scudder, J.R. 1990. *The practical, moral, and personal sense of nursing: A phenomenological philosophy of practice.* Albany: SUNY Press.

Bishop, A. and Scudder, J. 2001. *Nursing ethics: Holistic caring practice.* 2nd edition. Boston: Jones and Bartlett.

Blum, L.A. 1994. *Moral perception and particularity.* Cambridge, UK: Cambridge University Press.

Botes, A. 2000a. A comparison between the ethics of justice and the ethics of care. *Journal of Advanced Nursing, 32*(5), 1071–1075.

Botes, A. 2000b. An integrated approach to ethical decision-making in the health care team. *Journal of Advanced Nursing, 32*(5), 1076–1082.

Bowden P. 2000. An "ethic of care" in clinical settings: Encompassing "feminine" and "feminist" perspectives. *Nursing Philosophy, 1*, 36–49.

Browne, A.J. and Smye, V. 2002. A postcolonial analysis of health care discourses addressing Aboriginal women. *Nurse Researcher, 9*(3), 28–41.

Cahoone, L. 1996. *From modernism to postmodernism: An anthology.* Cambridge: Blackwell.

Cameron, M.E. 1991. Justice, caring and virtue. *Journal of Professional Nursing, 7*(4), 206.

Campbell, M.L. 2001. Textual accounts, ruling action: The intersection of knowledge and power in the routine conduct of community nursing work. *Studies in Cultures, Organizations and Societies, 7*, 231–250.

Canadian Nurses Association. 2002. *Code of Ethics for Registered Nurses.* Ottawa: Canadian Nurses Association.

Chally, P.S. 1992. Moral decision-making in neonatal intensive care. *JGNN, 21*(6), 475–482.

Chambers-Evans, J. 2002. The family as window onto the world of the patient: Revising our approach to involving patients and families in the decision-making process. *Canadian Journal of Nursing Research, 34*(3), 15–32.

Chambliss, D.F. 1996. *Beyond caring: Hospitals, nurses, and the social organization of ethics.* Chicago: The University of Chicago Press.

Cooper, M.C. 1988. Convenantal relationships: Grounding for the nursing ethic. *Advanced Nursing Science, 10*(4), 48–59.

Cooper, M.C. 1989. Gilligan's different voice: A perspective for nursing. *Journal of Professional Nursing, 5*, 10–16.

Cooper, M.C. 1991. Principle-oriented ethics and the ethic of care: A creative tension. *Advances in Nursing Science, 14*(2), 22–31.

Corley, M.C. and Goren, S. 1998. The dark side of nursing: Impact of stigmatizing responses on patients. *Scholarly Inquiry for Nursing Practice, 12*(2), 99–118.

Cortis, J.D. and Kendrick, K. 2003. Nursing ethics, caring and culture. *Nursing Ethics, 10*(1), 77–88.

Curtin, L. 1979. The nurse as advocate: A philosophical foundation for nursing. *Advances in Nursing Science, 1*(3), 1–10.

Curtin, L. 1982. Human problems: Human beings. In L. Curtin and M.J. Flaherty (Eds.), *Nursing ethics: Theories and pragmatics* (pp. 37–42). Maryland: Robert J. Brady.

Curzer, H. 1993. Is care a virtue for health care professionals? *The Journal of Medicine and Philosophy, 18*, 51–69.

Daniels, N. 1996. Wide reflective equilibrium in practice. In L.W. Sumner and J. Boyle (Eds.), *Philosophical perspectives on bioethics* (pp. 96–114). Toronto: University of Toronto Press.

David, B.A. 2000. Nursing's gender politics: Reformulating the footnotes. *Advances in Nursing Science, 23*(1), 83–93.

Edwards, S.D. 2001. *Philosophy of nursing: An introduction.* Hampshire, UK: Palgrave.

Flaherty, M.J. 1982. Nursing's contract with society. In L. Curtin and M.J. Flaherty (Eds.), *Nursing ethics: Theories and pragmatics* (pp. 67–78). Maryland: Robert J. Brady.

Flanagan, O. 1991. *Varieties of moral personality.* Cambridge, MA: Harvard University Press.

Flanagan, O. and Jackson, K. 1993. Justice, care, and gender: The Kohlberg-Gilligan debate revisited. In M.J. Larrabee (Ed.), *An ethic of care: Feminist and interdisciplinary perspectives* (pp. 69–84). New York: Routledge.

Fox, R. 1990. The evolution of American bioethics: A sociological perspective. In G. Weisz (Ed.), *Social science perspectives on medical ethics* (pp. 201–217). Netherlands: Kluwer Academic.

Frost, L.J. 2003. *The paradox of a caring profession.* Unpublished masters thesis, Simon Fraser University, Burnaby, British Columbia.

Fry, S.T. 1987. Research on ethics in nursing: The state of the art. *Nursing Outlook, 35*(5), 246.

Fry, S.T. 1989. Toward a theory of nursing ethics. *Advances in Nursing Science, 11*(4), 9–22.

Fry, S.T. 1991. A theory of caring: pitfalls and promises. In D.A. Gaut and M. Leininger (Eds.), *Caring: The compassionate healer* (pp. 161–172). New York: National League for Nursing.

Fry, S.T. 1999. The philosophy of nursing. *Scholarly Inquiry in Nursing Practice, 13*(1), 5–15.

Fry, S. and Johnstone, M.J. 2002. *Ethics in nursing practice: A guide to ethical decision making.* 2nd edition. Oxford, UK: Blackwell.

Gadow, S. 1985. Nurse and patient: A caring relationship. In A.H. Bishop and J.R. Scudder (Eds.), *Caring, curing, coping: Nurse, physicain, patient relationships.* Alabama: University of Alabama Press.

Gadow, S. 1990. Existential advocacy. In T. Pence and J. Cantral (Eds.), *Ethics in nursing: An anthology* (pp. 41–51). New York: National League for Nursing.

Gadow, S. 1999. Relational narrative: The postmodern turn in nursing ethics. *Scholarly Inquiry in Nursing Practice, 13*(1), 57–70.

Gaudine, A.P. and Beaton, M.R. 2002. Employed to go against one's values: Nurse managers' accounts of ethical conflict within their organizations. *Canadian Journal of Nursing Research, 34*(2), 17–34.

Gaul, A.L. 1995. Casuistry, care, compassion, and ethics data analysis. *Advances in Nursing Science, 17*(3), 47–57.

Georges, J.-J. and Grypdonck, M. 2002. Moral problems experienced by nurses when caring for terminally ill people: A literature review. *Nursing Ethics, 9*(2), 155–178.

Gandhi, L. 1998. *Postcolonial theory: A critical introduction.* New York: Columbia University Press.

Gillett, G. 1995. Virtue and truth in clincial science. *Journal of Medicine and Philosophy, 20*(3), 285–298.

Gilligan, C. 1982. *In a different voice.* Cambridge, MA: Harvard University Press.

Gilligan, C. 1988. Remapping the moral domain: New images of self in relationship. In C. Gilligan, J.V. Ward, J. McLean Taylor and B. Bardige (Eds.), *Mapping the moral domain: A contribution to women's thinking to psychological theory and education* (pp. 3–19). Cambridge, MA: Harvard University Press.

Godkin, M.D. 2002. *Apprehending death: The older adult's experience of preparing an advance directive.* Unpublished doctoral dissertation. University of Alberta, Edmonton.

Greipp, M.E. 1995. Culture and ethics: A tool for analyzing the effects of biases on the nurse-patient relationship. *Nursing Ethics: An International Journal for Health Care Professionals, 2*(3), 211–221.

Hartrick Doane, G. 2002a. In the spirit of creativity: The learning and teaching of ethics in nursing. *Journal of Advanced Nursing, 39*(6), 521–528.

Hartrick Doane, G. 2002b. Am I still ethical? The socially-mediated process of nurses' moral identity. *Nursing Ethics, 9*(6), 623–635.

Heckman, S.J. 1995. *Moral voices, moral selves.* University Park, PA: Pennsylvania State University Press.

Hewitt, J. 2002. A critical review of the arguments debating the role of the nurse advocate. *Journal of Advanced Nursing, 37*(5), 439–445.

Hiltunen, E.F., Medich, C., Chase, S., Peterson, L. and Forrow, L. 1999. Family decision making for end-of-life treatment: The SUPPORT nurse narratives. *The Journal of Clinical Ethics, 10*(2), 126–134.

hooks, b. 1995. Postmodern blackness. In W.T. Anderson (Ed.), *The truth about the truth* (pp. 117–124). New York: G.P. Putnam's Sons.

Houston, B. 1989. Prolegomena to future caring. In M.M. Brabeck (Ed.), *Who cares? Theory, research, and educational implications of the ethic of care* (pp. 84–100). New York: Praeger.

Huggins, E. and Scalazi, C. 1988. Limitations and alternatives: Ethical practice theory in nursing. *Advances in Nursing Science, 10,* 43–47.

Jameton, A. 1984. *Nursing practice: The ethical issues.* Upper Saddle River, NJ: Prentice Hall.

Jezewski, M.A. 1994. Do-not-resuscitate status: Conflict and culture brokering in critical care units. *Heart & Lung, 23*(6), 458–465.

Johnstone, M.-J. 1999. *Bioethics: A nursing perspective.* 3rd edition. Sydney, Australia: Harcourt.

Johnstone, M.-J. 2002. Poor working conditions and the capacity of nurses to provide moral care. *Contemporary Nurse, 12*(1), 7–15.

Kanitsaki, O., Newman, J. and Davidhizar, R. 2000. Diversity in caring. In J. Crisp and C. Taylor (Eds.), *Potter & Perry's fundamentals of nursing* (pp. 114–137). Sydney, Australia: Mosby.

Kikuchi, J.F. and Simmons, H. (Eds.).1992. *Philosophical inquiry in nursing.* Newbury Park, CA: Sage.

Kikuchi, J.F. and Simmons, H. (Eds.). 1994. *Developing a philosophy of nursing.* Thousand Oaks, CA: Sage.

Kohnke, M.F. 1990. The nurse as advocate. In T. Pence and J. Cantral (Eds.), *Ethics in nursing: An anthology* (pp. 56–58). New York: National League for Nursing.

Kottow, M.H. 2001. Between caring and curing. *Nursing Philosophy, 2,* 53–61.

Kuhse, H. 1997. *Caring: Nurses, women and ethics.* Oxford: Blackwell.

Kvale, S. 1995. Themes of postmodernity. In W.T. Anderson (Ed.), *The truth about the truth* (pp. 18–15). New York: G.P. Putnam's Sons.

Levi, B.H. 1996. Four approaches to doing ethics. *The Journal of Medicine and Philosophy, 21,* 7–39.

Levine, M. 1977. Ethics: Nursing ethics and the ethical nurse. *American Journal of Nursing, 77*(5), 845–849.

Liaschenko, J. 1993. *Faithful to the good: Morality and philosophy in nursing practice.* Unpublished doctoral dissertation. University of California, San Francisco.

Lipp, A. 1998. An enquiry into a combined approach for nursing ethics. *Nursing Ethics, 5*(2), 122–138.

Lyotard, J.F. 1984. *The postmodern condition: A report on knowledge.* Manchester, UK: Manchester University Press.

Lützén, K. 1997. Nursng ethics into the next millennium: A context-sensitive approach for nursing ethics. *Nursing Ethics, 4,* 218–226.

Lützén, K. and Nordin, C. 1993. Structuring moral meaning in psychiatric nursing practice. *Scandinavian Journal of Caring Sciences, 7,* 175–180.

MacDonald, C. 2002. Nurse autonomy as relational. *Nursing Ethics, 9*(2), 194–201.

Mann, P.S. 1994. *Micro-politics: Agency in a postfeminist era.* Minneapolis, MN: University of Minnesota Press.

May, W. 1983. *The physician's covenant.* Philadelphia: Westminster Press.

May, W.F. 1989. Code, covenant, contract, or philanthropy. In R.M. Veatch (Ed.), *Cross cultural perspectives in medical ethics: Readings* (pp. 156–173). Boston: Jones & Bartlett.

Mackenzie, C. and Stoljar, N. 2000. Autonomy refigured. In C. Mackenzie and N. Stoljar. (Eds.), *Relational autonomy: Feminist perspectives on autonomy, agency and the social self* (pp. 3–31). New York: Oxford University Press.

McConaghy, C. 1997. *What constitutes today's colonialism? Reconsidering cultural relevance and mainstreaming in Indigenous social and educational policy.* Reading 4. Unpublished manuscript. Armidale Department of Educational Studies.

McMahah, E.M., Hoffman, K. and McGee, G.W. 1994. Physician–nurse relationships in clinical settings: A review and critique of the literature, 1966–1992. *Medical Care Review, 51*(1), 83–112.

Melia, K. 1994. The task of nursing ethics. *Journal of Medical Ethics, 20*(1), 7–11.

Mitchell, G.J. 2001. Policy, procedure and routine: Matters of moral influence. *Nursing Science Quarterly, 14*(2), 109–114.

Morse, J.M., Bottorff, J.L., Neander, W. and Solberg, S. 1992. Comparative analysis of conceptualizations and theories of caring. In J.M. Morse (Ed.), *Qualitative health research* (pp. 69–90). Newbury Park, CA: Sage.

Nagle, L.M. 1999. A matter of extinction or distinction. *Western Journal of Nursing Research, 21*(1), 71–82.

Nelson, H.L. 1992. Against caring. *The Journal of Clinical Ethics, 3*(1), 8–15.

Noddings, N. 1984. *Caring: A feminine approach to ethics and moral education.* Berkeley, CA: University of California Press.

Nortvedt, P. 1998. Sensitive judgement: An inquiry into the foundations of nursing ethics. *Nursing Ethics, 5*(5), 385–392.

Nortvedt, P. 2001. Clinical sensitivity: The inseparability of ethical perceptiveness and clinical knowledge. *Scholarly Inquiry of Nursing Practice, 15*(3), 1–19.

Noureddine, S. 2001. Development of the ethical dimension in nursing theory. *International Journal of Nursing Practice, 7,* 2–7.

Nussbaum, M.C. 2001. *Upheavals of thought: The intelligence of emotions.* New York: Cambridge University Press.

Olsen, D.P. 1992. Controversies in nursing ethics: A historical review. *Journal of Advanced Nursing, 17,* 1020–1027.

Omery, A. 1989. Values, moral reasoning and ethics. *Nursing Clinics of North America, 24*(2), 499–509.

Omery, A., Kasper and C.E., Page, G.G. (Eds.). 1995. *In search of nursing science* (pp. 72–80). Thousand Oaks, CA: Sage.

Paterson, J.G. and Zderad, L.T. 1988. *Humanistic nursing.* New York: National League for Nursing.

Pellegrino, E.D. and Thomasma, D.C. 1993. *The virtues in medical practice.* New York: Oxford University Press.

Pellegrino, E.D., Veatch, R.M. and Langan, J.P. 1991. Preface. In E.D. Pellegrino, R.M. Veatch and J.P. Langan (Eds.), *Ethics, trust, and the professions: Philosophical and cultural aspects* (pp. vii–ix). Washington, DC: Georgetown University Press.

Peter, E. and Morgan, K. 2001. Explorations of a trust approach for nursing ethics. *Nursing Inquiry, 8*, 3–10.

Polaschek, N.R. 1998. Cultural safety: A new concept in nursing people of different ethnicities. *Journal of Advanced Nursing, 27,* 452–457.

Puka, B. 1989. The liberation of caring: A different voice for Gilligan's "Different Voice." In M.M. Brabeck (Ed.), *Who cares? Theory, research, and educational implications of the ethic of care* (pp. 19–44). New York: Praeger.

Purkis, M.E. 1994. Entering the field: Intrusions of the social and its exclusion from studies of nursing practice. *International Journal of Nursing Studies, 31*(4), 315–336.

Quayson, A. 2000. *Postcolonialism: Theory, practice or process?* Cornwall: Polity.

Ramsden, I. 1993. Kawa Whakaruruhau. Cultural safety in nursing education in Aotearoa (New Zealand). *Nursing Praxis in New Zealand, 8(3)*, 4–10.

Ramsden, I. and Spoonley, P. 1993.The cultural safety debate in nursing education in Aotearoa. *New Zealand Annual Review of Education, 3*, 161–174.

Reed, P. 1989. Nursing theorizing as an ethical endeavor. *Advances in Nursing Science, 11*(3), 1–9.

Reimer Kirkham, S., Smye, V., Tang, S., Anderson, J., Blue, C., Coles, R., Henderson, A., Lynam, J., Perry, J., Shapero, L. and Semeniuk, P. In review. Waiting for the field: Rethinking cultural safety. (Manuscript submitted to *Research in Nursing and Health*).

Reynolds, W., Scott, P.A. and Austin, W. 2000. Nursing, empathy and perception of the moral. *Journal of Advanced Nursing, 32*(1), 235–242.

Roberts, S.J. 1983. Oppressed group behaviour: Implications for nursing. *Advances in Nursing Science 5*, 21–30.

Rodney, P., Varcoe, C., Storch, J. L., McPherson, G., Mahoney, K., Brown, H., Pauly, B., Hartrick, G., and Starzomski, R. 2002. Navigating toward a moral horizon: A multisite qualitative study of nurses' enactment of ethical practice. *Canadian Journal of Nursing Research, 34*(3), 75–102.

Rodney, P. 1991. Patients in shock: Some questions about resource allocation. *Canadian Critical Care Nursing Journal, 8*(3), 13–15.

Rodney, P.A. 1997. *Towards connectedness and trust: Nurses' enactment of their moral agency within an organizational context.* Unpublished doctoral dissertation. University of British Columbia, Vancouver, BC.

Rodney, P.A. and Varcoe, C. 2001. Toward ethical inquiry in the economic evaluation of nursing practice. *Canadian Journal of Nursing Research, 33*(1), 35–57.

Rorty, R. 1999. *Philosopy and social hope.* London: Penguin.

Salsberry, P.J. 1992. Caring, virtue theory, and a foundation for nursing ethics. *Scholarly Inquiry for Nursing Practice: An International Journal, 6*(2), 155–168.

Sawchuk, P.J. and Ross-Kerr, J. 2000. Choices, decisions and control: Older adults and advance care directives. *Canadian Nurse, 96*(7), 16–20.

Seigfried, C.H. 1989. Pragmatism, feminism, and sensitivity to context. In M.M. Brabeck (Ed.), *Who cares? Theory, research, and educational implications of the ethic of care* (pp. 63–83). New York: Praeger.

Shogan, D. (Ed.). 1992. *A reader in feminist ethics.* Toronto: Canadian Scholars' Press.

Sher, G. 1987. Other voices, other rooms? Women's psychology and moral theory. In E.V. Kittay and D.T. Meyers (Eds.), *Women and moral theory* (pp.178–189). Rowan & Littlefield.

Sherblom, S., Shipps, T.B. and Sherblom, J.C. 1993. Justice, care, and integrated concerns in the ethical decision making of nurses. *Qualitative Health Research, 3*(4), 442–464.

Sherwin, S. 1992a. Feminist and medical ethics: Two different approaches to contextual ethics. In H. Bequaret Holmes and L. Purdy (Eds.), *Feminist perspectives in medical ethics* (pp. 17–31). Indianapolis, IN: Indiana University.

Sherwin, S. 1992b. *No longer patient: Feminist ethics and health care.* Philadelphia: Temple University Press.

Sherwin, S. 1998. A relational approach to autonomy in health care. In S. Sherwin (Ed.), *The politics of women's health: Exploring agency and autonomy* (pp. 19–47). Philadelphia: Temple University Press.

Simpson, C. 2002. Hope and feminist care ethics: What is the connection? *Canadian Journal of Nursing Research, 34*(2), 81–94.

Smith, K.V. and Godfrey, N.S. 2002. Being a good nurse and doing the right thing: A qualitative study. *Nursing Ethics, 9*(3), 301–312.

Smye, V., and Browne, A.J. 2002. Cultural safety and the analysis of health policy affecting aboriginal people. *Nurse Researcher, 9*(3), 42–56.

Squires, J. 1993. Introduction. In J. Squires (Ed.), *Principled positions: Postmodernism and the rediscovery of value* (pp. 1–13). London: Lawrence and Wishart.

Starzomski, R. 1997. *Resource allocation for solid organ transplantation: Toward public and health care provider dialogue.* Unpublished doctoral dissertation, University of British Columbia, Vancouver, BC.

Stenberg, M.J. 1979. The search for a conceptual framework as a philosophic basis for nursing ethics: An examination of code, contract, context, and covenant. *Military Medicine, 144*(1), 9–22.

Stephenson, P. 1999. Expanding notions of culture for cross-cultural ethics in health and medicine. In H. Coward and P. Ratanakul (Eds.), *A cross-cultural dialogue on health care ethics* (pp. 68–91). Waterloo, ON: Wilfrid Laurier University Press.

Storch, J.L. 1992. Ethical issues. In A.J. Baumgart and J. Larsen (Eds.), *Canadian nursing faces the future,* 2nd ed. (pp. 259–270). St. Louis, MO: Mosby Year Book.

Storch, J. 1999. Moral relationships between nurse and client: The influence of metaphors. In E.-H. Kluge (Ed.), *Readings in biomedical ethics: A Canadian focus* (pp. 145–154). Scarborough, ON: Prentice Hall.

Storch, J., Rodney, P., Pauly, B., Brown, H. and Starzomski, R. 2002. Listening to nurses's moral voices: Building a quality health care environment. *Canadian Journal of Nursing Leadership, 15*(4), 7–16.

Strum, D. 1998. *The politics of relationality.* New York: State University of New York Press.

Taylor, C. 1992. *Multiculturalism and the politics of recognition.* Princeton: Princeton University Press.

Taylor, C. 1995. Medical futility and nursing. *Image, 27*(4), 301–306.

Taylor, C. 1997. Everyday nursing concerns: Unique? Trivial? Or essential to healthcare ethics? *HEC Forum, 9*(1), 68–84.

Thompson, I.E., Melia, K. and Boyd, K.M. 1994. *Nursing ethics.* Edinburgh, UK: Churchill Livingstone.

Tilden, V.P., Tolle, S.W., Nelson, C.A., Thonpson, M. and Eggman, S.C. 1999. Family decision making in foregoing life-extending treatments. *Journal of Family Nursing, 5*(4), 426–442.

Tong, R. 1997. *Feminist approaches to bioethics: Theoretical reflections and practical applications.* Boulder, CO: Westview.

Tronto, J.C. 1993. *Moral boundaries: A political argument for an ethic of care.* New York: Routledge.

Tuhiwai Smith, L. 1999. *Decolonizing methodologies: Research and indigenous peoples.* London: Zed.

Varcoe, C. 1997. *Untying our hands: The social context of nursing in relation to violence against women.* Unpublished doctoral dissertation. University of British Columbia, Vancouver, BC.

Varcoe, C. 2001. Abuse obscured: An ethnographic account of emergency nursing in relation to violence against women. *Canadian Journal of Nursing Research, 32*(4), 95–115.

Varcoe, C. and Rodney, P. 2002. Constrained agency: The social structure of nurses work. In B.S. Bolaria and H.D. Dickinson (Eds.), *Health, illness and health care in Canada,* 3rd ed. (pp. 102–128). Scarborough, ON: Nelson Thomson Learning.

Varcoe, C. and Rodney, P. 2003. Trends and new thinking. In G. Doane (Ed.), *Rethinking ethics education in nursing* (pp. 40–59). Unpublished manuscript. University of Victoria School of Nursing, Victoria, BC.

Varcoe, C., Rodney, P. and McCormick, J. In press. Health care relationships in context: An analysis of three ethnographies. *Qualitative Health Research.*

Veatch, R. 1981. Nursing ethics, physician ethics, and medical ethics. *Law, Medicine and Health Care, 9,* 17–19.

Veatch, R.M. and Fry, S.T. 1987. *Case studies in nursing ethics.* London: J.B. Lippincott.

Volbrecht, R.M. 2002. *Nursing ethics: Communities in dialogue.* New Jersey: Prentice Hall.

Watson, J. 1988. *Nursing: Human science and human care.* New York: National League for Nursing.

Winslow, G.R. 1990. From loyalty to advocacy: A new metaphor for nursing. In T. Pence and J. Cantral (Eds.), *Ethics in nursing: An anthology.* New York: National League for Nursing.

Weiss, S.M., Malone, R.E., Merighi, J.R. and Benner, P. 2002. Economism, efficiency, and the moral ecology of good nursing practice. *Canadian Journal of Nursing Research, 34*(2), 95–119.

Wolf, S.M. 1994. Shifting paradigms in bioethics and health law: The rise of a new pragmatism. *American Journal of Law & Medicine, 20*(4), 395–415.

Wood, P. and Schwass, M. 1993. Cultural safety: A framework for changing attitudes. *Nursing Praxis, 8*(1), 4–15.

Woods, M. 1999. A nursing ethic: The moral voice of experienced nurses. *Nursing Ethics, 6*(5), 423–433.

Wurzbach, M.E. 1999. The moral metaphors of nursing. *Journal of Advanced Nursing, 30*(1), 94–99.

Yarling, R.R. and McElmurry, B. J. 1986. The moral foundation of nursing. *Advances in Nursing Science, 8*(2), 63–73.

Yeo, M. 1989. Integration of nursing theory and nursing ethics. *Advances in Nursing Science, 11*(3), 33–42.

Zoucha, R. and Husted, G.L. 2000. The ethical dimensions of delivering culturally congruent nursing and health care. *Issues in Mental Health Nursing, 21,* 325–340.

chapter eight

Moral Agency: Relational Connections and Trust

Patricia Rodney,
Helen Brown, and
Joan Liaschenko

The dominant rationalist view... has given us a model of ourselves as disengaged thinkers (Charles Taylor 1995, 63).

The dominant rationalist view with its focus on disengaged thinkers, which Canadian philosopher Charles Taylor critiques, has not served nursing well. It tends to reduce moral problems to binary solutions,[1] thereby diminishing the interface of moral problems with the human experiences of nurses, their clients, and their colleagues in other disciplines. Moreover, it provides a limited conceptual vantage point from which to understand the interface of nurses with the complex—and increasingly problematic—sociopolitical health care environments in which they practice.[2] This has rendered nurses' moral agency largely invisible.[3] In this chapter, we will argue that understanding the intersection between nursing knowledge and nursing work helps us to better appreciate the moral situation of nurses. We will further argue that nurses' enactment of their moral agency is influenced by gender and context and is profoundly dialogical and relational. Lastly, we will argue that authentic presence and trust are important elements of the network of relationships within which nurses enact their moral agency. We close by reflecting on the implications of our arguments for collaborative practice. Throughout the chapter, it is our premise that unless nurses are able to enact their moral agency, they will have difficulty fulfilling their professional responsibilities. Such difficulty is to the detriment of patient/family/community care and to the detriment of nurses and other health care providers.[4]

Nurses are not disengaged thinkers, and neither are the rest of the persons they encounter in their practice. It is encouraging to note that our current scholarship is increasingly reflecting this realization.[5] Here we wish to contribute to the growing dialogue by providing our own analyses of nurses as moral agents. In the next section of this text—specifically Chapters 10, 11, and 12—Rodney and other authors will say more about how nurses' moral agency is constrained by the moral climate of their workplaces, with some suggestions as to how we might improve that climate and hence nursing practice.

We start this chapter with two accounts of practice from nurses in direct care. We then visit the everyday nature of nursing knowledge, linking this knowledge to nurses' work. This leads us to a more detailed explication of nurses' moral agency, including the influence of gender, context, and relationships. We subsequently look at nurses' relational connections, including moral agency in a collaborative context. In so doing, we draw on research focused on nursing ethics to show how nurses work in an interconnected web (matrix) of relationships with their colleagues in nursing and other disciplines. We conclude by emphasizing the importance of trust in sustaining relationships with colleagues. Overall, this chapter identifies theoretical themes that are picked up in different ways through the remaining chapters of the book. In the subsequent chapters, these themes are enriched by the diverse theoretical and practice backgrounds of the various authors.

CONCEPTUALIZING MORAL AGENCY

Before we proceed, we will make more explicit what we mean by **moral agency.** Within the overall field of ethics, the traditional view of an agent is that of a person who is capable of deliberate action and/or who is in the process of deliberate action (Angeles 1981, 6). An agent may engage in deliberate action with or without moral overtones. It is the former variety that we are interested in, which we will term "moral agency." Characteristics that have been used by philosophers to define moral agency include rationality, autonomy, and (limited) self-interest (Sherwin 1992b, 41). Thus, traditional perspectives on moral agency reflect a notion of individuals engaging in self-determining or self-expressive choice (Taylor 1992, 57). Those perspectives have been greatly influenced by Immanuel Kant, who had human dignity and rationality at the centre of his moral view (Taylor 1989, 364).[6]

Over the past two decades or so, critics within philosophy and health care ethics[7] have raised concerns about theories of moral agency. Feminist and other contextual theorists have come to understand agency as enacted through **relationships** in particular **contexts** (Mackenzie and Stoljar 2000a; McNay 2000; Mann 1994; Sherwin 1992; 1998; Taylor, 1992).[8] For instance, Sherwin (1992a; 1992b; 1998) critiques traditional perspectives on moral agency that arise in the form of ethical theory dominating contemporary Anglo-American philosophy—that is, Kantian deontology, consequentialism (one form of which is utilitarianism), and contractarianism.[9] Sherwin notes that Kantian theory "does not direct us to make our ethical assessments in terms of particular details of the lives of... individuals," and that utilitarianism "discounts some important features," such as the particulars of relationships and the positions of the oppressed (1992a, 20–21). Sherwin notes similar problems with contractarianism. She claims that contractarianism has an individualistic bias such that "individuals are encouraged to consider themselves and their interests as independent from others" (Sherwin 1992a, 23).[10]

Thus, one problem with traditional perspectives on moral agency is that they presuppose a "level playing field" (Rodney 1997). This misses the multiple kinds of relationships that exist within society in which there is an asymmetry of **power** between agents; for instance, it misses parent-child relationships and nurse-patient relationships (Baier 1994; Sherwin 1992b). Such asymmetries are not unusual in health care and have diverse causes. Moral agents in health care (patients, families, and professionals/providers) are not as "equal" and autonomous as the traditional perspectives might assume.

Second, the traditional focus on rationality and self-interest neglects the relational, contextual nature of moral agency (Rodney 1997). This abstract neutrality is particularly objectionable from the perspective of feminist ethics, which demands an explicit focus on the social and political contexts of individuals in its moral deliberations (Sherwin 1992b, 40). Women "are assumed to fall under the general rubric of 'the agent,' but the moral concerns that are examined are always those most salient from the male perspective" (Sherwin 1992b, 44).

In fact, feminists are especially interested in **constraints** on women's agency:

> On the most general level, a revised understanding of agency has long been the explicit or implicit concern of feminist research devoted to the uncovering of the marginalized experiences of women. These experiences attest to the capacity for autonomous action in the face of often overwhelming cultural sanctions and structural inequities (McNay 2000, 10).

While there are various forms of feminist theory that pursue questions about agency in different ways (McNay 2000; Sherwin 1998), in this chapter, we are particularly interested in *relational* approaches. Such approaches "focus attention on the need for a more fine-grained and richer account of the autonomous *agent* [italics in original]" (Mackenzie and Stoljar 2000b, 21). As Mackenzie and Stoljar (2000b) explain,

> ... [A]n analysis of the characteristics and capacities of the self cannot be adequately undertaken without attention to the rich and complex social and historical contexts in which agents are embedded; they point to the need to think of autonomy as a characteristic of agents who are emotional, embodied, desiring, creative and feeling, as well as rational, creatures; and they highlight the ways in which agents are both psychically internally differentiated and socially differentiated from others (21).

Agents are seen as relational "because their identities or self-conceptions are constituted by elements of the social context in which they are embedded" and "because their natures are produced by certain historical and social conditions" (Mackenzie and Stoljar 2000b, 22).

As can be seen from the above, there is an important reciprocity between agency and **autonomy.** Sherwin (1998) explains that "[t]o exercise agency, one need only exercise reasonable choices" (32), while to be autonomous means, minimally, "to resist oppression" (Sherwin 1998, 33). This requires us to consider not only the kinds of choices that agents make, but also the circumstances and relationships that are affecting their ability to make those choices. *For the purposes of this chapter, then, our conceptualization of moral agency includes rational and self-expressive choice, notions of identity, social and historical relational influences, and autonomous action.* When autonomy is threatened, we will speak of moral agency as being constrained.[11]

Theorists from other contextual perspectives also expand our understanding of moral agency for this chapter. For instance, Charles Taylor (1995) critiques the old epistemological idea of a single agent engaged in monological acts, claiming instead that some actions (for example, log sawing or ballroom dancing) "require and sustain an integrated agent" (171–172). What we take Taylor to mean here is that many acts require the co-ordinated action of more than one agent, which is congruent with our interest in relational connections.

There are some resonances here with the feminist theorist Patricia Mann (1994), who claims that "individual moral agency is typically interactive, necessarily understood in terms of relations between two or more individuals" (14). Mann also claims that moral agency refers to "those individual or group actions deemed significant within a particular social or institutional setting" (14).

Taylor (1995) further posits moral agency as engaged, where "the world of the agent is shaped by one's form of life, or history, or bodily existence" (62; see also Benner 2000). Taylor (1995) goes on to explain:

> Our body is not just the executant of the goals we frame, nor just the locus of causal factors shaping our representations. Our understanding itself is embodied. That is, our bodily know-how, and the way we act and move, can encode components of our understanding of self and world (170).

Adding Taylor's (1992; 1995) conceptualization of moral agency to what we have distilled from feminist theorists,[12] we see moral agency as inclusive of rational and self-expressive choice, notions of identity, social and historical relational influences, autonomous action, and embodied engagement.[13]

NURSES' VOICES

In an ethnographic study of nurses practising on two acute medical units, nurses spoke of the importance of the relationships they had with their colleagues in nursing and other disciplines, as well as with patients and their family members. A sense of **connectedness** and **trust** in these relationships enabled them to feel more able to deal with ethical problems in their practice (Rodney 1997). In Ethics in Practice 8-1, two nurses from the study talk in separate interviews about the ethics of their practice. While they do not explicitly use the language of ethics, they say a great deal about how they operate as moral agents—that is, how they act to promote what they see as "the good" of patients and patients' families.[14] The first nurse participant, a relatively inexperienced nurse, talks of how much she relies on her experienced nurse colleagues to help her with patient crises. The second participant, who has years of nursing experience on an acute medical unit, talks of how she continues to rely on her colleagues to help her "see a pattern."

Ethics in Practice 8-1	Working Together

First Nurse Participant: You know, the thing is that you often get ways of working around [dealing with a patient crisis].... [O]ther nurses have lots of experience and so you work together to figure out what to do. There's some things written in the policy and procedure, but yet, that's not really [enough]. I mean it works out fine in the end, but if you come up with a situation that you've never seen before or nobody has seen before then you can run into a problem.

Second Nurse Participant: I think you know, [with] really critically ill people and really anxious scenarios we, we have to take our leads from what is being said... by the family and that and go from there till we can see a pattern, and the pattern may not show up for a week or two sort of thing,... especially

where we have so many of our own personnel involved because we're all
[working eight hour shifts] and so
there's a lot of turnover and everybody
works and sees things through different
eyes.... Well what we also do... is ask for
feedback among ourselves like "What
do you think...?" or "How do you see

this?"... [S]ometimes you wonder if its
your own perception or maybe it's... a
pattern that's coming up in [the perception of]... other staff members as well
and that's... why we have conferences
too sometimes or... why we leave notes
for one another... just so that we don't
get misled (Rodney 1997, 142).

Both nurses in Ethics in Practice 8-1—and every other nurse in the study—emphasized
the importance of their relationships with their colleagues. We will say more about this as
we proceed in this chapter and revisit these nurses' words periodically throughout our
analyses. At this point, we turn to examine the relationships between nursing knowledge
and nurses' work as essential for understanding nurses' enactment of moral agency and
ethical nursing practice.

NURSES' KNOWLEDGE AND NURSES' WORK

Knowledge is a critical aspect of morality (Audi 1997; Flanagan 1991). We act in accordance with what we know or believe to be the case about the material and social world.
Responsibility for our actions can be influenced by the knowledge we have about the situation and moral agents involved. A moral agent can be released from responsibility for
their actions, or held less responsible for them, if they lacked knowledge that would have
led them to judge and act differently. On the other hand, we can be held responsible for
knowledge we should have had in specific situations. This sounds straightforward and
uncomplicated enough. However, as the two nurse participants in Ethics in Practice 8-1
indicated, acquiring knowledge is a process fraught with uncertainty ("if you come up with
a situation that you've never seen before or nobody has seen before" and "everybody works
and sees things through different eyes"). We can appreciate that acquiring knowledge is
complicated and involves appreciation of cultural norms, experience, the particular circumstances, consequences, and other features. And when moral agents are set in highly
complex social organizations with multiple moral agents in multiple relational networks,
the relations between knowledge and morality are even more complex (Liaschenko 1997;
Liaschenko and Fisher 1999).

Knowledge is always distributed in societies—that is, some groups have knowledge of
some things and not others, or the knowledge may vary by degree between groups. This
knowledge may be formal or informal. To provide an example, a registered nurse in a rehabilitation setting knows how to organize the activity, rest, socialization, medication, and
other regimes for residents. He or she also has knowledge of the occupational therapy and
physiotherapy treatments the residents are receiving. However, specialized rehabilitation
knowledge is required for a number of treatments (e.g., treatment for swallowing difficulties, work on regaining balance and neuromuscular tone). While the nurse participates in
the ongoing implementation of the residents' programs of treatment and care, he or she
also relies on the expert knowledge of his or her colleagues in rehabilitation. And, of
course, the reverse is also true.

This is what we mean by saying that knowledge is distributed. When many people are involved in working to produce an outcome, the knowledge is typically distributed along a continuum that depends not only on formal divisions specified by educational requirements and licensing, but also on other features. These other features include, for example, experience and location. Experience is necessary for the transformation of a novice to an expert (Benner 1984; 1991; Benner and Wrubel 1989; Benner, Tanner and Chesla 1996). Location of the work is relevant because locations bind knowledge in particular ways (Stein-Parbury and Liaschenko in review). All the health care professionals working in a rehabilitation setting, for instance, will know more about rehabilitation than their colleagues working in critical care—this is the whole point of specialization. Indeed, the nurses in Ethics in Practice 8-1 emphasized the importance of experience ("other nurses have lots of experience and so you work together to figure out what to do"), and they were speaking from their specialized location of an acute medical unit. Understanding how knowledge is distributed therefore helps us to understand some of the social and historical contexts in which nurses as moral agents are embedded, and it helps us to understand some of their differentiation from moral agents in other disciplines.

In direct patient care the key moral agents involved are those closest to the patient and the patient's family: nurses, physicians, and their colleagues in other disciplines. Knowledge essential to patient care includes (but is not limited to) knowledge of anatomy and physiology, the pathophysiology of disease, therapeutics, and human responses to illness (*case knowledge*). It also requires knowledge of how the disease is manifest in this particular patient, any unique features of anatomy and physiology in this patient, and how this patient responds to treatments (*patient knowledge*). It may require knowledge of the patient's unique biography and how they understand the meaning of the disease and its treatment in their lives (*person knowledge*) (Liaschenko and Fisher 1999). None of this knowledge is exclusive to any particular discipline among health care providers. If it were, the work could not be done. However, there are clearly levels of emphasis, focus, and legal parameters in how the knowledge is distributed. Patient care also typically requires knowledge about how to get things done within an institutional setting—or a relational network that may involve many institutions or settings, such as in-patient practices programs and community care networks (Liaschenko 1998).

Critical to case, patient, and person knowledge is *social knowledge*. By social knowledge we mean knowledge of human beings in situations in which the individual is a subject, (that is, a moral actor) and not an object. In other words, it includes knowledge about social relations. The difference is particularly relevant to patient knowledge because patient knowledge can be knowledge of the patient primarily as an object or primarily as a subject. For example, certain kinds of measures of a patient's response to treatment, such as blood oxygenation or hematocrit, are knowledge of the patient as an object. However, knowledge of the patient as a subject would be, for example, knowing that the patient does not take medication in the way prescribed because the patient is resisting the establishment of a routine that disrupts his or her previously known life. Even case knowledge is social in the important sense that human beings work together to produce case knowledge. *Who* the people are is critical. In nursing, for instance, knowing the individual physician is an important piece of knowledge that nurses use in caring for surgical intensive care unit patients (Liaschenko and Fisher 1999). Knowing the physician provides nurses with various kinds of knowledge: preferred techniques and drugs, the latitude nurses have in exercising their discretionary judgment about when to call and when to take a "watch and see" attitude. For nurses, all forms of knowledge are central to their location within a complex system. This knowledge both informs and arises from moral action and makes it possible. For instance, nurses have and require knowledge of other moral agents, the routines which make up the everyday flow of activities that are health care work, and how to get things done.

If we are to understand the nature of nurses' moral work, we must better understand the nature of knowledge used by nurses in their practice (Liaschenko and Fisher 1999; see also Manias and Street 2001). Looking at the connection between knowledge and work, as we have begun to sketch above, allows us to pay attention to more than what has traditionally been described as knowledge in nursing. Everyday nursing knowledge does not necessarily resonate with what has been constructed in the past as knowledge for practice—nursing theories, nursing diagnoses, outcome measures, and the nursing process may actually have little meaning for nurses in practice (Liaschenko and Fisher 1999). The work of nursing can best be captured in an integration of the language of the everyday work of caring for patients and the language of science. Similarly, the nature of knowledge is inseparable from nursing work—reflective of the historical invisibility and silencing of what counts as nursing knowledge (Liaschenko 1997).[15] For example, the "witnessing and telling" that make up the ways in which nurses "know how" in their practice does not fit with many previously established accounts of nursing knowledge (Liaschenko 1997; 1998).

NURSES' MORAL AGENCY

The previous description of the intersection between nursing knowledge and nursing work helps us to understand the moral situation of nurses, since both nursing knowledge and nursing work are socially-mediated processes that are part of the contextual realities of nursing practice. Here we would like to further explore the notion of nurses' moral agency.[16] Health care professionals such as nurses are considered to have a particular kind of moral agency because of the unique knowledge and skills—and hence power—they hold (Danis and Churchill 1991; Fowler 1990; Jennings, Callahan and Wolf 1987; Poff and Waluchow 1991; Rodney 1997; Starzomski and Rodney 1997). Yet our knowledge of the ethics of professional practice is far from complete (Brunk 1991; Pellegrino, Veatch and Langan 1991; Liaschenko and Peter in review; Saks 1995). As Pellegrino, Veatch, and Langan explain, "the whole edifice of ethics in the professions has become problematic. Professionals themselves are confused about the nature of their obligations and the moral values that ought to govern their relationships with those who seek their help" (vii). Although Pellegrino and his colleagues made this observation over a decade ago, we still do not know a great deal about how nurses and other health care professionals/providers *enact* their moral agency.[17] We need to have a better sense of this if we are to support the ethical practice of nurses and our colleagues in other disciplines, and so we will say more here about nurses.

Nurses' actions arise from a primary commitment to patients. This commitment is therefore an important site for inquiry about moral agency and ethical practice. Nursing has as its foremost mandate a professional and ethical commitment to promoting the health and well-being of patients. Since nurses' primary ethical and professional commitment is to patients, the nurse-patient relationship is often viewed as the moral foundation of nursing practice (Peter and Morgan 2001) and, therefore, represents a central site of nursing work (Bishop and Scudder 1990; 1999; 2001; Gadow 1980; Yarling and McElmurry 1986; see also Chapter 7). This commitment means that nursing by its very nature is a moral endeavour (Bishop and Scudde 1990; Liaschenko 1995; Paterson and Zderad 1988; Smith and Godfrey 2002). A commitment to patients, coupled with the fact that nurses are the largest group of health care providers consistently with patients, helps to delineate the importance of nurses' status as moral agents (Georges and Grypdonack 2002; Yarling and McElmurry 1986). Yet that status is contested.

Contested Agency

Gender and Context

The nature of nursing work is mediated by the social location of nursing as a predominately women's profession. As will be highlighted in different ways in several chapters in this text, this social location has a profound impact on nurses' enactment of their moral agency. We will argue here that **gender** problems threaten nurses' autonomy as moral agents.[18] In so doing, we will be taking up feminist concerns about the marginalized experiences of women.

Questions about the social status of women and nursing mark the landscape of what nursing is about, both historically and for the future. Many of the contemporary assumptions regarding nursing work have their roots in the cultural tradition of the 19th century—a century marked by highly differentiated status between women and men, reflecting hierarchical social organization and authoritarian lines of command (Kuhse 1997).[19] Nursing has been described as a metaphor for subordinated femininity and most often described as a "natural" extension of a woman's role such that the status afforded to women and nurses has been and continues to be compared (David 2000). Women's historic invisibility and the language that sustains such invisibility are long-standing problems for nursing as a female-dominated profession. Kuhse asserts that a lack of women's visibility has contributed to the undervaluing of nursing care as part of socially assigned women's work. The language of women's work shapes the way in which nursing work is valued on personal, professional, institutional, and societal levels. David (2000) adds that language and power intersect to perpetuate the insidious nature of nurses' oppression. Since nursing has a history of subordination in health care settings, and of being composed primarily of women, we believe that any analysis of the socialization and practice of nursing work must thoughtfully attend to nurses' historically constructed experiences. Attending to such experiences can expose how language and power intersect, which can facilitate a language of social change in nursing (David 2000; Latimer 2000). The latter goal will be picked up in the next section of this text.

Social discourses shaping nursing work that are particularly relevant in an exploration of nurses' moral agency are the textual and social conversations arising from locating **caring** as *the* moral foundation for nursing.[20] Caring language, as it is taken up in nursing, both legitimizes and marginalizes different subject positions (David 2000). The texts of caring in nursing have frequently constructed caring as evolving from a nurse's character and individual motivation for caring while ignoring both the material conditions and power relations in the particular contexts where nurses work (MacPherson 1991). As the feminist theorists whom we cited at the outset of this chapter have claimed, the material conditions and power relations matter. For example, the nurses in Ethics in Practice 8-1 were attempting to provide (even basic) nursing care for elderly and critically ill patients on the acute medical unit where they worked, yet the nursing staffing was such that their work was characterized by a race against the clock (Rodney 1997). The nurses themselves had almost no say in administrative decisions about their **conditions of work.**[21] Care, with its gendered connotation in Western culture, is all too easily, in our view, reduced to feminine character and virtue and evaluation of what it means to be a "good nurse." For instance, the concept of "burnout" in nursing locates the "problem" in the hands of the professional nurse as one who fails to have the personal resiliency necessary for work-related demands. Attention is neither paid to the sociopolitical context of that work nor to the apparent unreasonableness of being overworked. For these reasons, care and the related social practices it entails become problematic as the moral foundation for nursing when issues of power, social justice, and domination remain obscured and unaccounted for (Bowden 1997; 2000; Liaschenko and Peter 2003).[22]

Finally, it is clear that since nursing is a profession predominantly (although not exclusively) pursued by women, a disciplinary, social, cultural, political, *and* gender-based analysis of nursing is necessary when examining the moral work of nursing and nurses' moral agency. In other words we will not be able to understand—and hence support—nurses' enactment of their moral agency if we think of nurses as isolated, rational individuals who are discharging their professional ethical obligations. Nurses' sociopolitical position greatly influences what they are able to accomplish. A body of emerging nursing research is emphasizing the **contextual** as well as the relational nature of nurses' enactment of their moral agency.[23]

Moral Sequelae

We have argued that nurses' sociopolitical position influences what they are able to accomplish as moral agents. While nurses have great capacity and resilience—and are quite skilful in navigating the complexities of the practice world (Rodney et al. 2002; Varcoe and Rodney 2002)—they are too often limited in their autonomy as moral agents. There are significant moral sequelae for such problems with autonomy. And there is an expanding theoretical and empirical literature in nursing that is tracking sequelae such as moral distress.

Moral distress is a concept that started to gain prominence in the nursing literature as a result of the work of the American ethicist Andrew Jameton (1984). The concept was later used by an American nurse researcher, Judith Wilkinson (1985), in her qualitative study of nurses in a variety of practice areas. *Essentially, we have come to understand moral distress as being what nurses (or any moral agents) experience when they are constrained from moving from moral choice to moral action.* In nursing, it is associated with experiences of anger, frustration, guilt, and powerlessness.[24] Reflecting back to the nurses in Ethics in Practice 8-1, for instance, we said earlier that they were attempting to provide nursing care for elderly and critically ill patients on the acute medical unit where they worked, yet their work was characterized by a race against the clock (Rodney 1997). This often left them feeling frustrated and inadequate, especially as the nurses themselves felt powerless to affect their conditions of work. In other words, they were experiencing moral distress. It is our contention that constraints to nurses' autonomy as moral agents, and their resultant moral distress, threaten the well-being of nurses and the well-being of patients and families.

In recent years, there has been growing interest in the theoretical development of moral distress as a concept and empirical measurement of that concept. Empirical studies continue to identify moral distress in nursing practice (for example, Corley 2002; Hefferman and Heilig 1999; Fry et al. 2002), and nurse theorists continue to express concern about the prevalence of moral distress (e.g., Hamric 2000; Mitchell 2001; Redman and Fry 2000). Definitional work has been taking place to explore related phenomena such as ethical distress and stress (e.g., Lützén et al. 2003; Raines 2000).[25] There is also work being done to develop and evaluate a moral distress scale (Corley et al. 2001). And models describing the moral phenomena leading to moral distress are being developed and tested (e.g., Corley 2002; Fry et al. 2002).To illustrate, Fry et al. (2002) have developed a model of a military moral distress phenomenon that includes *initial* moral distress, associated with perceptions of barriers and feelings, and *reactive* moral distress, associated with experiences, effects, and consequences of moral distress over time. All of this work on the theoretical development and measurement of the concept is important. As is explained in Chapter 10, while there is compelling empirical work linking the quality of nurses' workplaces to patient and nurse outcomes, we do not yet have a way to statistically correlate these outcomes with moral phenomena. Yet the empirical and experiential data we have to date indicates that moral phenomena have a profound effect on the quality of nurses' workplaces and therefore work.

We still have a great deal to learn about moral distress and the phenomena associated with it. For one, it is probably not a linear process of cause (constraints) and effect (moral distress). In a qualitative meta-analysis of three ethnographic studies[26] that one of us (Rodney) was involved in, our understanding of moral distress shifted. Rather than focusing on just individual action, we came to see a network of individuals acting in relation to one another, sometimes in ways that worsened moral distress and sometimes in ways that resolved it (Varcoe, Rodney and McCormick in press). It was not just external constraints such as excessive workloads that got in the way of moral action. It was also how interconnected individuals acted in relation to each other to facilitate or constrain moral action—nurses sometimes exercised coercive power over each other as well as over the patients and families they worked with (Varcoe, Rodney and McCormick in press). We need to understand more about this "dark side" of nursing (Corley and Goren 1998) so as to promote more ethical practice.[27]

Regardless of the particular conceptualization, the cumulative effects of moral distress are being recognized as a serious concern. Two Canadian ethicists, Webster and Baylis (2000), have claimed that unresolved moral distress can lead to moral compromise and **moral residue**—moral residue being what we carry with us when we knew how we should act but were unwilling and/or unable to do so (see also Mitchell 2001; Varcoe, Rodney and McCormick in press). Webster and Baylis acknowledge that the experience of moral residue can encourage the moral agent to reflect on and improve his or her practice, but they also warn that the moral agent may move toward denial, trivialization, or unreflective acceptance of the incoherence between beliefs and action (224–226).

Nurses' Relational Connections

Nurses' moral work is profoundly embedded in the interconnectedness and relationships of everyday health care encounters—sometimes to the detriment of the autonomy of nurses as moral agents, as we have discussed above. *Based our analysis so far, we can say that moral agency is a construct that focuses on nurses as engaged actors who draw on their various sources of knowledge as they live their nursing work.*

Such a claim about the moral situation of nurses means that we locate embodied, empathic relations as an essential site in which moral agency arises—embodied relations with their support for the moral relevance of personal involvement, values, emotions, inter-subjectivity, moral sensitivity, and experience (Benner 2000; Nortvedt 1998; 2001; Scott; see also Chapter 21 and Chapter 22). A **relational** turn in nursing ethics (Gadow 1999) means that the notion of nurses as moral agents can be articulated within the dialectic of nurses' normative and particular commitment to doing good in nursing practice. For instance, nurses' work is about both being with and doing for/with patients at times when they are made vulnerable by illness, suffering, and treatment. Yet, the **emotional work** of nursing has been rendered invisible and has been systematically devalued while the more technical work becomes visible and valued (Duncan 2003; Henderson 2001; Rodney and Varcoe 2001; Yylelland 1994). The important paradox here is that the emotional work of nursing and the technical work both affect one another. In other words, expertise in nursing practice is about being both humanly involved in relationships and responsive and capable to respond to the emotional, physiologic, and treatment needs of another. The moral situation of nurses is about striving to do good when responding to the needs of the other—both a personal and technical response. The person and the knowledge, skills, and techniques are a coherent whole in ethical nursing practice.

Let us illustrate by saying more about the ethnographic study of nurses practising on an acute medical unit that we introduced at the outset of this chapter (Ethics in Practice 8-1). In this study, Rodney (1997) came to understand that moral agency was not just enacted by individual nurses per se, but was enacted by a matrix of individual nurses working in inter-dependent relationships (see also McCormick, Rodney and Varcoe in press; Varcoe, Rodney and McCormick in press). For instance, as one of the nurses in Ethics in Practice 8-1 said, "What we also do... is ask for feedback among ourselves." Rodney used the concept of **relational matrix** to illustrate the connectedness and interdependence of individuals working in relationship with each other in an organizational context. The connectedness was not linear.[28] Further, it was embedded in the particularities of the patient care context, and, when working well, lent support to the work of individuals. For example, one of the nurse participants on the acute medical unit told the story of a distraught family trying to decide whether or not to continue treatment with their mother, whose condition was irreversible (Rodney 1997). The nurse was on an evening shift and was not able to reach the attending physician and so reached the physician on call, whom she had never met. The physician came to see the nurse and the family immediately. Over the course of the evening, the family, nurse, and on-call physician worked together in (what the nurse described as) an egalitarian manner to try to make sense of the best interests of the dying woman. While the experience was emotionally draining, the nurse reported that the family, she, and the physician felt that they had arrived at the best possible decision for the patient. In this situation, the individuals involved (including the family) were connected and interdependent in a manner that was based only in part on their roles. They came together on the basis of a shared concern and were able to work around formal and informal hierarchies (for instance, on the unit being studied, norms about on-call physicians being less involved in family support and team decision-making, and the common trend for physicians not to consult with nurses).

Rodney (1997) found that the matrix may or may not be supportive of nurses' efforts to effect their moral intentions, and it seemed that the nature of the relationships between individuals in the matrix made a significant difference. Disrupted and/or conflicted relationships between even a few individuals were problematic. Moreover, *who* was part of the matrix was not a given. Individuals from a variety of disciplines were involved depending on the particular practice context—in the example above, the family, the on-call physician, and the evening nurse. Counter to this example, though, despite their shared responsibility in patient care, physicians were often not perceived to be part of the relational matrix. In particular, they were often not accessible to help nurses deal with ethical problems in their practice, and/or their absence created ethical problems for the nurses.

However, as our earlier discussion of moral distress has foreshadowed, the problems nurses experienced in the relational matrix were also caused by fellow nurses (Rodney 1997). And when physicians *were* available and *were* perceived to be supportive and respectful, nurses described the positive impact that this had on the care of patients and families (as in the evening nurse's story). Knowing each other was beneficial, though not required, as the on-call physician illustrates. There were also accounts where individuals were well known but seemed to have a profoundly negative impact on the relational matrix—for instance, a physician who "yelled at" nursing staff regularly and a group of nurses on a shift opposite a nurse participant's who were difficult to approach for help. It seemed that being *authentically present* for each other made a tremendous difference for the quality of relationships within the matrix.[29] Authentic presence meant being respectful and listening as well as being willing to be available to help (whether in person or over the telephone or through other means).[30]

What Rodney's (1997) study illustrated was that who was in the relational matrix changed over even short periods of time. In other words, the boundaries of the relational matrix were not fixed but were fluid. Significantly, Rodney (1997) found that the relationships in the relational matrix worked best when they were founded on trust. Furthermore, it appeared that authentic presence helped trust to flourish.[31] The nurses in Ethics in Practice 8-1, for instance, clearly identified that in order for them to draw on their colleagues' expertise, they had to trust that those colleagues were both knowledgeable and approachable.

Trust

The feminist philosopher Annette Baier (1994) defines trust as "reliance on others' competence and willingness to look after, rather than harm, things one cares about which are entrusted to their care" (128).[32] Rodney (1997) came to think of trust as the "glue" that holds the relational matrix together and authentic presence as a major constituent of that glue. She saw the relational matrix in terms of the connectedness and interdependence of individuals working in relationship with each other in an organizational context. The connectedness was not linear, but was, rather, embedded in particular contexts and lent support to the work of individuals.

In continuing to reflect on the relational matrix, we do not wish to say that when there is trust between most individuals the relational matrix will support every health care professional's/provider's or patient's/family member's enactment of their moral agency. Nor is it to deny that there could be some trusting matrices where individuals are authentically present for each other, but where the resultant standards of care are unethical. And, of course, not all individuals uphold the knowledge, skill, or other attributes they are being trusted to. These are questions that Baier (1994) takes up in her writing about trust.[33] What we want to underscore here is the importance of trust for its influence on nurses' abilities to enact their moral agency.

Peter and Morgan (2001) further emphasize the importance of trust. They claim that little work has been done on trust as a dimension of nurse-patient relationships from a normative perspective that has the potential to inform nursing ethics.[34] Specifically, they examine how approaches to the nurse-patient relationship based on contracts, paternalism, and care are not adequate. While identifying the limitations of each of these approaches, Peter and Morgan also use Baier's (1994) theory of trust that incorporates both love and obligation and points towards how justice and care have similarly been reconciled. All three authors describe an ethic of trust as feminist, thereby attending to the concerns raised about a feminine ethic of care as apolitical and potentially exploitative. Foregrounding an ethic of trust, they argue, politicizes trust as a moral concept by identifying the potential for oppression and other harms in trusting relationships.

In summary, we started this chapter with a conceptualization of moral agency as inclusive of rational and self-expressive choice, notions of identity, social and historical relational influences, autonomous action, and embodied engagement. We have contributed some details to adapt this conceptualization for nursing, first by locating our analysis within the nature of nurses' knowledge and nurses' work. We identified nurses as engaged actors who draw on their various sources of knowledge as they live their nursing work. Following this, we commented on constraints to nurses' autonomous agency. We then posited that nurses and other individuals operate within a relational matrix as moral agents, and that this matrix flourishes with authentic presence and trust. In other words, to work together as moral agents requires more than just sharing information and using a decision-making process to arrive at solutions (Rodney 1997). It requires that we come closer to what is meaningful in each other's experiences and that such proximity become the basis for enacting moral agency in nursing practice. This is true within and between nursing and other disciplines.

TOWARD COLLABORATIVE PRACTICE

How does focusing on authentic presence and trust as essential for enactment of nurses' moral agency point toward particular implications for practice? Carol Taylor (1997) describes everyday nursing work as essential to ethical deliberations. She emphasizes the nature of **interdisciplinary teamwork** and philosophical questions about human well-being. In Carol Taylor's work the concrete illustration of everyday nursing knowledge can be seen in nurses' respect for human dignity and commitment to both holistic care and individualized care. This care is responsive to unique needs of patients and entails responsibility for continuity of care, demarcation of scope of authority, identification of the limits of caregiving, and the balance of competing agendas. Such a commitment to responding to the unique needs of patients requires that nurses collaborate with multidisciplinary teams. Collaboration with physicians, social workers, dieticians, physiotherapists, and others is a significant feature of nursing work as nurses engage in a primary commitment to patients—a commitment shared by others in practice (Forbes and Fitzsimons 1993; Jones 1997; McClelland and Sands 1993). Nurse-patient relationships and interactions between nurses and other professionals are activities whose meanings are dependent on context (McMahah, Hoffman and McGee 1994).

To illustrate, the nurses in Ethics in Practice 8-1 identified that for them to draw on their colleagues' expertise, they had to trust that those colleagues were knowledgeable as well as approachable. Trust is an attitude of optimism about the goodwill and competence of another that leads us to think we can count on the other person for something (Jones

1996). Knowledge involves trust, and trust, knowledge. "Trust and distrust are not beliefs, but emotional attitudes with perceptual, behavioral, and cognitive dimensions" (McLeod 2002, 85). What this meant for the situation in Ethics in Practice 8-1 was that nurses in the relational matrix needed case knowledge as well as the situated or particular knowledge of the patient, person, and social context (Liaschenko and Fisher 1999). All these forms of knowledge were tied to context and, therefore, reflected differences in time and space, or geography. And all required interdisciplinary collaboration. For instance, nurses needed case knowledge (e.g., the resistance of a particular strain of pneumococcus to antibiotics), patient knowledge (e.g., the progression of this patient's pneumonia and response to the antibiotic), person knowledge (e.g., the meaning that the patient and family attached to the pneumonia and subsequent hospitalization), and social knowledge (e.g., how to get physician assistance quickly if the patient's oxygenation dropped). From this illustration we can say that for nurses to be able to acquire and work with all these forms of knowledge as moral agents, they need to have a supportive relational matrix of colleagues for collaboration within and outside of nursing.

Collaboration is typically understood as a style of interaction characterized by mutual respect for different perspectives. In health care, we have known for a while that nurse-physician collaboration improves patient outcomes (Baggs and Schmitt 1988; Baggs et al. 1992; Fisher and Peterson 1993; Northouse and Northouse 1992). When there is civil communication and no conflict over the meaning or interpretation of knowledge, collaboration can be said to be occurring. *Yet the theoretical and practical barriers to collaboration are pervasive.* Current research tells us that physicians and nurses operate from quite different forms of knowledge and quite different interpretations of what ethical practice is (Botes 2000a; 2000b; Lützén, Johansson and Nordström 2000; Manias and Street 2001). Moreover, under conditions of uncertainty—when the uncertainty has diagnostic and management work that is split between disciplines—collaboration can break down (Stein-Parbury and Liaschenko in review). This leaves us with a number of challenges if we are to foster nurses' enactment of their moral agency within the context of interdisciplinary teams, especially in today's cost-constrained health care environment. As we said earlier in this chapter, the sociopolitical context matters. And, as the next section of this text will illustrate, that sociopolitical context is currently fraught with problems such as short staffing, loss of clinical leadership, and inadequate services for patients and families, to name a few.

While we certainly need more inquiry about *how* to foster collaborative practice, we can posit a number of conclusions and subsequent recommendations here. Individuals, we have said, must be present to be effective moral agents—present in the sense that they are involved in the here-and-now of the actual patient care situation, and present in the sense that they are trying to understand what their colleagues and/or patients and family members are experiencing. Individuals need to be authentically present for each other so that their relationships can be built on a foundation of trust. In order for this to happen—or be sustained in places where it is already occurring—it is our belief that at least the following changes are required:[35]

1. Workload and staffing patterns in all areas of practice must provide *time* for nurses, physicians, and other health care providers to meet regularly, share perspectives, and engage in planning for treatment and care. Time also needs to be built in for patients/clients and their family members to engage in regular dialogue with members of the health care team. While electronic and other media can supplement such meetings, they should not replace face-to-face contact if at all possible.

2. Time is necessary but it is not sufficient in itself. Nurses, physicians, and other health care providers also need help to *reflect critically on the quality of their interactions* within and between disciplines and with patients/clients and their family members. In order to enhance their ways of being with each other, they ought to be cognizant of the implicit and explicit power relationships that are always at play in health care encounters, with the aim of being more authentically present for each other. Skills in communication techniques can be helpful but must arise from a philosophical stance of mutual respect. There must be awareness of the vulnerability that arises in relationships of unequal power.

3. Health care providers should be *more proactive in engaging patients/clients and their family members* in discussions about the *meaning* of their treatment and care, related concerns, expectations and aspirations, and so forth. It is difficult to build or retrieve trust with patients/clients and their family members if such discussions are fragmented, late, or non-existent.

4. *Leadership in clinical practice* is required to ensure the successful implementation of these first three changes. Most health care providers require some mentoring in how to be more present for their colleagues, patients/clients, and family members. Clinical leadership is also required to ensure that the structure of the work environment makes it possible for individuals to be able to connect with each other and find ways to collaborate in taking moral action. Further, if clinical leaders are to be effective, they must also be *authentically present* for providers, patients/clients, and family members. This means that their management portfolios ought not to be so huge that they are inaccessible.

5. *Education about collaboration, authentic presence, and trust* ought to be built into preparatory and continuing education programs for all health care providers. Ethics committees are well situated to take some leadership in continuing education for practice agencies. As well, they can foster a moral climate that makes all of these recommendations more likely to flourish.

Although it is not difficult to articulate the recommendations above on paper, it is, of course, much more difficult to sustain and/or implement such action in practice. The chapters in the next section of this text, Moral Climate, will offer some insights into the current sociopolitical climate within which nurses enact their moral agency, including some ideas about how to improve that climate.

FOR REFLECTION

1. Think of an area of clinical practice you are familiar with and identify examples of the case, patient, person, and social knowledge used.

2. We have argued that embodiment is an important part of moral agency. Identify some examples of how that plays out in clinical practice.

3. What actions can nurses take as individuals to strengthen their autonomy as moral agents? As members of organizations? In professional groups?

4. Remember (or imagine) a policy initiative that was meant to improve collaborative practice. What are the most important characteristics of the initiative? What helped it to work or not work?

ENDNOTES

1. By binary solutions we mean, for example, yes/no or treat/do not treat. See also Chapter 4.

2. See also Chapter 5 and Chapter 7.

3. Carnevale (2002); Chambliss (1996); Johnstone (1999); Liaschenko (1993a); Mitchell (2001); Rodney (1997); Rodney and Varcoe (2001); Rodney et al. (2002); Varcoe and Rodney (2002).

4. This is a premise that is provided with empirical support in Chapter 10.

5. See, for example, Benner (2000); Bergum (2002); Corley et al. (2001); Gadow (1999); Hamric (2000); Hartrick Doane (2002a; 2002b); Nortvedt (1998); Raines (1994; 2000); Reynolds, Scott, and Austin (2000); see also Chapters 19, 21, 22, and 24 in this text.

6. As Taylor explains, Kant's moral view was that

   > Rational beings have a unique dignity. They stand out against the background of nature, just in that they are free and self-determining (Taylor 1989, 364).

   See also Chapter 4.

7. See Chapter 5.

8. See also Rodney (1997); Rodney et al. (2002); and Varcoe and Rodney (2002) for related analyses.

9. See Chapter 4 for definitions of these theories.

10. See also Fox (1990) for a sociological analysis of ethics. For other feminist and related critiques of the traditional approach to moral agency, see Baier (1994); Blum (1994); Flanagan (1991); Mackenzie and Stoljar (2000a); McNay (2000); and Sherwin (1998).

11. This remains a tentative conceptualization and one that will continue to evolve. It is important to note that we are departing from Sherwin (1998) by viewing autonomy as part of moral agency—her conceptual approach is to see agency as part of relational autonomy. Nonetheless, Sherwin (1998) also notes that the "language of agency and autonomy is quite varied within feminist (and other) discourses" (47).

12. There are, of course, significant similarities between the conceptualizations. Feminist theorists emphasize power inequities more than most other contextual theorists (Charles Taylor included) though.

13. See also Chapter 21.

14. Our use of the term "the good" is congruent with an Aristotelian notion of ethics, where ethics is seen as integral with character and action and with practice (Aristotle c.320 BC/1985; Benner, Tanner and Chesla 1996; Sher 1987). As Benner and her colleagues claim,

    > even in clinical situations, where the ends are not in question, there is an underlying moral dimension: the fundamental disposition of the nurse toward what is good and right and action toward what the nurse recognizes or believes to be the best good in a particular situation (Benner, Tanner and Chesla, 6).

    Nurses' notions of the good therefore provide a value-based direction for their practice. See also Rodney (1997); Rodney et al. (2002); and Varcoe and Rodney (2002) for related discussions in nursing and Pellegrino (2001) for a related discussion in medicine and other helping and healing professions.

15. See also Chapter 7.

16. For other analyses of moral agency in nursing, see Benner (2000); Georges and Grypdonck (2002); and Raines (1994; 2000).

17. As an anonymous reviewer of this chapter has noted, we need to understand more about what "enactment" entails. Embeddedness, relational knowledge, and (as we will argue later) trust are important, but so are virtues, professional values, experience, and other qualities. Answering this question about enactment more fully requires the kind of composite approach to ethical theory argued for in Chapter 5 and Chapter 6. While we realize that there is more to say on enactment than we have articulated in this chapter, we hope that our colleagues in nursing and other disciplines will continue to take up the question. In the interim, we have found the writings of Edmund Pellegrino (e.g., Pellegrino 2001; Pellegrino, Veatch and Langan 1991) and Barry Hoffmaster (e.g., Hoffmaster 1991; 1993; 1999; 2001) helpful.

18. See also MacDonald (2002) for a discussion of nurse autonomy as relational.

19. Chapter 2 provides an interesting analysis of the history of nursing and the implications for nursing ethics.

20. See also Chapter 7.

21. See Chapter 10 for an overview of related research findings.

22. These are not the only reasons. Locating caring as the main (or only) theory for nursing ethics would have the potential to overlook the importance of caring in other disciplines and in other societal roles. The relationship of care to justice is also significant and problematic. The authors of Chapter 7 have laid out some of these concerns more explicitly. While we do not want to argue that conceptualizations of care do not have a role, we believe that nursing ethics needs more than just care theory, and that the care theory we do employ ought to come from feminist theorists. This is argued in Chapter 7.

23. See, for example, Benner (2000); Bergum (2002); Gadow (1999); Georges and Grypdonck (2002); Hartrick Doane (2002b); Liaschenko (1995); Liaschenko and Peter (2003); Raines (1994; 2000); and Varcoe and Rodney (2002); see also Chapters 21 and 24.

24. Erlen and Frost (1991); Fenton (1988); Gaul (1995); Holly (1993); Jameton (1984); Ketefian and Ormond (1988); Millette (1994); Rodney (1988; 1997); Rodney and Starzomski (1993); Rodney and Varcoe (2001); Rushton (1992); Wilkinson (1985, 1987/1988, 1989); Yarling and McElmurray (1986); Yeo and Ford (1996).

25. There are a variety of related terms describing associated moral pheneomena that Jameton (1984) and others articulate. For example, Australian nurse ethicist Megan-Jane Johnstone (1999) articulates moral unpreparedness, moral blindness, moral indifference, amoralism, immoralism, moral complacency, moral fanaticism, moral disagreements and controversies, and moral dilemmas, as well as moral stress, moral distress, and moral perplexity (163–183).

26. In this meta-analysis we "re-read" the findings across our three ethnographic studies to arrive at newly synthesized interpretations (McCormick, Rodney and Varcoe In press).

27. Looking at the history of nursing can help us to take seriously—and hopefully prevent— the "dark side" of our practice. For instance, Steppe (1992) has provided insightful analyses of nurses' collaboration with the Nazis in Germany and their complicity with crimes against humanity. See also Lagerway (1999).

28. The notion of "matrix" was used rather than "team" because team often implies a linear hierarchy. The matrix had multiple intersecting connections that shifted according to the exigencies of the patient care context (Rodney 1997). Rodney's adaptation of the concept of matrix was thus somewhat different from the notion of matrix organizations that has been articulated in organizational theory. Matrix organizations are seen to incorporate lateral and vertical hierarchical structure (Huse and Cummings 1985, 177–178), which implies a more linear arrangement than she was describing. Instead, the use of the term "relational matrix" was closer to one of the earliest attempts to define a matrix organization, which suggested that it functioned as "a 'web of relationships' rather than a line and staff relationship of work performance" (Mee 1964; cited in Huse and Cummings, 178). This was congruent with how Mann (1994), a feminist philosopher, locates moral agency—that is, in terms of a "complex nexus of social relationships" (1).

29. See Sørlie, Lindseth, Uldén and Norberg (2000) for an interesting study of female physicians' accounts of the importance of supportive relationships in their practice.

30. For a thoughtful critique of authenticity, see Aranda and Street (1999).

31. Charles Taylor's (1991; 1995) writing on authenticity has influenced this conceptualization. He describes authenticity, for instance, as "being true to myself and my own particular way of being" (Taylor 1995, 227). See also Bishop and Scudder (2001) for a discussion of authenticity in nurse-patient relationships.

32. Baier (1994) builds her conceptualization of trust on Hume's theory of moral sentiment and Gilligan's theory of care.

33. See also Liaschenko (1994); Corley and Goren (1998); Varcoe and Rodney (2002); and Varcoe, Rodney, and McCormick (in press).

34. See also Hupcey, Penrod and Morse (2000); Peter and Watt-Watson (2002); see also Chapters 7 and 12 in this text.

35. These recommendations are based on the analysis provided in this chapter as well as on the authors' experiences in practice, education, research, and ethics consultation. Furthermore, the recommendations have also been distilled from a variety of sources in nursing, medicine, and ethics, including: Calam and Andrew (2000); Calam, Far, and Andrew (2000); Chinn (1995; 2001); Corley and Goren (1998); DeRenzo and Strauss (1997); Hartrick Doane (2002); Hiltunen et al. (1999); Hupcey, Penrod, and Morse (2000); King (1992); Kuhl (2002); Liaschenko (1994); Liaschenko and Fisher (1999); Marsden (1988); Nisker (2001); Peter and Watt-Watson (2002); Quill (2000); Robinson (2000); Rodney (1997); Rodney et al. (2002); Rodney and Howlett (in press); Rodney and Varcoe (2001); Söderberg, Gilje, and Norberg (1999); Solomon (1995); Solomon et al. (1993); Sørlie et al. (2000); Storch (1999); Storch et al. (2002); Taylor, Carol (1995; 1997); Thorne (1993); Tilden et al. (1999); Varcoe et al. (in press); Varcoe and Rodney (2002); and Varcoe, Rodney, and McCormick (in press).

REFERENCES

Angeles, P.A. 1981. *Dictionary of philosophy*. New York: Barnes & Noble.

Aranda, S.K. and Street, A.F. 1999. Being authentic and being a chameleon: Nurse–patient interaction revisited. *Nursing Inquiry, 6*, 75–82.

Aristotle. 1985. *Nicomachean ethics*. Translator: T. Irwin. Indianapolis, IL: Hackett. (Original work published c. 320 B.C.)

Audi, R. 1997. *Moral knowledge and ethical character*. New York: Oxford University Press.

Baggs, J.G. and Schmitt, M.H. 1988. Collaboration between nurses and physicians. *Image, 20*(3), 145–149.

Baggs, J.G., Ryan, S.A., Phelps, C.E., Richeson, J.F. and Johnson, J.E. 1992. The association between interdisciplinary collaboration and patient outcomes in a medical intensive care unit. *Heart & Lung, 21*(1), 18–24.

Baier, A.C. 1994. *Moral prejudices: Essays on ethics*. Cambridge, MA: Harvard University Press.

Benner, P. 1984. *From novice to expert: Excellence and power in clinical nursing practice.* Menlo Park, CA: Addison-Wesley.

Benner, P. 1991. The role of experience, narrative, and community in skilled ethical comportment. *Advances in Nursing Science, 14*(2), 1–21.

Benner, P. 2000. The roles of embodiment, emotion and lifeworld for rationality and moral agency in nursing practice. *Nursing Philosophy, 1,* 1–14.

Benner, P.A., Tanner, C.A. and Chesla, C.A. (with contributions by H.L. Dreyfus, S.E. Dreyfus and J. Rubin). 1996. *Expertise in nursing practice: Caring, clinical judgment, and ethics.* New York: Springer.

Benner, P. and Wrubel, J. 1989. *The primacy of caring: Stress and coping in health and illness.* Menlo Park, CA: Addison-Wesley.

Bergum, V. 2002. Ethical challenges of the 21st century: Attending to relations. *Canadian Journal of Nursing Research, 34*(2), 9–15.

Bishop, A. H. and Scudder, J. R. 1990. *The practical, moral and personal sense of nursing: A phenomenological philosophy of practice*. Albany: State University of New York Press.

Bishop, A.H. and Scudder, J.R. 1999. A philosophical interpretation of nursing. *Scholarly Inquiry for Nursing Practice, 3*(1), 17–27.

Bishop, A. and Scudder, J. 2001. *Nursing ethics: Holistic caring practice.* 2nd edition. Boston: Jones and Bartlett.

Blum, L.A. 1994. *Moral perception and particularity*. Cambridge, MA: Cambridge University Press.

Botes, A. 2000a. A comparison between the ethics of justice and the ethics of care. *Journal of Advanced Nursing, 32*(5), 1071–1075.

Botes, A. 2000b. An integrated approach to ethical decision-making in the health care team. *Journal of Advanced Nursing, 32*(5), 1076–1082.

Bowden, P. 1997. *Caring: Gender-sensitive ethics*. London: Routledge.

Bowden, P. 2000. An "ethic of care" in clinical settings: Encompassing "feminine" and "feminist" perspectives. *Nursing Philosophy, 1*(1), 36–49.

Brunk, C.G. 1991. Professionalism and responsibility in the technological society. In D.C. Poff and W.J. Waluchow (Eds.), *Business ethics in Canada,* 2nd ed. (pp. 122–137). Scarborough, ON: Prentice Hall.

Calam, B. and Andrew, R.F. 2000. CPR or DNR? End-of-life decision making on a family practice teaching ward. *Can Fam Physician, 46*, 340–346.

Calam, B., Far, S. and Andrew, R. 2000. Discussions of "code status" on a family practice teaching ward: What barriers do family physicians face? *Canadian Medical Association Journal, 163*(10), 1255–1259.

Carnevale, F.A. 2002. Betwixt and between: Searching for nursing's moral foundations. *Canadian Journal of Nursing Research, 34*(2), 5–8.

Chambliss, D.F. 1996. *Beyond caring: Hospitals, nurses, and the social organization of ethics.* Chicago: University of Chicago Press.

Chinn, P.L. 1995. *Peace & power: Building communities for the future.* 4th edition. New York: NLN Press.

Chinn, P.L. 2001. *Peace & power: Building communities for the future.* 5th edition. Boston: Jones & Bartlett.

Corley, M.C. 2002. Nurse moral distress: A proposed theory and research agenda. *Nursing Ethics, 9*(6), 636–650.

Corley, M.C., Elswick, R.K., Gorman, M. and Clor, T. 2001. Development and evaluation of a moral distress scale. *Journal of Advanced Nursing, 33*(2), 250–256.

Corley, M.C. and Goren, S. 1998. The dark side of nursing: Impact of stigmatizing responses on patients. *Scholarly Inquiry for Nursing Practice, 12*(2), 99–118.

Danis, M. and Churchill, L.R. 1991. Autonomy and the common weal. *Hastings Center Report, 21*(1), 25–31.

David, B.A. 2000. Nursing's gender politics: Reformulating the footnotes. *Advances in Nursing Science, 23*(1), 83–93.

DeRenzo, E.G. and Strauss, M. 1997. A feminist model for clinical ethics consultation: Increasing attention to context and narrative. *HEC Forum, 9*(3), 212–227.

Duncan, R. 2003. *Shaped to care: A study of the subjectivity and emotional labour in nursing theory and practice.* Unpublished doctoral dissertation. University of Melbourne, Melbourne, Australia.

Erlen, J.A. and Frost, B. 1991. Nurses' perceptions of powerlessness in influencing ethical decisions. *Western Journal of Nursing Research, 13*, 397–407.

Fenton, M. 1988. Moral distress in clinical practice: Implications for the nurse administrator. *Canadian Journal of Nursing Administration, 1*, 8–11.

Fisher, B.J. and Peterson, C. 1993. She won't be dancing much anyway: A study of surgeons, surgical nurses, and elderly patients. *Qualitative Health Research, 3*(2), 165–185.

Flanagan, O. 1991. *Varieties of moral personality: Ethics and psychological realism.* Cambridge, MA: Harvard University Press.

Forbes, E.J. and Fitzsimons, V. 1993. Education: The key to holistic interdisciplinary collaboration. *Holistic Nursing Practice, 7*(4), 1–10.

Fowler, M. 1990. Social ethics and nursing. In N.L. Chaska (Ed.), *The nursing profession: Turning points* (pp. 24–31). St. Louis, MO: Mosby.

Fox, R.C. 1990. The evolution of American bioethics: A sociological perspective. In G. Weisz (Ed.), *Social science perspectives on medical ethics* (pp. 201–217). Philadelphia: University of Pennsylvania Press.

Fry, S.T., Harvey, R.M., Hurley, A.C. and Foley, B.J. 2002. Development of a model of moral distress in military nursing. *Nursing Ethics, 9*(4), 373–387.

Gadow, S. 1980. Existential advocacy: Philosophical foundation of nursing. In S.F. Spiker and S. Gadow (Eds.), *Nursing: Ideals and images, opening dialogue with the humanities* (pp. 79–101). New York: Springer-Verlag.

Gadow, S. 1999. Relational narrative: The postmodern turn in nursing ethics. *Scholarly Inquiry for Nursing Practice, 13*(1), 57–69.

Gaul, A. L. 1995. Casuistry, care, compassion, and ethics data analysis. *Advances in Nursing Science, 17*(3), 47–57.

Georges, J.J. and Grypdonck, M. 2002. Moral problems experienced by nurses when caring for terminally ill people: A literature review. *Nursing Ethics, 9*(2), 155–178.

Hamric, A.B. 2000. Moral distress in everyday ethics. *Nursing Outlook, 48*, 199–201.

Hartrick Doane, G. 2002a. In the spirit of creativity: The learning and teaching of ethics in nursing. *Journal of Advanced Nursing, 39*(6), 521–528.

Hartrick Doane, G. 2002b. Am I still ethical? The socially-mediated process of nurses' moral identity. *Nursing Ethics, 9*(6), 623–635.

Hefferman, P. and Heldig, S. 1999. Giving "moral distress" a voice: Ethical concerns among neonatal intensive care unit personnel. *Cambridge Quarterly of Healthcare Ethics, 8*, 173–178.

Henderson, A. 2001. Emotional labor and nursing: An under-appreciated aspect of caring work. *Nursing Inquiry, 8*(2), 130–138.

Hiltunen, E.F., Medich, C., Chase, S., Peterson, L. and Forrow, L. 1999. Family decision making for end-of-life treatment: The SUPPORT nurse narratives. *The Journal of Clinical Ethics, 10*(2), 126–134.

Hoffmaster, B. 1991. The theory and practice of applied ethics. *Dialogue, 30*, 213–234.

Hoffmaster, B. 1993. Can ethnography save the life of medical ethics? In E.R. Winkler and J.R. Coombs (Eds.), *Applied ethics: A reader* (pp. 366–389). Oxford: Blackwell.

Hoffmaster, B. 1999. Secular health care ethics. In H. Coward and P. Ratanakul (Eds.), *A cross-cultural dialogue on health care ethics* (pp. 139–145). Waterloo, ON: Wilfrid Laurier University Press.

Hoffmaster, B. 2001. Introduction. In B. Hoffmaster (Ed.), *Bioethics in social context* (pp. 1–11). Philadelphia: Temple University Press.

Holly, C.M. 1993. The ethical quandaries of acute care nursing practice. *Journal of Professional Nursing, 9*(2), 110–115.

Hupcey, J., Penrod, J. and Morse, J.M. 2000. Establishing and maintaining trust during acute care hospitalizations. *Scholarly Inquiry for Nursing Practice, 14*(3), 227–242.

Huse, E.F. and Cummings, T.G. 1985. *Organizational development and change.* 3rd edition. St. Paul, MN: West Publishing Company.

Jameton, A. 1984. *Nursing practice: The ethical issues.* Englewood Cliff, New Jersey: Prentice Hall.

Jennings, B., Callahan, D. and Wolf, S.M. 1987. The professions: Public interest and common good. *Hastings Center Report, 17*(1), 3–10.

Jones, K. 1996. Trust as an affective attitude. *Ethics, 107*(1), 4–25.

Jones, R.A. 1997. Multidisciplinary collaboration: Conceptual development as a foundation for patient-focused care. *Holistic Nursing Practice, 11*(3), 8–16.

Johnstone, M.J. 1999. *Bioethics: A nursing perspective.* 3rd edition. Sydney, Australia: Harcourt.

Ketefian, S. and Ormond, I. 1988. *Moral reasoning and ethical practice in nursing: An integrative review.* New York: National League for Nursing.

King, N.M.P. 1992. Transparency in neonatal intensive care. *Hastings Center Report, 22*(3), 18–25.

Kuhl, D. 2002. *What dying people want: Practical wisdom for the end of life.* Toronto: Doubleday.

Kuhse, H. 1997. *Caring: Nurses, women, and ethics.* Oxford: Blackwell.

Lagerway, M.D. 1999. Nursing ethics at Hadamar. *Qualitative Health Research,* (6), 759–772.

Latimer, J. 2000. *The conduct of care: Understanding nursing practice.* Cornwall, UK: Blackwell Science.

Liaschenko, J. 1993a. *Faithful to the good: Morality and philosophy in nursing practice.* Unpublished doctoral dissertation. University of California, San Francisco.

Liaschenko, J. 1994. Making a bridge: The moral work with patients we do not like. *Journal of Palliative Care, 10*(3), 83–89.

Liaschenko, J. 1995. Ethics in the work of acting for patients. *Advances in Nursing Science, 18*(2), 1–12.

Liaschenko, J. 1997. Knowing the patient? In S.E. Thorne and V.E. Hayes (Eds.), *Nursing praxis: Knowledge and action* (pp. 23–38). Thousand Oaks, CA: Sage.

Liaschenko, J. 1998. The shift from the closed to the open body—ramifications for nursing testimony. In S.D. Edwards (Ed.), *Philosophical issues in nursing* (pp. 1–16). London: Macmillan.

Liaschenko, J. and Fisher, A. 1999. Theorizing the knowledge that nurses use in the conduct of their work. *Scholarly Inquiry for Nursing Practice: An International Journal, 13*(1), 29-41.

Liaschenko, J. and Peter, E. 2003. Feminist ethics. In V. Tschudin (Ed.), *Ethics in Nursing: Issues in advanced practice*. Oxford: Butterworth Heinemann.

Liaschenko, J. and Peter, E. In review. Nursing ethics and conceptualizations of nursing: Profession, practice, work. (Manuscript in review with *Journal of Advanced Nursing.*)

Lützén, K., Cronqvist, A., Magnusson, A. and Andersson, L. 2003. Moral stress: Synthesis of a concept. *Nursing Ethics, 10*(3), 312–322.

Lützén, K., Johansson, A. and Nordström, G. 2000. Moral sensitivity: Some differences between nurses and physicians. *Nursing Ethics, 7*(6), 520–530.

MacDonald, C. 2002. Nurse autonomy as relational. *Nursing Ethics, 9*(2), 194–201.

Mackenzie, C. and Stoljar, N. (Eds.). 2000a. *Relational autonomy: Feminist perspectives on autonomy, agency and the social self.* New York: Oxford University Press.

Mackenzie, C. and Stoljar. N. 2000b. Autonomy refigured. In C. Mackenzie and N. Stoljar (Eds.), *Relational autonomy: Feminist perspectives on autonomy, agency and the social self* (pp. 3–31). New York: Oxford University Press.

MacPherson, K. I. 1991. Looking at caring and nursing through a feminist lens. In R.M. Neil and R. Watts (Eds.), *Caring and nursing: Explorations in feminist perspectives* (pp. 25–42). New York: National League for Nursing.

Manias, E. and Street, A. 2001. The interplay of knowledge and decision making between nurses and doctors in critical care. *International Journal of Nursing Studies, 38*, 129–140.

Marsden, C. 1988. Care giver fidelity in a pediatric bone marrow transplant team. *Heart & Lung, 17*(6), 617–625.

Mann, P.S. 1994. *Micro-politics: Agency in a postfeminist era.* Minneapolis: University of Minnesota Press.

McClelland, M. and Sands, R. G. 1993. The missing voice in interdisciplinary communication. *Qualitative Health Research, 3*(1), 74–90.

MacLeod, C. 2002. Deconstructive discourse analysis: Extending the methodological conversation. *South African Journal of Psychology, 32*(1), 17–25.

McCormick, J., Rodney, P. and Varcoe, C. In press. Re/Interpretations across studies: An approach to meta-analysis. (Manuscript accepted for publication with *Qualitative Health Research.*)

McMahah, E.M., Hoffman, K. and McGee, G.W. 1994. Physician-nurse relationships in clinical settings: A review and critique of the literature, 1966–1992. *Medical Care Review, 51*(1), 83–112.

McNay, L. 2000. *Gender and agency: Reconfiguring the subject in feminist and social theory.* Cambridge: Polity.

Mee, J.F. 1964. Ideational items: Matrix organization. *Business Horizons,* (Summer), 70–72.

Millette, B.E. 1994. Using Gilligan's framework to analyze nurses' stories of moral choices. *Western Journal of Nursing Research, 16*(6), 660–674.

Mitchell, G.J. 2001. Policy, procedure and routine: Matters of moral influence. *Nursing Science Quarterly, 14*(2), 109–114.

Nisker, J.A. 2001. Chalcedonies. *Canadian Medical Association Journal, 164*(1), 74–75.

Northouse, P.G. and Northouse, L.L. 1992. *Health communication: Strategies for health professionals.* 2nd edition. Norwalk, CT: Appleton & Lange.

Nortvedt. P. 1998. Sensitive judgement: An inquiry into the foundations of nursing ethics. *Nursing Ethics, 5*(5), 385–392.

Nortvedt, P. 2001. Clinical sensitivity: The inseparability of ethical perceptiveness and clinical knowledge. *Scholarly Inquiry of Nursing Practice, 15*(3), 1–19.

Paterson, J.G. and Zderad, L.T. 1988. *Humanistic nursing.* New York: National League for Nursing.

Pellegrino, E.D. 2001. The internal morality of clinical medicine: A paradigm for the ethics of the helping and healing professions. *Journal of Medicine and Philosophy, 26*(6), 559–579.

Pellegrino, E.D., Veatch, R.M. and Langan, J.P. 1991. Preface. In E.D. Pellegrino, R.M. Veatch and J.P. Langan (Eds.), *Ethics, trust, and the professions: Philosophical and cultural aspects* (pp. vii–ix). Washington, DC: Georgetown University Press.

Peter, E. and Morgan, K.P. 2001. Exploration of a trust approach for nursing ethics. *Nursing Inquiry, 8*(3), 3-10.

Peter, E. and Watt-Watson, J. 2002. Unrelieved pain: An ethical and epistemological analysis of distrust in patients. *Canadian Journal of Nursing Research, 34*(2), 65–80.

Poff, D.C. and Waluchow, W.J. 1991. Part three: Morality and the professions. In D.C. Poff and W.J. Waluchow (Eds.), *Business ethics in Canada,* 2nd ed. (pp. 117–120). Toronto: Prentice Hall.

Quill, T.E. 2000. Initiating end-of-life discussions with seriously ill patients: Addressing the "elephant in the room." *JAMA, 284*(19), 2502–2507.

Raines, D.A. 1994. Moral agency in nursing. *Nursing Forum, 29*(1), 5–11.

Raines, M.L. 2000. Ethical decision making in nurses: Relationships among moral reasoning, coping style, and ethics stress. *JONA's Healthcare Law, Ethics, and Regulation, 2*(1), 29–41.

Redman, B.K., and Fry, S.T. 2000. Nurses' ethical conflicts: What is really known about them? *Nursing Ethics, 7*(4), 360–366.

Reynolds, W., Scott, P.A. and Austin, W. 2000. Nursing, empathy, and perception of the moral. *Journal of Advanced Nursing 32*(1), 235–242.

Robinson, C.A. 2000. Response to "Establishing and maintaining trust during acute care hospitalizations." *Scholarly Inquiry for Nursing Practice, 14*(3), 243–248.

Rodney, P. 1988. Moral distress in critical care nursing. *Canadian Critical Care Nursing Journal, 5*(2), 9–11.

Rodney, P.A. 1997. *Towards connectedness and trust: Nurses' enactment of their moral agency within an organizational context.* Unpublished doctoral dissertation. University of British Columbia, Vancouver, BC.

Rodney, P. and Howlett, J. In press. Elderly patients with cardiac disease: Quality of life, end of life, and ethics. In D. Fitchett (Ed.), *Canadian Cardiovascular Society Consensus Document on Care of the Elderly with Cardiac Disease.*

Rodney, P. and Starzomski, R. 1993. Constraints on the moral agency of nurses. *Canadian Nurse, 89*(9), 23–26.

Rodney, P.A. and Varcoe, C. 2001. Toward ethical inquiry in the economic evaluation of nursing practice. *Canadian Journal of Nursing Research, 33*(1), 35–57.

Rodney, P., Varcoe, C., Storch, J.L., McPherson, G., Mahoney, K., Brown, H., Pauly, B., Hartrick Doane, G. and Starzomski, R. 2002. Navigating toward a moral horizon: A multi-site qualitative study of nurses' enactment of ethical practice. *Canadian Journal of Nursing Research, 34*(3), 75–102.

Rushton, C.H. 1992. Care-giver suffering in critical care nursing. *Heart & Lung, 21*(3), 303–306.

Saks, M. 1995. *Professions and the public interest: Medical power, altruism and alternative medicine.* London: Routledge.

Scott, P.A. 2000. Emotion, moral perception, and nursing practice. *Nursing Philosophy 1*, 123–133.

Sher, G. 1987. The nature of moral virtue: Aristotle. In G. Sher (Ed.), *Moral philosophy: Selected readings* (p. 67). San Diego: Harcourt Brace.

Sherwin, S. 1992a. Feminist and medical ethics: Two different approaches to contextual ethics. In H.B. Holmes and L.M. Purdy (Eds.), *Feminist perspectives in medical ethics* (pp. 17–31). Bloomington, IN: Indiana University Press.

Sherwin, S. 1992b. *No longer patient: Feminist ethics & health care.* Philadelphia: Temple University Press.

Sherwin, S. 1998. A relational approach to autonomy in health care. In S. Sherwin and the Feminist Health Care Ethics Research Network (Eds.), *The politics of women's health* (pp. 19–47). Philadelphia: Temple University Press.

Smith, K.V. and Godfrey, N.S. 2002. Being a good nurse and doing the right thing: A qualitative study. *Nursing Ethics, 9*(3), 301–312.

Söderberg, A., Gilje, F. and Norberg, A. 1999. Transforming desolation into consolation: The meaning of being in situations of ethical difficulty in intensive care. *Nursing Ethics, 6*(5), 357–373.

Solomon, M.Z. 1995. The enormity of the task: SUPPORT and changing practice. *Hastings Center Report, 25*(6), S28–S32.

Solomon, M.Z., O'Donnell, L., Jennings, B., Guilfoy, V., Wolf, S.M., Nolan, K., Jackson, R., Koch-Weser, D. and Donnelley, S. 1993. Decisions near the end of life: Professional views on life-sustaining treatments. *American Journal of Public Health, 83*(1), 14–23.

Sørlie, V., Lindseth, A., Uldén, G. and Norberg, A. 2000. Women physicians' narratives about being in ethically difficult care situations in paediatrics. *Nursing Ethics, 7*(1), 47–62.

Starzomski, R. and Rodney, P. 1997. Nursing inquiry for the common good. In S.E. Thorne and V.E. Hayes (Eds.), *Nursing praxis: Knowledge and action* (pp. 219–236). Thousand Oaks, CA: Sage.

Stein-Parbury, J. and Liaschenko, J. (Manuscript in review with *Social Science and Medicine*.)

Steppe, H. 1992. Nursing in Nazi Germany. *Western Journal of Nursing Research, 14*(6), 744–753.

Steppe, H. 1996. The war and nursing in Germany. *IHNJ, 1*(4), 61–71.

Storch, J.L. 1999. Ethical dimensions of leadership. In J.M. Hibberd and D.L. Smith (Eds.), *Nursing management in Canada*, 2nd ed. (pp. 351–367). Toronto: W.B. Saunders.

Storch, J.L., Rodney, P., Pauly, B., Brown, H. and Starzomski, R. 2002. Listening to nurses' moral voices: Building a quality health care environment. *Journal of Nursing Leadership, 15*(4), 7–16.

Taylor, Carol. 1995. Medical futility and nursing. *Image, 27*(4), 301–306.

Taylor, Carol. R. 1997. Everyday nursing concerns: Unique? Trivial? Or essential to health care ethics? *HEC Forum, 9*(1), 68–84.

Taylor, Charles. 1989. *The sources of the self: The making of the modern identity.* Cambridge, MA: Harvard University Press.

Taylor, Charles. 1991. *The malaise of modernity.* Concord, ON: Canadian Broadcasting Corporation (CBC).

Taylor, Charles. (with A. Gutmann, S.C. Rockefeller, M. Walzer and S. Wolf). 1992. *Multiculturalism and "The politics of recognition."* Princeton: Princeton University Press.

Taylor, Charles. 1995. *Philosophical arguments.* Cambridge, MA: Harvard University Press.

Thorne, S. 1993. *Negotiating health care: The social context of chronic illness.* Newbury Park, CA: Sage.

Tilden, V.P., Tolle, S.W., Nelson, C.A., Thonpson, M. and Eggman, S.C. 1999. Family decision making in foregoing life-extending treatments. *Journal of Family Nursing, 5*(4), 426–442.

Varcoe, C., Hartrick Doane, G., Pauly, B., Rodney, P., Storch, J., Mahoney, K., McPherson, G., Brown, H. and Starzomski, R. In press. Ethical practice in nursing: Working the in-betweens. (Manuscript accepted for publication with *Journal of Advanced Nursing.*)

Varcoe, C. and Rodney, P. 2002. Constrained agency: The social structure of nurses' work. In B.S. Bolaria and H.D. Dickinson (Eds.), *Health, illness and health care in Canada,* 3rd ed. (pp. 102–128). Toronto: Nelson.

Varcoe, C., Rodney, P. and McCormick, J. In press. Health care relationships in context: An analysis of three ethnographies. (Manuscript accepted for publication with *Qualitative Health Research.*)

Webster, G.C. and Baylis, F.E. 2000. Moral residue. In S.B. Rubin and L. Zoloth (Eds.), *Margin of error: The ethics of mistakes in the practice of medicine* (pp. 217–230). Hagerstown, MD: University Publishing Group.

Wilkinson, J.M. 1985. *Moral distress in nursing practice: Experience and effect.* Unpublished Master's thesis. University of Missouri, Kansas City, Missouri.

Wilkinson, J.M. 1987/1988. Moral distress in nursing practice: Experience and effect. *Nursing Forum, 23,* 16–28.

Wilkinson, J.M. 1989. Moral distress: A labor and delivery nurse's experience. *JOGNN, 18*(6), 513–519.

Yarling, R. and McElmurray, B. 1986. The moral foundation of nursing. *Advances in Nursing Science, 8*(2), 63–73.

Yeo, M. and Ford, A. 1996. Integrity. In M. Yeo and A. Moorhouse (Eds.), *Concepts and cases in nursing ethics,* 2nd ed. (pp. 267–306). Peterborough, ON: Broadview.

Yyelland, B. 1994. Structural constraints, emotional labour and nursing work. In B.S. Bolaria and R. Bolaria (Eds.), *Women, medicine and health* (pp. 231–240). Saskatoon: University of Saskatchewan.

section II

Moral Climate

Janet L. Storch

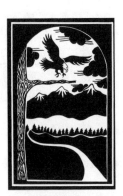

Assertions of the basic elements of care and social responsibility might seem naive and sentimental in the contemporary world of health care and public policy... [But] they are fundamental to the very structure, not only of health care, but also society as a whole (Byock 2003, S41).

Nursing literature is replete with rich descriptions of the need for quality practice environments for nurses and the threat that poor work environments pose to nurses' ability to practice in a safe, competent manner. The lack of quality environments has serious implications for those who receive nursing care—the *persons* in health care. Yet, in spite of high-level (national and international) calls for attention to the nursing shortage and worsening working conditions for nursing, the climate of health care continues its downward trend as we write this book. In this section, the six selected chapters provide both practical and theoretical understandings of the significance of the moral climate—at the macro, meso, and micro levels of health care.

In Chapter 9, Bernadette Pauly provides ideological reasons for the health care system's slowness to change. She argues that despite evidence indicating that for-profit–funded and operated services have not been shown to be more efficient or effective, the press to replace public services with private for-profit services is a continued tension in health care planning and delivery at provincial—and to some extent national—levels. She emphasizes that nurse leaders need to have more detailed information about health care funding and delivery in order to enhance their ability to recognize and debate health care options (and the assumptions underlying each option). Acting upon an informed understanding of these options, nurses can make a substantial contribution by identifying for, and with, others the *ethical choices* involved.

Patricia Rodney and Annette Street, in Chapter 10, carry this theme forward in a critique of how changes (called "health care reforms") have been managed—that is, with limited consultation and evaluation. Focusing on the moral climate created by a corporate ethos, these authors highlight Canadian and Australian examples, augmented by international insights. They close by suggesting how to take action to change that climate, particularly in dealing with power inequities in health care, and how to build a moral community and thereby recover a sense of possibilities in health care. Their approach is pragmatic and visionary.

In Chapter 11, Patricia Marck provides fresh insights through the lens of an ecological understanding of health care. Marck speaks about the depletion of natural resources with parallel lessons for depletion of human resources in health care. Through practical examples and relatively new (to nursing) but powerful theoretical language, she underscores the need for healing the health care system itself.

As one tangible illustration of the need for healing of the health care system, Elizabeth Peter focuses on the ethics of home health care policy and practice in Chapter 12. With reforms in health care (such as earlier discharge of hospitalized patients), the current state of home care in Canada is, she argues, inadequate and unethical. As a "non-system," home care harbours numerous inequities. Passing the buck to families and friends may often mean that no one is able to provide the needed care for those who are chronically ill, acutely ill, or dying. Peter emphasizes the need to develop trust at all levels in health care to effect meaningful change.

Reflecting on the numerous ethical concerns at the end of life in Chapter 13, Janet Storch asks how people lost control over their dying and how they have tried to regain control. She highlights an, as yet, somewhat under-emphasized point in this literature—

that living wills (advance directives) are really about living, that is, living one's final days well. This, she maintains, imposes on nurses and other health professionals a moral imperative to pay attention to all that makes for good final days, including encouraging those who are dying to reflect on their life and their dying in a way that allows for moral engagement, learning, and meaningfulness.

Jeffrey Nisker is a physician who teaches ethics using narratives. His Chapter 14 will be a treat for all who seek to understand ethics in order to develop and promote moral sensitivity in health care. Through a narrative approach, Nisker helps us see how we can gain insights into our moral climate and its meaning for those in our care. He suggests that through those insights, health care professionals can gain mutual understandings, make the invisible apparent, and promote ethical policies and practices.

It is the Editors' hope that readers can take from this section critical sensitivity to the sources of moral distress rising from current sociopolitical changes. Such changes have diminished the moral agency of nurses and other health care providers and have had seriously negative impacts on the quality of patient/family/community care. This section should also help readers to envision possibilities for action that will create a healing health care environment.

REFERENCE

Byock, I. 2003. Rediscovering community at the core of the human condition and social convenant. *Access to hospice care: Expanding boundaries, overcoming barriers. Hastings Center Report Special Supplement, 33*(2), S40–S41.

chapter nine

Shifting the Balance in the Funding and Delivery of Health Care in Canada

Bernadette Pauly

Decisions to embrace certain health care reforms over others reflect ethical choices about how we want to live together as a society (Kenny, 2002).

We are experiencing an intense period of debate about the future of the Canadian health care system (Commission of Study on Health and Social Services 2001; Saskatchewan Commission on Medicare 2001; Premier's Advisory Council on Health for Alberta 2001; British Columbia Standing Committee on Health 2002; Standing Senate Committee on Social Affairs, Science and Technology 2002; Commission on the Future of Health Care in Canada 2002). A recurrent theme in the debate surrounds the public/private balance in the funding and delivery of health care. Should public sources of funding be increased? Is there a need to increase the role of private health care insurance? Should user fees be implemented? Should services be delivered publicly on a not-for-profit or for-profit basis?

While the questions above may seem far removed from ethics and the everyday practice of nurses, the action or inaction of policy-makers in the development and implementation of health care policy will shape the context of the health care system and the delivery of health care in subtle and invisible ways. Registered nurses, because of their location in the health care system, have first-hand knowledge and experience of the impact of potential and actual health care reforms on patients and ethical nursing practice (Stevens 1992). Understanding the tensions, debates, and dialogues at the macro level can provide insight into current developments in practice and provide a foundation from which to raise questions about shifting the balance in health care funding and delivery, and from which to take informed action within the professional and public arena to ensure continued access to health care for all patients. The purpose of this chapter is to provide some beginning background about the funding and delivery of health care in Canada and to discuss the ethical implications involved in shifting the public/private balance in the funding and delivery of health care. In particular, I address the ethics of increasing private funding and the role of for-profit delivery in health care. I begin with some thoughts about the significance of health policy decisions for registered nurses and ethical practice. Then, I discuss the importance of values to health policy decision-making and the values of Canadians on the health care system. Next, I review and discuss how introducing more sources of private funding and shifting to for-profit health care delivery impacts access to health care. Finally, I discuss the roles and responsibilities of nurses and nursing organizations at the micro, meso, and macro levels for taking ethical action.

SIGNIFICANCE FOR ETHICAL PRACTICE IN NURSING

On a daily basis, registered nurses and nurse leaders are navigating through ethical challenges in practice. These challenges result from dialogues, debates, decisions, and trends at the macro level in the funding and delivery of health care. Registered nurses, acting from an ethical perspective, will raise different questions for consideration in the policy process. Some of these considerations include asking who will be affected by the reforms, how reforms will affect those with the least resources and poorest health, who will benefit from the reforms, and whether those most at risk are likely to receive an increased benefit. In order to highlight the impact of health policy decision-making on the funding and delivery of health care, it may be useful to look at scenarios from nursing practice. These scenarios illustrate some of the subtle and invisible ways that issues related to shifting the public/private balance in the funding and delivery of health care permeate nursing practice and patient care.

Ethics in Practice 9-1	Access to Private Home Care Service

A registered nurse working in acute care is concerned because there is no longer funding to cover post-acute home care services for patients being discharged following surgery. Based on her nursing assessment for several of her patients, she is concerned that nursing care to assist with dressing changes will not be available, increasing the risk for complications. In her practice, she has frequently seen such patients readmitted for post-operative wound complications. She is aware of the option to use private home care services. However, she is also aware that private home care services would not be financially accessible to several of her patients and would pose significant financial burdens for several others.

The registered nurse in Ethics in Practice 9-1 highlights the difficulties of a lack of universal funding for home care, issues related to private payment and private for-profit delivery of services. Currently, each province is responsible for making decisions about the degree and scope of funding available for home care services. At present, there is no national program for home care.[1] The Commission on the Future of Health Care (2002) suggested that a national program to fund home care services in three areas is needed (for post-acute home care, palliative care, and mental health). However, this does not address issues related to funding other home nursing care services, personal care services, and the home support necessary to maintain people living in their own home.

Ethics in Practice 9-2	**Access to Private Surgical Clinics**

A clinical nurse specialist caring for people experiencing chronic pain is distressed at the increased waiting time for patients requiring orthopedic surgery that might alleviate pain for some of her clients. Many of her clients have indicated that if they had the financial resources they would access a private clinic in another large city for their surgery. They believe this would decrease the waiting list in the public system. This nurse wonders about the need for private options for those who can afford it but wonders what impact this will have on the publicly funded health care system.

Private surgical clinics are seen to provide an option for those with financial resources, and they offer the hope that waiting times will be reduced for surgery for both those who access private services and those obtaining services in the public system. This approach assumes that there are adequate numbers of providers available to provide the needed services and that publicly funded services will not be negatively affected by increasing private for-profit surgical care.

Ethics in Practice 9-3	**Access to Community Health Centres**

A nurse practitioner working in an inner-city clinic has observed that many of her clients have benefitted from access to primary health care services within the clinic. Clients at the clinic often see a nurse practitioner for urgent, non-complex concerns, for ongoing monitoring of complex health problems, and for assessment of or intervention in complex social issues. As part of an interdisciplinary team, the nurse facilitates access to other providers and programs to address complex health issues for clients, both individually and in groups. Services available include physiotherapy, dental care, and mental health counselling. The nurse knows that this approach to care has resulted in decreased emergency room visits and hospitalizations as well as better health for patients. However, provincial funding cuts mean that the availability of the community health centre services and programs will be affected. Additionally, discussions about the introduction of user fees for patients using the local emergency department will significantly affect the ability of her clients to access services after hours and on weekends in a timely and appropriate manner.

Public funding for health care services other than those provided by physicians and hospitals is at the discretion of the provinces. While many have promoted the benefits of the community health centre approach to comprehensive client-focused care, restructuring of primary care service delivery has been very slow, and access to a team of practitioners as an effective and efficient strategy for the provision of comprehensive care has not been fully realized. This has limited the possibilities for promotive and preventative care at the point of entry into the system and reduced opportunities for interdisciplinary collaboration and intervention. User fees, although in contravention of the Canada Health Act, continue to be raised as an option for increasing revenue and deterring unnecessary use of services by patients.

Ethics in Practice 9-4	**Public-Private Partnerships**

A clinical nurse specialist in a large urban hospital has recently been asked to be part of a chronic disease management program. This program will involve a public-private partnership with a large corporation that produces diabetic medication and equipment. The nurse recognizes that this will provide an important source of funding for a much needed program to address care of people with chronic diseases such as diabetes. However, she feels a sense of uneasiness about the initiative because of the for-profit motives of the partner corporation. The nurse is concerned that she will be expected to promote the products of this company to her patients.

As Ethics in Practice 9-4 indicates, public-private partnerships have the potential to provide new sources of revenue for developing patient services, building new facilities, and buying much needed equipment. At the level of policy, however, there are few guidelines for how public-private partnerships can be implemented to ensure appropriate and ethical practices. In some areas, public-private partnerships might be workable; in other areas, they might be contraindicated. A constant concern is that for-profit motives might influence clinical advice and decision-making.

Although each of these situations raises different issues related to the funding and delivery of health care in Canada, the relevance of health care policy decision-making to practice is evident in each situation. In each Ethics in Practice scenario, it is clear that registered nurses have first-hand knowledge of the concerns, the unanswered questions, and the potential effects of shifting the balance between public and private funding in the delivery of health care in Canada. In order to more fully address the implications for ethical practice in each of these situations, it is important to consider the relationship between values, ethics, and health policy as a framework for the discussion of shifting the public-private balance in the funding and delivery of health care in Canada.

VALUES, ETHICS, AND HEALTH POLICY

Beginning with Values

Societal values outline what we believe is good and how we choose to live and relate to one another in society (Kenny 2002; Beauchamp and Childress 1994). Good public policy is a reflection of public and common values that reflect our identity as a society (Stone 1997).

While some might argue that values are too general and/or too subjective to be meaningful (for example, see Fraser 2003), "a social consensus about values, even if only rough and incomplete, is required for a practical system" (Beauchamp and Childress 1994, 356). Values serve as important guides to action (Blue et al. 1999; Marmor, Okma and Latham 2002). "The fact that values are general and may compete with one another does not, after all, render them meaningless. Values are no policy straitjacket, but there are certain choices they rule out" (Marmor, Okma and Latham, 2002, 2). From an examination of data from OECD countries including Canada, these authors conclude:

> Values may serve as a foundation for social programs... but they do not supply those programs' architecture. Differences in social institutions are reflective not only of fundamentally different ideological positions, but of subtle historical (and contingent) differences in those programs' initial construction, and in the subsequent play of political and social interests (17).

While there clearly are other influences on the structure of social programs, it is our values that determine how we frame the problems in health care and which solutions we endorse (Kenny 2002). In the following paragraphs, I will briefly discuss the influence of the Canadian public on the values of Canadian health care.[2]

In Canada, our health care system has become symbolic of what it means to be Canadian (Baylis et al. 1995; Conference Board of Canada 2000; Marmor, Okma and Latham 2002; Mendelsohn 2002; Schafer 2002). The principles of the Canada Health Act reflect our belief that health care in Canada is "regarded as a common good to which all of us, as moral equals, are entitled. Our public system of health care displays our shared concern and responsibility for one another and differentiates Canada from the United States, where health care is regarded more as a commodity" (Baylis et al. 1995, 75). In the most recent public consultations conducted by the Commission on the Future of Health Care (2002), Canadians continue to affirm the belief that health care is a common good that should be accessible to all, not a commodity to be bought and sold.

Numerous public opinion polls and surveys have concluded that Canadians clearly support a publicly funded universally accessible system of care in which need, not ability to pay, is the basis on which care is, and should be, provided. (Peters 1995; Conference Board of Canada 2000; Canadian Medical Association 2001; Graves, Beauchamp and Herle 1998). Canadians tend to rank universality and accessibility as the most important of the five principles of the Canada Health Act (Peters 1995; Conference Board of Canada 2000).

In two separate comprehensive reviews of Canadian public opinion over the past two decades, equality of access and quality of care emerged as the most important values of Canadians in the reform of the health care system (Conference Board of Canada 2000; Mendelsohn 2002). In the final report of the Commission on the Future of Health Care (2002), the values of universality, equity, and solidarity were identified as the dominant values of Canadians (Commission on the Future of Health Care 2002). For Canadians, equity is understood as equality (fairness) in access to health care, and it is embedded in the principles of universality, accessibility, and comprehensiveness. Equality of access is often given priority over quality. As Schafer (2002) observes, "Equality of access is probably the defining value of our health care system. It is clearly the moral value in which most Canadians are most heavily invested" (4).

Moving to Ethics

While values reflect our beliefs, ethics, as a discipline, is concerned with the normative dimension of decisions and actions. Arras, Steinbock, and London (1999) define bioethics as "inquiries about the rightness or wrongness of various actions, character traits, and social policies" (2). All public policy has a moral dimension because it involves decisions that affect others who may or may not be involved in the process of deciding how a particular problem should be addressed (Malone 1999). As Kenny (2002) observes,

> These moral and ethical dimensions are not always visible in our public policies; health care is a notable exception. Here, our intuitions of vulnerability and our personal experiences of illness, disease and disability, both for us and for our loved ones, evoke strong convictions that health care policy is about things that really matter (45).

Theories of justice such as libertarian and egalitarian theories contain general principles to "determine how social burdens and goods, and services, including health care goods and services, should be distributed—or, as some insist, redistributed" (Beauchamp and Childress 1994, 334; Daniels 1985). Libertarians adopt the free market ideal in the distribution of health care goods and services. In the United States, a libertarian system of health care has predominated, and individual self-reliance is highly valued. Health care is treated more like a commodity (something to be bought and sold in a market) rather than a social good accessible to all and equally distributed (Daniels 1985).[3]

In the United States, where there is a greater portion of private health insurance and for-profit health care,[4] approximately 41 million people did not have any type of health insurance at any time during the year 2001 (U.S. Census Bureau 2002). "Further analysis in a report by Families USA (2003) estimates that approximately 74.7 million people under the age of 65—*nearly one out of three (30.1 percent)*—were without health insurance for all or part of 2001 and 2002. Of these 74.7 million uninsured individuals, almost two-thirds were uninsured for six months or more" (1).[5] The emphasis on private health care in the United States and the corresponding lack of access to health care have been identified as a serious ethical concern by several American bioethicists (Daniels 1985; Buchanan 1995; Caplan, Light and Daniels 1999).

"Egalitarian theories of justice propose that persons be provided an equal distribution of certain goods such as health care...." (Beauchamp and Childress 1994, 339). Fairness, in an egalitarian sense, assumes that everyone is of equal value or worth and that fairness is achieved by seeking to "reduce the differences in health and health care between groups" (Caplan, Light and Daniels 1999, 854). In this sense, health care is a public or common good which everyone has a right of access. "More commonly, a right of access to health care refers to a right to obtain specified goods and services to which every entitled person has an equal claim" (Beauchamp and Childress 1994, 353).

Several authors have argued that a fairer, more just system of health care would incorporate an egalitarian rather than libertarian theory of justice (Buchanan 1995; Daniels 1985; Beauchamp and Childress 1994). Within an American context, Buchanan (1995) and Caplan, Light, and Daniels (1999) have proposed that criteria for a more just system of health care would include: (1) universal access to an adequate level of health care services in which financial and non-financial barriers to health care would be minimized, (2) fair distribution of the costs of health care among societal members, (3) rationing fairly on the basis of need, (4) an emphasis on primary health care to address social determinants of health, including health promotion and disease prevention, (5) clear public accountability, (6) generation and maintenance of a sustainable workforce, and (7) a focus on health research and utilization of research. Lastly, as Buchanan (1995) observes, the system should have the capacity for reform and improvement toward achieving the previously identified criteria. Canadian values, as discussed previously, are more closely aligned with egalitarian rather than libertarian views of justice and fairness. Next, I will examine the ethical stance of professional nursing in Canada.

Ethical Commitments of Nursing

The Canadian Code of Ethics for Registered Nurses "is a statement of the ethical commitments of nurses to those they serve" and "sets forth the ethical standards by which nurses are to conduct their nursing practice (Canadian Nurses Association 2002, 2). In addition to providing guidance for ethical care, the code clearly points to an active role for nurses in the health policy process to improve ethical nursing practice for the benefit of the public. The Canadian Nurses Association (2002) states:

> The ability of nurses to engage in ethical practice in everyday work and to deal with ethical situations, problems, and concerns can be the result of decisions made at a variety of levels—individual, organizational, regional, provincial, national and international. Differing responsibilities, capabilities, and ways of working toward change also exist at these various levels. For all contexts and levels of decision-making, the code offers guidance on providing care that is congruent with ethical practice, and for actively influencing and participating in policy development, review and revision (5).

The values and related responsibilities which outline nurses' commitment to participation in health policy decision-making and development can be found in a variety of places in the code (Canadian Nurses Association 2002). The clearest statement is under the value of justice. This value is defined by the statement that "Nurses uphold principles of equity and fairness to assist persons in receiving a share of health services and resources proportionate to their needs and promoting social justice" (15). Each of the responsibilities under this value point to the involvement of nurses in health care policy at the micro, meso, and macro level for the purposes of ensuring equity of access, equity of resource allocation (including addressing the broader determinants of health), and policies that are ethically sound and based on current knowledge and research. An additional responsibility identifies the obligation of nurses to address broader social issues that require action in order to contribute to social change both as a professional and a citizen. However, the degree to which moral commitments can be enacted is affected by the nurses' relative positions of power and authority within the health care system (Rodney et al. 2002; Storch et al. 2002; Varcoe et al. in press).

Nursing values, as embodied in the ethical commitments outlined in the Canadian Nurses Association Code of Ethics (Canadian Nurses Association, 2002), are consistent with Canadian values and an egalitarian system of health care. As a registered nurse, support for a strong, publicly funded system of health care in which access is based on need, not ability to pay, is consistent with professional ethical values. Clearly, equality of access is an important value for nurses. Nurses are ethically committed to actively advocating for social justice in health care reforms. Social justice requires that group differences be addressed and the criteria of social justice demand assessment of the impact of reforms on those who are the most vulnerable (Lebacqz 2002; Young 1990). Given this ethical stance, it is extremely difficult to ethically endorse strategies for reform that reduce access to care for those with limited financial resources or those unable to pay. Reforms that create conflicts for providers between professional ethical commitments to the well-being of patients and for-profit motives would be ethically unacceptable (Schafer 2002).

In the next section, the ethics of shifting the public-private balance in funding and delivery of health care in Canada will be discussed. In this discussion, the focus is on the *ethics* rather than the *economics* of shifting the balance in public-private funding and delivery of health care. Economic analysis will be discussed as it supports the ethical analysis presented here. While there are important benefits to be gained from a fuller integration of economic and ethical analysis of health policy options (Fuchs 1996; Hurley 2001), a full economic analysis of the options for shifting the public-private balance in health is beyond the scope of this chapter. Furthermore, a primary question in the public-private debate should be, "Is privatization likely to move us closer to a just health care system?" (Buchanan 1995, 221).[6] Lastly, although one might wish for a more balanced approach in the discussion of private health care options, this is difficult unless one completely abandons egalitarian values in favour of more libertarian values. However, from the discussion above, it is evident that neither a majority of the general public nor professional nurses have adopted libertarian values in relation to the health care system in Canada. Furthermore, American bioethicists have argued for a change from a libertarian to an egalitarian system of health care in the United Stated (Buchanan 1995; Caplan, Light and Daniels 1999).

FUNDING AND DELIVERY OF HEALTH CARE

Although the funding and delivery of health care are closely related, in this chapter these aspects will be examined separately. "Funding" or "financing" refers to the source of payment for services. "Delivery" refers to the way in which services are organized, managed, and provided (Deber 2002; Evans 2000; 2002; Kolderie 1986). Funding may be from public or private sources. Services may be delivered publicly, for-profit, or not-for-profit. In the next section, I provide a brief overview of the primary sources of funding in Canada and discuss the ethical implications of shifting the public-private balance in health care funding. This will be followed by a discussion of health care delivery and the implications of shifting the balance in health care delivery.

Funding of Health Care

There are essentially four sources of funding for health care systems: general taxation, social insurance, out-of-pocket payment, and private insurance (Evans 2002). General taxation and social insurance are considered to be public sources of funding (Evans 2002;

Evans et al. 2000). In a tax-financed system of funding, contribution is based on income and there is a pooling of collective risk (Evans 2002). According to Evans (2000), social insurance is achieved through employment deductions and can be distinguished from private insurance.

> Social insurance is compulsory, with contributions based largely or wholly on income, not on risk status. Private insurance may be more or less voluntary, from commercial or not-for-profit firms. In competitive insurance markets, premiums will be based on risk status, not on income (2).

Direct out-of-pocket payment and user charges require that individuals using services pay at the point of service. Payment for services is tied to usage not income (Evans 2002). As Evans observes, health systems are funded by a combination of several funding sources.

Canada is characterized primarily by a tax-financed system supplemented by private sources (Evans 2002).[7] In 2003, 72 percent of the health care system was publicly funded through taxation (CIHI 2003).[8] Private sources of funding include private insurance and out-of-pocket expenses, which account for most of the remaining 28 percent of health care funding (CIHI 2003).[9] "In Canada, the term 'private health care' is generally understood to describe care that is paid for by private sources: private insurance plans, employer-provided health plans, deductibles and other out-of-pocket expenses" (DeCoster and Brownell 1997, 301). From 1975 to 1998, private sector funding of health care increased from 23.8 percent to 29.9 percent (CIHI 2000).

There has been considerable pressure to increase sources of private funding. Proponents of increasing private sources of funding argue that health care costs are spiralling out of control and that the current publicly funded system is unsustainable (Boychuk 2002).[10] The proposed solution is to open health care to the market and introduce greater sources of private funding. At the same time, we are experiencing increasing global pressure both internationally and from the United States to open health care to the market (Fuller 1998; Price, Pollack and Shauol 1999; Schafer 2002; Kenny 2002). While Canadians remain committed to a publicly funded system of health care that ensures equality of access, fear of escalating costs and growing concerns about the quality of health care have influenced public opinion and have generated support for some privatization options (Schafer 2002; Mendolsohn 2002). "This is a crucial value tension: Canadians want to nurture the public system but they fully sympathize with someone who wants to spend their own money to get the care they need" (Mendelsohn 2002, viii). Although, Evans (2002) does not frame the issue as values or ethics; he does acknowledge that the underlying issue in all modern health care systems is the tension created when those with health and wealth contribute more to the collective than those who are unhealthy and not wealthy but are more likely to reap the benefits of a social system of health care. As Schafer (2002) observes, this is the middle-class bargain, which has the potential to break down in the face of perceived concerns about the quality of health care such as increased waiting time for certain procedures and diagnostic tests. Thus, an ethical tension exists. This tension calls for a balance between individual rights and freedoms and collective interests. An examination of potential options for shifting the balance to increase private sources of funding in the Canadian health care system will now be critically examined.

Shifting the Balance to Increase Private Sources of Funding

In Canada, a number of strategies have been proposed which would increase private funding for health care. Increased private funding of health care can occur through reductions in federal funding, user fees, medical savings accounts, and public-private partnerships. Each of these options will be discussed and examined in the following section.

REDUCTIONS IN FEDERAL FUNDING

Although not necessarily an active attempt to increase private sources of funding, reductions in federal funding indirectly encourage an increase in private funding. In the 1990s, reductions in federal spending on health care resulted in provinces delisting services—that is, cutting back services that fell outside of the Canada Health Act (Deber, Mhatre and Baker 1994; Tholl 1994; RNAO 2000). For example, in some provinces, eye examinations were delisted, and in other provinces, the frequency of eye exams was reduced (Armstrong and Armstrong 1996). At the same time, hospital beds were closed and hospital services reduced. According to Taft and Steward (2000), delisting services heightens the need for private insurance and creates a climate that encourages the growth of private insurance. Indeed, as identified by the nurses in Ethics in Practice 9-1 and 9-2, many clients who are in need of health care services would not be able to afford private insurance or to pay for service directly. Decreased public funding creates new challenges in rationing health care at all levels. Although not always recognized in formal discussions of resource allocation, registered nurses compelled to practise with fewer resources are faced with increasingly difficult ethical choices in the rationing of their time and care to patients (Rodney et al. 2002; Rodney and Varcoe 2001).

Federal reductions in funding for health have been accompanied by a growing movement to deinstitutionalize care and dehospitalize patients through greater use of day surgery, short stays, and outpatient services. While community care has considerable advantages, the Canada Health Act does not require provinces to cover home care services, long-term care, or pharmaceuticals (Health Canada 2003; RNAO 1999; RNAO 2000). It is at the discretion of the provinces to determine to what extent these services will be funded. When appropriate publicly funded community services are not in place, the cost of care is transferred to the individuals, and responsibility is shifted from the public to the private sector (RNAO 2000). Many people have experienced the growing financial and personal costs of home care and the added costs of pharmaceuticals as a result of early discharge. Furthermore, a greater move to community care generally has the effect of shifting the burden of care to family caregivers, particularly women, when adequately funded community services are not in place (Armstrong and Armstrong 1996; Marshall 1994; Angus, Auer, Cloutier and Albert 1995; OWN and RNAO 1998).

USER FEES

User fees continue to surface as a solution for improving the health care system (Rachlis and Kushner 1994; Kenny 2002; Evans, Barer and Stoddart 1993). User fees refer to direct payments for care received from a physician or hospital (Commission on the Future of Health Care, June 2002).[11] Those who advocate user fees primarily argue that such fees would decrease inappropriate use and abuse of the system (Commission on the Future of Health Care, June 2002; Canadian Health Services Research Foundation 2001). However, much of the cost of health care is not within the control of patients (Canadian Health Services Research Foundation 2001; Commission on the Future of Health Care, June 2002; Kenny 2002). According to the Commission on the Future of Health Care,

Big-ticket items in healthcare—like hospital admissions, drugs, and surgery—must all be ordered by doctors, so user fees for patients won't do much to discourage use. And services like visits to the family doctors, which the public has some choice in and thus might use frivolously, just don't cost a lot (June 2002, 5).

User fees have been found to decrease use, but only among those who are poor and at higher risk for health problems (Beck and Horne 1980; Canadian Health Services Research Foundation 2001; Commission on the Future of Health Care in Canada, June 2002; Evans, Barer and Stoddart 1993; Moorhouse 1993; Rachlis and Kushner 1994).

User fees for physician or hospital services have been utilized in several provinces in Canada since the introduction of Medicare. Two notable examples were the introduction of user fees in Saskatchewan and Quebec. In Saskatchewan, when physician user fees were introduced, overall health care costs did not decrease, and usage did not decrease except among the poor and elderly who were often in need of service (Beck and Horne 1980). In Quebec, introducing user fees into the pharmacare program resulted in the elderly taking about 90 percent less of their needed medication and needing more emergency room visits (Tamblyn et al. 2001).

The Commission on the Future of Health Care in Canada (2002) concluded,

> There is overwhelming evidence that direct charges such as user fees put the heaviest burden on the poor and impede their access to necessary health care. This is the case even when low income exemptions are in place. The result may be higher cost in the long run because people delay treatment until their conditions gets worse. In addition, user fees and co-payments also involve significant administrative costs that directly reduce the modest amount of revenue generated from the fees (28).

Based on the evidence, numerous other authors have concluded that user fees are not an acceptable means for controlling health care expenditures or raising revenues as they unfairly penalize the sick and the poor (Evans, Barer and Stoddart 1993; Armstrong and Armstrong 1996; Canadian Health Care Association 2002; Moorhouse 1993; Rachlis and Kushner 1994; RNAO 1999; Rich 2001). As Kenny (2002) states, "They [user fees] go against the fundamental Canadian understanding of equity, because they focus on the ability to pay rather than on response to need" (146). Both economic and ethical analyses result in the conclusion that user fees will not achieve the goals of health care in Canada.[12]

MEDICAL SAVINGS ACCOUNTS

In order to address issues related to the funding of health services, some have proposed the introduction of medical savings accounts (Gratzer 1999; Migue 2002). A medical savings account would be a yearly health care allowance given to individuals to buy health care services (Forget, Deber and Roos 2002; Hurley 2002; Commission on the Future of Health Care 2002; Migue 2002). Although medical savings accounts are a way to allocate funds rather than finance health care, they have the effect of introducing private payment for health care. There are numerous ways to design medical savings accounts, but all are based upon the belief that medical savings accounts would save money in the system by encouraging more appropriate use and would increase patient choice.[13]

Medical savings accounts are grounded in values of personal responsibility and self-reliance (Ham 2001; Barr 2001; Shortt 2002; Hurley 2002). From an analysis of the introduction of medical savings accounts in Singapore, several authors have raised concerns about the shortcomings of medical savings accounts related to equity (Shortt 2002; Ham 2001; Hsiao 2001). In terms of equality of access, medical savings accounts provide some advantages over private insurance, but they do not score as well in terms of fair financing as health care systems funded through taxation or social insurance (Ham 2001). Shortt (2002) explains:

> MSAs, especially when coupled with tax advantages, are attractive to the healthy and wealthy, leaving the pooled unwell either to seek higher cost comprehensive insurance or to bear increased out-of-pocket expenses (162).[14]

It should be noted that the overall cost of health care would be increased if catastrophic insurance was provided publicly (Shortt 2002; Commission on the Future of Health Care 2002). Equally concerning is the shift in values needed to support the introduction of medical savings accounts. As Shortt concludes, "The introduction of MSAs would challenge a half century of Canadian belief that health care costs are a shared responsibility rather than a burden to be borne by unwell individuals" (162). At this point, both economic and ethical analyses have raised more questions than answers about the role of medical savings accounts in a publicly funded health care system.

Public-Private Partnerships[15]

More recently, public-private partnerships have been embraced in British Columbia and other Canadian provinces as a potential source of additional capital funding. In essence, public-private partnerships are not a source of general revenue but a way of funding particular projects and initiatives. Public-private partnerships can take a variety of forms, such as providing capital for building projects or funding a health care provider's position. While it may seem innovative to access capital from the private sector in order to finance health care projects and initiatives, it should be remembered that unless it is a philanthropic project, the expectation of the private sector is always to make a profit. Further, if money must be borrowed, the public sector is normally able to borrow capital at a cheaper rate than is the private sector (Deber 2002). At present, there is a lack of government regulation to ensure that such ventures are undertaken in the best interest of the public and not solely for the benefit of for-profit corporations. Ethical analysis of this policy direction is needed. Without such analysis, nurses are left to navigate a minefield of potential ethical issues that might be created by the demands of for-profit partners. For example, nurses may be challenged to promote products and services of the for-profit partner rather than provide services based on needs.

Shifting the Balance, Shifting Equity

The significant difference between the four sources of funding (taxation, social insurance, private insurance, and out-of-pocket payment) is "the way they apportion the total cost of health care among the national population" (Evans 2002, 4). Therefore, the particular mix of financing mechanisms

> must involve a balance of benefits and harms in which different people's interests are weighed differently. The very permanence of the controversy should tell us that it arises from a permanent conflict of embedded interest, not from a simple inability to find the "right mix" for everyone. In that sense, the choice of financing mechanisms is a matter of values, not a technical question (Evans 2002, 3).

In a primarily tax-funded system, those with higher incomes contribute the same or a greater share of their incomes than do those with lower incomes. Evans (2000; 2002) maintains that tax financing is the most progressive form of health care funding because it places the heaviest financial burdens on those who are the wealthiest. However, this burden is in proportion to their income. Access to health care is based on need, not on ability to pay. In contrast, private insurance (when purchased directly),[16] user charges, and out-of-pocket expenditures place a greater financial burden on those with greater risk and/or lower incomes (Evans 2002). This is particularly significant since those with lower incomes are at greater risk for health problems and more likely to require health services (Aday 1993; Daniels 1985; Hall, Stevens and Meleis 1994; Hall 1999; Kreiger 1999).The primary benefit of moving towards more private sources of funding is increased consumer choice and better access to health care for those able to afford it (Deber et al. 1997; Evans 2002). In a paper commissioned by the National Forum on Health, Deber et al. (1997) examined several models for organizing health care and concluded that "public financing of medically necessary services seems to be the optimal model for health systems" and that public funding for medically necessary services increases both equity and efficiency (Part II, 1). "It is widely recognized that divorcing access to a comprehensive mix of health services from ability to pay inherent in public financing enhances equity. As one moves along the public/private continuum to include more private sector involvement, equity decreases" (4). These authors concluded that the only justification for mixing public and private sector funding of health care is to provide greater consumer and provider choice.

Canadians have placed a high value on equality of access. In a just health care system, individuals need to have a fair opportunity to access health care (Daniels 1985; Buchanan 1995; Beauchamp and Childress 1994). The increasing financial burden of illness for individuals, diminished access for those with the least health and wealth, and delays in care associated with increased private funding of health care are not only contrary to Canadian values but raise ethical concerns about the maintenance of a just health care system. Fortunately, both the Commission on the Future of Health Care (2002) and the Standing Senate Committee report (2002) recommended maintaining a strong publicly funded system based on the view that it reflects the values of Canadians and is the most efficient system. I now move to a discussion of the delivery of care and the ethics of increasing for-profit delivery of health care.

Delivery of Health Care

While the final report on the Commission on the Future of Health Care (2002) and Standing Senate Committee Report (2002) both recommended public funding of the health care system, they did not agree on the delivery of health care services. Romanow, in the Commission on the Future of Health Care (2002) report, made a clear distinction between clinical and non-clinical services, proposing that only non-clinical services could be provided on a for-profit basis. Kirby, in the Standing Senate Committee on Social Affairs, Science and Technology report (2002), advocated for a range of delivery models. There continues to be an enduring belief that for-profit delivery of health care services will be more efficient. These recommendations, combined with the growing public concern about waiting lists, will create continual pressure to increase the private for-profit provision of health care.

Deber (2002) also completed a comprehensive review of the evidence related to different models of health care delivery (public, private not-for-profit, and private for-profit). In Canada, many publicly funded health services are delivered privately (either on a not-for-profit or for-profit basis). For example, physician services are publicly funded and operated as a for-profit small business. Many hospitals and service agencies are operated on a private not-for-profit basis.[17] The difference between the for-profit and not-for-profit delivery of services is an important distinction in the discussion of the delivery of services. Deber further distinguished between for-profit small business and for-profit corporations. In small for-profit services, profits return to the owners directly, and they may choose to reinvest such profits to enhance the service. However, for-profit corporations expect to make a profit, which is distributed as dividends to company shareholders. Next, I will discuss some of the options for increasing for-profit delivery of care that are evident in Canadian health care.

Shifting the Balance in the Delivery of Health Care

Options for increasing the private for-profit delivery of health care include closing facilities and selling public assets, reducing services, contracting out, and developing a parallel for-profit system of care. When health care facilities are closed, the opportunity is created for the delivery of private for-profit services within the health care system (Taft and Steward 2000). Furthermore, delisting and cutbacks in service starve the system; thus, private for-profit provision of health was not only encouraged but needed to meet the demand for health care (Taft and Steward 2000). As Taft and Steward observe, drastic cuts in hospital services in Alberta led to the growth of private for-profit institutions in the delivery of health care, without the benefit of increased access to health care or a decrease in waiting lists for certain procedures.

A popular option for increasing for-profit provision of service is to contract out non-clinical and/or clinical services. In 1985, Stoddart and Labelle examined the benefits of contracting out non-clinical services, such as laundry and food services, in an attempt to realize cost savings. They concluded that the cost savings and quality of these strategies were questionable. However, provinces have continued to pursue the contracting out of clinical and non-clinical services in spite of concerns about safety, quality, and efficiency. The SARS (Sudden Acute Respiratory Syndrome) epidemic highlighted the importance of maintaining well-trained housekeeping staff. Since continuing in-service education is essential for the maintenance of quality, the accountability for such preparedness is an important matter. Provision of sound orientation and continuing education have frequently been sacrificed to cost-cutting—a worrisome trend in regard to contracting out such services.

Throughout the 1990s, the contracting of clinical services, such as laboratory services in Ontario and surgical services in Alberta, has increased without decreases in cost or increases in access to service (Canadian Health Services Research Foundation 2002; Fuller 1998; RNAO 2000). Bill 11 in Alberta, which legislated the contracting out of surgical services to for-profit facilities, has caused significant concern on several fronts. In two different analyses of Bill 11, the authors concluded that the contracting out of surgical services would likely affect access as those able to pay for enhanced services would be able to jump the queue and gain faster access, thus reducing access for those unwilling or unable to pay (Rachlis 2001; Donaldson and Currie 2000). A second significant concern is the potential for the activation of potentially irreversible provisions within NAFTA and world trade agreements that would force Canada to open our health care system to the market as a result of contracting out (Rachlis 2000; Deber 2002; Evans et al. 2000; Price, Pollack and Shaoul 1999). Other concerns related to private contracting include creaming (drawing the most profitable clients into the private system), transparency, appropriateness of service, and extra-billing (Evans et al. 2000).

Lastly, there is growing pressure from some private corporations, some health professionals, and some consumers to make services that are now exclusively provided by the public sector available in the private sector. In other words, there is pressure to develop a parallel private system in which the private for-profit sector is in direct competition with the public sector (some might refer to this as a two-tiered system of health care) (Lowry 1996; Dirnfield 1996). A primary motivation is the belief that this will reduce waiting lists in the public system. However, waiting lists are more likely the result of decreased federal funds to operate existing facilities at full capacity, lack of adequately trained personnel, and lack of management and centralized co-ordination of waiting lists (Commission on the Future of Health Care 2002; Deber 2002). A parallel private system might well promote creaming of the least complicated low-risk patients, draw health human resources from the public system, and decrease quality of care in the public system. Deber et al. (1997) conclude that private clinics that operate parallel to the public system charge more for similar services and are inadvertently subsidized by the public because the private sector has the ability to send patients with complications back to the public system. This has been confirmed by others (Canadian Health Services Research Foundation 2002).

SHIFTING THE BALANCE IN THE PRIORITIES FOR CARE

Almost two decades ago, Kolderie (1986) suggested that privatized delivery of services, when operated on a not-for-profit basis, does not appear to pose a threat to publicly funded health care as long as the government maintains a strong policy-making and regulating role. This remains true today. It is the greater role of private *for-profit* delivery of health care that is of serious concern because of the introduction of the *profit motive* (Taft and Steward 2000; Evans et al. 2000). In her review, Deber (2002) states that for-profit firms have the potential to make profits because of economies of scale and better management, but she raises the following caution:

> [S]avings frequently arise from more contentious measures, including freedom from labor agreements (and different wage levels and skill mixes), evasion of cost controls placed on other providers, sacrifice of difficult-to-measure intangibles, risk selection/cream skimming, and even dubious practices (vii).

She acknowledges that efficiency in the private sphere rests on the assumption of competition, which is not always possible or even desirable in health care. Although there are difficulties in comparing for-profit and not-for-profit agencies and organizations, Deber concludes that not-for-profit delivery is often the best choice "because NFP providers are less sensitive to bottom-line incentives and hence are more likely to deliver the desired level of quality in such complex environments" (vii).

According to Buchanan (1995), proponents and adversaries of increasing the private provision of health care argue that the application of market principles in health care will increase efficiency and the choices available to consumers and providers and will result in a higher quality of care. In general, economic evaluations have not found that private for-profit delivery of services increases efficiency, enhances choice, or increases quality of care (Silverman, Skinner and Fisher 1999; Deber et al. 1997; Himmelstein and Woolhander 1999; Woolhander and Himmelstein 1997; Garg et al. 1999).[18]

For-profit motives in the delivery of health care have the potential to foster discrimination in the provision of services to certain groups of people who have greater health needs, to decrease the quality of service in order to realize a profit, and to increase the cost of health care because of the need to make a profit. For practitioners, for-profit care has the potential to create conflicts between professional and corporate values that may lead to the sacrifice of quality care and the patient's best interest in the face of corporate profit-making priorities (Schafer 2002; Evans et al. 2000). In the next section, I return to a discussion of the role of nurses and the nursing profession.

WHERE IS THE PROFESSION OF NURSING?

Nurses' work is socially, historically, and contextually situated and must be understood in relation to organizational and societal forces (Fisher 1995; Chambliss 1996; Liaschenko 1995; Street 1992; Olson 1995; Rodney and Varcoe 2001; Varcoe 2001; Varcoe in press). Nurses often experience constraints on their practice that are a result of decisions made at other levels. For example, in the past, nurses have had to navigate the move to a more corporate, business-oriented approach in which organizational values of efficiency and effectiveness have marginalized values related to quality of care and patient good (Storch et al. 2002). In the current health care context of scarcity, corporatization, and shortages, the ability of nurses to practise ethically and safely is being jeopardized (Varoce et al. in press; Rodney and Varcoe 2001). Macro decisions force difficult micro-level resource allocations when nurses at the bedside are faced with increasing workloads and pressures as a result of reductions and cutbacks. The endorsement of public-private partnerships in the funding of health care at federal, provincial, and regional levels has meant that nurse leaders are in the position of implementing these directives, often without the legitimate power and authority to raise questions about the ethical implications of such directives. Individual nurses involved in implementation of such initiatives have not been involved in the decision to pursue particular directions, but are responsible and involved in the implementation of these initiatives that will ultimately shape practice.

It is the norm that policy directions and trends in reforming the health care system are taken up without consideration of the ethical consequences for practitioners or the public. In fact, the implications of policy decision-making for ethical practice and the public have largely been ignored in the policy process. Only recently have nursing authors begun to articulate the importance of ethical evaluations of proposed reforms. As Rodney and Varcoe (2001) observe, nursing work is often overlooked and invisible when the sole focus is on economic evaluations of nursing practice in health care policy development and evaluation. They urge us to complement economic evaluation with ethical inquiry in health care decision-making and health policy development in order to ensure a health care system that is humane, effective, and efficient. This means that it is imperative for nurses to be engaged in policy development at all levels and to raise questions about the ethical implications of policies for practitioners and the public. Specifically, nurses must urge that policy directives be examined to determine exactly how such directions will affect the delivery of health care and the particular individuals and groups who are the recipients of care. It is important to examine the ethical obligations of nurses to take this kind of action at the micro, meso, and macro levels of health care decision-making.

The Role of Nursing Organizations

Both national and provincial nursing organizations (professional associations and unions) have been active in raising the visibility of nursing issues and concerns at the policy level and in influencing the development of health policy for nurses and the public. At the national level, the Canadian Nurses Association has actively sought to influence the federal government in maintaining and restoring federal funding for health care to the provinces through submissions to the Minister of Health and the Romanow Commission and as a member of the Health Action Lobby (HEAL). The Canadian Nurses Association has continued to strongly reject greater private for-profit reforms and has embraced moving to a system of primary health care as the means for reforming the system. Similarly, provincial nursing associations and unions have taken a strong stance against further privatization in health care and have taken an active role in efforts to preserve medicare and to ensure the provision of publicly funded services by the provinces.

In Alberta, the Alberta Association of Registered Nurses and the United Nurses of Alberta actively lobbied against legislation promoting private for-profit provision of health care in Alberta, such as Bill 37, which would have granted tax concessions to private health care corporations, and the more recent Bill 11, which allows for the contracting of surgical services to private facilities. These groups have taken a stance against privatization, and they are promoting primary health care as a better alternative. In Ontario, nurses have actively spearheaded a campaign to warn the public about increasing the provision of private for-profit health care and they have stressed the importance of primary health care reforms (RNAO 2000). The British Columbia Nurses' Union (BCNU) has actively advocated for a strong publicly funded health care system in BC, rejecting private for-profit solutions (BCNU 2001). Such actions are consistent with the ethical duties and obligations outlined in the Canadian Nurses Association Code of Ethics, Canadian values, and a just system of health care.

It is the obligation of the professional association to promote the best interests of the public. However, it should be remembered that the best interests of the public are closely tied to the best interests of nurses in their ability to provide safe, competent, and ethical care. Professional associations are vehicles for bringing the voice of registered nurses into the policy arena at the macro level of health care. This requires strong knowledge of policy and politics among nursing leaders in all nursing organizations and moral courage on behalf of nursing organizations to articulate their values and positions. The Canadian Nurses Association, with representation from the provinces and territories, provides a unique forum for debate and discussion of professional values and positions on particular issues. The Canadian Nurses Association Code of Ethics also provides a strong moral basis for supporting reforms that are consistent with social justice. Registered nurses should continue to advocate for a system of public funding for health care, which is more likely to result in a fairer distribution of costs and to ensure equality of access to health care. Additionally, registered nurses should support collaborative research, which further explicates the values of Canadians and fosters the development of ethical frameworks for health policy analysis.

Through professional associations and unions, registered nurses can bring to the awareness of politicians, administrators, and the public the implications of for-profit health care for individuals who receive care. Registered nurses at national, provincial, and local levels can continue to bring to debates about privatization the recognition that privatization may enhance choice but is often inconsistent with Canadian values and the principles of universality, accessibility, and comprehensiveness.[19] Additionally, registered nurses can develop and speak to alternatives for enhancing the publicly funded system of health care.

As an alternative to private for-profit health care, the Canadian Nurses Association has endorsed a system of primary health care as a strategy for health care reform. This approach has long been advocated in their policy statements and positions as well as in submissions to the Hall Commissions of 1964 and 1980 (Canadian Nurses Association 1992; 1996). Reforms based on primary health care do have the capacity to create a more just system of care. Registered nurses need to continue to endorse and support a system of primary health care. As Judith Shamian observed at the February 2001 Nursing Leadership Conference in Ottawa, registered nurses need to clearly articulate the definition and principles of primary health care and to continue to educate politicians, the public, and other health care providers that *primary care* is not the same as *primary health care*. Primary health care means equitable access, maximum community involvement, increased emphasis on promotive and preventative services, appropriate use of technology, and multi-sectoral collaboration (Canadian Nurses Association 1988; 1993). In contrast, primary care reform is often a form of alternate funding mechanisms for physician services and is only one aspect of primary health care. From his analysis of health care funding mechanisms, Evans (2002) concludes that an efficient and effective health care system "requires reform of the delivery system, of how providers are organized and funded, rather than merely distributing the burdens and benefits of the present system" (vi).

While nursing organizations can clearly articulate values, develop and communicate policy positions, provide key messages, and mobilize nurses, individual nurses have an ethical commitment to be informed and to take action where possible at local, provincial, and national levels on health care reform issues that promote distributive and social justice in both personal and professional capacities.

Nursing leaders within health care organizations at the meso and micro levels of health care delivery have a different but equally important role to play in health care policy. These nurses are at the forefront of health care policy decision-making in practice and are increasingly well positioned to raise ethical questions and to call for ethical analysis. Nursing leaders can monitor their workplaces for changes to care and restructuring that promote further for-profit privatization. In the face of such proposals, registered nurses can ask, What will these changes mean for clients, especially those who already face barriers to access, including those from other cultures, the mentally ill, women, and those living in poverty?

Nurses cannot remain aloof from the politics of the policy process, either professionally or personally, because the result will be health care policy shaped *for* nursing but not *by* nursing (Chinn 1992; Cohen et al. 1996; Grant 1995; Pender 1992; Porter O'Grady 1997; Spurgeon 1997; Wakefield 1999; Whitman 1998). As Grant (1995) observes, the result of not taking action is that nurses remain an invisible, voiceless, and silent majority. Bernstein (1991) uses the term "ethical-political" to recall the classical Greek understanding of the "symbiotic relation" between ethics and politics. "Ethics is concerned with *ethos*, with those habits, customs and modes of response that shape and define our *praxis*. Politics is concerned with our public lives in the *polis*—with the communal bonds that at once unite and separate us as citizens" (9). Although distinguishable, ethics and politics are inseparable as disciplines concerned with praxis and as "aspects of a unified practice philosophy" (9). Ethics requires that we think through our political commitments and responsibilities, and understanding politics should bring us back to ethics. As Bernstein observes, this broadens our understanding of morality and brings ethics and policy into our practice.

It is clear that nurses often face ethical challenges in acting politically because of organizational and social constraints (Storch et al. 2002). While nurses have been called to take up their role in the development of health policy, nurses often feel unprepared and lacking in the knowledge and skills needed to take on this role. Several authors have suggested that health policy content needs to be integrated into nursing education programs (Buerhaus 1992; Choudry and Callahan 1993; Murphy 1999). Other authors have suggested that, at the graduate level, health policy internships or fellowships are an important strategy for enhancing nursing knowledge and skills and for making the impact of nursing visible in the health policy process (Lefort 1993; Raudonis and Griffith 1991; Stimpson and Hanley 1991). It is critical that nurses, through formal education or involvement in professional activities, develop skills for the ethical analysis of health policy and the ability to articulate their ethical concerns for the benefit of the profession and the public.

TOWARDS INFORMED ETHICAL CHOICES

Decisions to embrace certain health care reforms over others reflect ethical choices about how we wish to live together as a society (Kenny 2002). Canadian values have remained remarkably clear, unchanged and consistent with an egalitarian system of health care, with nursing values, and with criteria for a just health care system. However, Canadian beliefs about how to *achieve* these values have recently been strongly influenced by a number of sociopolitical forces. There is considerable pressure both within and outside of Canada to reduce spending on health care as a means of deficit reduction, and to treat health care as a commodity rather than a public good. As a result, privatization of the Canadian health care system is occurring by default and by design (Tholl 1994). The underlying beliefs driving this trend towards greater privatization are that opening health care to the market will correct the perceived problem of the ever-increasing costs and inefficiencies associated with a publicly funded and delivered health care system. However, this is clearly at odds with Canadian values, nursing values, and the criteria for a just health care system. The shifts in public-private funding and delivery of care within the health care system have created an ethical dissonance in which justice and fairness in health care are at risk of being undermined and eroded (Kenny 2002). Canadian values that embrace universality, equity, and solidarity are in danger of being replaced by competing values that endorse individual choice and the efficiency of the market (Commission on the Future of Health Care 2002; Kenny 2002).

If we believe in equity of access and fair opportunity in accessing the goods of society for everyone, then it is clear that we should embrace a universal publicly funded system in which everyone has the opportunity to access health care because need, not ability to pay, determines access. Proposed solutions that flow from this value system are more likely to focus on improving the organization and delivery of care than to encourage private sources of funding or for-profit care. However, if we fundamentally believe that the demand for health care will increase in perpetuity and that health care is a market good (a commodity to which those who can afford should have the privilege of access), then we are much more likely to endorse market reforms that introduce a greater private for-profit role into the funding and delivery of health care (Kenny 2002).

It is essential that nurse leaders understand the way in which health care is funded and delivered in order to assess the ethical consequences of introducing particular health care reform strategies. The choice to support publicly funded health care and to refuse to allow further private for-profit health care in Canada is a value choice Canadians have made and can continue to make. These values are morally sound and consistent with nursing values and current research. There is *no strong economic or ethical evidence* to support moving to greater private funding or private for-profit delivery of health care. There *is good evidence* to support adequate funding for a publicly funded universally accessible system of care, and a need to reorganize and improve the delivery of care (Buchanan 1995; Taft and Stewart 2000). If we are to maintain a system of publicly funded health care that is responsive and available to meet the needs of all, especially those who are most vulnerable to health problems and are often excluded or marginalized in the process of obtaining health care, it is imperative that nurses participate in the health policy process at all levels and advocate for ethical analysis of proposed reforms. All registered nurses within the scope of their power and authority have a role to play in maintaining the fabric of a fair and just health care system that meets the needs of Canadians and provides a context for safe, competent, and ethical care in nursing.

FOR REFLECTION

1. Are Canadian values shifting, and, if so, what is responsible for this shift?

2. What are the ethical tensions associated with greater private for-profit health care funding and delivery in Canada?

3. What are the ethical responsibilities of individual nurses in response to these tensions at the micro, meso, and macro levels of health care?

4. What are the ethical responsibilities of nursing collectives in response to these trends towards increasing private sources of funding and for-profit delivery in health care?

5. What constraints or facilitators might nurses experience in taking action consistent with their ethical duties and obligations in the development of health care policy?

ENDNOTES

1. The Canada Health Act only requires that coverage be provided for hospital and physician services. It is important to note that the Canada Health Act was developed and passed at a time when the scope of services such as home care, diagnostic texts, and pharmaceuticals did not exist to the same degree as they do today (Kenny 2002). The intent was to cover the most costly services so that those in need would not be bankrupted. Also, the original vision of Tommy Douglas was much broader than that of doctors and hospitals. However, due to opposition of powerful interests in the business and medical community, this was the compromise. For a more comprehensive discussion of the development of the Canada Health Act see Fuller (1998) and Kenny (2002).

2. In talking about Canadian values, I am explicitly referring to the values articulated by the Canadian public in a variety of polls and surveys conducted over the past thirty years. However, it should be noted that not all Canadians share the values articulated by the majority. There is a strong and powerful minority of Canadians who favour individual self-reliance and personal responsibility for health over communitarian values such as universality, equity, and solidarity (Schafer 2002). Values such as self-reliance and personal responsibility are more consistent with market-driven approaches to health care such as increasing private insurance, adoption of user fees, and medical savings accounts. These underlying values are consistent with a libertarian notion of justice in which health care is a commodity and individuals are responsible for their own care (Schafer 2002). However, the majority of Canadians continue to embrace the notion of social justice in which health care is a fundamental human right and common good to which all should have access. "According to this social justice tradition, every citizen—regardless of ability to pay—is part of the same moral community. In consequence, all are entitled, as a matter of justice rather than charity, to receive the medical treatment they need" (Schafer 2002, 5).

3. A fundamental point of disagreement in discussions of health care reform has focused on the introduction of market principles into the Canadian health care system. Proponents of increasing private sources of funding and greater for-profit care have argued that introduction of the market is necessary for the sustain-

ability of the Canadian health care system. Alternatively, opponents of private health care have argued that the introduction of the market will erode a strong publicly funded system of health care and that the solution is to reorganize the health care delivery system and increase the emphasis on primary health care. (See Kenny 2002; Malone 1999). The intent in this chapter is to look expressly at the ethical implications of increasing private sources of funding and introducing greater for-profit care.

4. In the United States, approximately 44 percent of the system is funded from public sources while the remaining 56 percent is funded privately through private insurance or other means of direct payment (OECD 2000). In Canada, approximately 70 percent of health care is publicly funded and all Canadians are insured through our system of public insurance.

5. Himmelstein, Woolhandler, and Wolfe (1992) state that "The number of people without health insurance is an important indicator of the adequacy of our health care system" (381). In Canada, the Canada Health Act ensures that every citizen has access to physician and hospital care. This system of public insurance means that all citizens have health insurance for physician, hospital, and other public health care services such as home care. Some estimates suggest that the cost of insuring every person in Canada is less than in the United States.

6. As Buchanan (1995) observes, "If, as I shall argue, a preponderant reliance on private insurance is likely to produce a system that scores poorly on criteria of justice, then the case for such a system is not strong on grounds of efficiency, choice, and quality, which makes criticisms on grounds of justice all the more telling" (223).

7. Taxation financing means that tax dollars are used to pay for most of the health care expenditures or are the largest source of funding (Evans 2002).

8. Public health, hospital services, services to status Indians, and physicians' services are funded through public sources. Home care rehabilitative services, residential long-term care, ambulances, and prescription drugs are funded through a mixture of public and private funding sources (CIHI 2000).

9. The most common expenditure of private funds is on drugs and dental services. Other privately funded services include optometry, non-prescription drugs, and non-physician health care providers such as physiotherapy and complementary medicine. Extended health care, purchased through employers, is an example of private insurance in Canada (CIHI 2000).

10. Many have argued that a better assessment of the costs of health care is to examine the portion of the Canadian Gross Domestic Product (GDP) spent on health care (e.g., Kenny 2002; Boychuk 2002; Schafer 2002). Health care spending as a portion of the GDP has remained remarkably stable at about 9 percent for the past ten years (CIHI 2000). This rate of expenditure is consistent with other countries in which publicly funded health is the norm and is considerably less than countries such as the United States, where there is a greater balance of private health care. The United States spends about 13 percent of their GDP on health care (CIHI 2003; OECD 2000). It should be remembered that while health care spending has been stable as a percent of GDP, there are clear fluctuations in terms of who bears the cost of health care, overall revenues in relation to expenditures, and spending in other governmental sectors (Boychuk 2002). When federal spending on health care decreased, a greater burden was placed upon the provinces in terms of the cost of health care. At the same time, the provinces were faced with rising costs. Some provinces reduced taxes, which had the effect of reduced revenues and a perception of growing expenditures in relation to shrinking revenues. Additionally, when spending is reduced in other public sectors, the percent of budget spent on health care will automatically increase even though the actual costs of health care have not increased. The fact is that health care accounts for a greater portion of a steadily shrinking budget. As Boychuk (2002) observes, this is why it is inaccurate to project that health care costs are unsustainable and spiralling out of control. He argues that we are not in a funding crisis, nor is there an impending funding crisis. However, we are in a crisis in terms of federal-provincial relationships and sustainability of the health care system (Boychuk 2002). Kenny (2002) contends that this is a crisis in which we are at risk of losing the fundamental values related to justice and equity in health care.

11. It should be noted that user fees already exist in Canada for items such as prescription drugs (Commission on the Future of Health Care in Canada 2002). The Commission states that outside of hospitals drugs, "may be partially covered by provincial health insurance plans or private coverage, or not covered at all" (4). Another example in British Columbia is the provision of physiotherapy services on the basis of user pay. Currently, user fees for hospital and physician services are not permitted under the Canada Health Act. According to the Commission, Canadians have mixed responses to the idea of introducing user fees for hospital and physician services.

12. It has previously been noted that there is much to learn from the integration of ethical and economic analysis in assessment of health care policy. Also, as indicted previously, a full economic analysis is beyond the scope of this chapter. However, it is important to note that when one examines the economic evidence, there is, as several authors have observed, congruence between ethical and economic analysis of private options for reforming health care (Schafe 2002; Hurley 2001). As Buchanan (1995) has observed, the fact that the economic evidence goes against the belief that private is more efficient makes the ethical analysis all the more telling.

13. Based on an analysis of physician and hospital costs of individual Manitoba residents, Forget et al. (2002) point out that allowing people to keep the money allocated to them but not spent may have the effect of increasing choice but would actually increase health care costs significantly without any gains in equity.

14. It should be noted that if catastrophic insurance was provided publicly, "costs could actually increase because governments would not only provide the initial allowance but also continue to pay for catastrophic insurance to protect people against very high costs" (Commission on the Future of Health Care 2002, 29). In other words, as Shortt (2002) observes, "If coverage were provided by a public source, it would require subsidy by tax revenues, which is exactly what MSA's are intended to avoid" 162.

15. Many countries have engaged in public-private partnerships or P3s. In particular, there has been considerable experience with P3s in Britain. For an overview and discussion of the Private Finance Initiative, see Deber (2002).

16. The concern is when private insurance must be purchased directly by the individual. This is a particular concern for those who would not have the benefit of employer-provided health programs. Many Canadians have private insurance for drugs or dental care as an employee benefit through an individual agreement or union contract.

17. It could be argued that most of health care is already privately delivered. Clearly, physicians provide health services on a private for-profit basis. Deber (2002) has argued that health authorities could be considered to be private not-for-profit providers. However, given that health authorities in most provinces are appointed by legislation, carry out a public mandate, allocate public funds, operate in a not for-profit basis, and are accountable to government, it can be argued that they are becoming more like public sector bodies, although not necessarily government bodies (M. Prince, personal communication, April 28, 2003). However, for the purposes of this chapter, regional health authorities will be considered to be private not-for-profit entities.

18. Each of the four studies cited here have been carefully evaluated (see, for example, Deber 2002; Taft and Steward 2000). The results of these studies are an important source of data in understanding the implications of for-profit health care in terms of efficiency and quality.

19. As well, as has been noted previously, economic evaluations reveal that private options for reforming health care are not likely to result in a more efficient use of resources or to be more cost effective.

REFERENCES

Aday, L. 1993. *At risk in America: The health and health care needs of vulnerable populations in the United States*. San Francisco: Jossey-Bass.

Angus, D.E., Auer, L. Cloutier, J. E. and Albert, T. 1995. *Sustainable health care for Canada: Synthesis report*. Queen's–University of Ottawa Economic Projects.

Armstrong, P. and Armstrong, H. 1996. *Wasting away: The undermining of Canadian health care.* Toronto: Oxford University Press.

Arras, J.D., Steinbock, B. and London, A. J. 1999. Moral reasoning in the medical context. In J.D. Arras and B. Steinbock (Eds.), *Ethical issues in modern medicine*, 5th ed. (pp. 1–40). Toronto: Mayfield Publishing Company.

Barr, M.D. 2001. Medical savings accounts in Singapore: A critical inquiry. *Journal of Health Politics, Policy and Law, 26*(4), 709–726.

Baylis, F., Downie, J., Freedman, B., Hoffmaster, B. and Sherwin, S. (Eds.). 1995. *Health care ethics in Canada*. Toronto: Harcourt Brace.

BCNU (British Columbia Nurses Union). 2001. *Submission to the select standing committee on health.* Retrieved May 28, 2003 from www.bcnu.org/submisson_nov_01.htm

Beauchamp, T. and Childress, J. 1994. *Principles of biomedical ethics.* 4th edition. New York: Oxford University Press.

Beck, R.G. and Horne, J. M. 1980. Utilization of publicly insured health services in Saskatchewan before, during and after copayment. *Medical Care, 18*(8), 787–800.

Bernstein, R.J. 1991. *The new constellation: The ethical–political horizons of modernity/postmodernity.* Cambridge, MA: MIT Press.

Blue, A., Keyserlingk, E., Rodney, P. and Starzomski, R. 1999. A critical view of North American health policy. In H. Coward and P. Ratanakul (Eds.), *A cross-cultural dialogue on health care ethics* (pp. 215–225). Waterloo, ON: Wilfred Laurier University Press.

Boychuck, G. 2002. *The changing political and economic environment of health care in Canada.* Commission on the Future of Health Care Discussion. Retrieved July 15, 2002 from : www.healthcarecommission.ca/Suite247/Common/GetMedia_WO.asp?MediaID=878&Filename=Boychuk_E.pdfReference

British Columbia Select Standing Committee on Health. 2002. *Patients first 2002: The path to reform.* Victoria: Office of the Clerk of Committees.

Buchanan, A. 1995. Privatization and just care. *Bioethics, 9*(3/4), 220–239.

Buerhaus, P. 1992. Teaching health care public policy. *Nursing and Health Care, 13*(6), 304–309.

Canadian Health Care Association. 2002. *A responsive, sustainable, publicly funded health system in Canada—the art of the possible. CHA's ten-point plan for moving from discussion to action.* Ottawa: Canadian Health Care Association. Available online: www.canadian-healthcare.org/documents/romanow.doc

Canadian Health Services Research Foundation. 2001. *Mythbusters: User fees would stop waste and ensure better use of the healthcare system.* Ottawa: Canadian Health Services Research Foundation. Available online: www.chsrf.ca

Canadian Health Services Research Foundation. 2002. *Mythbusters: For-profit ownership of facilities would lead to more efficient health care system.* Ottawa: Canadian Health Services Research Foundation. Retrieved from www.chsrf.ca.

Canadian Medical Association. 2001. *National Report Card.* Available online: www.cma.ca/national_report_card2001.pdf.

Canadian Nurses Association. 1988. *Health for all Canadians: A call for health care reform.* Ottawa: Canadian Nurses Association.

Canadian Nurses Association. March, 1992. *Health promotion (Policy Statement).* Ottawa: Canadian Nurses Association.

Canadian Nurses Association. 1993. Five guiding principles for Primary Health Care. *Journal of Nursing Administration, 23*(5), 4, 10.

Canadian Nurses Association. March, 1996. *The comprehensiveness of Canada's health care system (Policy Statement).* Ottawa: Canadian Nurses Association.

Canadian Nurses Association. 2002. *Code of Ethics for Registered Nurses.* Ottawa: Canadian Nurses Association.

Caplan, R. Light, D. and Daniels, N. 1999. Benchmarks of fairness: A moral framework for assessing equity. *International Journal of Health Services, 29*(4), 853–869.

Chambliss, D. 1996. *Beyond caring.* Chicago: University of Chicago Press.

Chinn, P. 1992. Where and when does change begin? *Nursing Outlook, 40*(3), 102–103.

Choudry, U. and Callahan, P. 1993. Integrating health policy into the nursing curriculum. *Registered Nurse, 5*(4), 10–11, 38.

CIHI (Canadian Institute of Health Information). 2000. *Total health expenditure, Canada summary 1975–1999*. Available online: www.cihi.ca

CIHI (Canadian Institute of Health Information). 2003. *Health care in Canada*. Retrieved May 29, 2003 from: www.cihi.ca.

Cohen, S., Mason, D., Kovner, C. Leavitt, J., Pulcini, J. and Sochalski, J. 1996. Stages of nursing's political development: Where we've been and where we ought to go. *Nursing Outlook, 44*(6), 259–266.

Commission on the Future of Healthcare in Canada. 2002. *Sustainability of Canada's healthcare system*. Retrieved July 15, 2002 from: www.healthcarecommission.ca/Suite247/common/GetMedia_WO.asp?MediaID=763&Filename=sustainability.pdf.

Commission on the Future of Health Care in Canada. 2002. *Building on values: The future of health care in Canada*. Final Report. Ottawa: Commission on the Future of Health Care in Canada.

Commission of Study on Health and Social Services. 2001. *Emerging solutions: Report and recommendations*. Quebec: Government of Quebec. Retrieved May 20, 2003 from www.cessss.gouv.qc.ca/pdf/en/01-109-01a(pdf)

Conference Board of Canada. 2000. *Canadians' values and attitudes on Canada's health care system: A synthesis of survey results*. Ottawa: Conference Board of Canada.

Daniels, N. 1985. *Just health care*. Cambridge: Cambridge University Press.

Deber, R.B., Mhatre, S. L. and Ross Baker, G. 1994. A review of provincial initiatives. In A. Blomqvist and D. Brown (Eds.), *Limits to care: Reforming Canada's health system in an age of restraint*. Toronto: C.D. Howe Institute.

Deber, R., Narine, L., Baranek, P., Hilfer Sharpe, N., Masnyk Duvalko, K., Zlotnik-Shaul, R., Coyte, P., Pink, G. and Williams, A.P. 1997. *National forum on health: Summary of the public/private mix in health care* (Parts I and II). Available online: wwwnfh.hc-sc.gc.ca/publicat/issuesum.

Deber, R. 2002. *Delivering health care services: Public, not-for-profit, or private?* Discussion Paper No. 17. Ottawa: Commission on the Future of Health Care in Canada.

DeCoster, C. and Brownell, M. 1997. Private health care in Canada: Saviour or siren? *Public Health Reports, 112*(4), 298–305.

Dirnfield, V. 1996. The benefits of privatization. *Canadian Medical Association Journal, 155*(4), 407–410.

Donaldson, C. and Currie, G. 2000. *The public purchase of private surgical services: A systematic review of the evidence on efficiency and equity*. Institute of Health Economics Working Paper 00-9. Retrieved May 15, 2003 from: www.ihe.ca/publications/papers/pdf/2000-09paper.pdf.

Evans, R., Barer, M. and Stoddart, G. 1993. The truth about user fees. *Policy Options, 14*(8), 4–9.

Evans, R.G., Barer, M.L, Lewis, S. Rachlis, M. and Stoddart, G. 2000. *Private highway, one-way street: The deklein and fall of Canadian Medicare?* Centre for Health Services and Policy Research. Retrieved July 15, 2002 from: www.chspr.ubc.ca

Evans, R.G. 2000. *Financing health care: Taxation and the alternatives*. University of British Columbia: Centre for Health Services and Policy Research.

Evans, R.G. 2002. *Raising the money: Options, consequences, and objectives for financing health care in Canada*. Discussion Paper No. 27. Ottawa: Commission on the Future of Health Care in Canada.

Families USA. 2003. *Going without health insurance: Nearly one in three non-elderly Americans*. Report released by the Robert Wood Johnson Foundation. Retrieved from: www.familiesusa.org/site/DocServer/Going_without_report.pdf?docID=273

Fisher, A. 1995. The ethical problems encountered in psychiatric nursing practice with dangerous mentally ill persons. *Scholarly Inquiry for Nursing Practice, 9*, 193–208.

Forget, E., Deber, R. and Roos. 2002. Medical savings accounts: Will they reduce costs? *Canadian Medical Association Journal, 167*(2), 143–147.

Fraser, R. 2003. The exploitation of Canadian values—'Building on values' the Romanow Report. *Health Ethics Today, 13*(1), 2–4.

Fuchs, V. 1996. Economics, values and health care reform. *American Economic Review, 86*(1), 1–23.

Fuller, C. 1998. *Caring for profit: How corporations are taking over Canada's health care system.* Vancouver: New Star Books.

Garg, P.P., Frick, K.D., Diener-West, M. and Powe, N.R. 1999. Effect of theownership of dialysis facilities on patients' survival and referral fortransplantation. *New England Journal of Medicine, 341*(22), 1653–1660.

Grant, A. 1995. Flex your muscle. *Canadian Nurse, March*, 37–41.

Gratzer, D. 1999. *Code Blue: Reviving Canada's health care system.* Toronto: ECW Press.

Graves, F.L., Beauchamp, P. and Herle, D. 1998. Research on Canadian values in relation to health and the health care system. In *Canada Health Action: Building on the legacy: Papers commissioned by the National Forum on Health. Making decisions: Evidence and Information,* volume 5 (pp. 351–437). Sainte-Foy: Editions MultiMondes.

Hall, J.M., Stevens, P. and Meleis, A.I. 1994. Marginalization: A guiding concept for valuing diversity in nursing knowledge development. *Advances in Nursing Science, 16(4)*, 23–41.

Hall, J.M. 1999. Marginalization Revisited: Critical, postmodern, and liberation perspectives. *Advances in Nursing Science, 22*(2), 88–102.

Health Canada. 2003. *Canada Health Act.* Retrieved May 28, 2003 from: www.hc-sc.gc.ca/medicare/home.htm

Hsiao, W. 2001. Commentary: Behind the ideology and theory: What is the empirical evidence for medical savings accounts? *Journal of Health Politics, Policy and Law, 26*(4), 739–745.

Ham, C. 2001. Commentary: Values and health policy: The case of Singapore. *Journal of Health Politics, Policy and Law, 26*(4), 739–745.

Himmelstein, D., Woolhandler, S. and Wolfe, S. 1992. The Vanishing health care safety net: New data on uninsured Americans. *International Journal of Health Services, 22*(3), 381–396.

Himmelstein, D. and Woolhandler, S. 1999. Quality of care in investor-owned vs. not-for-profit HMO's. *Journal of the American Medical Association, 282*(2), 159–163.

Hurley, J. 2001. Ethics, economics and public financing of health care. *Journal of Medical Ethics, 27*(4), 234–239.

Hurley, J. 2002. Medical savings accounts will not advance Canadian health care objectives. *Canadian Medical Association Journal, 167*(2), 152–152.

Kenny, N.P. 2002. *What good is health care? Reflections on the Canadian experience.* Ottawa: CHA Press.

Kolderie, T. 1986. The two different concepts of privatization. *Public Administration Review, 46*(4), 285–291.

Kreiger, N. 1999. Embodying inequality: a review of concepts, measures, and methods for studying health consequences of discrimination. *International Journal of Health Services, 29*(2), 295–352.

Lebacqz, K. 2002. Plenary presentation to the Canadian Bioethics Society Conference, October, 2002. Victoria, BC.

LeFort, S. 1993. Shaping health care policy. *Canadian Nurse, 89*(3), 23–27.

Liaschenko, J. 1995. Ethics in the work of acting for patients. *Advances in Nursing Science, 18*(2), 1012.

Lowry, F. 1996. Larger private-sector role in health needed now, think tank warns. *Canadian Medical Association Journal, 154*(4), 549–551.

Malone, R. 1999. Policy as product: Morality and metaphor in health policy discourse. *Hastings Center Report, 29*(3), 16–22.

Marmor, T.R., Okma, K.G. and Latham, S.R. 2002. *National values, institutions and health policies: What do they imply for medicare reform?* Commission on the Future of Health Care in Canada. Discussion paper No. 5. Retrieved September 2002 from: www.healthcarecommission.ca

Marshall, V. 1994. A critique of Canadian aging and health policy. In V. W. Marshall and B.D. McPherson (Eds.), *Aging: Canadian perspectives* (pp. 232–244). Peterborough: Broadview Press.

Mendelsohn, M. 2002. *Canadians' thoughts on their health care system: Preserving the Canadian Model through innovation.* Commission on the Future of Health Care in Canada. Retrieved November 20, 2002 from: www.healthcarecommission.ca

Migue, J.L. 2002. *Funding and production of heath services: Outlook and potential solutions.* Discussion Paper No. 10. Ottawa: Commission on the Future of Heath Care in Canada.

Moorhouse, A. 1993. User fees: Fair cost containment or a tax on the sick? *The Canadian Nurse, 89,* 21–24.

Murphy, N.J. 1999. A survey of health policy content in Canadian graduate programs in nursing. *Journal of Nursing Education, 38*(2), 88–91.

OECD (Organization for Economic Development and Cooperation). 2000. *Public expenditures on health.* Retrieved May 15, 2002 from: www.oecd.org

OECD (Organization for Economic Development and Cooperation). 2000. *Total Expenditures on health—%GDP.* Retrieved May 15, 2002 from: www.oecd.org

Olson, L. 1995. Ethical climate in health care organization. *International Council of Nurses, 42*(3), 85–95.

OWN (Older Women's Network) and RNAO (Registered Nurses Association of Ontario). 1998. Joint statement: *The impact of health care restructuring on older women.* Toronto: OWN and RNAO.

Pal, L 1997. *Beyond policy analysis: Public issue management in turbulent times.* Scarborough: Nelson Thomson Learning.

Peters, S. 1995. *Exploring Canadian values: A synthesis report.* Ottawa: Canadian Policy Research Networks.

Pender, N. 1992. Making a difference in health policy. *Nursing Outlook, 40*(3), 104–105.

Porter-O'Grady, T. 1997. Influencing policy: Foreign territory for nurses. *Advanced Practice Nursing Quarterly, 3*(32), 79–80.

Price, D., Pollock, A.M. and Shaoul, J. 1999. How the World Trade Organization is shaping domestic policies in health care. *Lancet, 354,* 1889–1892.

Premier's Advisory Council on Health for Alberta. 2001. *A framework for reform: Report of the Premier's Advisory Council on Health.* Government of Alberta. Retrieved May 20, 2003 from: www.premieradvisory.com/pdf/PACH_report_final.pdf

Rachlis, M. and Kushner, C. 1994. *Strong medicine: How to save Canada's health care system.* Toronto: HarperCollins.

Rachlis, M. 2000. *A review of the Alberta private hospital proposal.* Ottawa: Caledon Institute of Social Policy.

Raudonis, B. and Griffith, H. 1991. Model for integrating health services research and health care. *Nursing and Health Care, 12*(1), 32–36.

Rich, P. 2001. User fees if necessary but not necessarily user fees. *Canadian Medical Association Journal, 165,* 1526 [Electronic version]. Retrieved July 15, 2002 from Health Source (Nursing/Academic Edition).

Rodney, P., Varcoe, C., McPherson, G., Storch, J., Mahoney, K., Brown, H., Pauly, B., Hartrick, G. and Starzomski, R. 2002. Navigating a Moral Horizon: A multi-site qualitative research study of nurses' enactment of ethical practice. *Canadian Journal of Nursing Research, 34*(3), 75–102.

RNAO (Registered Nurses Association of Ontario). 1999. *Nurses warn about privatization: Backgrounder.* Toronto: RNAO.

RNAO (Registered Nurses Association of Ontario). 2000. *The Canada Health Act: To preserve and protect.* Toronto: RNAO.

Rodney, P. and Varcoe, C. 2001. Toward ethical inquiry in the economic evaluation of nursing practice. *Canadian Journal of Nursing Research, 33*(1), 35–57.

Saskatchewan Commission on Medicare. 2001. *Caring for medicare: Sustaining a quality system.* Retrieved May 20, 2003 from: www.health.gov.sk.ca/info_center_pub_commission_on_medicare_bw.pdf

Schafer, A. 2002. *Waiting for Romanow: Canada's health care values under fire.* Ottawa: Canadian Center for Policy Alternatives. Retrieved January 15, 2003 from: www.policyalternatives.ca

Shortt, S.E. 2002. Medical savings accounts in publicly funded health care systems: Enthusiasm versus evidence. *Canadian Medical Association Journal, 167*(2), 159–162.

Silverman, E. Skinner, J. and Fisher, E. 1999. The association between for-profit hospital ownership and increased medicare spending. *New England Journal of Medicine, 34*(6), 420–426.

Spurgeon, P. 1997. How nurses can influence policy. *Nursing Times, 93*(45), 34–35.

Standing Senate Committee on Social Affairs, Science and Technology. 2002. *The health of Canadians—The Federal role. Final report on the state of the health care System in Canada. Volume Six: Recommendations for reform* (M.J.L. Kirby, Chair). Ottawa: Standing Senate Committee on Social Affairs, Science and Technology. Retrieved May 20 from: www.parl.gc.ca/37/2/parlbus/commbus/senate/come-e/soci-e/rep-e/report02vol6-e.pdf

Stevens, P. 1992. Who gets care? Access to health care as an arena for nursing action. *Scholarly Inquiry for Nursing Practice, 6*(3), 185–200.

Stimpson, M. and Hanley, B. 1991. Nursing policy analyst: Advanced practice role. *Nursing and Health Care, 12*(1), 10–15.

Stoddart, G. and Labelle, R. 1985. *Privatization in the Canadian Health Care System: Assertions, evidence, ideology and options.* Ottawa: Minister of Supply and Services Canada.

Stone, D. 1997. Policy paradox: *The art of political decision-making.* New York: W.W. Norton and Co.

Storch, J., Rodney, P., Pauly, B., Brown, H. and Starzomski, R. 2002. Listening to nurses' moral voices: Building a quality health care environment. *Canadian Journal of Nursing Leadership, 15*(4), 7–16.

Street, A. 1992. *Inside nursing: A critical ethnography of clinical nursing practice.* Albany: State of New York Press.

Taft, K. and Steward, G. 2000. *Clear answers: The economics and politics of for-profit medicine.* Edmonton: Duval House Publishing, University of Alberta Press, and Parkland Institute.

Tamblyn, R. et al. 2001. Adverse events associated with prescription drug cost-sharing among poor and elderly persons. *Journal of the American Medical Association, 285*(4), 421–429.

Tholl, W.G. 1994. Health care spending in Canada: Skating faster on thinner ice. In A. Blomqvist and D. Brown (Eds.), *Limits to care: Reforming Canada's health system in an age of restraint* (pp. 53–89). Ottawa: Renouf Publishing Company Limited.

United States Census Bureau. 2002. *Number of Americans with and without health insurance rise, Census Bureau Reports.* September 30, 2002 press release retrieved May 28, 2003 from: www.census.gove/Press-release/www/2002/cb02-127.html

Varcoe, C. 2001. Abuse obscured: An ethnographic account of emergency nursing in relation to violence against women. *Canadian Journal of Nursing Research, 32*(4), 95–115.

Varcoe, C., Doane, G., Pauly, B., Rodney, P., Storch, J., Mahoney, K., McPherson, G., Starzomski, R. and Brown, H. In press. Ethical practice in nursing: Working the in-betweens. *Journal of Nursing Scholarship.*

Wakefield, M. 1999. Canaries in the mine. *Journal of Professional Nursing, 15*(4), 205.

Whitman, M. 1998. Nurses can influence public health policy. *Advanced Nursing Practice Quarterly, 3*(4), 67–71.

Woolhandler, S. and Himmelstein, D. 1997. Costs of care and administration at for-profit hospitals in the United States. *New England Journal of Medicine, 336,* 769–774.

Young, I.M. 1990. *Justice and the politics of difference.* Princeton, N.J.: Princeton University Press.

chapter ten

The Moral Climate of Nursing Practice: Inquiry and Action

Patricia Rodney
and Annette Street

Recommended as a rational method of improving nurse productivity, I argue that objective needs assessment and staffing procedures result in decisions that are neither as rational as they seem nor more trustworthy than those made on nurses' judgement alone. The objective decisions do, however, mean that nursing-care time can be limited and nurses' work intensified. Such outcomes add stress to nurses' working conditions that, combined with reductions in the scope and level of services able to be offered under new time constraints, threaten the quality of care for hospital patients (Campbell 1987, 463).

Over the past decade and more, the economic, political, and social contexts of Western health care delivery have undergone rapid and often devastating changes. In Canada and other Western countries, this has led to an era in which there is a widely held assumption that actions to save money in health care and other social services are inherently justifiable. Efficiency considerations have come to trump considerations of quality of care in the implementation of a great deal of health policy. Thus, patients, families, and communities are experiencing increasing difficulty accessing services appropriate for their needs, and the impact on health care providers—especially nurses—has been close to catastrophic.[1] In this chapter it is our intent to discuss some of the implications of contemporary policy shifts for nursing, particularly in terms of the **moral climate** of nursing practice. It is also our intent to point towards directions nursing can take (and is beginning to take) to improve that moral climate.

Let us start by laying out some of our premises. First, we assume that changes in health care policy per se are not necessarily problematic. Indeed, the changes are usually driven by positive goals such as making health care delivery more patient centred, reducing over-treatment, and having more input from regions and communities about what they need. A number of policy initiatives have, no doubt, been beneficial. However, as we will explain in this chapter, our primary concern is that the *processes* by which changes are planned, the processes by which changes are implemented, and the lack of evaluation of the effects of the changes are problematic. A **corporate ethos**[2] has infused health care policy processes, with resultant power inequities that have generated a number of (presumably unintended) negative consequences. Secondly, we assume that **power inequities** in contemporary health care policy processes are interfering with nurses' abilities to provide good quality patient/family/community care. This is an assumption that we support with data as we proceed. Thirdly, we assume that nurses' difficulties in providing good quality care constitute a serious ethical problem. Providing quality care to patients, families, and communities is an important ethical good—important because it underpins the entire health care enterprise. Therefore, allowing nurses to provide care in a manner that is respectful to the nurses themselves and to the values of the nursing profession is also an important ethical good—instrumentally important because it helps to preserve the health and well-being of the public.[3] We will profile some research data warning what happens to the health and well-being of the public when nurses are unable to provide quality care.

In expanding on our premises we commence with illustrations of relevant nursing research from Canada, Australia, and a recent international outcomes project. This will lead us to a reflection on the impact of Western economic, political, and social changes on health care delivery, and particularly on nursing practice. Following this we will link power inequities in health care policy processes to the moral climate of nursing practice. In concluding, we will posit a number of strategies that can help to improve that climate. We will also point to areas for future nursing inquiry.

INQUIRY INTO THE MORAL CLIMATE OF NURSING PRACTICE

Early nursing ethics research tended to focus on naming ethical issues and on understanding nurses' patterns of moral reasoning (Rodney 1997). Thus, as Chapter 8 on nurses' moral agency pointed out, our understanding of the complex **sociopolitical contexts** in which nurses enact their **moral agency** is still relatively underdeveloped. Our profession has a burgeoning body of research on the serious challenges to nurses' workplaces arising from the sociopolitical contexts in which we practise—including some of nursing's strengths in negotiating these contexts. We will highlight some relevant nursing research here and then reflect on the implications for the moral climate of nursing practice.

Canadian Illustrators

As we indicated at the outset of this chapter, Canadians have witnessed a progressive deterioration in the conditions of **nurses' work** and a simultaneous deterioration in the health care received by patients/clients, families, and communities. Across Canada, nurses face excessive workloads, a shortage of skilled colleagues, a decimated cadre of nurse leaders, and the increasing acuity/distress of those for whom they provide care (Rodney and Varcoe 2001,

35).[4] For example, nurses on acute medical wards report that they are not staffed well enough to properly assess and intervene with critically ill patients (Rodney 1997), nurses in emergency units report that they do not have time to talk or listen to patients even in situations where conversation is essential (such as when patients receive life-threatening diagnoses or experience violence by their partners) (Varcoe 1997; 2001), and community nurses report that they cannot always offer their clients and families the health programs that they need (MacPhail 1996; Oberle and Tenove 2000; Peter and Morgan 2001; see also Chapter 12).

To further illustrate, in a recent study that one of us was engaged in (Rodney), a research team undertook a qualitative study of the meaning of ethics for nurses providing direct care, for nurses in advanced practice positions in nursing, and for students in nursing (Rodney et al. 2002; Storch et al. 2002; Varcoe et al. in press; see also Appendix A).[5] Our research team was also interested in how these three groups of nurses/student nurses described their enactment of ethical practice. Our findings included insights about how the organizational context influenced nurses' abilities to uphold the ethics of their practice— that is, their ability to work towards a moral horizon (Rodney et al. 2002). Throughout our study, nurses in every practice context identified their practice as frequently constrained— and, fortunately, also assisted—by influences outside of their immediate control. We came to understand such influences as currents affecting navigation and, thus, affecting progress towards the moral horizon.

Ethics in Practice 10-1 provides a sample of a focus group interview with nurses practising on an acute medical unit, which highlights some of our findings. The nurses are discussing end-of-life care.

Ethics in Practice 10-1	On the Medical Unit

First Medical Unit Nurse:... [I]n the last few cases... I said [to the doctor], "Well, they've got a hospital bed now, they're not going to get a hospice bed, that's the way the system works."... And in a very rare case, the squeaky wheel does get greased and they get a hospice bed, but it's a very rare case. Those two that we had both died on the ward, waiting and wanting to go to hospice. I'm not saying that we didn't make them comfortable. Because we do a lot of hospice care on our floor, just like they do in [the hospice]. But you know, they [the patients] really, in their mind, they'd gone through the hospice program, they got the [information], they wanted to die in hospice, they had the tour, that's where they wanted to spend their last

days and they couldn't do that because somewhere in the communication they ended up getting sent to the hospital.

Second Medical Unit Nurse: I think everyone's so busy, that everyone's running around. And that's why it's too bad there's not one person on the unit looking over all of it. I think that would be wonderful. I don't know, I think things would run so much smoother... because from casual nurse to part-time to full-time... you're not as familiar as you would like to be. But if there was one designated person on the unit that could oversee that...

Third Medical Unit Nurse: There used to be the head nurse to do all the discharge planning....

First Medical Unit Nurse: There's nothing more frustrating, and we've all done it, it's going in to see a patient in the morning and they say, "Okay, I'm supposed to see L," or whoever [the] social worker happens to be that day, "at 2:15 today and meet with so-and-so." And you have no clue. Let alone why.... And so then they [the patient] think, "Oh, this one's stupid."

Second Medical Unit Nurse: Yeah, I often sometimes feel very stupid. Like in the last two days that it's been so busy on the unit. I don't know their names and I don't know their diagnosis.

First Medical Unit Nurse: All of a sudden they become a bed: "[Bed 4] and he wants...." I know... I think a lot of that has to do with the fact that there's so much going on. And we try, I mean we make these new forms... and here's a new discharge planning form and a new form for this and that's fine, it might put everything together, but unless we use them and have the time to use them, they're useless (Storch et al. 2001).

In Ethics in Practice 10-1, the medical unit nurses were trying to navigate to a place where they could offer their patients meaningful choices in **end-of-life care** and help to coordinate activities with other colleagues (such as social workers). However, the corporate ethos meant that nurses' time to communicate or plan was not valued, and they were required to care for as many patients as they could as quickly as possible—findings that Rodney (1997) also came up with in her ethnography on two acute medical units and that Varcoe (1997; 2001) came up with in her ethnography on two emergency units (see also Varcoe, Rodney and McCormick in press). Thus, the corporate emphasis on efficiency trumped considerations of patient/family well-being, interdisciplinary team cohesion, and nurse satisfaction. Time for quality nursing care became a prized and contested commodity (Rodney et al. 2002). In the transcript above, for instance, the paperwork required to implement a new discharge planning process was felt to be too time consuming to implement, especially in the absence of unit-based nursing leadership. The consequences of not being able to move towards a moral horizon were more than just dissatisfaction. The nurses felt exhausted and demoralized ("stupid"), which they spoke of more as the focus group interview progressed.

Significantly, we heard similar concerns echoed in every focus group with nurses involved in direct care (Rodney et al. 2002; Storch et al. 2002; Varcoe et al. in press). Fortunately, there were also situations in which the prevailing currents facilitated nurses' attempts to navigate towards a moral horizon (Rodney et al. 2002). Supportive colleagues in nursing and other disciplines were a major positive influence, as were professional guidelines and standards and access to ethics education. While our focus in this chapter is primarily the problems that nurses encounter, understanding such assets is also important.

The impact of the constrained organizational context on patients, families, and communities is not yet well documented, but the evidence we do have indicates that it is profound. In an ethnographic study with 60 patients and 56 health care professionals in a large teaching hospital in a major Canadian city, for instance, nurses found "difficulties in ensuring patients' basic care needs were met," particularly "when care needs of patients changed unexpectedly, when new care needs arose, when patients did not follow the 'usual' progression of recovery or when they had needs that had not been considered" (Lynam et al. 2003, 123). Furthermore, researchers noticed that while patients generally expressed satisfaction with the care they received in hospital, rapid discharge from hospital left many of them vulnerable when they returned home. Patients and families were not prepared, there were often inadequate resources in the home, and the families were not sure whom to call if they ran into difficulty. Families who did not speak English and who were not well off economically were especially vulnerable (Lynam et al. 2003). Another researcher (Stajduhar 2003) raised similar concerns about the impact on patients and families in an ethnographic study of home-based palliative caregiving (with 12 dying patients, 13 family members, and 47 caregivers as well as 28 health care providers and 10 administrators). She warned that "restructuring of home support resulted in some caregivers losing familiar home support workers they trusted" and that "policy changes to accommodate provincial standards for home support resulted in reduced numbers of subsidized home support hours for families" (31). Stajduhar shed light on a chilling picture in the following interview segment from a retired woman on a small pension:

> I was told that if he wasn't dead before November 1st that I wouldn't have any more support hours left.... If he's not dead before November 1st, I don't know what I'll do (Stajduhar 2003, 31).

What **policy processes** have led to the kinds of problems for nurses, patients, and families we have illustrated above? The nurses in Ethics in Practice 10-1 also spoke of the absence of nursing leadership on their unit. Let us look at another recent Canadian illustration. Gaudine and Beaton (2002) focused on ethical practice and leadership in their qualitative study of 15 nurse managers in an eastern Canadian province. Their findings add a disturbing overlay to the concerns expressed in the other studies we have cited so far.

Gaudine and Beaton (2002) articulated four themes of ethical conflict arising between nurse managers and their organizations, including voicelessness, where to spend the money, rights of individuals versus needs of the organization, and unjust practices on the part of senior administration and/or the organization. Significantly, the theme of voicelessness was identified in every interview. It reflected a widespread sense of powerlessness on the part of the nurse managers. Ethics in Practice 10-2 provides a transcript quotation from one of the nurse managers.

Ethics in Practice 10-2 | **The Manager**

There doesn't seem to be knowledge [by senior administration] with regards to why we need nursing, why we need to have a good float pool, why we need to have permanent staff versus casual staff.... The bottom line is always the dollar and the cents and I keep going back saying, "Well, you know, this is a business, but it's a health care business, and when you forget that you have forgotten why we're here." And of course everybody looks at me like I'm from another planet.... I really don't think that they want to get it (Gaudine and Beaton 2002, 23).

Given that supportive nursing leadership is prerequisite to a safe and competent work-place (Canadian Nurses Association 1998; Health Canada Office of Nursing Policy 2001; Health Canada 2002; Storch 1999), the absence and/or demoralization of nurse leaders portrayed in Ethics in Practice 10-1 and Ethics in Practice 10-2 (and also portrayed in Lynam et al. 2003 and Stajduhar 2003) is a major concern. In fact, Gaudine and Beaton's (2002) entire study is a graphic portrayal of the power inequities inherent in the corporate ethos that have come to dominate health care delivery. Nurses' voices are apparently not heard in the planning, implementation, or evaluation of health care policy.

Ethics in Practice 10-2 is a bleak contrast to the finding over 20 years ago from research with **"magnet hospitals"** in the United States that

> Nursing... has a voice at the top decision-making level of the hospital, and there is a perception that others at that same level fully understand and value the contribution that the profession makes not only to patient care but also to the institution's reputation in the community (McClure, Poulin, Sovie and Wandelt 1983, 85).

What happened? Our colleagues in the United States have certainly been experiencing the same erosion and demoralization of nursing leadership (and attendant problems for nurses, patients, and families) that we have in Canada in the two decades since McClure et al. pub-lished their findings.[6] Understanding the values shifts that have created such problems requires stepping back to do a broader analysis of Western health care. While we are not offering an exhaustive comparison between Canada and other Western countries, the reso-nance of research findings between countries is instructive. We will therefore turn to an illustration from Australia.

An Australian Illustration

Like their counterparts in countries with similar health care systems (such as Canada), Australian nurses are consistently ranked in public opinion polls as the most ethical pro-fessionals, ahead of other helping professions such as medicine, education, pharmacy, and law (Australian Nursing Journal 2002). Yet nurses in Australia also share with their col-leagues from Western countries a range of concerns: nursing shortages, poor **retention** rates, and a corporate ethos with low **morale** and low **job satisfaction** (Aiken et al. 2001; Auditor General Victoria 2002; Heath 2002). In other words, the policy and power shifts that have hit Canadian nurses are shared across national borders.

One of us (Street) has been working with a colleague in an **action research** study directed at assisting nurses to improve the health of elderly residents of a residential aged care facility. Strategies in this study are aimed at improving the quality of use of medicines and the reduction of inappropriate polypharmacy (Street 1999; 2002). The nurses involved in this research were morally distressed when they discovered that the high-fibre diet and exercise program they had successfully implemented to wean patients off laxatives was abruptly discontinued by management arrangements to have food supplies outsourced (contracted out). The bulk food delivered by the contract kitchen was uniformly bland and easily swallowed, but this meant that the individualized diets that had been developed to meet specific resident requirements could not be continued. In this instance the good of the patient was overruled by economic considerations (see also Chapter 9).

The undesirable effects of moral distress on nurses[7] are illustrated in another incident that came to light in the project outlined above. Nurses reflected on their practice in terms of providing adequate pain relief and promoting comfort for older residents with cognitive dysfunction. The nurses had been concerned about an elderly woman who whimpered and curled up on her bed whenever anyone tried to provide care. The nurses were certain the woman was engaging in this behaviour due to pain. Yet her community physician would not prescribe adequate analgesic support. After repeated requests to the community physician, the nurses became distressed that they were unable to provide the woman with enough pain relief and that she had been put on a behavioural management regime. This moral distress affected their interactions with the woman. Nurses reported that they avoided caring for her as they disliked touching her and adding to her evident discomfort. They felt powerless to change the situation. A senior nurse with a background in palliative care and a strong knowledge of analgesia—a nurse whom the community physicians respected—was able to initiate a review of the pain management that improved the situation both for the woman and the nurses. This example highlights the difficulties that nurses have in negotiating toward a moral horizon in a hierarchical ethos that privileges the medical knowledge of a visiting physician, (or a senior nurse not involved in the patient's care) over that of the team of nurses who provide 24-hour care.

International Insights

Thus far, the research we have cited from Canada and Australia portrays significant constraints and power inequities in the organizational contexts within which nurses work and raises worrisome questions about the negative impacts on patients, families, and communities. There is an important emerging body of international research that adds other relevant insights. This international research is looking at the quality of nurses' **work environments** and the impact of those environments on nurses and the patients they serve. Although not conceptualized in moral or ethical terms, the research has a great deal to say about the moral climate of nurses' work, which we will pick up in the next section of this chapter.

In 1998, an international team of investigators led by Dr. Linda Aiken from the United States launched a program of research to better understand the impact of health care restructuring on the nursing workforce and patient outcomes. There are seven sites in the research program, including Pennsylvania in the United States, British Columbia, Alberta, and Ontario in Canada, Scotland and England in the United Kingdom, and Germany in the European Union (Clarke at al. 2001, 51). The conceptual framework of Aiken et al.'s research was based on the earlier research with magnet hospitals that we mentioned above. While the results are continuing to be disseminated as we write this chapter, the findings to date are consistent and alarming. They show that the **cost constraint** measures that have swept through Western health care since the late 1980s—which include rapid restructuring with limited nursing input, increased registered nurse/patient ratios, casualization of the nursing workforce, loss of nurse leaders, and limited continuing education opportunities—have harmed patients as well as nurses. More specifically, the results show increased **morbidity and mortality** of patients (including "failure to rescue," or failure to stop a preventable complication), reduced patient satisfaction, reduced nurse satisfaction, skyrocketing nurse illness and injury, and widespread nurse attrition (Aiken, Clarke and Sloane 2000; Aiken et al. 2002; Clarke et al. 2001; Dunleavy, Shamian and Thomson 2003; Duncan et al. 2001; Shamian et al. 2002; Sochalski et al. 1998).

Perhaps one of the most significant insights from the program of research is the researchers' observation that *so little* research has been done in the planning or evaluation of the reforms that have swept through health care. Aiken and her colleagues warn:

What we know about changes in organization and structure and the potential for those changes to affect patient outcomes pales by comparison to what we do not know. However, this is itself an important finding: we are subjecting hundreds of thousands of very sick patients to the unknown consequences of organizational reforms that have not been sufficiently evaluated before their widespread adoption (Aiken, Clarke and Sloane 2000, 463).

The Moral Climate of Nursing Practice

While the international research by Aiken and her colleagues on nurses' workplaces does not include an explicit moral or ethical analysis, it does greatly inform value-based inquiry.[8] That is, it tells us about problems in the moral climate for nursing practice that make it difficult for nurses to enact their moral agency. By "moral climate," we mean the implicit and explicit **values** inherent in nurses' workplaces. Those values operate at individual, organizational, and societal levels and affect the structural and interpersonal resources available for nursing practice.

It is important to note that the constraints nurses experience in accessing structural and interpersonal resources are not just external features of the environment but are also part of the **culture** of the organizational context in which they practise. As was identified in Chapter 5 and 6, culture is more than just ethnicity. It permeates health care delivery and influences implicit and explicit values. The long-standing disempowerment of nurses as a cultural group within health care is remarkable given the extent of our professional responsibilities and the importance of nursing care for patient well-being (Campbell 1994; Canadian Nurses Association 1998; Chambliss 1996; Keddy et al. 1999; Jameton 1990; Liaschenko 1993; Picard 2000; Stelling 1994a; 1994b; Street 1992; Varcoe and Rodney 2002; Yylelland 1994). For instance, in Ethics in Practice 10-1, it was taken for granted that the nurses would work largely without the benefit of access to other members of the health care team (e.g., social workers) because of the lack of mechanisms such as regular interdisciplinary rounds (see also Rodney 1997). Such rounds were not a part of the culture of the unit they worked on, whereas dying patients in the culture of a palliative care unit would have had access to an interdisciplinary team that met regularly. The reason for the difference was not patient needs—the patient needs were often equivalent in both places. The resultant sense of powerlessness of the nurses on the so-called non-specialty (medical) unit is not new. But coupled with erosions in staffing, loss of nursing leadership, and high turnover, it has certainly become more problematic. In other words, long-standing cultural problems in health care delivery have been exacerbated by the current corporate ethos, which has come with its own set of power inequities.

Our illustrations of ethical research from Canada and Australia and workplace studies from international research indicate that problems with the moral climate for nursing practice have become endemic in Western health care and that we are only beginning to grasp their consequences. While our illustrations are drawn from a limited number of studies, they are by no means idiosyncratic. Similar findings of situational constraints interfering with nurses' ability to practise according to the ethical standards of their practice are increasingly evident in the research literature throughout Western health care, especially in North America.[9] This is not to say that the *only* constraints nurses face in enacting their moral agency are external and out of their control. Nurses are sometimes complicit in reinforcing situational constraints (e.g., by undermining their colleagues' attempts to provide emotional support to patients), and they sometimes engage in unjust rationing of their care (e.g., because of judgments that a patient is not worthy) (Aroskar 1995; Corley and Goren 1998;

Liaschenko 1994; Rodney and Varcoe 2001; Rodney et al. 2002; Varcoe and Rodney 2002; Varcoe, Rodney and McCormick in press). But it is to say that the moral climate to support nursing practice has deteriorated significantly over the past two decades. Nurses experience moral stress, moral distress, and moral outrage when they find themselves in situations where they know what the right thing to do is but where institutional constraints make it difficult, if not impossible, to follow through (Corley et al. 2001; Jameton 1984; Johnstone 1999; Raines 2000). Moral distress is a pervasive problem that can cause unwanted moral residue for nurses and impact the quality of care they provide (Erlen 2001; Mitchell 2001; Storch et al. 2002; Varcoe and Rodney 2002; Webster and Baylis 2001; see also Chapter 8).

Nursing's historical position as a (primarily) women's occupation in a gender-biased culture has rendered it vulnerable to the economic forces sweeping through health care. And our long-standing difficulties with physicians have not helped.[10] Because nurses are the most numerous professionals and are the professionals who are most consistently present with the recipients of health care, their ability to practise ethically has a profound effect on the health and well-being of patients/clients, families, and communities. And their ability to practise ethically has a profound effect on the functioning of the entire health care team. Clearly, any deterioration in the quality of nursing and health care received by the recipients of health care is of concern. What is also of concern is the impact on nurses as professionals and as human beings.

Thus, nurses, as well as other health care providers, administrators, and policy-makers, need to strive for a more ethical work environment. The ideology that health care is a commodity, in which nurses are discussed in terms of scarcity and supply, must be challenged (Varcoe and Rodney 2002). Right now a significant proportion of nurses are trying to provide ethical care to patients in an under-resourced, severely strained, and poorly managed health care system. Moreover, nurses are trying to maintain their moral integrity in environments that are becoming increasingly characterized by conflict and disagreement (Johnstone 2002).

We turn now to some ideas about how a more positive moral climate can be fostered—and defended where it currently exists. This is new and important territory for nursing inquiry. While we now have fairly extensive documentation of problems in the moral climate of nursing practice, we do not yet have a great deal of research about how to *deal with* those problems.

TAKING ACTION

Perhaps the first step to improve the moral climate for nursing practice (and, hence, for health care delivery) is to *name* it as a goal. That is, "we want, as participants in institutional culture, to be able to notice our moral problems and to cope with them with sensitivity and integrity and to keep our health care institutions responsive to their moral goals" (Jameton 1990, 450). Thinking of ourselves as members of a **moral community** is a way of linking the goal to action. As one nurse ethicist explains,

> Nurses and others who contribute to delivery of nursing care should identify themselves as citizens of a moral community, a specialized community of individual moral agents with shared values and goals within the broader community of health care (Aroskar 1995, 134).

A moral community is a place where ethical values are made explicit and shared, where ethical values direct action, and where individuals feel safe to be heard (Aroskar 1995; Canadian Nurses Association 2002; Corley and Goren 1998; Erlen 2001; Jameton 1990;

McDaniel 1998; Olson 1998; Pask 2001; Rodney et al. 2002; Webster and Baylis 2000).[11] Fostering a moral community is going to involve organizational, political, and research-based action.

Organizational Action

It is clear that the moral climate for nursing practice has suffered from economically driven reductions in staffing and leadership and rapid, repeated changes with little nursing input. The program of research from Aiken and her colleagues tells us that "the most important hospital characteristics predictive of nurses' emotional exhaustion and [dis]satisfaction with their jobs are nurses not having control over their work environment, including not having sufficient resources, and not having effective nursing leadership" (Clarke et al. 2001, 54). They add that good nurse-physician collaboration and sufficient length of nursing experience on the hospital unit are also significant (54). *A minimal requirement for improving the moral climate for nursing practice and fostering the development of nursing as a moral community is to turn these negative characteristics around and strengthen the positive characteristics.* Thus, nurses' workplaces require better resources, including adequate staffing, regular work schedules, job security, positive interdisciplinary relationships, educational support, and available nurse leaders (Canadian Health Services Research Foundation 2001; Canadian Nurses Association 1998; Clarke et al. 2001; Health Canada 2002; Health Canada Office of Nursing Policy 2001; Laschinger et al. 2000; Storch 1999; Storch et al. 2002).

Resources will certainly help, but part of the challenge is also to tackle the taken-for-granted values that have helped to disenfranchise nurses as well as other health care providers, patients, families, and even communities. For example, the nurses in the Australian long-term care agency in the study cited above had trouble being heard because their expertise was not valued. And the nurse managers in Ethics in Practice 10-2 also felt disvalued—sometimes even by the nurses they were supposed to represent. Weiss et al. (2002) note that "besides the physical dimensions, the... moral dimensions of institutions can increase or decrease the likelihood that a community of practitioners, organized around common goals, will adopt the standards and visions of good practice" (115).[12] In other words, structural organizational changes are necessary but not sufficient. We also need to have positive values-based changes if nursing is to move forward as a moral community.

How to promote values-based change is by no means entirely clear. But a starting point is to help nurses to find their **moral voices** (Liaschenko 1993; Rodney et al. 2002; Storch et al. 2002). This means helping them to use the language of ethics in a way that supports the values in their practice. Ethics education for nurses is essential for this to happen (Hartrick Doane 2002a; 2002b; Varcoe et al. in press). While much of this education needs to happen in the preparatory nursing programs, a great deal can also be done in the workplace (see Exhibit 10-1).

Political Action

Organizational resources will not be liberated, and positive value shifts will not happen, however, without **political action.** What do we mean by political action? Clearly, we are not just talking about lobbying local and national governments, essential though such activities are. We are talking about a notion of politics that includes individual as well as

---

Exhibit 10-1	Promoting Nurses' Moral Voices in the Workplace

Strategies from Raines (2000, 40)

1. Start a nursing ethics library and/or a nursing ethics journal club;
2. Sponsor a nursing ethics committee and/or a nursing research committee;
3. Support a nursing ethics grand round and plan for interdisciplinary participation;
4. Provide an annual ethics educational program for all staff;
5. Circulate a nursing ethics article of the month and foster related discussion;
6. Do a biannual survey of staff to assess the ethical issues they are facing;
7. Send representatives of nursing staff to other agencies to learn about their strategies; and

8. Ensure that there are nurse representatives on the agency's ethics committee and research review board.

To this list we (the authors) would add

9. Encourage networking between community, hospital, long-term care, and other health care agencies to share nursing ethics resources;
10. Promote discussion of nursing ethics at regional, national, and international nursing association meetings; and
11. Work to ensure that nursing has a strong presence on regional, national, and international interdisciplinary ethics bodies.

---

group action. "Political theory tells us what can happen when people act in concert in certain ways" (McGowan 1998, 178). Acting in concert takes place, for instance, every day at the bedside, in a client's home, in a primary school office, in a hospital administrative meeting, at a regional health board meeting, and at a nursing association conference as well as in a national government house (see also Chapter 5).

Political action should foster respect for all individuals so that they can have meaningful participation in decisions that will affect the community that they live and/or work in (Galarneau 2002; Mann 1994; McGowan 1998). This means promoting a constructive dialogue that embraces diverse viewpoints—a process that equalizes power and is at the heart of democracy (Chinn 2001; Mouffe 1993). What we have presented about the moral context of nurses' practice indicates that democratic processes are not functioning all that well in health care policy construction and health care delivery throughout Western health care. The nurse manager quoted in Ethics in Practice 10-2, for example, found that rather than having her expertise valued and her perspective incorporated in senior administrative meetings, she felt as if everybody was looking at her like she was "from another planet."[13]

How can nurses engage in concerted political action? Every one of us in the profession has a role to play, and many have embarked upon significant political work throughout nursing's history. It is important to note that our codes of ethics can be political as well as ethical tools—they serve "as an ethical basis from which to advocate for quality practice environments with the potential to impact the delivery of safe, competent and ethical nursing care" (Canadian Nurses Association 2002, 2). Waving a copy of the Canadian Nurses Association's Code of Ethics at administrative meetings might not help the nurse manager in Ethics in Practice 10-2, but the knowledge that she has a professional ethical obligation to advocate for better nursing workplaces can help her to feel more confident about the validity of her moral stance. This confidence may also help her to seek support from peers, professional nursing associations, academic colleagues, and other sources.

Political action takes place at all levels of health care. At the macro level, we ought to be more proactive in challenging sociopolitical ideologies that disenfranchise nurses and those for whom they provide care—for instance, by hosting national and international conferences on health reform and cultivating strong media support. The current corporate ideology, with its prevalent marketplace metaphors, needs to be challenged (Annas 1995; Hiraki 1998). At the meso level, we especially need to improve the moral foundations of health policy, which takes nursing expertise and nursing leadership (Johnstone 2002; Malone 1999; Mitchell 2001; Rodney et al. 2002; Storch et al. 2002). The need for such expertise was evident, for instance, in the Canadian nurses' concerns about patient and family choices at the end of life and the Australian nurses' concerns about the diet and well-being of residents in long-term care.

At the micro level, we should learn to listen to diverse viewpoints and treat all others with respect—whether they are managers, other health care providers, patients, family members, or nursing colleagues. Interpersonal conflict, especially if it is demeaning, has an important interactive effect on the moral climate. Such conflict is worsened by problems with resources and power inequities but, in turn, exacerbates resource constraints and power inequities (Corley and Goren 1998; Rodney et al. 2002; Varcoe and Rodney 2002). In Ethics in Practice 10-2, for example, the managers in Gaudine and Beaton's (2002) study claimed that feeling unsupported by staff nurses made it much harder for them to do their job.

Research Action

We can also use the growing expertise in **philosophical inquiry** and **research** methodologies in nursing (and in other disciplines such as philosophy and sociology) to support nursing's evolution as a moral community. This can take place in at least three ways. First, we can use philosophical inquiry[14] as well as empirical inquiry to continue to articulate the nature (and importance) of nursing. At the heart of nursing's disempowerment in current health care policy processes lie implicit assumptions about the nature of nursing—that it can be reduced, parcelled out, and directed by non-nurses. To rebut these assumptions we need to better articulate the unique nature of nursing; that is, we need to better articulate what we do and why it matters (Mitchell 2001; Nagle 1999; see also Chapter 3). Secondly, we can do some conceptual work to further our research about nurses' work environments and the moral climate of nursing practice. In their work with a measurement tool for the international nursing outcomes research project, Estabrooks et al. (2002) note that such clarification is needed in future. They argue that

> A longer-range and more ambitious goal involves the systematic examination of the concepts of organizational culture, organizational climate, and practice environment from both conceptual and measurement perspectives (267).

We agree. And we would add that the concepts of moral agency, moral climate, and moral community ought to be considered at the same time. *Problems in nurses' workplaces have a significant moral dimension.*

Thirdly, we can promote action research to help to improve the moral climate of nursing practice. Action research is an umbrella term for a range of research methodologies that share: (1) a common commitment to political and strategic action that values human flourishing; (2) a focus on the relationship between knowledge and action; (3) inclusion of the participation of all relevant stakeholders in the conduct and decision-making of the research; and (4) the goal of addressing practical problems to improve a situation (Reason and Bradbury 2001; Street 2002). Drawing on the work of Habermas (1971), Park (2001) argues that the "full realisation of human life in society requires the mobilization of rationality that includes knowledge of moral values relevant in everyday living" (86). Action research is a process that is increasingly being adopted by nurses interested in identifying shared values and working together to improve a health care situation, particularly one characterized by injustice (Kelly and Simpson 2001). It offers significant promise in helping to redress some of the power dynamics that have led to our current moral climate, and so we will say more about it here.

The research process begins with a preliminary investigation to explore the literature and the politics of the health care context (Street 1995). Strategic action is planned, implemented, and monitored. Analysis of the findings is followed by collaborative critical reflection on the success of the plan or the need to modify it and begin another cycle of planning, implementation, data collection, analysis, and reflection. Nurses continue to work through this cyclical process until the situation has improved (Street 1999). The outcomes of action research in health care are context specific (Dickson 2000; Tobin 2000) and may be focused on improving a clinical situation (Rose et al. 1999), addressing policies (Roy and Cain 2001), or informing changes in the health care culture (Kelly and Simpson 2001; Wadsworth 2001).

The knowledge gained through these processes provides practical moral criteria for comprehending the complexity of health care situations and discerning appropriate, acceptable, and feasible plans to implement change (Park 2001). In consequence, co-researchers (involved stakeholders) reflect on their own values and on the consistency between these values and the action they have implemented through a process of critical reflection (Goodson 1997). In turn, this group deliberation leads to opportunities to uncover the exercise of power relations and its consequences for the nurses and those for whom they provide care.

For example, the movement from a negative moral climate towards a moral community was apparent in the Australian study we cited earlier. This action research was designed to improve the professional relationship between a multidisciplinary aged care community assessment team (ACAT) and nurses working in acute services (Robinson 2001). The intention of the study was to enhance collaboration in assessment, referral, and discharge planning of older people. Nurses working in both contexts had expressed dissatisfaction with their working relationships, which were characterized by ignorance of each other's roles, distrust of each other's motives, and a culture of apathy and blame. This culture had arisen in a context where biomedical and economic imperatives governed the way that the nurses structured their role, limiting their understanding of their responsibilities to the biomedical "here and now" rather than recognizing their moral responsibility to ensure that their patients were appropriately assessed and placed after discharge. A prevailing ethic existed within each ward that if clients experienced problems following discharge, "it would be picked up in the community." Meanwhile, the members of the ACAT were concerned with meeting their "core business" targets of numbers of assessments and the time between referral and assessments. This was despite the ACAT guidelines (Commonwealth Department of Health and Ageing 2002) that indicate a clear responsibility to work with other providers to facilitate client access (Robinson and Street In press).

The members of the ACAT identified that this dysfunctional climate was present in their team relationships. They met regularly to develop a moral climate in which they had an agreed position on their values and implementation strategies consistent with them. They moved from strategies to improve their own practice to establishing a collaborative working relationship with nurses in acute care. Interactive forums were established to explore shared values and collaborative strategies to improve care. These strategies found an answering response in the nurses on acute wards. As one ACAT nurse reported,

> They want the contact because when you turn up there [on the ward] they often troubleshoot with you. They often sit you down and things will come up, whereas they probably wouldn't have bothered to phone,... even if it's just to debrief... Now they know you're there when a crisis arises... but they also need to know there is support there as well (Robinson 2001, Participant A2).

The nurses on the acute wards supported this finding. For example, one of the nurses commented, "[I] feel much more comfortable ringing ACAT now I can put faces to names" (Robinson 2001, Participant RN4), while another stated that participation in the interactive forums "familiarizes ACAT and nursing staff so that we feel more comfortable in dealing with each other" (Robinson 2001, Participant RN8). The nature of this changed relationship and its effects were in part captured by the comments of one participant who noted, "They [ACAT] have become allies and co-workers instead of an outside dominating force" (Robinson 2001, Participant RN3). These changes were leading towards the development of a moral community in which shared values were discussed, which subsequently directed action.

As can be seen from the previous example, action research therefore gives us the chance to learn more about *how* to foster the development of nursing as a moral community. Such research generates organizational as well as political action. While we still have a lot to learn, the voices of the Australian ACAT nurses show us that there is hope.

LOOKING AHEAD

In this chapter we have argued that power inequities in contemporary health care policy processes have interfered with nurses' abilities to provide good quality patient/family/community care. We have claimed that those power inequities have worsened the moral climate of nursing practice and have been harmful to nurses as well as patients/families/communities. We have further claimed that fostering a stronger sense of moral community—in which ethical values are made explicit and shared, direct action is valued, and individuals feel safe to be heard—can help us to improve the moral climate of nursing practice. And we have posited some organizational, political, and research-based strategies that can help us to move towards a healthier moral community.

While not exhaustive, the strategies nonetheless mark an important turning point for nursing inquiry. A growing number of nurse researchers, nurse leaders, and colleagues in other disciplines are beginning to focus more on *how* to improve nurses' workplaces.[15] Our profession and, most especially, our patients and their families and communities need much more of this kind of work. We ought to continue to imagine and work towards a moral community that values nursing expertise for patient/family/community well-being, has a strong nursing leadership presence, is supportive of continuing education, and has a commitment to adequate staffing as well as good retention and recruitment programs. And we ought to continue to imagine and work towards equitable access to resources for those we serve regardless of attributes such as age, gender, sexual orientation, ability, ethnicity, and language fluency. Let us close with the words of some American nursing colleagues:

> We believe it is essential to recover the vision of what is possible in actual practices today in order to discover the mandates for reshaping our institutional structures, environments, and economics to serve attentive, sustaining, and healing relationships (Phillips and Benner 1994, vii).

FOR REFLECTION

1. What is it about "non-specialty" contexts (such as acute medical wards) that make them especially vulnerable to contemporary cost constraints?

2. Think back to the quotation from the nurse manager (from Gaudine and Beaton's [2002] study) in Ethics in Practice 10-2. How could the staff on the units for which the manager was responsible support the manager in her attempts to advocate for improving their conditions of work?

3. How do you think that nurses ought to use evidence about bad outcomes for patients/clients and nurses to make a political argument for improved resources? Include some ideas at the micro, meso, and macro levels of health care policy.

4. Participatory action research is built on democratic processes of participation. How might the insights we gain about such processes help nurses to become more involved in health policy work?

ENDNOTES

1. Canadian sources chronicling this include Anderson, Dyck and Lynam (1997); Anderson and Reimer-Kirkham (1998); Armstrong and Armstrong (2003); Blue et al. (1999); Brown (1996); Bolaria (2002); Burgess (1996); Carniol (1995); Cassidy, Lord and Mandell (1995); Commission on the Future of Health Care in Canada (2002); Dunleavy, Shamian and Thomson (2003); Fuller (1998); Gallagher et al. (2002); Gallagher and Hodge (1999); Gregor (1997); Health Canada (2002); Health Canada Office of Nursing Policy (2001); Kenny (2002); Kingwell (2000); Laxer (1996; 1998); Lynam et al. (2003); McQuaig (1993; 1999); Picard (2000); Rachlis and Kushner (1994); Saul (1995; 1997; 2001); Stephenson (1999); Stein (2001); Storch (1996; 2003); and Varcoe and Rodney (2002). See Storch (2003) for an insightful overview of the history of economic, political, and social changes in Canada and their impact on health care delivery. Chapters 9, 11, and 12 in this text also address a number of these changes and the resultant impact.

2. By corporate ethos (or ideology) we mean the taken-for-granted acceptance that a market approach to health care is best. The values of the marketplace come to dominate such that hierarchy, efficiency, and "the bottom line" implicitly replace values related to human well-being, personal integrity, and social justice (see also Annas 1995; Commission on the Future of Health Care in Canada 2002; Hiraki 1998; Kenny 2002; Mohr 1997; Rodney and Varcoe 2001; Varcoe and Rodney 2002). This is not to say that corporations are without positive human values—indeed, there is a thriving literature on, and a growing practice in, business ethics. Rather, it is to say that the taken-for-granted acceptance of a limited (and misapplied) set of marketplace values for health care policy processes is highly problematic.

3. The authors wish to thank an anonymous reviewer for an initial draft of these premises.

4. See also Campbell (1994); Canadian Nurses Association (1998); Dunleavy, Shamian and Thomson (2003); Health Canada (2002); Health Canada Office of Nursing Policy (2001); Keddy et al. (1999); Lynam et al. (2003); Nagle (1999); Picard (2000); Rodney et al. (2002); Varcoe and Rodney (2002); and Woodward et al. (1999).

5. This research did not employ one particular conceptual framework. Rather, the researchers used a composite approach to ethical theory that is consistent with Daniels' (1996) notion of wide reflective equilibrium (see also Chapters 4, 5, and 6). Ethical practice was defined in terms of Benner, Tanner and Chesla's (1996) Aristotelian notion of the "good" in practice. In exploring the meaning of ethics with nurses we therefore asked them to tell us about what helped or hindered them in "doing good" in their practice. See also Rodney et al. (2002).

6. See, for example, Adams and Bond (2000); Aiken, Clarke and Sloane (2001); Aiken et al. (2002); Barry-Walker (2000); Curran and Miller (1990); Hiraki (1998); Mohr (1997); Mohr and Mahon (1996); Olson (1998); Shindul-Rothschild, Berry and Long-Middleton (1996); and Weiss et al. (2002).

7. Chapter 8 provides a discussion of moral distress and moral residue.

8. We are using the terms "ethical" and "moral" interchangeably here. See Chapter 4 for definitions of each.

9. See, for example, Chambliss (1996); Corley et al. (2001); Georges and Grypdonck (2002); Kuhse (1997); Lipp (1998); Marck (2000); Oberle and Tenove (2000); Penticuff and Walden (2000); Raines (2000); Redman and Fry (2000); Rodney and Varcoe (2001); Street (1992); van der Arend and Remmers-van den Hurk (1999); Weiss et al. (2002); and Woodward et al. (1999); see also Chapter 11 and Chapter 12 in this text.

10. For insightful analyses of the gender-based history of nursing, including conflicts with physicians, see Ashley (1976); Corley and Mauksch (1988); David (2000); Gregor (1997); Kelly (2000); Roberts (1983); Street (1992); and Thompson, Allen and Rodrigues-Fisher (1992).

11. Terms used in the literature to discuss "moral community" sometimes include "moral or ethical climate" and "moral or ethical environment."

12. In an American research study involving 63 registered nurses from obstetrical units and 64 nurses from neonatal intensive care units, Penticuff and Walden (2000) had findings that support Weiss et al.'s (2002) conclusion. Penticuff and Walden determined that "nursing ethical practice is influenced not only by nurses' values and concern about ethics, but also by the settings in which they practice" (70). More specifically, nurses' dissatisfaction with their practice environment and perceptions that administrators did not support staff nurses' involvement in resolving ethical dilemmas made them less likely to act ethically (70).

13. Whether that was actually the perspective of the nurse manager's administrative colleagues is an empirical question. Nonetheless, the other studies we have cited also consistently portray the disempowerment of nurses in organizational decision-making.

14. Chapter 3 provides an overview of philosophy in nursing, including philosophical inquiry. See also Chapter 7 on the evolution of nursing ethics.

15. For instance, Laschinger et al. (2000) have done an insightful research study about the effects of organizational trust and empowerment in restructured health care settings on staff nurse commitment.

REFERENCES

Adams, A. and Bond, S. 2000. Hospital nurses' job satisfaction, individual and organizational characteristics. *Journal of Advanced Nursing, 32*(3), 536–543.

Aiken, L.H., Clarke, S.P. and Sloane, D.M. 2000. Hospital restructuring: Does it adversely affect care and outcomes? *JONA, 30*(10), 457–465.

Aiken, L.H., Clarke, S.P., Sloane, D.M., Sochalski, J.A., Busse, R., Clarke, H. et al. 2001. Nurses' reports on hospital care in five countries. *Health Affairs, 20*(3), 43–53.

Aiken, L.H., Clarke, S.P., Sloane, D.M., Sochalski, J. and Silber, J.H. 2002. Hospital nurse staffing and patient mortality, nurse burnout, and job dissatisfaction. *Journal of the American Medical Association, 288* (916), 23–30.

Anderson, J.M., Dyck, I. and Lynam, J. 1997. Health care professionals and women speaking: Constraints in everyday life and the management of chronic illness. *Health, 1*(1), 57–80.

Anderson, J. and Reimer Kirkham, S. 1998. Constructing nation: The gendering and racializing of the Canadian health care system. In V. Strong-Boag, S. Grace, A. Eisenberg and J. Anderson (Eds.), *Painting the maple: Essays on race, gender, and the construction of Canada* (pp. 242–261). Vancouver: UBC Press.

Annas, G.J. 1995. Reframing the debate on health care reform by replacing our metaphors. *New England Journal of Medicine, 332*(11), 744–747.

Armstrong, P. and Armstrong, H. 2003. *Wasting away: The undermining of Canadian health care.* 2nd edition. Don Mills, ON: Oxford University Press.

Aroskar, M.A. 1995. Envisioning nursing as a moral community. *Nursing Outlook, 43*(3), 134–138.

Ashley, J.A. 1976. *Hospitals, paternalism, and the role of the nurse.* New York: Teacher's College Press.

Auditor General Victoria. 2002. *Nurse workforce planning.* Melbourne, Australia: State of Victoria.

Australian Nursing Journal. 2002. Nurses top ethics poll again. *Australian Nursing Journal, 9*(7), 6.

Barry-Walker, J. 2000. The impact of systems redesign on staff, patient, and financial outcomes. *Journal of Nursing Administration, 30*(2), 77–89.

Benner, P.A., Tanner, C.A. and Chesla, C.A. (with contributions by H.L. Dreyfus, S.E. Dreyfus and J. Rubin). 1996. *Expertise in nursing practice: Caring, clinical judgment, and ethics.* New York: Springer.

Blue, A.W., Keyserlingk, E.W., Rodney, P. and Starzomski, R. 1999. A critical view of North American health policy. In H. Coward and P. Ratanakul (Eds.), *A cross-cultural dialogue on health care ethics* (pp. 215–225). Waterloo, ON: Wilfrid Laurier University Press.

Bolaria, B.S. 2002. Income inequality, poverty, food banks, and health. In B.S. Bolaria and H.D. Dickinson (Eds.), *Health, illness, and health care in Canada,* 3rd ed. (pp. 131–143). Scarborough, ON: Nelson Thomson Learning.

Brown, M.C. 1996. Changes in Alberta's Medicare financing arrangements: Features and problems. In M. Stingl and D. Wilson (Eds.), *Efficiency vs equality: Health reform in Canada* (pp. 137–151). Halifax: Fernwood.

Burgess, M. 1996. Health care reform: Whitewashing a conflict between health promotion and treating illness? In M. Stingl and D. Wilson (Eds.), *Efficiency vs equality: Health reform in Canada* (pp. 153–162). Halifax: Fernwood.

Campbell, M.L. 1987. Productivity in Canadian nursing: Administering cuts. In D. Coburn, C. D'Arcy, G.M. Torrance and P. New (Eds.), *Health and Canadian society: Sociological perspectives,* 2nd ed. (pp. 463–475). Markham, ON: Fitzhenry & Whiteside.

Campbell, M. 1994. The structure of stress in nurses' work. In B.S. Bolaria and H.D. Dickinson (Eds.), *Health, illness and health care in Canada* (pp. 592–608). Toronto: Harcourt Brace.

Canadian Health Services Research Foundation. 2001. *Commitment and care: The benefits of a healthy workplace for nurses, their patients and the system.* Ottawa: Canadian Health Services Research Foundation.

Canadian Nurses Association. 1998. *The quiet crisis in health care.* Paper submitted to the House of Commons Standing Committee on Finance and the Minister of Finance. Ottawa: Canadian Nurses Association.

Canadian Nurses Association. 2002. *Code of Ethics for Registered Nurses.* Ottawa: Canadian Nurses Association.

Carniol, B. 1995. *Case critical: Challenging social services in Canada.* 3rd edition. Toronto: Between the Lines.

Cassidy, B., Lord, R. and Mandell, N. 1995. Silenced and forgotten women: Race, poverty, and disability. In N. Mandell (Ed.), *Feminist issues: Race, class, and sexuality* (pp. 32–66). Scarborough, ON: Prentice Hall.

Chambliss, D.F. 1996. *Beyond caring: Hospitals, nurses, and the social organization of ethics.* Chicago: The University of Chicago Press.

Chinn, P.L. 1995. *Peace and power: Building communities for the future.* 4th edition. New York: NLN Press.

Chinn, P.L. 2001. *Peace and power: Building communities for the future.* 5th edition. Boston: Jones and Bartlett.

Clarke, H.F., Laschinger, H.S., Giovannetti, P., Shamian, J., Thomson, D. and Tourangeau, A. 2001. Nursing shortages: Workplace environments are essential to the solution. *Hospital Quarterly,* (Summer), 50–57.

Commission on the Future of Health Care in Canada. 2002. *Building on values: The future of health care in Canada.* ["The Romanow Report."] Ottawa: Commission on the Future of Health Care in Canada.

Commonwealth Department of Health and Ageing. 2002. *Aged care assessment program operational guidelines.* Authors: Australia.

Corley, M.C., Elswick, R.K., Gorman, M. and Clor, T. 2001. Development and evaluation of a moral distress scale. *Journal of Advanced Nursing, 33*(2), 250–256.

Corley, M.C. and Goren, S. 1998. The dark side of nursing: Impact of stigmatizing responses on patients. *Scholarly Inquiry for Nursing Practice, 12*(2), 99–118

Corley, M.C. and Mauksch, H.O. 1988. Registered nurses, gender, and commitment. In A. Statham, E.M. Miller, and H.O. Mauksch (Eds.), *The worth of women's work: A qualitative synthesis* (pp. 135–149). Albany, NY: State University of New York Press.

Curran, C.R. and Miller, N. 1990. The impact of corporate culture on nurse retention. *Nursing Clinics of North America, 25*(3), 537–549.

Daniels, N. 1996. Wide reflective equilibrium in practice. In L.W. Sumner and J. Boyle (Eds.), *Philosophical perspectives on bioethics* (pp. 96–114). Toronto: University of Toronto Press.

David, B.A. 2000. Nursing's gender politics: Reformulating the footnotes. *Advances in Nursing Science, 23*(1), 83–93.

Dickson, G. 2000. Aboriginal grandmothers' experience with health promotion and participatory action research. *Qualitative Health Research, 10*(2), 188–213.

Dunleavy, J., Shamian, J. and Thomson, D. 2003. Workplace pressures: Handcuffed by cutbacks. *Canadian Nurse, 99*(3), 23–26

Duncan, S.M., Hyndman, K., Estabrooks, C.A., Hesketh, K., Humphrey, C.K., Wong, J.S., Acorn, S. and Giovannetti, P. 2001. Nurses' experience of violence in Alberta and Brtish Columbia hospitals. *Canadian Journal of Nursing Research, 32*(4), 57–78.

Erlen, J.A. 2001. When the family asks, "What happened?" *Orthopedic Nursing, 19*(6), 68–71.

Estabrooks, C.A., Tourangeau, A.E., Humphrey, C.K., Hesketh, K.L., Giovannetti, P., Thomson, D., Wong, J., Acorn, S., Clarke, H. and Shamian, J. 2002. Measuring the hospital practice environment: A Canadian context. *Research in Nursing & Health, 25*, 256–268.

Fuller, C. 1998. *Caring for profit: How corporations are taking over Canada's health care system.* Vancouver, BC: New Star Books.

Galarneau, C.A. 2002. Health care as a community good: Many dimensions, many communities, many views of justice. *Hastings Center Report, 32*(5), 33–40.

Gallagher, E., Alcock, D., Diem, E., Angus, D. and Medves, J. 2002. Ethical dilemmas in home care case management. *Journal of Healthcare Management, 47*(2), 85–96.

Gallagher, E.M. and Hodge, G. 1999. The forgotten stakeholders: Seniors' values concerning their health care. *International Journal of Health Care Quality Assurance, 12*(3), 79–86.

Gaudine, A.P. and Beaton, M.R. 2002. Employed to go against one's values: Nurse managers' accounts of ethical conflict within their organizations. *Canadian Journal of Nursing Research, 34*(2), 17–34.

Georges, J. J. and Grypdonck, M. 2002. Moral problems experienced by nurses when caring for terminally ill people: A literature review. *Nursing Ethics, 9*(2), 155–178.

Gregor, F. 1997. From women to women: Nurses, informal caregivers and the gender dimension of health care reform. *Health and Social Care in the Community, 5*(1), 30–36.

Goodson, I. 1997. Action research and "The Reflexive Project of Selves." In S. Hollingsworth (Ed.), *International action research: A casebook for educational reform* (pp. 204–218). London: The Falmer Press.

Habermas, J. 1971. *Knowledge and human interests.* Boston: Beacon Press.

Hartrick Doane, G. 2002a. In the spirit of creativity: The learning and teaching of ethics in nursing. *Journal of Advanced Nursing, 39*(6), 521–528.

Hartrick Doane, G. 2002b. Am I still ethical? The socially-mediated process of nurses' moral identity. *Nursing Ethics, 9*(6), 623–635.

Health Canada. 2002. *Final report of the Canadian Nursing Advisory Committee.* Ottawa: Health Canada.

Health Canada Office of Nursing Policy. 2001. *Healthy nurses, healthy workplaces.* Ottawa: Health Canada Office of Nursing Policy.

Heath, P.C. 2002. *National Review of Nursing Education 2002: Our Duty of Care.* Melbourne, Australia: Commonwealth Department of Education, Science and Training,

Hiraki, A. 1998. Corporate language and nursing practice. *Nursing Outlook, 46,* 115–9.

Jameton, A. 1984. *Nursing practice: The ethical issues.* Englewood Cliffs, NJ: Prentice Hall.

Jameton, A. 1990. Culture, morality, and ethics: Twirling the spindle. *Critical Care Nursing Clinics of North America, 2*(3), 443–451.

Johnstone, M.-J. 1999. *Bioethics: A nursing perspective.* 3rd edition. Sydney, Australia: Harcourt.

Johnstone, M.-J. 2002. Poor working conditions and the capacity of nurses to provide moral care. *Contemporary Nurse, 12*(1), 7–15.

Keddy, B., Gregor, F,. Foster, S. and Denney, D. 1999. Theorizing about nurses' work lives: The personal and professional aftermath of living with healthcare "reform." *Nursing Inquiry, 6,* 58–64.

Kelly, C. 2002. *Nurses' moral practice: Investing and discounting self.* Indianapolis, IN: Sigma Theta Tau.

Kelly, D. and Simpson, S. 2001. Action research in action: Reflections on a project to introduce Clinical Practice Facilitators to an acute hospital setting. *Journal of Advanced Nursing, 33*(5), 652–659.

Kenny, N.P. 2002. *What good is health care? Reflections on the Canadian experience.* Ottawa: CHA Press.

Kingwell, M. 2000. *The world we want: Virtue, vice, and the good citizen.* Toronto: Penguin.

Kuhse, H. 1997. *Caring: Nurses, women and ethics.* Oxford: Blackwell.

Laschinger, H.K.S., Finegan, J., Shamian, J. and Casier, S. 2000. Organizational trust and empowerment in restructured healthcare settings: Effects on staff nurse commitment. *Journal of Nursing Administration, 30*(9), 413–425.

Laxer, J. 1996. *In search of a new left: Canadian politics after the neoconservative assault.* Toronto: Viking.

Laxer, J. 1998. *The undeclared war: Class conflict in the age of cyber capitalism.* Toronto: Penguin.

Lipp, A. 1998. An enquiry into a combined approach for nursing ethics. *Nursing Ethics, 5*(2), 122–138.

Liaschenko, J. 1993. Feminist ethics and cultural ethos: Revisiting a nursing debate. *Advances in Nursing Science, 15*(4), 71–81.

Liaschenko, J. 1994. Making a bridge: The moral work with patients we do not like. *Journal of Palliative Care, 10*(3), 83–89.

Lynam, M.J., Henderson, A., Browne, A., Smye, V., Semeniuk, P., Blue, C., Singh, S. and Anderson, J. 2003. Healthcare restructuring with a view to equity and efficiency: Reflections on unintended consequences. *Canadian Journal of Nursing Leadership, 16*(1), 112–140.

MacPhail, S.A. 1996. *Ethical issues in community nursing.* Unpublished Master's thesis. University of Alberta, Edmonton.

Malone, R.E. 1999. Policy as product: Morality and metaphor in health policy discourse. *Hastings Centre Report,* (May–June), 16–22.

Mann, P.S. 1994. *Micro-politics: Agency in a postfeminist era.* Minneapolis: University of Minnesota Press.

Marck, P.B. 2000. Nursing in a technological world: Searching for healing communities. *Advances in Nursing Science, 23*(2), 59–72.

McClure, M.L., Poulin, M.A., Sovie, M.D. and Wandelt, M.A. 1983. *Magnet hospitals: Attraction and retention of professional nurses.* Kansas City, MO: American Academy of Nursing.

McDaniel, C. 1998. Ethical environment: Reports of practicing nurses. *Nursing Clinics of North America, 33*(2), 363–372.

McGowan, J. 1998. *Hannah Arendt: An introduction.* Minneapolis: University of Minnesota Press.

McQuaig, L. 1993. *The wealthy banker's wife: The assault on equality in Canada.* Toronto: Penguin.

McQuaig, L. 1998. *The cult of impotence: Selling the myth of powerlessness in the global economy.* Toronto: Penguin.

Mitchell, G.J. 2001. Policy, procedure and routine: Matters of moral influence. *Nursing Science Quarterly, 14*(2), 109–114.

Mohr, W.K. 1997. Outcomes of corporate greed. *Image: Journal of Nursing Scholarship, 29*(10), 39–45.

Mohr, W.K. and Mahon, M.M. 1996. Dirty hands: The underside of marketplace health care. *Advances in Nursing Science, 19*(1), 28–37.

Mouffe, C. 1993. *The return of the political.* London: Verso.

Nagle, L.M. 1999. A matter of extinction or distinction. *Western Journal of Nursing Research, 21*(1), 71–82.

Oberle, K. and Tenove, S. 2000. Ethical issues in public health nursing. *Nursing Ethics, 7*(5), 425–438.

Olson, L.L. 1998. Hospital nurses' perceptions of the ethical climate of their work settings. *Image: Journal of Nursing Scholarship, 30*(4), 345–349.

Park, P. 2001. Knowledge and participatory research. In P. Reason and H. Bradbury (Eds.), *Handbook of action research: Participative inquiry and practice* (pp. 81–90). London: Sage.

Pask, E.J. 2001. Nursing responsibility and conditions of practice: Are we justified in holding nurses responsible for their behavior in situations of patient care? *Nursing Philosophy, 2,* 42–52.

Penticuff, J.H. and Walden, M. 2000. Influence of practice environment and nurse characteristics on perinatal nurses' responses to ethical dilemmas. *Nursing Research, 49*(2), 64–72.

Peter, E. and Morgan, K. 2001. Explorations of a trust approach for nursing ethics. *Nursing Inquiry, 8,* 3–10.

Phillips, S.S. and Benner, P. 1994. Preface. In S.S. Phillips and P. Benner (Eds.), *The crisis of care: Affirming and restoring caring practices in the helping professions* (pp. vii–xi). Washington, DC: Georgetown University Press.

Picard, A. 2000. *Critical care: Canadian nurses speak for change.* Toronto: HarperCollins.

Rachlis, M. and Kuschner, C. 1994. *Strong medicine: How to save Canada's health care system.* Toronto: HarperCollins.

Raines, M.L. 2000. Ethical decision making in nurses: Relationships among moral reasoning, coping style, and ethics stress. *JONA's Healthcare Law, Ethics, and Regulation, 2*(1), 29–41.

Reason, P. and Bradbury, H. 2001. Introduction: Inquiry and participation in search of a world worthy of human aspiration. In P. Reason and H. Bradbury (Eds.), *Handbook of action research: Participatory inquiry and practices* (pp. 1–14). London: Sage.

Redman, B.K. and Fry, S.T. 2000. Nurses' ethical conflicts: What is really known about them? *Nursing Ethics, 7*(4), 360–366.

Roberts, S.J. 1983. Oppressed group behavior: Implications for nursing. *Advances in Nursing Science, 5*(4), 21–30.

Robinson, A.L. 2001. *At the interface: Developing inter-sectoral networks in aged care.* Unpublished doctoral dissertation. La Trobe University, Melbourne, Australia.

Robinson, A.L. and Street, A.F. In review. Improving networks between acute care nurses and an Aged Care Assessment Team. (Manuscript accepted by *Journal of Clinical Nursing*).

Rodney, P.A. 1997. *Towards connectedness and trust: Nurses' enactment of their moral agency within an organizational context.* Unpublished doctoral dissertation. University of British Columbia, Vancouver, BC.

Rodney, P. and Varcoe, C. 2001. Towards ethical inquiry in the economic evaluation of nursing practice. *Canadian Journal of Nursing Research, 33*(1), 35–57.

Rodney, P., Varcoe, C., Storch, J. L., McPherson, G., Mahoney, K., Brown, H., Pauly, B., Hartrick Doane, G. and Starzomski, R. 2002. Navigating toward a moral horizon: A multi-site qualitative study of nurses' enactment of ethical practice. *Canadian Journal of Nursing Research, 34*(3), 75–102.

Rose, K., Waterman, H., McLeod, D. and Tullo, A. 1999. Planning and managing research into day-surgery for cataract. *Journal of Advanced Nursing, 29*(6), 1514–1519.

Roy, C.M. and Cain, R. 2001. The involvement of people living with HIV/AIDS in community-based organizations: contributions and constraints. *AIDS Care, 13*(4), 421–432.

Saul, J.R. 1995. *The unconscious civilization.* Concord, ON: Anansi Press.

Saul, J.R. 1997. *Reflections of a Siamese twin: Canada at the end of the twentieth century.* Toronto: Penguin.

Saul, J.R. 2001. *On equilibrium.* Toronto: Penguin.

Shamian, J., Kerr, M.S., Laschinger, H.K.S. and Thomson, D. 2002. A hospital-level analysis of the work environments and workforce health indicators for registered nurses in Ontario's acute-care hospitals. *Canadian Journal of Nursing Research, 33*(4), 35–50.

Shindul-Rothschild, J., Berry, D. and Long-Middleton, E. 1996. Where have all the nurses gone? Final results of our patient care survey. *American Journal of Nursing, 96*(11), 25–39.

Sochalski, J., Aiken, L., Rafferty, A., Shamian, J., Muller-Mundt, G., Hunt, J., Giovannetti, G. and Clarke, H., 1998. Building multinational research. *Reflections, 24*(3), 20–23, 45.

Stajduhar, K.I. 2003. Examining the perspectives of family members involved in the delivery of palliative care at home. *Journal of Palliative Care, 19*(1), 27–35.

Stein, J.G. 2001. *The cult of efficiency.* Toronto: Anansi.

Stelling, J. 1994a. Nursing metaphors: Reflections on the meaning of time. In B.S. Bolaria and R. Bolaria (Eds.), *Women, medicine and health* (pp. 205–217). Saskatoon: University of Saskatchewan.

Stelling, J. 1994b. Staff nurses' perceptions of nursing: Issues in a woman's occupation. In B. Singh-Bolaria and H.D. Dickinson (Eds.), *Health, illness, and health care in Canada,* 2nd ed. (pp. 609–626). Toronto: Harcourt Brace.

Stephenson, P. 1999. Expanding notions of culture for cross-cultural ethics in health and medicine. In H. Coward and P. Ratanakul (Eds.), *A cross-cultural dialogue on health care ethics* (pp. 68–91). Waterloo, ON: Wilfrid Laurier University Press.

Storch, J.L. 1996. Foundational values in Canadian health care. In M. Stingl and D. Wilson (Eds.), *Efficiency vs equality: Health reform in Canada* (pp. 21–26). Halifax: Fernwood.

Storch, J.L. 1999. Ethical dimensions of leadership. In J.M. Hibberd and D.L. Smith (Eds.), *Nursing management in Canada,* 2nd ed. (pp. 351–367). Toronto: W.B. Saunders.

Storch, J. 2003. The Canadian health care system and Canadian nurses. In M. McIntyre and E. Thomlinson (Eds.), *Realities of Canadian nursing: Professional, practice, and power issues* (pp. 34–59). Philadelphia: Lippincott Williams & Wilkins.

Storch, J., Rodney, P., Pauly, B., Brown, H. and Starzomski, R. 2002. Listening to nurses' moral voices: Building a quality health care environment. *Canadian Journal of Nursing Leadership, 15*(4), 7–16.

Street, A.F. 1992. *Inside nursing: A critical ethnography of nursing practice.* Albany, NY: State University of New York Press.

Street, A.F. 1995. *Nursing replay: Researching nursing culture together.* Melbourne, Australia: Churchill Livingstone.

Street, A.F. 1999. Bedtimes in nursing homes: Exploring an action research approach for gerontic nursing. In R. Nay and S. Garrett (Eds.), *Nursing older people: Issues and innovations* (pp. 353–368). Sydney, Australia: MacLennan and Petty.

Street, A.F. 2002. Action research. In Z. Schneider, D. Elliott, C. Beanland, G. LoBiondo-Wood and J. Haber (Eds.), *Nursing research methods: Critical appraisal and utilisation.* 2nd edition. Sydney, Australia: Mosby.

Thompson, J.L, Allen, D.G. and Rodrigues-Fisher, L. (Eds.). 1992. *Critique, resistance, and action: Working papers in the politics of nursing.* New York: National League for Nursing Press.

Tobin, M. 2000. Developing mental health rehabilitation services in a culturally appropriate context: An action research project involving Arabic-speaking clients. *Australian Health Review, 23*(2), 177–184.

van der Arend, A.J.V. and Remmers-van den Hurk, C.H.M. 1999. Moral problems among Dutch nurses: A survey. *Nursing Ethics, 6*(6), 468–482.

Varcoe, C. 1997. *Untying our hands: The social context of nursing in relation to violence against women.* Unpublished doctoral dissertation. University of British Columbia, Vancouver, BC.

Varcoe, C. 2001. Abuse obscured: An ethnographic account of Emergency Unit nursing in relation to violence against women. *Canadian Journal of Nursing Research, 32* (4) 95–115.

Varcoe, C., Hartrick Doane, G., Pauly, B., Rodney, P., Storch, J., Mahoney, K., McPherson, G., Brown, H. and Starzomski, R. In press. Ethical practice in nursing: Working the in-betweens. (Manuscript accepted for publication with *Journal of Advanced Nursing.*)

Varcoe, C. and Rodney, P. 2002. Constrained agency: The social structure of nurses' work. In B.S. Bolaria and H. D. Dickinson (Eds.), *Health, illness and health care in Canada,* 3rd ed. (pp. 102–128). Scarborough, ON: Nelson Thomson Learning.

Varcoe, C., Rodney, P. and McCormick, J. In press. Health care relationships in context: An analysis of three ethnographies. (Manuscript accepted for publication with *Qualitative Health Research.*)

Wadsworth, Y. 2001. The mirror, the magnifying glass, the compass and the map: Facilitating participatory action research. In P. Reason and H. Bradbury (Eds.), *Handbook of action research: participatory inquiry and practice* (pp. 420–432). London: Sage.

Webster, G.C. and Baylis, F.E. 2000. Moral residue. In S.B. Rubin and L. Zoloth (Eds.), *Margin of error: The ethics of mistakes in the practice of medicine* (pp. 217–230). Hagerstown, MD: University Publishing Group.

Weiss, S.M., Malone, R.E., Merighi, J.R. and Benner, P. 2002. Economism, efficiency, and the moral ecology of good nursing practice. *Canadian Journal of Nursing Research, 34*(2), 95–119.

Woodward, C.A., Shannon, H.S., Cunningham, C., McIntosh, J., Lendrum, B. Rosenbloom, D. and Brown, J. 1999. The impact of re-engineering and other cost reduction strategies on the staff of a large teaching hospital: A longitudinal study. *Medical Care, 37*(6), 556–569.

Yyelland, B. 1994. Structural constraints, emotional labour and nursing work. In B.S. Bolaria and R. Bolaria (Eds.), *Women, medicine and health* (pp. 231–240). Saskatoon: University of Saskatchewan.

chapter eleven

Ethics for Practitioners:
An Ecological Framework

Patricia Marck

... [Y]ou have two more patients come in that are requiring one-to-one attention, so now you have one nurse looking after eight patients... our patients' safety could be so easily compromised, but it's seen as, "What do you mean you can't handle it? You have two empty spots—what do you mean you can't take two more patients, you have two empty spots. There's no nurses? Oh, you can look after the patients (Elva, in Marck 2000a, 189).

In a growing international body of research and reports, clear connections are drawn between the moral complexities of daily practice and the strained environments where nurses struggle to deliver care.[1] As the Canadian Nursing Advisory Committee observed in its final submission to the federal government: "Simply put, as nursing goes, so goes the rest of the system... What is evident in all of this work is not the need to repair nursing, but to repair the work environments in which nurses practise" (Health Canada 2002, 2, 25). The Canadian Nurses Association supports this call to improve the conditions of nurses' work, citing quality practice environments as one of eight core values for the profession (2002a; 2001). To strengthen our understanding of the ethical issues that nurses face in today's practice environments, this chapter outlines a framework for thinking ecologically (Orr 1992) about nurses' work. Ecological thinking draws on knowledge from several disciplines in order to re-imagine the scientific, ethical, and practical tensions which characterize modern health systems.[2] As with any ethical framework, an ecological approach is useful to the extent that it helps practitioners to question assumptions, critically incorporate new research, and keep faith with good practice in the course of their daily work.

To outline the features of the framework in question, several steps are required. First, knowledge is integrated from research and other work in two healing vocations, those of nursing and ecological restoration, in order to define what is good, healing, and adaptive in the context of modern health systems. In the discussion that flows from these initial definitions, three matters of ecological and moral significance for nurses' practice and practice environments are considered—those of integrity, residue, and healing capacities (Exhibit 11-1). Principles of relations, resistance, and response are also explored in order to examine tensions that arise between integrity, residue, and healing in nurses' work environments, and key questions for ethical reflection (Exhibit 11-2) are proposed. Throughout the discussion, ecological concepts and principles are integrated with exemplars and case scenarios from the source for this ethical framework—namely, research on technology and nurses' work in acute care.[3] The potential merits and limits of an ecological approach to nursing and health care ethics are considered, and suggestions for further inquiry are outlined. At the core of an ecological framework, one question remains central for practitioners and for those they serve. In today's troubled health system, what kind of ethical commitments and actions are needed in order to sustain practices and places that heal? To construct this ecological lens, we begin by learning to "think like" a living system.

"THINKING LIKE" A SYSTEM: MATTERS OF INTEGRITY

> ... [O]nce we moved... there were so many different people. Everybody doing their own thing, and not as much cohesiveness as a unit... [Y]ou are getting 15 surgeons coming to visit patients now and residents, you know you've got three different services, surgical services with three different senior residents in their entourage. Nobody could figure out what they wanted. So it took a lot more time to get comfortable with each other and just when you did, things would change (Ellen, in Marck 2000a, 235).

> ... [T]he greatest value of restoration as an ecological research technique is the power it has to draw attention to what is important in a system—in other words, to force an ecologist to an increasingly clear conception of the critical parameters governing the system with which he or she is dealing... Of course, different kinds or degrees of disruption elicit and bring into the foreground different aspects of the system (William R. Jordan III 1995, 377).

As a starting point for many disciplines, **ecology** may be thought of as "the study of the relation of living things" with each other and with their environment (Barnhart 1988, 313). In the field of **ecological restoration,** such study incorporates knowledge from philosophy, ethics, history, anthropology, economics, the biological and environmental sciences, and other fields to effect the lasting repair of damaged lands (Higgs 1999a). To assess the **ecological integrity** or overall health of a given ecosystem, restorationists gather information about a number of factors, including, but not limited to

- the diversity of life forms;
- the processes and structures for birth, growth, death, and renewal;
- the regional and historical context for economic development; and

- the cultural practices that sustain or erode ethical relations within communities and with the land (Society for Ecological Restoration 1996).

Restoration efforts are then directed at strengthening local and regional relations, practices, and structures that enable living systems and their inhabitants to thrive (Higgs in press; 1999a; Gunderson, Holling and Light 1995).

   To tap into the wisdom of restoration for our present health care environments, it is useful to recall the counsel of conservationist Aldo Leopold, who urged his fellow American citizens in 1949 to "think like the mountain" instead of "thinking like" a clear cut logging operation. Essentially, Leopold argued that when we "think like" instead of "look at" the over-harvested mountain, we regain a sense of a vulnerable, exploited home place that we need to reinhabit in ways that are more ethically and scientifically sound.[4] As we notice the deepening damage of excessive logging, including lost topsoil, declining species, proliferating pulp mills, and polluted rivers, we recognize the complex connections between our own health and the health of the land. Principles of good restoration therefore stimulate us to ask, What relations, practices, and conditions foster the integrity and sustainability of a particular living system and its inhabitants? As we explore that question for nurses' environments, however, critical distinctions between technically proficient as opposed to good restorations become important.[5] Specifically, Higgs (1999a) notes that in technically efficient restoration projects, such as cosmetic repairs to an industrial park, practitioners tend to "green" the landscape of a damaged ecosystem without actually arresting environmental decay. In contrast, he argues, practitioners who seek good, lasting restorations must work to address fundamental ethical issues of excessive industrialization and pollution, over-extraction of natural resources, and consumptive human habits. At the same time, however, Higgs proposes that several technological tendencies within contemporary society favour transient technical repairs over the completion of restorations that are more ethically and scientifically sound. These tendencies include

- a pervasive "cult of efficiency" that automatically favours the achievement of short-term efficiencies over more sustainable levels of production and benefit for the longer term;
- a relentless "speed-up" of activity characterized by an excessive pace, volume, and fragmentation of human work; and
- an insidious form of "reverse adaptation" (Winner 1977) to the pressures of efficiency, speed-up, and fragmentation where people focus more on the rapid performance of disjointed tasks than on the fundamental goals that the work was originally intended to achieve.

   Arguing that good restorations demand the development of stronger ethical relations with each other and with the places we inhabit, Higgs notes, "To restore an ecosystem or an ecological process or many ecosystems within a larger landscape requires at the outset a clarity about goals: What are we after?" (1999a, 19). Urging resistance to the toxic effects of technological tendencies on restoration practice, Higgs calls for an "ethical counterpoise" that includes more communal management of the land, a tempered consumption of available resources, and the redevelopment of cultural practices that sustain each other and the places we call home (1999a). In the face of a depleted health care workforce, an unsustainable pace and volume of work, and increasingly fragmented delivery systems, the parallel technological tendencies that characterize the corporate greening of degraded ecosystems and the corporate redesigns of today's health systems become apparent. Practitioners who work with the short-lived efficiencies of re-engineered health systems can use Higgs' observations about restoration work to ask, What are we after in health care? How do we foster and sustain a system that heals? What kinds of structures, resources, and relations sustain its optimum functioning? and What actions and repairs are therefore most likely to produce the healing environments we seek? With these questions in mind, the definitions that anchor the present framework are as follows:

- The central **good** or goal of ethical nursing practice is viewed as the strengthened capacity or potential of individuals, families, and communities to heal.
- **Healing** encompasses a range of adaptive responses to the experiences of birth, growth and reproduction, suffering and decline, and inevitable death in a technologically complex and ecologically compromised world.
- **Adaptive responses** arise from interactions between relations, processes (including processes of resistance), and structures that synergistically foster individual, communal, and ecological integrity within our health system, and in our world.

In the context of these definitions, several kinds of integrity are foundational to ethical practice. For example, the **personal integrity** of practitioners, the **professional integrity** of their practices, and the **ecological** or **systemic integrity** of their practice environments are all requisites for safe, healing systems and morally sufficient nursing care. Principles of individual and environmental integrity also intersect with principles of **scientific integrity** that are core to the ethical conduct and application of scientific research. For example, the links between systemic, professional, and scientific integrity are deficient when patients and families are not given sufficient opportunity to consider the merits of experimental research protocols relative to those of other treatment options. In such cases, nurses need to actively question whether the research design and current organizational practices provide for non-coercive and adequately informed consent and then take the necessary steps to protect the decision-making of those in their care (CNA 2002b). Practitioners also serve these forms of integrity when they question treatment decisions that amount to unethical experimentation when inappropriately applied to patients who are irreversibly ill. As one critical care nurse indicates,

> I find now that I'll stand up for my patients more than I would have in the past. I will ask, "Why are you doing this with this patient?" "... we are going to dialyze your patient? Well, why?" (Marck 2000a, 226)

In such instances, practitioners can mount informed resistance by encouraging their colleagues to consult a variety of guidelines that address end-of-life issues for professionals and persons receiving care.[6]

In addition to questioning such technological toxins as inappropriate life-extending treatments, practitioners need to confront a variety of other toxins or residues that threaten the integrity of safe practice environments and good nursing care. For example, Webster and Baylis (2000) argue that disabling forms of **moral residue** can linger on in people, and within organizations, as a result of situations where questionable actions and outcomes unfold. One obstetrical nurse revealed moral residue, for instance, in her haunting recollection of a frightened teen who laboured alone on a chaotic shift. Pulled away to an emergency Caesarean section and unable to secure more staff for the floor, this nurse never made it back to the young woman until just before the onset of birth. Even though mother and baby were physically unharmed, she noted months later that "I felt like I had betrayed her trust" (Marck 2000, 95). The unsafe staffing policy that fed this situation also illustrates the contaminating effects of **theoretical residue** (Mitchell 2001) that occur when non-nursing knowledge from business, engineering, or other disciplines is inappropriately applied to the practice of nursing. Recent studies of re-engineered health care environments also confirm the presence of several related **environmental residues,** including an increased incidence of abusive relations within the workplace (Duncan et al. 2001), a lethal suppression of mistakes (Sinclair 2000; Zoloth and Rubin 2000), and excessive demands on shrinking numbers of nursing staff.[7]

Exhibit 11-1	Ecological Matters for Ethics in Practice

- Matters of **integrity** refer to the individual and environmental wholeness or soundness, the unimpaired or uncorrupted conditions (Barnhart 1988) that are necessary for health and healing.
- **Moral** (Webster and Baylis 2000), **theoretical** (Mitchell 2001), and **environmental** residues (Marck 2000a, b, c) are persistent deficiencies in character, thought, and systemic supports that threaten the individual and environmental integrity essential for healing.
- The **healing capacities** of people and their environments are those synergistic relations, processes, and structures that enable adaptive responses to a variety of threats in ways that continually restore towards a condition that is more whole.

The devastating effects of moral, theoretical, and systemic **residues** on both individual and systemic integrity are clearly outlined in Justice Sinclair's report (2000) of 12 deaths within the restructured Winnipeg Health Sciences Centre pediatric cardiac surgery program. Specifically, the use of external consultants in 1993–1994 was followed by rapid cost-cutting, disruptive reorganization, a loss of cohesive team work and clinical mentorship, and dysfunctional decision-making that corroded the team's ability to provide safe cardiac surgical care (Hardingham, Marck, McKneally and Read 2001; Sinclair 2000; Sibbald 1997). Principles of work redesign originated with for-profit business principles rather than local practitioners' knowledge of safe surgical protocols, and the persistent efforts of nurses, anesthetists, and eventually families to question unacceptable practices were repeatedly ignored. The Winnipeg experience teaches us the first ecological principle of **relation** by reminding us that neither a health system nor any of its local settings can be redesigned for short-term efficiencies alone. Instead, a complex web of relations within each environment, as well as the larger system, needs to be treated and supported as a living network that carries the secrets of survival for good patient care. It becomes obvious that the sudden loss of seasoned practitioners can lead to a critical deficit of practice wisdom and that the smallest daily measures in a well-tended environment can mean the difference between life and death. An operating room (OR) nurse demonstrates this ecological approach to relations when she recounts her actions at change of shift, saying,

> ... often the wards were really busy and that's your clue when you are a nurse to know okay, if we are busy, that means that some things weren't checked or that maybe equipment needs to be put back in place... you need to follow up on some things on your shift. Then they also report on any important factors per theater per list of patients, particularly to keep things in order. It's important for all of the rooms to know, because we have to coordinate equipment... (Kara, in Marck 2000a, 243).

The Winnipeg experience also demonstrates the importance of the second principle of healing systems, which is that nurses and others need to mount steadfast **resistance** when moral, theoretical, or systemic toxins threaten their capacity to maintain good nursing care. In their work on ecosystems management and human organizations, Gunderson, Holling, and Light (1995) assert that the thoughtful resistance of "loyal heretics" plays a vital role in alerting decision-makers to significant problems and necessary reforms (1995, xii). The OR nurse who insists that "We are short today and we cannot run these rooms, for the safety of the patients" is a loyal heretic, as is the obstetrical nurse who won't "take no for an answer" from a sceptical physician trying to avoid examining a patient she is concerned about (Marck 2000a, 228, 229). In this sense, the actions of "loyal heretics" shore up the healing capacities of damaged environs in modern health care. Other examples of necessary heresy include the courage to counter a toxic unit culture by speaking up when patients or co-workers are abused or the commitment to intervene with an impaired or incompetent co-worker to preserve the safety of patient care (AARN 2001; Wilkin 1999; CNA 1996). These examples underscore the critical links between nurses' resistance and the integrity of patient care, but our knowledge of today's over-burdened practice environments also indicates that these linkages are at risk. As the following account of a team meeting in an out-patient setting conveys, nurses' resistance therefore requires the commitment to speak up regardless of who is "in charge":

> ... [T]hey were talking about the budget for next year and the capital equipment that they want to buy... [T]hey want to buy this new machine, they want to buy that one... I said "Well, what we need is better monitoring equipment in the rooms for the nurses."... [T]hey looked at me like I had two heads... I said "I think that needs to be a priority. We have very poor blood pressure cuffs, two of the rooms don't have ECG monitoring equipment when we have bad bleeds" (Michelle, in Marck 2000a, 227).

Michelle's comments also underscore that the development and maintenance of effective forms of relation and resistance require a wider foundation of environmental structures and processes that enable sufficiently adaptive **responses** to the ecological conditions of modern health care. Forums for interdisciplinary teamwork must be provided, communications need to easily move across an organization's layers and roles, and leaders need to create environments that respect and attend to the concerns of loyal heretics. Mechanisms for self-monitoring and self-correction need to be encouraged, and rewards for reporting individual and systemic vulnerabilities need to be transparently rewarded. The guiding questions that flow from ecological principles and matters (see Exhibit 11-2) are therefore intended to **guide** practitioners towards the kinds of responses that strengthen integrity, minimize the residues that threaten integrity, and optimize the capacities of individuals, communities, and systems to heal.

Exhibit 11-2	An Ecological Framework: Guiding Questions for Reflection

1. **What are the goals of healing care** for the patient and family, practitioners, and the system as a whole?
2. **What forms of integrity are at stake** (personal, professional, ethical, scientific, systemic) in this situation or could be at risk?
3. **Where's the residue** (personal moral, communal or systemic moral, or theoretical) that threatens to contaminate or dilute our moral character, judgments, and actions?
4. **What moral violations must be prevented** to safeguard the integrity of the individuals and the situation?
5. **What strengthens our capacities** to maintain individual and systemic integrity, recognize and resolve individual and systemic residue, prevent or redress moral violations, and further the goals of healing care?

In Ethics in Practice 11-1, an experienced critical care nurse describes a chaotic night on a cardiac unit in which her unintentional neglect of a dying patient still haunts her. Using the questions for reflection in Exhibit 11-2, it becomes evident that this nurse and her colleagues take steps to resist environmental practices that threaten the integrity of their care.

Ethics in Practice 11-1	"She Fell to the Bottom of the Pile"

... [T]hey were so short of staff that there were things missed at the desk, orders missed at the desk because the charge nurse had to take over the medication giving [because there was] the orderly and then one other nurse around. They couldn't answer phones. It was just like chaos... the previous nurse was overwhelmed when she gave me her report, and then I walk into the guy that was confused. There was one medication linked in with another medication in the IV that shouldn't have been connected. They were going together.... I had to quickly check the blood sugars because it was insulin and some other medica-tion that shouldn't have been going together... I tried to get my medications out. I tried to go through all of the orders to see where I was at... a lot of things that weren't completed or weren't done quite right or follow-ups... They did the best they could under the circumstances and the nurse that was in charge... was just about in tears... I said... oh man this is a real hellhole tonight. You are doing the best you can and I want you to know that... I was given four patients of which one was basically terminally ill, esophageal cancer... She was basically a palliative care patient that hadn't been put on that list yet. I felt so sick that she was just in the wrong place. I couldn't provide her with the kind of care that I felt was critical for a dying woman... she just fell to the bottom of the pile.... I like to make myself available, okay I'm yours, I've finally got this time... [I]n this particular situation I had to go immediately to things, the biggest problems... the squeakiest wheel first. I never even got in to see her. I never even really got in to see her and ask her how she was doing until probably an hour or two later (Smoky, in Marck 2000a, 93, 129, 138, 229).

Nominated by her peers for excellence in clinical practice and certified in her critical care specialty, Smoky took great pride in maintaining good care for her patients under almost any set of circumstances. She valued both new and experienced colleagues, and she recalled that she and her co-workers had tried to build teamwork on the night in question by "calling each other Smoky the Bear" because they seemed to be putting out one forest fire after another. Faulty organizational assumptions about efficiency resulted in a continual baseline staffing deficit and the chronic overuse of floats and casual staff, and every form of integrity was at stake. Despite her knowledge, efforts, and esprit de corps, Smoky could not get past the urgent needs of her critically ill patients to adequately nurse her dying patient, a failure that constituted abandonment in her view. While she did not blame herself for this moral violation, she felt accountable to act and led her reluctant colleagues to complete a written report on the unsafe staffing for that night. Professional associations support these actions, providing guidelines that support nurses to make informed decisions about staffing, overtime requests, and other potential safety issues (Alberta Association of Registered Nurses 2001; Registered Nurses Association of British Columbia 2001).

Smoky's experience demonstrates that conscientious practitioners inevitably incur some degree of moral distress and moral residue in the course of their practice because there are times when preventable harms occur despite our best efforts. However, persistent resistance to unacceptable compromises is a necessary ethical counterpoise to organizational residues and deficiencies with the potential to cause real harms. Nurses therefore need to question a wide range of tensions that surface between various forms of integrity and residue because these points of strain guide us to ethical turning points that demand reflection (see Exhibit 11-3). Webster and Baylis argue that if we undertake such reflection and critique of events, the experience of moral residue can be "a profound teaching moment... even healing" (2000, 228).

In Ethics in Practice 11-2, several of these turning points are apparent as a nurse struggles for moral resolution long after the original, devastating event. Sarah's story is one of being caught up in an ever-deepening morass of things gone wrong. The chain of events was initiated three days prior when one of their elderly patients with a fractured hip was originally transferred to ICU for a 48-hour stay required by hospital policy after special diagnostic tests. When the minimum required ICU stay expired as of that Saturday morning, a pressured critical care unit made it plain to Sarah that they needed their bed back immediately for another patient.

As Sarah's narrative unfolds, we enter a hectic Saturday morning on an orthopaedic unit full of fresh post-op patients, many of whom are elderly and have multiple comorbidities. As the only experienced nurse on shift, Sarah assumed charge duty plus a heavy patient load in order to lessen the strain for a younger, much less experienced float nurse. When the patient and chart arrived on Sarah's unit with the documentation that this patient was "stable to transfer," Sarah looked at her limited staffing resources and assigned the float nurse with the lighter load to admit the woman and provide care. However, Sarah soon recognized that the younger nurse was struggling with her assignment and promptly responded to her request to assess the patient. Even though she couldn't discern the exact nature of the woman's condition, she was convinced that something was wrong. Her cumulative nursing wisdom fed her vigilance, and she started trying to contact the resident right away. He did not arrive in a timely fashion, so she started to try to contact the woman's staff physician. The physician was in the OR, however, and did not appreciate the level of her concern. Even though Sarah spent much of her shift reassessing the patient and trying to obtain what she viewed as necessary medical attention, things deteriorated into irreversible harm.

Ethics in Practice 11-2	**"Stable to Transfer"**

... [S]he comes back to us and again we have part-time staff, we have full-time, we have casuals. It was a casual girl who was working with her that day and she came out to me, I was in charge, and she said Sarah, I don't know this woman, can you tell me anything about her?... When I went in to help sit her up, I was appalled... I called the resident back, because it was a dramatic change. Called the physician... but he was in the operating room. It took sort of all morning. I had talked to the resident, I had talked to the doctor—and he said well, he didn't have time... [B]y 4 o'clock he came back, well then it hit the fan, because there was a definite shift and the next thing we know, the lady is being rushed off to ICU and entubated... it was a series of miscommunication, not enough information, not enough documentation. She should never have come to us. She should have stayed under neuro for that sort of a thing, but the politics came in there that they needed that neuro bed for somebody, so send her back to us... [W]e did everything we could, I did the best I could to get people there... a totally different resident to look at her... Totally different nurses... I mean, I looked over the chart and it said, you know, stable to transfer... [T]he lady died (Sarah, in Marck 2000c, 147, 158).

In Sarah's experience, one good nurse's professional integrity is not able to overcome the degraded environmental conditions that led her patient into fatal and possibly avoidable harm. Her moral anguish leads us to ask: When compromises to nurses' practice environments increasingly fragment the safety and continuity of care, at what point is the margin for error reduced to an unacceptable degree? Sarah's story is particularly disturbing because she identifies her nursing unit as one with strong clinical leadership and a respect for the value of nursing care. Her head nurse encourages Sarah's other roles of clinical teaching and troubleshooting the unit's computerized charting system. Learning is valued, and considerable effort is made to provide adequate numbers of qualified staff for care. Yet her story reveals that experienced weekend staffing was minimal, and, in combination with a brimming ICU, questionable transfer criteria, and an unresponsive medical staff, an essential web of relations and structures fragmented to the point where there was no remaining margin for error. The ecology of nurses' work environments tells us that to preserve a viable margin of safety for practitioners and patients, we must increase our ability to recognize and address the toxic residues that threaten the integrity of healing places.

Exhibit 11-3	Integrity and Residue: Sample Questions to Identify Ethical Turning Points

Personal Integrity: Do I refrain from actions at work that unacceptably compromise who I am as a person?

Professional Integrity: Do I exercise honesty with co-workers, patients, and families in the handling of mistakes?

Systemic Integrity: Are the processes and structures for the prevention and management of errors fair and transparent?

Ethical Integrity: Do I use professional codes of conduct to reflect upon my practice?

Scientific Integrity: Do I ensure that my own practice does not enable or cover up the unethical conduct of clinical research?

Moral Residue: Do we encourage critical feedback from patients and staff, or do we discount critics by labelling them "resistant to change?"

Theoretical Residue: Are we using nurses' knowledge and experience to design and evaluate the outcomes of nurses' work?

Systemic Residue: Do short-term "efficiencies" such as minimal staffing contribute to excessive longer term costs in rising staff overtime and increased adverse events for patients?

PRESERVING ETHICAL MARGINS: RE-INHABITING PLACES THAT HEAL

> I had a fellow who was diagnosed with lung cancer... I remember just sitting there and saying to myself, "I'm going to do this"... [H]e needed to talk with someone... I did close the curtain around me so nobody saw me sitting there, because someone would probably criticize the fact that I was "doing nothing" (Ellen, in Marck 2000a, 218).

> Restoration is about accepting the brokenness of things, and investigating the emergent properties of healing. It's the closing of the frontier—ceasing our demand for open land to "develop"—and the re-inhabiting of exploited or abandoned places (Mills 1995, 2).

An ecological ethic encourages nurses to watch over each other, their patients and clients, and the places where they work with deep ethical commitment to the *raison d'être* of nursing, which is to strengthen the capacity to heal. Nurses' exemplars, relations, resistance, and response illustrate necessary ethical counters to the toxic effects of moral, theoretical, and systemic residues on the integrity of their practice and practice environments. This ethical counterpoise assists nurses, their co-workers, and the patients in their care to reside within a tolerable margin of error. Ellen (above) keeps faith with the healing goals of good nursing care by responding to her patient's need after the receipt of devastating news. She resists a unit culture of breakneck, fragmented care, she overrules her first inclination to move onto the next task, and she sits down instead to support a lonely, frightened man.

As nurses navigate the hazardous tenements of today's practice environments and an international shortage of qualified health care practitioners deepens, we cannot discount the ecological lessons of nurses' work. At the margins of integrity, only one way leads forward. The promise of an ecological ethic for nursing is the recovery of foundational relations, processes, and structures that enable the practices of nursing to thrive and create openings to heal (Cameron 1998). One corresponding danger to this promise is that by offering much needed hope for our damaged practice environments, any form of ecological ethic could be under-critiqued and inappropriately applied. The interplay between technology, nursing, and ecology cannot be thoroughly examined within the confines of one chapter, and over-simplification can foster misconceptions. The worst fate for ecological ethics would be for it to become the next bandwagon in an overly reactive health system. Various schools of ecology, environmental ethics, and ecosystems management emphasize different principles or priorities than those of this work, and many traditional principles of health care ethics could also be better integrated into an ecological framework with additional effort.

Writing about the ongoing struggle to repair damaged wilderness, Higgs notes that "a quantity of engaging work" awaits (1991, 97). Research in ethics, ecological restoration, and nursing all indicate that to repair and strengthen the integrity of our care and care environments, we too must get on with some essential healing work. Adequate evaluation of this ecological ethic, as with most contemporary ethical frameworks, is pending, and most of its potential applications await further inquiry. The proposed framework requires ongoing research and refinement if it is to contribute to the moral development of health care practitioners and organizations in a lasting way. In the meantime, a hasty consumption of an ecological ethic is far less advisable than a more careful consideration of its healing goals.

FOR REFLECTION

1. Critique the strengths and limits of an ecological framework for analyzing an ethical issue in your own nursing practice. What aspects of an ecological approach assist your thinking? What are the limitations? Can you see the framework operating equally well for a variety of ethical problems in your practice setting? Why or why not?

2. Consider an alternative framework for ethical analysis, either from this text or from another source of your choice. Where does it exceed the ecological approach for analyzing the issue of your choice? Where is it equivocal or less helpful, and why? What happens if you combine the best of both approaches into a different, hybrid framework of your own? For example, are there potential relationships between the concepts of integrity, residue, and healing that this framework proposes and the concepts of ethical fitness (see Chapter 1), moral climate (see Chapter 10), and relational ethics (see Chapter 24)?

3. Reflect upon a situation in your own practice where, despite everyone's best intentions, things went wrong and real harms occurred. What learning—for better or worse— occurred from the way that the situation was handled? Given how things turned out,

how would you handle a similar adverse event today, and with what intended outcomes in mind? What steps can nurses independently take to strengthen the integrity of their own environments for care, and what partnerships are needed to enhance their efforts?

ENDNOTES

1. For recent research reviews and comprehensive reports on nurses' practice environments and health system safety issues, see the Final Report of the National Steering Committee on Patient Safety (2002); the Canadian Nurses Advisory Committee Final Report to Health Canada (2002); Aiken, Clarke, Sloane, Sochalski and Silber (2002); Leape, Berwick and Bates (2002); Shojania, Duncan, McDonald and Wachter (2002); Zwarenstein and Reeves (2002); Aiken, Clarke, Sloane, Sochalski, Busee, Clarke, Giovannetti, Hunt, Rafferty and Shamian (2001); Baker and Norton (2001); Blythe, Baumann and Giovannetti (2001); the World Health Organization Secretariat (2001); Australian Council for Safety and Quality in Health Care (2001); National Health Service (2001); Aiken, Clarke and Sloane (2001); and the Institutes of Medicine (1999).

2. For further discussion of the research which guides this framework, see Marck (2000a, b, c, d). For related work in restoration see Cowell (1993); Higgs (1991; 1999a; 1999b; in press,); Jordan III (1995); Leopold (1949); Meekison and Higgs (1998); Mills (1995); and Wierwille (1994); in ecosystems management see Gunderson, Holling and Light (1995); Woodley, Kay and Francis (1993); and Orr (1992); in philosophy see Higgs, Light and Strong (2000); Borgmann (1999; 1992; 1984); and Feenberg (1995; 1991); and in health care ethics see Bergum and Dossetor (in press); Whitehouse (1999); Donnelly (1998); and Potter (1990).

3. Practice exemplars and case scenarios are excerpted from the author's doctoral research (Marck 2000a; Alberta Heritage Foundation for Medical Research Incentive Grant and University of Alberta Dissertation Fellowship, 1998–2000) and nursing experience. The research was conducted with 10 nurses working in acute care and guided by Dr. Vangie Bergum, Dr. Marion Allen, and Dr. Eric Higgs, University of Alberta. Additional critiques of this research were provided by the Relational Ethics Project, University of Alberta and by Carol Gahan R.N., Deliah Robinson R.N., and Dr. Albert Borgmann, University of Montana. At the time of the study, participants possessed between 10 and 34 years of nursing practice and were employed at one or more of seven large tertiary care hospitals in Alberta.

4. Relevant work on caring for the environments where we live and work as we would our homes is found in Rowe (1990); Buell (1995; 2001); Mills (1995); Donnelly et al. (1998); Higgs (1999a); and Marck (2000a).

5. For elaboration on the challenges facing restoration work in the technologically mediated culture of a global marketplace, see especially Cypher and Higgs (1997); Higgs (1999a; 2003; in press); Light and Higgs (1996); and Strong (1995). All of these scholars draw on philosopher Albert Borgmann's extensive inquiry into the nature of technology in contemporary life (1999; 1992; 1984).

6. In addition to other chapters in this text, see further discussion of treatment decisions and other ethical issues at the end of life in Bergum and Dossetor (in press); Lanuke, Fainsinger, deMoissac and Archibald (2003); Neumann (2001); Valente (2001); CNA (2001; 2000; 1998); Fainsinger and Te (1999); Cassell (1999); Voth and Fainsinger (1999); Canadian Healthcare Association et al. (1999); and CNA et al. (1995).

7. For further relevant discussion of the ethical nature or climate of health care organizations in re-engineered health systems, see, for example, Varcoe and Rodney (2001); Storch (1998); Storch et al. (2002; 1998); Rodney et al. (2003); Goodstein and Potter (1999); and Corser (1998).

REFERENCES

Aiken, L.H., Clarke, S.P. and Sloane, D.M. 2001. Hospital restructuring: Does it adversely affect care and outcomes? *Journal of Health & Human Services Administration, 23*(40), 416–442.

Aiken, L.H., Clarke, S.P., Sloane, D.M., Sochalski, J.A., Busee, R., Clarke, H., Giovannetti, P., Hunt, J., Rafferty, A.M. and Shamian, J. 2001. Nurses reports on hospital care in five countries. *Health Affairs, 20*(3), 43–53.

Aiken, L.H., Clarke, S.P., Sloane, D.M., Sochalski, J. and Silber, J.H. 2002. Hospital nurse staffing and patient mortality, nurse burnout, and job dissatisfaction. *Journal of the American Medical Association, 288*(16), 1987–1993.

Alberta Association of Registered Nurses. 2001. *Working extra hours: Guidelines for registered nurses on fitness to practice and the provision of safe, competent, ethical nursing care.* Edmonton: Alberta Association of Registered Nurses.

Australian Council for Safety and Quality in Health Care. 2001. *Safety in practice: making health care safer.* Second Report to the Australian Health Ministers' Conference. Retrieved December 1, 2002, from: www.safetyandquality.org/articles/Publications/med_saf_rept.pdf

Baker, G.R. and Norton, P. 2001. Making patients safer! Reducing error in Canadian health care. *HealthCare Papers*, *2*(1), 10–31.

Barnhart, R.K. and Steinmetz, S. (Eds.). 1988. *The Barnhart dictionary of etymology.* New York: H.W. Wilson Co.

Bergum, V. and Dossetor, J.B. (In press, 2004) *Relational ethic: The full meaning of respect.* Hagerstown, MD: University Publishing Group.

Blythe, J., Baumann, A. and Giovannetti, P. 2001. Nurses' experience of restructuring in three Ontario hospitals. *Journal of Nursing Scholarship*, First Quarter, 61–68.

Borgmann, A. 1984. *Technology and the character of contemporary Life.* Chicago: University of Chicago Press.

Borgmann, A. 1992. *Crossing the postmodern divide.* Chicago: University of Chicago Press.

Borgmann, A. 1999. *Holding on to reality. The nature of information at the turn of the millennium.* Chicago: University of Chicago Press.

Buell, L. 1995. *The environmental imagination. Thoreau, Nature Writing and the Formation of American Culture.* Cambridge, Mass: The Belknap Press of Harvard University Press.

Buell, L. 2001. *Writing for an endangered world. Literature, culture, and environment in the U.S. and beyond.* Cambridge, Mass: The Belknap Press of Harvard University Press.

Cameron, B.L. 1998. Understanding nursing and its practices. Unpublished doctoral dissertation. University of Alberta, Edmonton.

Canadian Healthcare Association, Canadian Medical Association, Canadian Nurses Association, and Catholic Health Association of Canada. 1999. *Joint statement on preventing and resolving ethical conflicts involving health care providers and persons receiving care.* Ottawa: Canadian Nurses Association, Canadian Medical Association, Canadian Nurses Association, and Catholic Health Association of Canada.

Canadian Nurses Association, Canadian Healthcare Association, Canadian Medical Association, Catholic Health Association of Canada, with the Canadian Bar Association. 1995. *Joint statement on resuscitative interventions.* Ottawa: Canadian Nurses Association.

Canadian Nurses Association. 1996. Substance misuse and chemical dependency in nursing. Ottawa: Canadian Nurses Association.

Canadian Nurses Association. 1998. "Ethics in practice" paper: *Advance directives: The nurse's role.* Ottawa: Canadian Nurses Association.

Canadian Nurses Association. 2000. *End-of-life issues.* Ottawa: Canadian Nurses Association.

Canadian Nurses Association. 2001. *Quality professional practice environments for registered nurses.* Ottawa: Canadian Nurses Association.

Canadian Nurses Association. 2002a. *Code of ethics for registered nurses.* Ottawa: Canadian Nurses Association.

Canadian Nurses Association. 2002b. *Ethical research guidelines for registered nurses.* Ottawa: Canadian Nurses Association.

Cassell, E.J. 1999. Commentary: Is this palliative care medicine? *Journal of Pain and Symptom Management, 17*(6), 450–451.

Corser, W. 1998. The changing nature of organizational commitment in the acute care environment. Implications for nursing leadership. *Journal of Nursing Management, 28*(6), 32–36.

Cowell, C.M. 1993. Ecological restoration and environmental ethics. *Environmental Ethics, 15*(1), 19–32.

Cypher, J. and Higgs, E.S. 1997. Colonizing the imagination: Disney's wilderness lodge. *Capitalism, Nature, Socialism. A Journal of Socialist Ecology, 8*(4), 107–130.

Donnelly, S. 1998. Civic responsibility and the future of the Chicago region. *Hastings Center Report, 28*(6), S2–S5.

Duncan, S.M., Hyndman, K., Estabrooks, C.A., Hesketh, K., Humphrey, C.K., Wong, J. S., Acorn, S., and Giovannetti, P. 2001. Nurses' experience of violence in Alberta and British Columbia hospitals. *Canadian Journal of Nursing Research, 32*(4), 57–78.

Fainsinger, R. and Te, L. 1999. Case presentation: When is palliative care alone appropriate? *Journal of Pain and Symptom Management, 17*(60), 446–447.

Feenberg, A. 1991. *Critical Theory of Technology.* New York: Oxford University Press.

Feenberg, A. 1995. *Alternative modernity. The technical turn in philosophy and social theory.* Berkeley: University of California Press.

Goodstein, J. and Potter, R.L. 1999. Beyond financial incentives: Organizational ethics and organizational integrity. *Healthcare Ethics Forum, 11*(4), 293–305.

Gunderson, L.H., Holling, C.S. and Light, S. S. (Eds.). 1995. *Barriers and bridges to the renewal of ecosystems and institutions.* New York: Columbia University Press.

Hardingham, L., Marck, P.B., McKneally, M. and Read, J. 2001. *Managing mistakes in modern health care: What can ecosystems teach us about sustainable margins of error?* Workshop for the Canadian Bioethics Society 13th Annual Conference. October 13, Winnipeg, Manitoba.

Health Canada. 2002. *Our health, our future. Creating quality workplaces for Canadian nurses.* Final report of the Canadian Nursing Advisory Committee. Ottawa: Health Canada. Available online: www.hc-sc. gc.ca/english/for_you/nursing/cnac_report/index.html

Higgs, E.S. 1991. A quantity of engaging work to be done: Ecological restoration and morality in a technological culture. *Restoration and Management Notes, 9*(2), 97–103.

Higgs, E.S. 1999a. What is good ecological restoration? *Conservation Biology, 11*(2), 338–348.

Higgs, E.S. 1999b. The Bear in the Kitchen. Ecological Restoration in Jasper Park Raises questions about wilderness in the Disney age. *Alternatives Journal, 25*(2), 30–35.

Higgs, E.S. In press. *Nature by design.* Chicago: University of Chicago Press.

Higgs, E.S., Light, A. and Strong, D. (Eds.). 2000. *Philosophy in the service of things: Devices, focal things and the quality of life.* Chicago: University of Chicago Press.

Hunter, G. 1995. An unnecessary death. *The Canadian Nurse, 91*(6), 20–25.

Institutes of Medicine. 1999. *To err is human: Building a safer system.* Washington: National Academy Press. Retrieved December 1 from: www.nap.edu/to_err_is_human

Jordan III, W.R., 1995. Restoration ecology: A synthetic approach to ecological research. In J. Cairns (Ed.), *Rehabilitating Damaged Ecosystems,* 2nd ed. (pp. 373–384). Boca Raton, Florida: Lewis Publishers.

Lanuke, K., Fainsinger, R., DeMoissac, D. and Archibald, J. 2003. Case reports: Sedation and two remarkable dyspneic men. *Journal of Palliative Medicine, 6*(2), 277–281.

Leape, L.L. i Berwick, D.M. and Bates, D.W. 2002. What practices will most improve safety? Evidence-based medicine meets patient safety. *Journal of the American Medical Association, 288*(4), 501–507. Available online: http://jama.ama-assn.org/issues/v288n4/rfull/jcv20002.html

Leopold, A. 1949. *A Sand County almanac: With essays on conservation from Round River.* New York: Oxford University Press.

Light, A. and Higgs, E.S. 1996. The politics of ecological restoration. *Environmental Ethics, 18*(4), 227–247.

Marck, P.B. 2000a. Technology and registered nurses' work in acute care: A healing inquiry. Unpublished doctoral dissertation. University of Alberta, Edmonton.

Marck, P.B. 2000b. Nursing in a technological world: Searching for healing communities. *Advances in Nursing Science, 23*(2), 59–72.

Marck, P.B. 2000c. Strengthening integrity: Ecological error management for ethical health care. *Provincial Health Ethics Network Newsletter In Touch*, December, 1–2.

Marck, P.B. 2000d. Recovering ethics after technics: Developing critical text on technology. *Nursing Ethics, 7*(1), 5–13.

Meekison, L. and Higgs, E. 1998. The rites of spring (and other seasons). The ritualization of restoration. *Restoration & Management Notes, 16*(1), 73–81.

Mills, S. 1995. *In service of the wild. Restoring and re-inhabiting damaged land.* Boston: Beacon Press.

Mitchell, G.M. 2001. Policy, procedure and routine: Matters of moral influence. *Nursing Science Quarterly, 14*(2), 109–114.

National Health Service. 2000. *An organization with memory: Report of an expert working group on learning from adverse events in the NHS.* London: Department of Health. Retrieved December 2 from: www.doh.gov.uk/orgmemreport.

National Steering Committee on Patient Safety. 2002. *Building a safer system. A national integrated strategy for improving patient safety in Canadian health care.* Ottawa: National Steering Committee on Patient Safety. Available online: http://rcpsc.medical.org/english/publications

Neumann, J.L. 2001. Ethical issues confronting oncology nurses. *Nursing Clinics of North America, 36*(4), 827–841.

Orr, D. 1992. *Ecological literacy: Education and the transition to a postmodern world.* Albany: SUNY Press.

Potter, V.R. 1999. Bioethics, biology, and the biosphere. Fragmented ethics and "bridge bioethics." *Hastings Center Report, 29*(1), 38–40.

Registered Nurses Association of British Columbia. 2001. Implications of the nurse shortage. Questions & Answers for Registered Nurses. Vancouver, B.C.: Registered Nurses Association of British Columbia.

Rodney, P.A., Varcoe, C., Storch, J.L., McPherson, G., Mahoney, K., Brown, H., Pauly, B., Hartrick-Doane, G. and Starzomski, R. 2002. Navigating toward a moral horizon: A multi-site qualitative study of nurses' enactment of ethical practice. *Canadian Journal of Nursing Research, 34*(3), 75–102.

Rowe, S. 1990. *Home place. Essays on ecology.* Canadian Parks and Wilderness Society Henderson Book Series No. 12. Edmonton: NeWest.

Shojania, K.G., Duncan, B.W., McDonald, K.M. and Wachter, R.M. 2002. Safe but sound. Patient safety meets evidence-based medicine. *Journal of the American Medical Association, 288*(4), 508–513. Retrieved December 8 from: http://jama.ama-assn.org/issues/v288n4/rfull/jcv20003.html

Sibbald, B. 1997. A right to be heard. *Canadian Nurse, 93*(10), 22–28, 30.

Sinclair, Justice Murray. 2000. *The report of the Manitoba pediatric cardiac surgery inquest.* Winnipeg: Government of Manitoba. Available online: www.pediatriccardiacinquest.mb.ca

Society for Ecological Restoration. 1996. Official definition of ecological integrity. Available online: http://ser.org

Storch, J. 1998. Casualization of nurses and unregulated workers impair ethical practice. *International Nursing Review, 45*(5), 140–141.

Storch, J.L., Rodney, P., Pauly, B., Brown, H. and Starzomski, R. 2002. Listening to nurses' moral voices: Building a quality health care environment. *Canadian Journal of Nursing Leadership, 15*(4), 7–16.

Strong, D. 1995. *Crazy mountains. Learning from wilderness to weigh technology*. New York: SUNY Press.

Valente, S.M. 2001. End-of-life issues. *Geriatric Nursing, 22*(6), 294–298.

Varcoe, C. and Rodney, P. 2001. Constrained agency: The social structure of nurses' work. In B.S. Singh and H.D. Dickinson (Eds.), *Health, illness and health care in Canada*, 3rd ed. (pp. 102–128). Scarborough, Ontario: Nelson Thomson Learning.

Voth, A.J. and Fainsinger, R. 1999. Commentary: Is this a palliative care patient? *Journal of Pain and Symptom Management, 17*(60), 448–449.

Webster, G.C. and Baylis, F.E. 2000. Moral residue. In L. Zoloth and S.B. Rubin (Eds.), *Margin of error: The ethics mistakes in the practice of medicine* (pp. 217–230). Hagerstown, MD: University Publishing Group.

Whitehouse, P.J. 1999. The Ecomedical Disconnection Syndrome. *Hastings Center Report, 29*(1), 41–44.

Wierwille, J.E. 1994. Remaking and restoring dare county. In A.D. Baldwin, J. De Luce and C. Pletsch (Eds.), *Beyond preservation: Restoring and reinventing landscapes*. Minneapolis: University of Minnesota Press.

Wilkin, G. 1999. Boundaries in nurse/client relationships. *Partners in Psychiatric Health Care Journal, 2*(1), 14–20.

Winner, L. 1977. *Autonomous technology: Technics-out-of-control as a theme in political thought*. Cambridge, Mass: MIT Press.

Woodley, S., Kay, J. and Francis, G. (Eds.). 1993. *Ecological integrity and the management of ecosystems*. Ottawa: St. Lucie Press.

World Health Organization Executive Board, EB 109/9, 109th Session, December 2001. Provisional Agenda Item 3.4. Quality of Care: Report on Patient Safety. Report of the Secretariat. Available online: www.who.int/gb/EB_WHA/PDF/EB109/eeb1099.pdf

Zoloth, L. and Rubin, S.B. (Eds.). 2000. *Margin of error: The ethics mistakes in the practice of medicine*. Hagerstown, MD: University Publishing Group.

Zwarenstein, M. and Reeves, S. 2002. Working together but apart: Barriers and routes to nurse-physician collaboration. *Journal of Quality Improvement, 28*(5), 242–247.

chapter twelve

Home Health Care and Ethics[1]

Elizabeth Peter

Home care nurses have had the privilege of coming to know their patients and families as they actually live their lives. Fiscal restraints, however, have constrained home care nurses' capacity to provide care holistically and have led to role conflict and confusion because the range of care activities deemed necessary by nurses is often not considered worthy of remuneration.

Many nursing services and other health services that were previously provided in institutional settings are now being offered in the homes of Canadians. This change in setting is the result of health system restructuring and health policy shifts. Technological advances have also allowed for more medical treatments and assistive and monitoring devices to be offered in the home. Today, home care can include acute care, long-term care, and end-of-life care services. It is not unusual for people to receive intravenous therapy, nutrition therapy, chemotherapy, dialysis, and respiratory services in the home. In addition, there is a range of people who receive assistance with homemaking and other activities of daily living because of disabling conditions or the frailties of age (CARP 1999; Commission on the Future of Health Care in Canada 2002; Standing Senate Committee on Social Affairs, Science and Technology 2002). The demand for home care services is expected to rise as more patients are discharged from hospital earlier and sicker and as the Canadian population ages.

Currently, however, Canadians are not entitled to home care services under the Canada Health Act (CHA) (1984). There exists tremendous variation among provinces and territories with respect to the availability of covered home care services. Some provinces provide extensive coverage for home nursing care, while others strictly limit nursing services to a fixed dollar or hourly amount. Wide variations also exist with respect to the provision of home medical supplies and home rehabilitation services. Therefore, no "floor," or basic set, of services is available to all Canadians (Commission on the Future of Health Care in Canada 2002). As a result, many people are without adequate resources and must rely on family members, when they are available, to provide care that is often extensive and highly sophisticated.

Health restructuring has also eroded the role of home care nurses, along with the associated autonomy of this role. Traditionally, home care nurses have embraced the importance of home and family as foundational to practice. Home care nurses have held a deep commitment to holistic and family-centred care that encompasses health promotion and disease prevention. As guests in the homes of their patients, home care nurses have valued collaborative relationships with patients and have striven to adapt to a never-ending variety of patient-controlled environments. Home care nurses have had the privilege of coming to know their patients and families as they actually live their lives. Fiscal restraints, however, have constrained home care nurses' capacity to provide care holistically and have led to role conflict and confusion because the range of care activities deemed necessary by nurses is often not considered worthy of remuneration (CHNAC 2003).

This lack of available resources and the transfer of responsibility for care from the state to the family are of great ethical importance, having major implications for patients and their families, health care organizations, health care professionals, and governments. In this chapter, I argue that this lack of resources is the result of shifting services to the home outside of the protection of the Canada Health Act. This shift has been made possible by a political ideology that is neo-liberal in nature. I then address some of the implications of current home care policy, particularly those that concern the well-being of patients, families, and home care workers and those that have an impact upon nurse-patient-family relationships. I then offer a counter-ethic that has its basis in a feminist ethic of trust in order to challenge neo-liberal values and beliefs.

THE POLITICAL CONTEXT: NEO-LIBERALISM AND GLOBALIZATION

Prior to the CHA, two federal acts—the Hospital Insurance and Diagnostic Services Act (1957) and the Medical Care Act (1968)—governed hospital and medical care insurance in such a way that all Canadians were entitled to medically necessary hospital and insurance programs. The passage of the CHA in 1984 replaced these acts but retained the basic principles underlying the existing national health insurance program and also eliminated extra-billing. The CHA contains five well-known requirements that the provinces and territories must meet to qualify for full federal funding, including public administration, comprehensiveness, universality, portability, and accessibility. These, however, apply to insured health care services only, that is, medically necessary hospital services, physician services, and surgical dental services provided in a hospital. They do not apply to extended health care services, that is, aspects of long-term residential care and the health aspects of home care (Health Canada 2002). Consequently, as home care becomes more prevalent, the CHA is becoming increasingly incapable of protecting the health care needs of Canadians. Today's health care involves more than the one privileged place (the hospital) and more than the one privileged provider (the physician), resulting in many health care services falling outside of the scope of the CHA (Coyte 2002). In fact, the Commission on the Future of Health Care in Canada (2002) names home care and pharmaceuticals as the two biggest areas of change since medicare was introduced 40 years ago.

The rise of neo-liberalism and globalization underlies these health care reforms that have left many without coverage, including those who require home care services. **Neo-liberalism,** as a political and social philosophy, has been characterized by Coburn (2000) as possessing the following assumptions:

1. that markets are the best and most efficient allocators of resources in production and distribution;
2. that societies are composed of autonomous individuals (producers and consumers) motivated chiefly or entirely by material or economic considerations; and
3. that competition is the major market vehicle for innovations (138).

With markets functioning as resource allocators, the lack of state intervention in the form of welfare and income redistribution can be justified from a neo-liberal perspective. Furthermore, the autonomous, economically motivated individual has little to no responsibility for the well-being of others. In this political culture, individuals are framed in terms of their rights and freedoms (Rose 1998). Others merely function as competition to material goods (Coburn 2000).

Neo-liberalism promotes a view of justice such that persons receive a fair distribution of goods according to free-market exchanges. Market inequalities are seen as "just" because what one puts into the market one gets out. "That is, the invisible hand doctrine implies some reasonable relationship between one's activities and subsequent rewards" (Coburn 2000, 138). Inequalities from this viewpoint, therefore, can be justified because it is presumed that individuals are equally equipped to compete for resources.

Adherents of neo-liberal ideologies view public and social expenditures, like health care, as a source of inefficiency and waste in this era of globalization. In the end, free-market forces and private profits are substituted for the collective public good (Williams et al. 2001; Navarro 1999). **Globalization** refers to a "specific form of internationalization that responds to specific financial and economic interests that are articulated in the class relations of each society" (Navarro 1999, 220). There is nothing inherently good or bad about this flow of capital, labour, and knowledge around the world, per se. The goodness or badness is dependent upon who governs and who benefits from it (Navarro 1999). Thus far, the evidence indicates that the high-income sectors of the population are benefiting as the welfare state's publicly supported commitment to social justice and equity among citizens declines (Austin 2001; Anderson 2001; Bjornsdottir 2002). Thus, neo-liberalism and globalization are mutually supporting and intimately intertwined discourses (Williams et al. 2001).

At the heart of neo-liberalism are two core ideals that threaten the values fundamental to the CHA and to Canadian identity and that are contrary to the stated values of home care nurses. The first is the belief that the free market is a just allocator of resources, such that each person fairly receives his or her share of resources by virtue of market exchanges. In contrast, the CHA is based largely on the belief that justice is served when each person receives his or her share of resources according to need, a central principle informing Canadian identity. As the Commission on the Future of Health Care in Canada (2002) states, "Canadians view medicare as a moral enterprise, not a business venture" (xx). The Canadian

Community Health Nursing Standards of Practice also do not support a market sense of justice. Instead, community nurses believe in advancing social justice by facilitating universal and equitable access to conditions for health and to health services. They recognize that sociopolitical issues may underlie individual and community problems (CHNAC 2002).

Social justice can be viewed as an opposing perspective to market justice (Beauchamp 1999). "Under social justice all persons are entitled equally to key ends such as health protection or minimum standards of income. Further, unless collective burdens are accepted, powerful forces of environment, heredity or social structure will preclude a fair distribution of these ends" (Beauchamp 1999, 105). Market justice is not appropriate for the distribution of health-related resources because factors such as disability, gender, age, and poverty impede people's abilities to access formal health care services and the determinants of health (Drevdahl et al. 2001).

The second related ideal is that of the self-interested and autonomous individual. With such an ideal, the neo-liberal vision is individualistic, not collectivist, in nature. Outside of immediate family and friends, others are viewed as competitors for scarce resources and are blamed and punished for their problems rather than helped. This individualistic market orientation elevates the level of social fragmentation and lowers the level of social cohesion and trust in a society. It also contributes to income inequalities, higher rates of violence, less community involvement, more chronic anxiety, and a lowered health status of citizens (Coburn 2000; Lynch 2000; Wilkinson 2000). This individualistic orientation is antithetical to the core values of equity, fairness, and solidarity that are central to a Canadian understanding of citizenship (Commission on the Future of Health Care in Canada 2002). It is also antithetical to the home care nurse's core belief in connecting with and caring for individuals, families, and communities (CHNAC 2002).

ETHICAL IMPLICATIONS: THE EVERYDAY LIVES OF PATIENTS, FAMILIES, AND HOME CARE NURSES

While only a few studies have examined ethical issues in home care in some depth (Liaschenko 1994; 1997; 2001; Liaschenko and Peter 2002; Holstien and Mitzen 2001; Arras and Dubler 1995; Kane and Caplan 1993; Collopy, Dubler and Zuckerman 1990), many studies have identified issues in home care that have arisen as a result of health reform. These issues have generally not been explicitly conceptualized as ethical in nature, but they are of ethical importance particularly on an everyday level because they affect the health and well-being of care recipients and caregivers alike. The following discussion will draw upon these issues to describe the ethical implications of neo-liberal health reforms. In addition, comments from home care nurses in Canada will be presented in Ethics in Practice narratives.[2]

Ethics in Practice 12-1	**Self-Care and Family Care**

Definitely in the community we're seeing a real challenge in terms of acuity of our clients that are coming out from the hospitals, from various ambulatory clinics, as well as even our clients that we are sending into the emergency departments because we feel that emergency is an appropriate place for them to be at that time. They come right back out and the onus is on community to somehow provide the resources to care for this person. I sometimes feel community is the dropping off point to the health care system. There are no beds, there's not room in the emergency department. You go home. We don't have the resources in the community to look after a lot of these people in terms of even providing non-professional supports. The home support agencies can't handle the amount that is out there and it comes right down to look after yourself or get your family to look after you. To a certain extent that's always been the case, but with the real level of acuity and illness that's out there now there's a real need and it's a real challenge to nursing. And it's probably where most of our frustration in the community lies, in our inability to help our clients because the resources are just not there.

In Ethics in Practice 12-1, a nurse describes many of the consequences of neo-liberal health reforms. As social expenditures for health decrease, only the most acutely ill people receive health services in hospitals. Yet, the community also does not have the resources to care for people adequately. Thus, many sick and disabled people must rely on themselves or their families, if available, to provide care. The moral distress of this home care nurse is evident as she or he describes the experience of wanting to provide care, but of being incapable of doing so because the resources are simply not available.

As this nurse suggests, others must be there to provide care when covered professional home care services are not available or are limited. High-income Canadians may be able to purchase their own professional services, but for most Canadians the onus falls on them to provide care for their loved ones. It is estimated that 80 to 90 percent of home care work is unpaid (Standing Senate Committee on Social Affairs, Science and Technology 2002). Low-income Canadians may be particularly affected because they often do not have extended health care benefits to cover the cost of pharmaceuticals and additional home care services, and many may not have the kinds of homes that are suitable for caregiving. As Anderson (2001) suggests, home care policy is dependent upon a particular notion of home that reflects the privileged middle class who are more likely to have the resources necessary to provide care.

The transfer of caregiving responsibilities from the state to the family also represents the state's reliance upon assumptions regarding women's availability and obligation to care for others in the home (Williams 2002). It is expected that women will provide this care in the home for their sick or disabled family members (Anderson 2001; Coyte and McKeever 2001) because caring for the home and the family has been the expected focus of many women's lives to the extent that "the house is identified as a place that is 'female' and caring as 'female' work" (Bowlby, Gregory and McKie 1997, 346). Indeed, in Canada, the greatest burden of both informal and formal care does fall upon women—generally wives, daughters, and daughters-in-law (Commission on the Future of Health Care in Canada 2002; Neysmith 2000).

The level of care provision can be extraordinary, encompassing both personal and high-tech care. It can include assistance with activities of daily living (e.g., bathing, eating, cooking, laundry, cleaning, and transportation) and also the provision and management of medications, injections, IVs, catheterizations, dialysis, tube feeding, and respiratory care. These informal caregivers are often responsible for 24-hour care with little available public support and often with inadequate training for the responsibilities they are expected to assume (CARP 1999). Approximately two thirds of Canadian home care recipients are women, largely because women have a greater life expectancy, often have chronic conditions, and can rely on less spousal assistance (Wilkins and Park 1998). In many instances, the resulting scenario is one of an old woman caring for a very old woman with only minimal formal home care support.

Ethics in Practice 12-2	**Working Conditions**

The home support worker is just another whole issue. No consistency, no licensure guidelines, no educational preparation. In the community, we grapple with knowing when do we delegate a function to our support worker. Sue identi- fied those home support workers as having no educational background, there are no standards—there's some minimum, I guess of standards there—but they're gone before they get to that level because of rate of pay, things like that.

In Ethics in Practice 12-2, the nurses share their concerns regarding home support workers. This brief account reveals a number of ethical concerns, including a concern over the quality of care that home care patients receive because the training of home support workers is inconsistent and, in some instances, limited. This nurse also draws attention to the interdependence of health care workers and the struggle to trust other workers whose qualifications are in question. The comment that home support workers leave before they become fully qualified because of "rate of pay, things like that" is most telling. It shows not only how money is a driving force in home care policy but also the poor working conditions of home support workers and other formal home care workers.

Formal home care workers in Canada are mainly women, many of whom are drawn from immigrant and visible minority populations. Although many community workers enjoy the autonomy and varied work environments that providing home care can offer, they generally work alone without the assistance and team support normally available in institutional settings. The requirement of round-the-clock services poses risks for all workers, but particularly for personal and home support workers who often rely on public transportation. While employers are required to comply with health and safety regulations, many of these rest on the premise that employers can exert control over the workplace. Employers, however, do not have this power when work is conducted off site, such as in private homes. Conditions in patients' homes can be highly variable and can fluctuate over time. It is not unusual for workers to face harassment, abuse, and exposure to illegal activities and domestic violence. Along with concerns regarding safety, home care work is poorly paid, is of low status, and must be completed within highly constrained amounts of time (Wojtak 2002; Aronson and Neysmith 1996; CARP 1999; CRIAW 1999; Liaschenko and Peter 2002).

Ethics in Practice 12-3	Nurse–Patient–Family Relationships

We've just started a home infusion programme in the community. Many of our nurses have been out of acute care for some time, and we had to say "you will be now doing acute infusion, antibiotics in the home. You'll be responsible for teaching these clients how to do it themselves and you'll be taking calls to trouble-shoot and problem solve." It's just one more thing that you add on. This is primarily our frustration.

The nurse in Ethics in Practice 12-3 describes the increasing responsibilities of home care nurses as patients in the community become more acutely ill. This adds to the nurses' already high workload and demands that some nurses redevelop their skills. The introduction of additional "high-tech" care also changes the relationship among the nurse, patient/client, and family. The nurse teaches the patient and family "how to do it themselves" and then takes "calls to trouble-shoot and problem solve." The patient/family becomes more self-sufficient and the nurse's role becomes less hands on. The relationship eventually takes place at a greater distance, the nurse acting as more of a resource than a direct caregiver. This type of relationship may or may not fully support the well-being of all involved depending on the resources of the patient and family. While home care nurses are enjoined to promote self-care, they must do so within certain parameters. The CHNAC (2002) standards state that home care nurses have the responsibility to "maximize the ability of an individual/ family to take responsibility for and manage their care according to resources and personal skills available" (11). In other words, the individual situations of patients and families must be taken into account. In our current system, however, these parameters cannot always be followed. Patients and their families must often take responsibility for their own care, even when they do not have the sufficient personal and other resources to do so.

In fact, many of the responsibilities of family caregivers are those that, until recently, would normally only have been held by regulated, formal caregivers. Families often assume the responsibilities and attain the skills of nurses but are not given the remuneration or the regulated working conditions and protections of formal providers. As nurses have enacted the role of physician extender, or the "Hamburger Helper" of medicine, when medical responsibilities have become inconvenient, too expensive, or otherwise unappealing to perform (Sandelowski 1999), so too have families become the "Hamburger Helper" of nursing. Because this transfer of responsibility is occurring in homes, it can easily be hidden and justified as merely an extension of "usual" family responsibility. Caregivers are profoundly affected by this work, to the extent that they experience increased morbidity and mortality (Flaskerud and Lee 2001; Schulz and Beach 1999).

These changes in policy have also had a profound effect upon nursing relationships. It is unclear whether the relationships that nurses have with family members should resemble those with co-workers rather than those with typical or traditional family members. It is difficult for home care nurses to negotiate professional boundaries and their scope of practice when family members occupy roles that obscure the distinction between formal and informal providers. In turn, it can also be difficult for family members and patients to determine their roles and responsibilities.

A Canadian study by Ward-Griffin and McKeever (2000) examined the relationships between community nurses and family members caring for frail elders. Four types of nurse–family caregiver relationships were identified: (1) nurse-helper, (2) worker-worker, (3) manager-worker, and (4) nurse-patient. The latter two were most frequent. The nurse-helper relationship was the least common relationship found. In this type of relationship nurses provided and co-ordinated most of the care, while family caregivers assumed a supportive role to nurses. Because of the cost of providing this type of care, nurses quickly moved to the second form of relationship—the worker-worker relationship. Care work was transferred to family caregivers, with nurses teaching them technical skills. These caregivers learned to assume much responsibility with little authority. Some family caregivers reported feeling afraid and unqualified to assume this level of responsibility. In time, these relationships moved to the manager-worker type, at the point which family caregivers had taken on virtually all of the care. At this stage, nurses no longer provided actual caregiving, but focused on the monitoring of family caregivers' coping skills and competence. Many family caregivers resisted this type of support, wanting assistance with actual caregiving instead. The final type of relationship, the nurse-patient relationship, occurred as frequently as the previous one. With this type of relationship, many caregivers, because of pre-existing health problems and the heavy demands of caregiving, became the nurse's patient too. The authors concluded that these family caregiver–nurse relationships were not partnerships, but were exploitative in character. The work of caring was transferred to family caregivers who were left socially isolated and without adequate resources to provide care.

The findings from this research illustrate well how current health policy is shaping the everyday lives of patients, families, and home care nurses. Home care recipients and their caregivers are often without the necessary resources to receive and provide care in such a way that the quality of care is maintained and individuals are not exploited. Every aspect of the work of home care nurses has been impacted, the well-being of all involved being threatened. This situation compromises the ability of nurses to enact one of nursing's most fundamental ethical values—the requirement to promote the health and well-being of persons (CNA 2002). Strategies must be sought to make changes in Canadian home care policy such that care recipients are protected and nurses can practise ethically.

A COUNTER-ETHIC: A FEMINIST ETHIC OF TRUST

Home care policy, like other forms of policy, expresses the values of the politically dominant group. Consequently, policy has a moral dimension in that it entails those with power making decisions about how others will be treated (Malone 1999; Cheek and Gibson 1997). Reflecting the interests of the most powerful, current Canadian home care policy upholds values and beliefs consistent with market justice and individualism. As such, home care policy constructs a neo-liberal notion of citizenship. This dominant vision of reality can be resisted, however. In recent years, a number of Canadian authors have offered alternative views.

Kenny (2002) presents the values of solidarity, equity, compassion, efficiency, and civility to supplant the market metaphor. She views health care not as a private commodity, but as a public and social good that must be distributed based on a communitarian sense of justice that embraces shared risk and collective responsibility.

The Romanow report (Commission on the Future of Health Care in Canada 2002) also explicitly puts forward alternatives to a market view of justice, offering the values of equity, fairness, and solidarity to challenge the view that health care is a business venture. Specifically, the report proposes that home care be targeted for additional funding in order to provide a foundation for a national home care strategy, and that the Canada Health Act be revised to include coverage for home mental health case management and intervention services, post-acute home care, and palliative home care. In addition, the report recommends that informal caregivers be given ongoing support through direct remuneration, tax breaks, job protection, caregiver leave, and respite. Yet the report falls short in leaving the provision of care for people with chronic illnesses and physical disabilities outside the focus of the report's priority areas. A danger exists that these individuals will become further marginalized and viewed as problems in the system.

In nursing, Rodney and Varcoe (2001), Varcoe and Rodney (2002), and Rodney et al. (2002) have described in rich detail how the underlying ideologies of globalization, corporatism, and scarcity have had a constraining influence on nurses' moral agency. They offer examples of how nurses have resisted these ideologies in a variety of ways, including through the negotiation of better care, relationship building among workers and patients, and rule bending. They suggest strategies of further resistance that involve tactics that go beyond the efforts of individuals, such as the restructuring of nurses' work in ways that aligns it with the goals of health and the common good instead of the goals of corporatism. They also recommend unmasking current ideologies in such a way that values can be laid bare so that nurses can become more conscious and deliberate about the values they are enacting in their practice.

Innovative and politically savvy nurse reformers may realize some of these goals. More likely, however, change will be made possible through the everyday activities of nurses who adopt these strategies. We must guard against the common tendency in nursing of either viewing nurses as powerless or of viewing power as somehow separate from the usual activities of nurses (Purkis 2001; Lunardi, Peter and Gastaldo 2002). With respect to home care nursing, Purkis (2001) suggests that the practice of home care nursing be re-conceptualized as a political practice that addresses and acknowledges the legitimacy of nurses' knowledge of the difficulties that they and their patients are experiencing. With this knowledge, nurses have the potential to resist managerial demands for efficiency by refusing to enact practices that exclude patients from the home care services they require. In my own previous work (Peter 2002), I have also examined the politics of home care by exploring how early 20th-century home care/private duty nurses exercised power. Despite the emphasis in nursing upon duty and obedience to physicians at that time, nurses also plainly expressed their capacity to influence their patients through education, role modelling, and the re-ordering of homes. These nurses also later played a significant role in the rise of hospitalization, as private duty nursing came to be viewed as a waste of nursing skill and money. Thus, nurses were not powerless. Their values left a mark not only on individual patients and families, but also on the health care system as a whole. Today our values also have influence. Therefore, purposefully explicating them may foster a much-needed awareness that can move us collectively forward to a more humane and ethical health care system.

In a previous publication, Morgan and I (Peter and Morgan 2001) explored the potential of Baier's (1985; 1986; 1994) work on trust in feminist ethics. We did this to inform the development of an ethic for nursing because of its capacity to draw together the values and beliefs of care, justice, and interdependence within a political perspective. Baier (1986) defines **trust** as "the reliance on others' competence and willingness to look after, rather than harm, things one cares about which are entrusted to their care" (259). She maintains that in trust relationships we expect others to love and care for us, but we also expect others to be just and to fulfill their obligations. Trust relationships also generally entail power differences and the potential for exploitation and other harms to come to those who trust. When we trust another, we become vulnerable to the other. Baier (1985; 1986; 1994) also goes beyond the analysis of dyadic trust relationships to include the idea of a network of trust relationships, thereby situating intimate relationships within a broader context of a community of trust.

Baier's (1985; 1986; 1994) work is relevant to nursing because it acknowledges the dimensions of vulnerability and power in trust relationships, and it integrates the ethics of care and justice. As a feminist perspective, it reconsiders the traditional boundary between politics and ethics and regards oppression as a focal moral and political wrong to be overcome (Tronto 1993; Liaschenko and Peter 2003; Brennan 1999). It also views persons as not wholly autonomous, as often vulnerable and interdependent and connected to others. Persons are viewed as unique, gendered, racialized, embodied and as existing within particular historical, political, economic, and cultural contexts. In these ways, an ethic of trust based on Baier's work is useful for situating nursing relationships within the broader society, including the health care system, and for understanding that we all exist in highly complex networks of interdependence and power. A recognition and acceptance of human interdependence and vulnerability exist at the core of an ethic of trust, making social cohesion a possibility.

A feminist ethic, such as trust, can function as an excellent counter-ethic to that currently informing home care policy. An ethic that is sensitive to gender, race, and class is necessary to oppose the dominant vision that constructs both the work of bodily caring as inferior and the place of women as in the home. Retaining care as a value is also important because it calls attention to the centrality of moral emotion and receptivity, the relief of suffering, the fostering of relationships, and the attention to particularity in everyday nursing practice. Home care nurses traditionally have had long-term, close relationships with their patients and have cared about the minutia of their patients' day-to-day lives. Nevertheless, an ethic of care is not sufficient on its own.

Feminist critics have argued that care approaches have the potential to perpetuate women's unrecognized and exploited caregiving (Bowden 1996; Tong 1996). They also can lead to a neglect of unknown others if those who are deeply engaged in caring for immediate others fail to address broader concerns of care. Considerations of justice, therefore, such as obligations, principles, and impartiality, are needed to ensure fairness both in situations concerning relationships with immediate others and in situations concerning distant/unknown others (Peter and Morgan 2001). It is important, however, to recognize that there are varying, and often competing, substantive principles of justice.

Instead of market justice, an ethic of trust demands a sense of social justice. Because social justice entails a belief in collectivism over individualism, it challenges neo-liberalism. Striving for social justice requires collective action to reduce the effects of factors such as age, disability, and poverty. Promoting awareness and action regarding human rights, homelessness, poverty, unemployment, stigma, and so on are ways of working toward social justice.

Opportunities exist for nurses to become vocal with respect to issues of social justice. Writing letters to local Members of Legislative Assemblies or Members of Parliament and participating in activities of professional organizations in nursing are realistic ways to have influence. Nursing curricula can also foster an understanding of social justice in future nurses. Students can become sensitized in the classroom and in clinical practice to the health concerns of marginalized groups and to the need not only to equitably distribute health care services, but also the determinants of health. The CNA's (2002) Code of Ethics for Registered Nurses can provide assistance in this manner, with its unequivocal stance on the requirement of nurses to promote social justice. It states,

> Nurses should be aware of broader health concerns such as environment pollution, violations of human rights, world hunger, homelessness, violence, etc. and are encouraged to the extent possible in their personal circumstances to work individually as citizens or collectively for policies and procedures to bring about social change (15).

In this chapter, I have described the current state of home care in Canada, revealing inadequacies and inequities in our system that privileges hospital and physician services. The rise of home care has been made possible not only through advances in technology, but also by neo-liberal beliefs in market justice and individualism that have informed the development of home care policy. I have recommended a counter-ethic, a feminist ethic of trust, to challenge neo-liberalism. It is a political ethic that rests on the values and beliefs of care, social justice, and interdependence/community.

FOR REFLECTION

1. How has neo-liberalism affected your nursing practice?

2. What are the ethical dimensions of health policy? How can nurses challenge unethical policies?

3. Is an emphasis upon social justice in nursing ethics compatible with the traditional ethical ideal of the caring nurse-patient relationship? Why or why not?

4. With the current emphasis upon acute care in home care provision, how can nurses ensure that the well-being of those with disabilities and chronic illnesses is protected?

ENDNOTES

1. This work was supported through the funding of the Social Sciences and Humanities Research Council of Canada.

2. The comments from the home care nurses come out of focus group data originally collected for a project entitled *Commitment and Care: The Benefits of a Healthy Workplace for Nurses, Their Patients, and the System* (2001) by A. Baumann, L. O'Brien-Pallas, M. Armstrong-Stasson, J. Blythe, R. Bourbonnais, S. Cameron, D. Irvine Doran, M. Kerr, L. McGillis-Hall, M. Vezina, M. Butt, and L. Ryan. This project was funded by the Canadian Health Services Research Foundation (CHSRF) and The Change Foundation. The report is available on the Web at: www.chsrf.ca and www.changefoundation.ca.

   The project was commissioned to study the impact of the working environment on the health of the nursing workforce and to develop solutions to improve the quality of the nursing work environment because there was recognition that work environments had become increasingly difficult through the reforms and cutbacks of the 1990s. Three resources were used in this project: a review of the published literature, an analysis of grey literature, and focus groups and interviews. Focus groups were held across Canada and included participants who were managers, front-line nurses, nursing association or nursing union representatives, government representatives, researchers, educators, and consultants. Participants were asked the following two questions: (1) "What are the major issues that affect nurses' well-being?" and (2) "What solutions are there to problems associated with these issues?"

Funding through the Nursing Effectiveness, Utilization, and Outcomes Research Unit, Faculty of Nursing, University of Toronto and ethics approval from the Health Science I Research Ethics Committee, University of Toronto were obtained to conduct a secondary analysis of the focus group data. The complete findings of this secondary analysis are forthcoming.

All names given in the Ethics in Practice narratives are pseudonyms.

I would like to acknowledge the support of Linda-Lee O'Brien Pallas who encouraged me to examine the ethical implications of these focus group data.

REFERENCES

Anderson, J.M. 2001. The politics of home care: where is "home"? *Canadian Journal of Nursing Research, 33*(2), 5–10.

Aronson, J. and Neysmith, S.M. 1996. "You're not just in there to do the work": Depersonalizing policies and the exploitation of home care workers' labor. *Gender and Society, 10*(1), 59–77.

Arras, J.D. and Dubler, N.N. 1995. Ethical and social implications of high-tech home care. In J.D. Arras (Ed.), *Bringing the hospital home: Ethical and social implications of high-tech home care* (pp. 1–31). Baltimore: Johns Hopkins University Press.

Austin, W. 2001. Nursing ethics in an era of globalization. *Advances in Nursing Sciences, 24*(2), 1–18.

Baier, A. 1985. What do women want in a moral theory? *Nous, 19*, 53–65.

Baier, A. 1986. Trust and antitrust. *Ethics, 96*, 231–260.

Baier, A. 1994. *Moral prejudices: Essays on ethics.* Cambridge: Harvard University Press.

Beauchamp, D. 1999. Public health as social justice. In D.E. Beauchamp and B. Steinbock (Eds.), *New ethics for the public's health* (pp. 101–109). New York: Oxford University Press.

Bjornsdottir, K. 2002. From the state to the family: reconfiguring the responsibility for long-term care at home. *Nursing Inquiry, 9*(1), 3–11.

Bowden, P. 1996. *Caring: Gender-sensitive ethics.* London: Routledge.

Bowlby, S., Gregory, S. and McKie, L. 1997. "Doing home": Patriarchy, caring, and space. *Women's Studies International Forum, 20*(3), 343–350.

Brennan, S. 1999. Recent work in feminist ethics. *Ethics, 109*, 858–893.

Canadian Association of Retired Persons (CARP). 1999. *Putting a face on home care.* Kingston: Queen's Health Policy Research Unit.

Canadian Nurses Association (CNA). 2002. *Code of ethics for Registered Nurses.* Ottawa: Canadian Nurses Association.

Cheek, J. and Gibson, T. 1997. Policy matters: Critical policy analysis and nursing. *Journal of Advanced Nursing, 25*(4), 668–672.

Coburn, D. 2000. Income inequality, social cohesion and the health status of populations: The role of neo-liberalism. *Social Science & Medicine, 51*, 135–146.

Collopy, B., Dubler, N. and Zuckerman, C. 1990. The ethics of home care: Autonomy and accommodation. *Hastings Center Report, 20*(2), 1–16.

Commission on the Future of Health Care in Canada. 2002. *Building on values: the future of health care in Canada.* Saskatoon: Commission on the Future of Health Care in Canada.

Community Health Nurses Association of Canada (CHNAC). 2002. *Canadian Community Health Nursing standards of practice* (Draft for Consultation).

Community Health Nurses Association of Canada (CHNAC). 2003. *Understanding home health nursing: A discussion paper*. Retrieved February 10 from: www.communityhealthnursescanda.org

Coyte, P.C. 2002. Expanding the principle of comprehensiveness from hospital to home. *Submission to the Standing Committee on Social Affairs, Science and Technology*.

Coyte, P.C. and McKeever, P. 2001. Home care in Canada: Passing the buck. *Canadian Journal of Nursing Research*, *33*(2), 11–27.

Canadian Research Institute for the Advancement of Women (CRIAW). 1999. *The changing nature of home care and its impact on women's vulnerability to poverty*. Ottawa: Status of Women Canada.

Drevdahl, D., Kneipp, S.M., Canales, M.K. and Dorcy, K.S. 2001. Reinvesting in social justice: A capital idea for public health nursing? *Advances in Nursing Science*, *24*(2), 19–31.

Flaskerud, J.H. and Lee, P. 2001. Vulnerability to health problems in female informal caregivers of persons with HIV/AIDS and age-related dementias. *Journal of Advanced Nursing*, *33*(1), 60–68.

Health Canada. 2002. *Canada Health Act overview*. Retrieved December 30 from: www.hc-sc.gc.ca/medicare/chaover.htm

Holstein, M.B. and Mitzen, P. 2001. *Ethics in community-based elder care*. New York: Springer.

Kane, R.A. and Caplan, A.L. 1993. *Ethical conflicts in the management of home care: The case manager's dilemma*. New York: Springer.

Kenny, N.P. 2002. *What good is health care? Reflections on the Canadian experience*. Ottawa: CHA Press.

Liaschenko, J. 1994. The moral geography of home care. *Advances in Nursing Science*, *17*(2), 16–26.

Liaschenko, J. 1997. Ethics and the geography of the nurse-patient relationship: Spatial vulnerabilities and gendered space. *Scholarly Inquiry for Nursing Practice: An International Journal*, *11*(1), 45–59.

Liaschenko, J. 2001. Nursing work, housekeeping ethics, and the moral geography of home care. In D.N. Weisstub, D.C. Thomasma, S. Gauthier and G.F. Tomossy (Eds.), *International library of ethics, law and the new medicine: Aging* (pp. 123–137). Boston: Kluwer Academic Press.

Liaschenko, J. and Peter, E. 2002. The voice of home care workers in clinical ethics. *Healthcare Ethics Committee Forum*, *14*(3), 217–223.

Liaschenko, J. and Peter, E. 2003. Feminist ethics. In V. Tschudin (Ed.), *Approaches to ethics: Nursing beyond boundaries* (pp. 33–43). Oxford: Butterworth, Heinemann.

Lunardi, V.L., Peter, E. and Gastaldo, D. 2002. Are submissive nurses ethical? Reflecting on power anorexia. *Revista Brasileira de Enfermagem*, *55*(2), 183–188.

Lynch, J. 2000. Income inequality and health: Expanding the debate. *Social Science & Medicine*, *51*, 1001–1005.

Malone, R.E. 1999. Policy as product: Mortality and metaphor in health policy discourse. *The Hastings Center Report*, *29*(3), 16–22.

Navarro, V. 1999. Health and equity in the world in the era of "globalization." *International Journal of Health Services*, *29*(2), 215–226.

Neysmith, S.M. 2000. *Restructuring caring labour: Discourse, state practice, and everyday life*. New York: Oxford University Press.

Peter, E. 2002. The history of nursing in the home: revealing the significance of place in the expression of moral agency. *Nursing Inquiry*, *9*(2), 65–72.

Peter, E. and Morgan, K. 2001. Explorations of a trust approach for nursing ethics. *Nursing Inquiry*, *8*(1), 3–10.

Purkis, M.E. 2001. Managing home nursing care: Visibility, accountability and exclusion. *Nursing Inquiry*, *8*(3), 141–150.

Rodney, P. and Varcoe, C. 2001. Towards ethical inquiry in the economic evaluation of nursing practice. *Canadian Journal of Nursing Research, 33*(1), 35–57.

Rodney, P., Varcoe, C., Storch, J.L., McPherson, G., Mahoney, K., Brown, H., Pauly, B., Hartrick, G. and Starzomski, R. 2002. Navigating towards a moral horizon: A multi-site qualitative study of ethical practice in nursing. *Canadian Journal of Nursing Research, 34*(3), 75–102.

Rose, N. 1998. *Inventing our selves: psychology, power, and personhood.* London: Cambridge University Press.

Sandelowski, M. 1999. Venous envy: The post-world war II debate over IV nursing. *Advances in Nursing Science, 22*(1), 52–62.

Schulz, R. and Beach, S.R. 1999. Caregiving as a risk factor for mortality: The caregiver health effects study. *Journal of the American Medical Association, 282*(23), 2215–2219.

Standing Senate Committee on Social Affairs, Science and Technology. 2002. *The health of Canadians—the federal role.* Ottawa: Standing Senate Committee on Social Affairs, Science and Technology.

Tong, R. 1996. An introduction to feminist approaches to bioethics: Unity in diversity. *Journal of Clinical Ethics, 7*(1), 13–19.

Tronto, J.C. 1993. *Moral boundaries: A political argument for an ethic of care.* New York: Routledge.

Varcoe, C. and Rodney, P. 2002. Constrained agency: The social structure of nurses' work. In B. Singh Bolaria and H.D. Dickinson (Eds.), *Health, illness, and health care in Canada* (pp. 102–128). Saskatoon: Nelson Thomson Learning.

Ward-Griffin, C. and McKeever, P. 2000. Relationships between nurses and family caregivers: Partners in care? *Advances in Nursing Science, 22*(3), 89–103.

Wilkins, K. and Park, E. 1998. Home care in Canada. *Health Reports, 10*(1), 29–37. Ottawa: Statistics Canada.

Wilkinson, R.G. 2000. Deeper than "neoliberalism": A reply to David Coburn. *Social Science and Medicine, 51*, 997–1000.

Williams, A. 2002. Changing geographies of care: Employing the concept of therapeutic landscapes as a framework in examining home space. *Social Science and Medicine, 55*, 141–154.

Williams, A.P., Deber, R., Baranek, P. and Gildiner, A. 2001. From medicare to home care: Globalization, state retrenchment, and the profitization of Canada's health-care system. In P. Armstrong, H. Armstrong and D. Coburn (Eds.), *Unhealthy times: Political economy perspectives on health and care* (pp. 7–30). New York: Oxford University Press.

Wojtak, A. 2002. Practice-based ethics: a foundation for human resource planning in community healthcare. *Healthcare Management Forum, 15*(3), 67–72.

chapter thirteen

End-of-Life Decision-Making

Janet L. Storch

... [E]nd-of-life care and decision-making continue to be very troubling moral issues for nurses.

Most ethical concerns about decision-making at the end of life are matters of recent history. Less than a generation ago, few decisions needed to be made beyond attending to the dying person's material affairs. Most people died at home, and matters of sustaining the lives of people through the use of technology were only possibilities on what seemed a distant horizon. But within a short time the possibilities became realities, and the locus of decision-making began to move away from the control of patient and family as specialists became involved in determining matters of life and death.

Over the past three decades people have worked to regain some degree of control over their final days and their end-of-life decisions. However, the balance of power and control remains an elusive goal. Too many people still spend their final days in a location that is not of their choosing, often in preventable pain and stripped of control over decision-making. Results of a study of hospital care in the United States in the mid-1990s indicated that aggressive care until death was still a norm in most hospitals (The SUPPORT Investigators 1995). A team of Canadian researchers also found that extensive use of hospitals by dying persons is the norm in Canada (Wilson et al. 2002), yet there was good evidence that many prefer to die at home (Wilson 2000). These trends mean that "slow dying" has increased over the years (Krisman-Scott 2000), and not always in the manner or place people would prefer. Additionally, too many health professionals experience severe moral distress when they cannot effect what they believe to be appropriate timing for termination of treatment (Doucet 1992; Georges and Grypdonck 2002). Findings of numerous studies that address ethical nursing practice provide clear evidence that end-of-life care and end-of-life decision-making raise some of the most ethically troubling situations for nurses (Gramelspacher, Howell and Young 1986; Corley 1995; Davis et al. 1995; Soderberg, Gilje and Norberg 1999; Raines 2000; White, Coyne and Patel 2001; Rodney et al. 2002)

In this chapter the moral uncertainties, moral dilemmas, and moral distress created by changes in technology and the shift in the locus of responsibility for decision-making will be analyzed. How we came to allow technology to gain such significance in end-of-life care will then be discussed, with a focus on dilemmas surrounding the determination of death, the apparent triumph of life-saving interventions, the tensions in judging medical futility, the use of "do-not-resuscitate" orders, and the moves to restore decision-making to people experiencing the end of their life. "Living wills" or "advance directives" and substitute decision-making will be reviewed, along with the challenges of introducing advance directives. The meaning of a "good death" and good care at the end of life will be described and discussed. The need to reframe our thinking about end-of-life care and nursing's interest, influence, and responsibilities in addressing ethical concerns at the end of life will be analyzed, with attention to emerging moral issues and new moral demands.

HOW DID PEOPLE LOSE CONTROL OF THEIR DYING?

Ivan Illich (1975), a prominent social critic in the 1970s, railed against the medicalization of life and death, suggesting that life and death in society had become like a game in which the chief function of the physician (as representative of the social body) was to serve as an umpire. The physician's job was to make sure everyone played the game according to the rules.

> The rules, of course, forbid leaving the game and dying in any fashion which has not been specified by the umpire. Death no longer occurs except as the self-fulfilling prophecy of the medicine man (148).

Illich also characterized death as the ultimate form of consumer resistance (149) and the movement towards medicalization of dying as the end of natural death. The development of bioethics and clinical ethics arose in part from recognition that technology had created seriously flawed and fractured decision-making, including decision-making at the end of life.

A number of medical advances made it possible to sustain life beyond normal human capability. These advances included ventilators, cardiac defibrillators, dialysis, new drugs, and other such additions to physicians' normal mechanisms to keep individuals alive. These developments led to a number of new ethical dilemmas: How do we determine death? How do we assess quality of life? How do we decide when and if treatment is futile or inappropriate? Who should make these apparently highly technical decisions?

Determining Death

Ethics in Practice 13-1	An Observer and Reporter of Death

As a student nurse in my six-month "probation" period, the author of this chapter was assigned to a busy surgical ward, with limited preparation to enable me to contribute to the work of the unit. Part way through my second day on the unit it became clear that an elderly man recently transferred to the unit was dying. Although he was not part of my patient assignment, I was seconded from my team to "observe" this man until he died. My instructions were to sit beside his bed, watch his respirations, await his Cheyne-Stokes respirations, and check his pulse. If I believed him to be dead, I was to hold a mirror to his mouth to determine if there was any sign of moisture on that mirror as a product of his breathing prior to calling a busy RN to let her know of my suspicions. I was to be an observer and reporter of death.

Until the early 1960s, determining death was fairly simple. A physician was required to verify a death but, in most instances, this was routine after a nurse had contacted the physician to report the death. If it was an expected death, the physician's visit to home or hospital to verify the death could wait until the morning. The main medical concern had been to ensure that people were not buried alive through faulty diagnosis (Alexander 1980). It was not until ventilators and cardiac resuscitation technologies came into widespread use that patterns of practice changed to make the determination of death a more troubling moral matter. Through the power of medical advances, the criteria to determine death became more complex and the moral dilemmas more convoluted. With the advent of organ transplantation capability, appropriate determination of death became yet more urgent a matter.

The sad part about the narrative in Ethics in Practice 13-1 is that the nursing students in this context were not taught to hold a dying person's hand or to stroke a brow to let a patient know he or she was not alone. For some, this might have been an intuitive act. But in the 1950s, 1960s, and into the 1970s, many nurses were still taught that to be professional was to maintain a professional distance from the patient. Emotion was not to be had or seen (if it should happen to be there), and the value of touch was not understood. Although pre-technology days are often recalled as ideal because machines and tests did not obstruct a focus on the person in care, that was not necessarily the case. It may be that one type of avoidance of death—that is, cool observation and reporting of the dying process and death itself—was simply replaced by another type: that of focusing on the machinery at the death bed instead of the person who is dying.

Over time, physicians around the world concentrated on establishing an agreed-upon set of criteria to determine death, and as medical technology has been refined, health professionals have a greater degree of confidence in these medical decisions (President's Commission 1981; Law Reform Commission of Canada 1979/1981). But the continuing concerns about determination of death prevail, as indicated by the frequent publications and conferences focusing on criteria to determine death (see, for example, Veatch 1993; Truog 1997; Morioka 2001). The concept of "brain death" has been replaced by the new language of "neurological determination of death" to address perceived shortcomings in the criteria for determining brain death. Families and friends do not always believe they can trust their caregivers in death-determining criteria and decisions. There continues to be an ongoing need to be present—that is, to be attentive, morally sensitive, and engaged with the survivors so that they might leave their loved one's deathbed with assurance and confidence that the appropriate time of death was a reality (Keenan et al. 2000). This is particularly so when the use of organs for transplant awaits the determination of death.

The technological imperative promoting the idea that if something can be done to preserve life, it should be done, contributes to the moral distress of the family, physicians, other care providers, and nurses. Families often feel uncertain and want to trust health professionals to make good judgments for their loved one. Nurses frequently feel caught between the family and friends and the physician's need to preserve the life. Often what the nurses witness during the 24-hour period of care gives them a growing conviction that the person is wanting and waiting to die. When the nurse's voice is not heard to convey that understanding to the physician, or when nurses are not included in end-of-life discussions and decisions, they experience a sense of moral distress (Storch et al. 2002b; Rodney et al. 2002b; Corley 1995; 2002).

Medical Futility

Toward the end of the 1980s a combination of enhanced life-sustaining technologies, an entrenched belief in patients' rights, and growing concerns about ethical resource allocation in health care led to academic discussions/debates and practice policies on medical futility. **Medical futility** is defined as "a medical treatment that is seen to be non-beneficial because it is believed to offer no reasonable hope of recovery or improvement of the patient's condition" (Canadian Nurses Association 2001). Perhaps it was the link of the word "utility" (understood to refer to a useful and productive life) with "futility" as its opposite that alerted many to the potential for an overemphasis on economics versus patient benefit in these debates. In 1997, Sharpe provided an analysis of the politics, economics, and ethics of "appropriateness," raising concerns about the misuse of the concepts of "futility" and "appropriateness." She pointed out that in the United States, "appropriate or necessary care is no longer simply assumed to be care that serves the health interests of the individual patient, but rather care that conforms to the economic goals of third-party payers" (340).

In any event, the term **inappropriate care** became the term invoked in discussions about a "way to set some reasonable boundaries to health care" that would be beneficial to the welfare of the patient and reasonable for society (Callahan 1991). There was a growing sentiment among administrators and policy-makers that it would be possible to collect good evidence about medical conditions and human responses to treatment at the end of life, as well as evidence related to socio-economic indicators, and that such evidence could lead to clearer decision-making about medical futility or inappropriate care. But as Callahan (1991) points out,

> ... [I]t turns out that there are facts and there are facts. Values, it soon became evident, can influence not only what facts are identified as facts, but also which ones are thought worth having and which are worth dismissing (300).

Since the anticipation of outcomes in beneficial patient care involves an interplay of physical well-being and improved overall well-being, information about both facts and values is involved. In considering the matter of medical futility, Carol Taylor (1995) suggests four classifications of futility:

1. not futile: beneficial to both physical and overall well-being;
2. futile: non-beneficial to both physical and overall well-being;
3. futile from the patient's perspective: medically indicated but not valued by the patient; and
4. futile from the clinician's perspective: valued by the patient but not medically indicated (301).

Clearly, these classifications have objective and subjective, quantitative and qualitative dimensions. Only some judgments, therefore, could rest with physicians and other health professionals, while a good many rest with the patient or family. Given that physicians may feel morally compromised by feeling obliged to provide treatment they believe will not benefit the person, the problem of who has priority in decision-making is very real for all involved. Carol Taylor (1995) presents a strong case for her recommendation

> that nurses play a leading role... by identifying patients, families and health care teams at risk of experiencing conflict about futile care, and then initiating dialogue that may prevent or resolve conflict. The focus in negotiation should be on everyone working together to obtain the best possible outcome for a particular patient, not on any person or group asserting their primacy of authority (303).

The difficulties of embarking upon such negotiation were recognized by professional bodies at the national level in Canada, leading to the *Joint Statement on Preventing and Resolving Conflicts Involving Health Care Providers and Persons Receiving Care* in 1999. Shortly thereafter, the Canadian Nurses Association issued a paper in their *Ethics in Practice* series to guide nurses in addressing the matter of futility (Canadian Nurses Association 2001). Varcoe and Rodney (2003) suggest that the problem identified as "inappropriate care" could be considered as a problem of unnecessary suffering resulting from dehumanizing practices (11).

The Canadian Pediatric Society (2000) reaffirmed its position on treatment decisions for infants and children, noting that "A primary role of medicine is to maintain life but not unthinkingly to prolong the dying process" (2). They outlined four exceptions to the general duty to provide life-sustaining (life-prolonging) treatment:

1. irreversible progression to imminent death;
2. treatment which is clearly ineffective or harmful;
3. instances where life will be severely shortened regardless of treatment and where non-treatment will allow a greater degree of caring and comfort than treatment; and
4. lives filled with intolerable and intractable pain and suffering (2).

These are sensitive guidelines for a very vulnerable group of young patients, but their application to treatment decisions for adults seems quite appropriate.

Meanwhile, the Canadian Critical Care Society has recently developed guidelines for withholding or withdrawing life support in critical care (Rocker and Dunbar 2000). This may seem a somewhat contradictory position since intensive care/critical care units are "designed to maintain life using maximum medical and nursing monitoring and advanced technology" (Nelson-Marten, Braaten and English 2001). With an emphasis on treatment and cure, the culture of the critical care unit can be seen as a battlefield where disease is regarded as the enemy, with doctors and nurses the staunch warriors dedicated to defeating disease, as noted earlier. Yet, these new guidelines urge physicians to carefully determine whether life support, for example, would simply prevent a natural and humane death (Rocker and Dunbar 2000; Truog et al. 2001). These practice guidelines are an important counterpoint to the assessment of intensive/critical care described by Illich earlier.

Do-Not-Resuscitate (DNR) Orders

One of the most dramatic ways in which decisions about medical futility are exercised is in documenting a "do-not-resuscitate" (DNR) decision as a physician's order, and in executing that order. While it should be recognized that DNR orders represent only one of the many decisions involved in declining technological prolongation of life, the majority of these types of decisions are difficult for caregivers and for families. Nurses, in particular, continue to experience the morally traumatic effects of the fateful dilemmas involved in the application of DNR policy. Over twenty years ago a group of nurses requested hospital administration to provide a DNR policy (MacPhail et al. 1981). That action and the decision of the hospital to support their request, in spite of Criminal Code directives[1], led to one of the first Canadian DNR policies developed. Subsequent to that action, hospitals across Canada adopted similar practices (Storch 1983). National guidelines were eventually developed to support appropriate DNR policies (Canadian Hospital Association, Canadian Medical Association, Canadian Nurses Association 1984) and were subsequently updated (Canadian Healthcare Association, Canadian Medical Association, Canadian Nurses Association, and the Catholic Health Association of Canada [in co-operation with the Canadian Bar Association] 1995). Yet, 25 years later, the tension remains within many hospitals regarding how a DNR policy should be framed to ensure appropriate actions are taken.

In many instances nurses have had to deal with verbal physician orders only, including a physician's directives calling for a "slow code."[2] Physicians' reticence to commit a DNR order to paper has centred on their (legitimate) concerns about being pressured into DNR decisions before they have an opportunity to adequately assess the individual and his or her wishes. This reticence may also be due to the physicians' own misinformation, misunderstanding, or fear of legal liability. Merely by being present with patients in hospital on a more constant basis than other health professionals, nurses are often in attendance when a cardiac arrest occurs.

> Nurses... often find themselves initiating or withholding cardiopulmonary resuscitation (CPR) in situations characterized by verbal orders, euphemistic documentation and poor communication, and when consultation with patients about their CPR choices often do not take place (Schultz 1997).

The importance of clarifying roles and responsibilities in CPR and DNR decision-making is critical (Kuhl 1998; Kuhl and Wilensky 1999). Patients and their families need to be well informed about the potential for CPR to make a difference for their health and life (Puopolo et al. 1997). Examination of various hospital policies about DNR suggest that variation continues to exist in who is allowed to make the DNR decision, what patients and families are told, whether health professionals are obligated to provide active life-sustaining treatments, and what the role of nurses might be in such decisions and actions.

In 2002, Rodney, Thompson, et al. reported on an evaluation of one hospital's DNR protocol. The researchers found that despite considerable effort directed at educating staff about the protocol as it was being developed and when it was completed (and although some progress was made), a number of factors led to difficulty in achieving a completely successful implementation of the DNR policy. Fluctuation in staff awareness due to high staff turnover, inundation of staff with other new initiatives, limited resources to continue the educational process, and significant hospital restructuring led to difficulties in implementation. Difficulties included both lack of awareness of the policy and failure to follow the policy. It is likely that most hospitals experience similar difficulties introducing revisions to DNR policies. The need for attention to sound policies supported by administrative structures, as well as continued education about DNR policies and processes, is critical to successful decision-making about, and implementation of, "do-not-resuscitate" orders. Included in this education is the importance of removing the widespread conflation of DNR with "no treatment"—a mistaken assumption which often hinders effective discussion and decision-making about DNR.

The actual mechanism, potential harms, and relative success rates of cardiopulmonary resuscitation are not always clearly stressed in providing information about CPR and DNR orders. The appropriateness of CPR, and the potential suffering it might engender, may be overlooked or minimized in communication with the patient and the family since the procedure itself has become a commonly used method of sustaining life. Or, staff may lack the time, energy, education, and/or resources to properly inform and consult with patients about this important issue (Kuhl and Wilensky 1999). Limited information about nontreatment is also common with regard to other life-preserving technologies such as renal dialysis. This is a serious oversight in the provision of full information to patients and may also represent a reluctance to entertain the idea of a natural death.

STRUGGLES TO REGAIN CONTROL

Many early attempts of patients and families to regain control of their dying process were initially fought in the courts. Some court decisions in the United States became highly publicized and were referred to by Canadian courts in subsequent cases. For example, in the United States, the cases of Karen Ann Quinlan in 1975–1986, Brother Fox in 1979–1980, and Nancy Cruzan[3] in 1983–1990 involved persons once competent but rendered unable to make decisions, whose end-of-life decisions were carried forward by friends and family and were contested in the courts (Annas 1980; Storch 1983; 1998; Pence 1995).

The struggle to locate the locus of decision-making for incompetent people was intense amongst families, physicians, the courts, and ethicists. The formation of ethics committees, consisting of a body of experts who could deal with these vexing issues, followed court decisions (Randal 1983; Veatch 1977). While in Canada ethics committees did not assume the legal significance of their U.S. counterparts, ethics committees were, and often continue to be, ideal forums in which to discuss difficult cases in end-of-life care (Storch et al. 1990; Storch and Griener 1992).

In Canada, different end-of-life stories emerged in two very public legal cases involving competent young women. Nancy B. was a 25-year-old woman who had been hospitalized for over two years due to Guillain-Barre syndrome, a condition that caused her to be bedridden and ventilator dependent and also caused the increasing decay of her motor nerves. Nancy requested that life-sustaining technology be withdrawn and that she be allowed to die. The Quebec Superior Court ruled in her favour and allowed the removal of her ventilator (Herbert 1996). Sue Rodriguez was a 42-year-old woman who was terminally ill with advanced amyotrophic lateral sclerosis (ALS). She faced the prospect of deterioration of her body to a state of total dependency unless a physician would end her life for her when she was ready for that end. She took her request, as her constitutional right, to the Supreme Court of Canada, but it was not supported by the Court[4]. As Moreno (1995) so well explains in *Arguing Euthanasia*, the obstacles to individuals' wishes to determine their time of death through medical intervention are health professionals' codes of ethics, the principles of bringing benefit and removing harm, and the ability of people to trust those who provide care for them.

Individuals like Nancy B. would want to know that life-support measures would be implemented when appropriate and discontinued when considered to not be in her best interests. At the same time, individuals, in particular the elderly and the disabled, need to trust that they would not become convenient subjects for early involuntary death through medical interventions (that is, be euthanized). The boundary of legal intervention drawn to exclude voluntary euthanasia and assisted suicide (Law Reform Commission of Canada 1982; Report of the Special Senate Committee 1995; Report of the Senate Subcommittee 2000) is intended to enable sustained commitments to autonomy and justice as well as beneficence and nonmaleficence in health care—although these, too, are contested by some, and the legal landscape is beginning to change (see, for example, Foley and Hendlin 1999; Battin 1995; McTeer 1999).

Living Wills and Advance Directives

One of the many outcomes of the legal cases cited above was to sensitize the public to the importance of an individual's letting others (family, friends, physicians, and others) know in advance what he or she would want if unable to make treatment decisions. Those who captured that idea early, even in advance of these high profile court cases, began to pen "living wills" by letter or will-type document as one way to communicate what they would want in regard to end-of-life decision-making (Baker 1980). Such living wills were considered of interest, but health professionals were not legally required to follow the wishes expressed in these documents. In 1977 California passed the Natural Death Act. Since that event, many other states, as well as provinces within Canada, enacted legislation to authorize and regulate these written documents and to provide a means for someone representing the individual to carry his or her wishes forward (Storch 1983). Provinces have entered this foray at various times with differently titled legislation and slightly different requirements for creating legally valid documents. For example, in British Columbia, the Representation Agreement Act provides for the creation of a means through which someone can become another individual's representative in end-of-life decision-making, and, in Alberta, the creation of a Personal Health Care Directive allows for a similar action.

The format of these documents, now commonly called advance directives, varies somewhat (for example, see Singer 1993; Molloy 2002). But most agree that the **advance directive** is "a written document containing a person's wishes about life-sustaining treatment" that "extend[s] the autonomy of competent patients to future situations in which the patient is incompetent" (Singer 1994, 111; see also Storch, Rodney and Starzomski 2002a,

413). This can be as simple as a letter or as complex as a many-page form. Most forms provide several direct situational categories of treatment decisions and/or some accompanying guidance to assist the individual to consider his or her wishes regarding treatment or no-treatment options.

After the individual is guided through the various interventions that can be taken to sustain life, the directives are often categorized under different levels of intensity. These levels can vary "from full acute care (including critical care) to palliative interventions only" (Rodney and Howlett in press). For example, some long-term care facilities have used a form that includes four levels of care: comfort care (palliation); limited care, which includes comfort care; surgical care, which includes limited care; and intensive care, which includes surgical care. These advance directives, which include provision for a proxy to represent the wishes of the individual if the person is unable to do so, should fulfill the need health professionals, families, and friends have for guidance at a time of personal anguish and allow the individual's wishes to be respected. Unfortunately, advance directives are not always followed.

Problems with Advance Directives

Despite the prevalence of talk about advance directives over the past three to four decades, in any group assembled to discuss advance directives only a handful of people will indicate that they have actually developed a directive. Studies have found the use of advance directives to be less than predicted or desired (Blondeau et al. 2000; Zronek et al. 1999). Why is implementation of this idea so elusive? What stops individuals from completing an advance directive? What limits health professionals in responding to advance directives? The subcommittee of the Standing Senate Committee on Social Affairs, Science and Technology, chaired by Carstairs and Beaudoin (2000), urged that advance directives "should not be viewed as purely legal documents" (12). Regardless of whether too much or too little detail is provided in an advance directive, there will always be challenges in interpretation of its contents and difficulties specifying in advance a person's wishes with regard to every possible medical situation. Instead, an advance directive should be only part of the communication and planning to help people prepare for death. If the people the dying person cares most about have been engaged in this communication, problems of interpretation are less likely to arise and "[the] passage to death is eased, the level of comfort rises, and the burden of care is lightened for the substitute decision-maker" (Report of the Senate Subcommittee 2000, 13).

Public Resistance

Some resistance resides within patients, families, and the general public. We are a death-denying society, or, at least, we are in denial that a situation requiring an advance directive will ever happen to us. Our societal mind-set is about living, with an assumption that we can leave death decisions until later. For some, this societal stance is augmented by an inability to personally face death. For others, doing the work of preparing an advance directive is too difficult to have to think through mentally and emotionally or is not considered a priority. Others may have difficulty trusting that the directives will be honoured. Some are unsure if they will be able to change the advance directive once made, and they fear making a lasting commitment. Many forms and guides for completion of an advance directive are complex and confusing. This means that one has to block off time to accomplish the task, and for many people time is a rare commodity. Some provinces also require legal certification in certain cases for the advance directive to be valid.

Health Professionals' Reluctance

A surprising number of health professionals are only vaguely aware of advance directives and may fail to see the relevance or worth of such directives. Often a barrier to health professionals' engagement with advance directives is their lack of knowledge and their reluctance to engage in "death talk" (Rodney and Howlett in press; Godkin 2002). Given that past practices discouraged doctors from conveying bad news to patients for fear of upsetting them and interfering in their recovery, it is not surprising that they might withhold information or be reluctant to engage in discussion of death with patients. Often those who do share the "bad news" are poorly prepared for the task and do not give themselves sufficient time to stay with the patient; such situations can lead to upset patients and distressed health care professionals. The mistaken assumption that withholding information is safer may in turn be reinforced, leading to further avoidance of end-of-life discussions. Ethics in Practice 13-2 provides one nurse's illustration of the type of difficulty health professionals might have in telling a patient about his or her impending death. (See Appendix A for details of the study that generated this narrative.)

Ethics in Practice 13-2	Moral Failure in Giving a Prognosis

We had a 94-year-old gentleman who was diagnosed and . . . he had quite advanced lymphoma. He had not been to a doctor for years and the doctor said, "This chemotherapy may prolong your life" and so he said "Okay." He wanted to try that.... [H]e had several rounds of chemotherapy over about a year . . . and he maxed out his chemo. He got to the point where every other day he would receive blood or platelets... and he would be so tired of being poked.... We would try to discuss it with the doctor and say you know, "What are you going to do with this gentleman, he's not going home." And she said, "I'll go and talk to him." Well, I listened to her talk to this patient. And her way of discussing it with him was, "Well, now, we're using the blood and platelets day by day, to sort of keep your levels up and that's going to keep you going, okay?" And that was her discussion.

All health professionals who work with patients at the end of life must see it as their role to ask patients about their wishes, listen to their responses, and urge them to document those wishes and communicate them to their family members or substitute decision-maker. When patients are unable to carry out this task without assistance, nurses and physicians should enable this work in whatever way they can. All health professionals need education about advance directives and about discovering an individual's wishes, transmitting those wishes to others, and respecting those wishes (Justin and Johnson 1989; Storch 1998; Blondeau et al. 2000).

The commitment of health professionals to attend to these expressed wishes is paramount. Such attention includes the exercise of sensitive clinical judgment when execution of the advance directive does not seem to match the intention of the patient. As Blondeau et al. (2000) remind us, the fact that an advance directive has been signed does not guarantee that the wishes stated will be respected. She urges that we should offset a false sense of security in these directives by paying more attention to developing relationships of trust between health professionals and patients.

Vulnerable Populations

One concern in end-of-life decision-making is that an over-reliance on advance directives for everyone might develop, without sufficient concern for vulnerable populations. How do advance directives affect the vulnerable in our society? The vulnerable include the disabled, the elderly, and street people in all our major cities. What do advance directives mean for them? Can they prepare an advance directive? Do they trust health professionals or their families to act in their best interests? Can they be sure their directive (should they have one) will not be used against them?

Ambrosio (1994) studied street people and advance directives in the early 1990s, pointing out the sociocultural and political contexts within which health care decisions are made. She noted how these realities serve to undermine the autonomy of individuals who are members of oppressed groups. Those with few social and economic resources tend to have access only to the options health professionals offer, and they may be denied some options (such as life-prolonging technologies) through the gate-keeping actions of physicians. Some have argued that, in addition to having unjustifiably restricted options offered to them, vulnerable patients may also feel coerced into choices leading to their premature death, or they might make "inauthentic choices because they have internalized others' oppressive choices about them" (Mayo and Gunderson 2002, 16).

Storch and Dossetor (1994; 1998) studied attitudes of Albertans regarding end-of-life decision-making. They found that those who were most vulnerable—for example, immigrants to Canada and those with limited education and economic resources—responded to questions about prolongation of life versus withdrawing from treatment differently than those who were less vulnerable. These vulnerable people expressed a strong determination to have everything done to preserve their life. Clearly, the meaning of advance directives to those most vulnerable may be very different than to those who have normally experienced greater control over their lives.

REFRAMING END-OF-LIFE DECISION-MAKING

Recent research has focused on the need to reframe our thinking about advance directives, away from negative connotations of refusal of this or that type of treatment (Storch 1998) to positive statements about how individuals would like to experience their death. Simply asking an individual about how and where he or she would like to die may provide opportunities to see dying in a different light (Kuhl 2002; Bailey 2003).

The Meaning of a "Good Death"

In his book, *What Do Dying Patients Want: Practical Wisdom at the End of Life*, David Kuhl (2002) details his research findings to answer the question posed by his study: What does it mean to have a "good death?" Because the term **euthanasia** in its simplest form also means "an easy and painless death" (deWolf et al. 1997), open discussions about a "good death" have often been avoided because there is so much confusion and anxiety about this controversial topic. The matter of euthanasia as "a painless killing, especially to end a painful and incurable disease, or mercy killing" (deWolf et al. 1997) was discussed briefly earlier in this chapter. At this juncture, the focus is on the meaning of a "good death," which is different from the meanings embodied in euthanasia.

According to Kuhl (2002), patients' perceptions of a good death include the relief of pain; being close to loved ones and being in good relationship with them; having the support of family and friends; feeling free to talk openly about death and about care; reflecting upon one's life and having those reflections valued by others; having trusting relationships with professional caregivers; and finding meaning in one's life and death. Each individual holds his or her own particular meaning of a "good death," and it is important to seek to understand that meaning. Not all individuals choose to use technology to prolong their life. Yet discussions about end-of-life decisions and narratives of individual struggles often feature language about fighting, conquering, and battling terminal illness. Such language may valorize patients' resistance in ways that imply that those who make other choices are falling short of what they ought to do. Sensitivity to the choices individuals make to fight—to "rage against the dying of the light" (Thomas 1969)—or *not* to fight, is critical. Nurses can be active in understanding the importance of this choice and in facilitating communication of it to patients and families.

Ethics in Practice 13-3 recounts the good death experience of one of the author's nursing colleagues, Sharon.[5]

Ethics in Practice 13-3	**A Good Death**

Sharon first learned about a potential life-threatening problem when her physician informed her during an office visit that biopsy tissue showed signs of melanoma. A referral to an oncologist led to the recommendation that surgery should be performed as quickly as possible. In preparation for her unanticipated absence from the workplace for a matter of weeks, she elected to ask for a meeting of the nursing staff to tell them directly of her lab results, to ask for their support, and to confirm that she wanted channels of communication to be honest and open with respect to her condition. Surgical findings meant that further treatment was required, involv-

ing more extensive time away from work. Throughout the months she was away, one nursing colleague had been selected by Sharon as the point of contact for staff in order to update them on her condition. She wanted all information to be available in order to give her colleagues an opportunity to help her with the moral and/or physical support she needed or might need. Telling her RN colleagues about her experience meant that she felt she could trust their response and their care.

During the weeks that stretched to a year, Sharon had many treatments, made many choices involving both traditional care and alternative therapies, and relied upon her family, her friends, members of her church, and her colleagues to support her will to live. At first her main discomfort was excessive fatigue from the treatments, but, as interferon therapy was replaced by chemotherapy, she experienced pain, nausea, and weakness. Home care nursing staff and her colleagues came to support her and to encourage her. All efforts were made to keep her as key decision-maker regarding her care, including making decisions about her pain control and management. To that end, she kept detailed notes in her journal, often referring back to previous entries to help keep track of medications and laboratory results.

Her family was very important to her, and her grandchildren gave her particular joy. Sharon and her closest friend (her husband Jack) planned that their children and grandchildren would come home on a more regular basis. Meanwhile, Sharon, her family, and her friends sought all advice possible about any potential for cure or hope for a remission. They also sought good information about her care. The time came when cancerous tumours had so thoroughly invaded her being that she had to succumb to further surgery. That surgical intervention took her to hospital for a matter of weeks. But when it was clear that nothing further could or should be done, her family brought her home where home care nurses, her nursing colleagues, her friends, and her family cared for her for several weeks. The day after Christmas Day it was clear that this would be her final day, and, surrounded by family and friends, she died in the evening. Her nursing colleagues gave her body its final care, and her family elected to have her rest in peace with them at home until the morning.

Good Care at the End of Life

The story of Sharon's final days (in Ethics in Practice 13-3) is unique to Sharon, as each life and death is unique. Others may not have the type of family, friends, or colleagues who are able to offer the level or kind of support Sharon received. Others may not have the will or ability to be as open and honest as Sharon was with those most significant to her. Respect is due to those who choose to be more private about their terminal condition and the choices they wish to make to deal with it. At the same time, nurses and other caregivers need to be aware that traditions surrounding "death talk" keep some people prisoners to custom, when what they may need most is openness and the support of their fellow human beings. With sensitivity to these individual needs, and awareness of the effect of societal constraints on actions, all caregivers need to engage with people at the end of their life. Such engagement allows caregivers to create situations for the dying that represent who they are and how they wish to spend their final days. All this should occur with careful attention to family wishes (Sahlberg-Blom, Ternestedt and Johansson 2000). What might that kind of care be like?

Research findings of both Singer et al. (1999) and Kuhl (2002), based upon interviews with people who were dying, were consistent in identifying the wishes of the dying. People want to have adequate pain and symptom management. They do not want to have their dying prolonged, to lose a sense of control, or to be a burden to others. They want to strengthen their relationships with loved ones. Godkin (2002), in particular, has emphasized that advance directives have important outcomes for older adults beyond controlling the dying process. Findings from her qualitative study point to the preparation of advance directives as affording people an opportunity to think about their life and its meaning and to be engaged with family and friends. Her research, along with Kuhl's, points to the reality that advance directives are not as much about dying as they are about living while one is entering one's final years and days. This suggests that advance directives really are "living wills"—that is, directions about planning for and living one's final days well.

Relief of Pain and Discomfort

Although nurses may well intend to provide relief of pain and discomfort at the end of life, there is good evidence that their efforts often fall short of that goal. White et al. (2001), in a study of the adequacy of nurses' preparation for end-of-life care, found that the highest ranked areas for additional education identified by nurses included pain control techniques and comfort care interventions. A fear of providing too much relief for pain through analgesics (particularly narcotics) seems pervasive in nursing for a number of reasons, including fear of creating an addiction, fear of prematurely ending a life, lack of understanding about pain relief through analgesia, poor pain assessment, and a belief that suffering serves an important purpose (Hunter 2000). Most of these fears and biases are both unfounded and misguided, and these motives of caregivers must be carefully discerned and corrected, with priority given to patients' needs and desires.

Furthermore, culturally sensitive care demands that differing views about the role of suffering and the acceptability of opioid analgesics be considered and respected. Tensions may be heightened when nurses must deal with particular family members' values and beliefs about pain relief, as illustrated in Ethics in Practice 13-4. (See Appendix A for details of the study that generated this narrative.)

Ethics in Practice 13-4	**Moral Distress in Pain Control**

And it was a horrible time for all the staff because this woman was terminal and she was in a lot of pain. And we had to play with that fine line between [having] the patient pain-free and keeping her awake so that her son could still see her. He did not want his mother to be unconscious or to not be able to respond to him; as far as he was concerned that was killing her. So we would have to justify all of the treatments that we were able to give her. And try as we might, by discussing with the husband, the other son, physicians, even managers... we could not get this young gentleman to change his mind, and we had horrible fears of coming into her room in the middle of the night and finding her dead and having to resuscitate her.

In addition to pain control through medication, a better understanding of alternative and complementary therapies is also important. Different cultural groups may have their own particular pain-relieving methods. For example, aboriginal elders may use prayer, or burn sage, sweet grass, or cedar (Fisher et al. 2000). Pain might be decreased through massage, hydrotherapy, music therapy, and other means (White, Coyne and Patel 2001). Moreover, sometimes the most distressing symptoms may not involve pain—for example, nausea, vomiting, breathlessness, hiccups, edema, dry mouth, pruritus, anorexia, fatigue, vertigo, insomnia, and many other physical conditions (Ferris et al. 2002). Alleviating these symptoms often takes nursing empathy and creativity, as well as the input of members of the entire health care team. Ethics in Practice 13-4 also raises the need for better family assessment and support.

Kuhl (2002) reminds us that pain in life and in dying extends beyond physical pain. His study findings suggest that the dying may experience unnecessary suffering because of the poor communication between caregivers and patients. This he describes as **iatrogenic suffering** because it is pain and suffering inflicted upon another person unintentionally but as a result of the way physicians and other health professionals speak to patients. Kuhl also underscores the fact that pain is comprised of psychological and spiritual features as well as physical. He maintains that too often physicians and nurses minimize the extent of pain an individual feels and neglect to provide the information and the support needed by those facing the end of their life.

Information and Truthfulness

Throughout his text, Kuhl (2002) emphasizes the importance of caregivers being honest with patients to facilitate the patients' control of their final days. Yet such truthfulness continues to be the exception in end-of-life care. Kristman-Scott (2000) provides an historical analysis of the "movement toward greater disclosure of health information to patients" (47) over the past half century. She notes that the cycle of pretense may rob an individual of power and control over what remains of his or her final days.

Interestingly, Kristman-White (2000) traces the belief of serious danger in disclosing a prognosis of terminal illness to patients back to the teachings of Hippocratic medicine. According to this tradition, patients will "take a turn for the worse" if they are told the truth. The halting efforts to change medical views on this dictum, based upon the principle of nonmaleficence, have lead to only modest changes in practice. Early studies by Glaser and Strauss (1965) and Kubler-Ross (1969) exposed the myth of harm (as opposed to benefit) in revealing a fatal prognosis. Even decades later, the practice of non-disclosure prevails in many settings. Struggles with levels of disclosure continue to exist, especially when family and/or the health care team is in conflict.

It is equally important that information not be forced upon patients. Cultural values vary with respect to truth-telling about serious and incurable illness, and this can be highly problematic for the health care team. Sometimes, too, there may be a gap between generations within a particular culture; younger members of the group may consider it important that seniors be told about a fatal prognosis while older members of the group may continue to believe that information about serious illness should not be shared with the individual who is dying (Fisher et al. 2000).

More difficult for patients and nurses is that physicians often believe that they tell patients the truth, even when the information given is considerably modified. This occurs, for example, when patients are given information about their treatment but blurred information about their prognosis, rendering a flexible meaning to the truth. To be fair, such vagueness—at least in the way patients understand what has been told to them—may occur for at least two additional reasons. Physicians may try to tell the truth about the person's condition in a sensitive and careful way that in fact has the effect of obscuring the message, or patients may not be able to comprehend the bad news at the first telling.

In 1984, Jameton raised yet another problem. He stated that, for nurses, sharing difficult news with people who are dying is not simply a matter of what to tell. Concomitant questions are who is to do the telling, and who *will* tell if those entrusted to tell do not make it their responsibility to do so. Unfortunately, some 20 years later, assurance that people will receive a full disclosure of their terminal condition is not yet universal (Krisman-Scott 2000).

Fostering Family and Friendship Support

Just as birth should be an event supported by family and friends, so should death be (Kuhl 2002; Chambers-Evans 2002). It is a time of "people needing people" to assist them in a significant life passage. Thus, for example, the protocol for decision-making at one major urban hospital emphasizes that end-of-life decisions require collaboration among the patient, family, family physician, and health professionals to fulfill an imperative to give appropriate and compassionate care (Rodney et al. 1999). By the same token, this protocol speaks to culturally sensitive end-of-life care that acknowledges different value systems in different cultures and ethnic groups. Urging that stereotyping be avoided, this directive includes the need for health professionals to recognize that "patients from other cultures and/or ethnic groups may defer to the wishes of their family to avoid conflict and to fulfill their duty to their family. Decisions may be made as a unit, rather than by the patient" and "families may decline to give permission to limit aggressive care, since this might be seen as a sign of disrespect for the patient" (Rodney et al. 1999, 30).

Related research emphasizes the importance of attending to cultural and personal meaning and support. For instance, in a study of ways in which patients participate in end-of-life decision-making, Sahlberg-Blom, Ternestedt, and Johansson (2000) found that patients' participation in care planning could be classified according to four main variations in participation with respect to decision-making: self-determination, co-determination, delegation, and nonparticipation. These authors suggest that their findings support the notion that people's dying and death are a reflection of the way they have lived.

Listening, Reflecting, and Developing Trust

Kuhl (2002) found that most people who are at the end of life need to know that someone is listening to them. Byock (2003) emphasizes that a core value for end-of-life care is community. She maintains that as a community we have certain commitments to each other, including keeping company with those who are suffering and dying so that they will not be alone (not be abandoned). She speaks of this type of obligation as a covenantal value involving trust and connection. Among our responsibilities to the dying is the enhancement of their quality of life and the life of the community by bearing witness and promoting opportunity. In bearing witness we promise to listen to their stories and to remember the stories of their passing. In promoting opportunity we remember that "some people change in ways that are valuable and important to them and their families during the time they are dying.... [In] reviewing their lives, sharing bad news, reconciling (when needed) and exploring existential and spiritual aspects of life, some people value assistance" (S41).

This may be the greatest gift that nurses and other caregivers can give to the dying. Attentive listening and reflecting back to an individual what we are hearing are powerful ways to assist another to understand him- or herself and others in new ways. It is in *hearing oneself talk*, and knowing what has been heard, that clarification occurs. And since attentive listening builds relationships, trust can develop between nurse and patient.

MORAL IMPERATIVES FOR NURSES

We know that in some parts of Canada the philosophy of hospice care in the community is well entrenched, and health services are provided to make a "good death" possible. But despite numerous calls for greater access to palliative care across Canada (Commission on the Future of Health Care in Canada 2002; National Health Forum 1997; Ferris et al. 2002; Report of the Special Senate Committee 1995; Report of the Special Senate Sub-Committee Report 2000), the majority of Canadians do not have access to such care as they enter their final months and days. The absence of end-of-life care attuned to the needs of the dying creates a moral imperative for nurses to become more sensitized to the dying (Canadian Nurses Association 1998) and more capable of doing their part to foster and provide care that leads to a good death. This is particularly important given the changing culture of health care organizations (with and without walls) where such care might be considered a frill rather than an evidence-based practice.

Nurse leaders have called upon nurses to be the "catalysts for improving end-of-life care" (Scanlon 1996). Scanlon challenges nurses to act upon their concerns that adequate and timely disclosure be given to persons who are dying. Similarly, Carol Taylor (1995) urges nurses to take a leading role in bringing clinicians, patients, and families together to negotiate end-of-life decision-making, particularly when conflict is beginning to be apparent and when the patient's prognosis is poor.

Many aspects of end-of-life care and decision-making fall squarely within the realm of nursing practice on an individual and collective level. Our research shows that these areas of practice continue to raise very troubling moral issues for nurses (Rodney et al. 2002b; Varcoe et al. in press; Storch et al. 2002b). Nurses must act on this knowledge to improve their own education in end-of-life care, to be better able to provide culturally sensitive end-of-life care, and to do so with confidence and comfort. In learning to listen to, to advocate for, and to support people who are dying, nurses will fulfill the mandate of care in a way that respects different views of a good death.

Trusting relationships are critical to ensuring that individuals' wishes are understood, that they receive their desired type of assistance in managing their discomfort, and that they receive full information to meet their needs. Moral imperatives for nurses underscore the need for nurses to enhance their education in end-of-life care and to be the catalysts to improve end-of-life care.

FOR REFLECTION

1. Consider situations you might describe as continuations of futile care at the end of life. Does the concept of "futility" assist or impede good decision-making in end-of-life care?

2. In your experience with DNR orders, what types of guidelines are most helpful to you and other nurses in sound implementation of such policies?

3. What are the predominant factors, in your experience, that have prevented greater attention to advance directives? What role do you see for advance nurse practitioners in creating a better environment for discovering, recording, and transmitting patients' wishes about their end-of-life care?

4. What role might nurses take in fostering better communication amongst health professionals, families, and individuals in end-of-life care?

ENDNOTES

The author of this chapter would like to acknowledge with gratitude Patricia Rodney's invaluable input and assistance in locating resources for the chapter and in critiquing drafts.

1. The Criminal Code of Canada includes several sections that operate to prohibit assisted suicide and euthanasia, which have served as barriers to the freedom to implement DNR policies. These sections include the following: 14, 219, 224, and 241. For example, section 14 states that "No person is entitled to consent to have death inflicted upon him...," and section 241 makes counselling someone to commit suicide illegal.

2. A "slow code" refers to an order (usually given verbally) from a physician to a nurse to indicate that if a nurse witnesses a cardiac arrest, that nurse should take his or her time in calling a code—that is, to take his or her time in bringing the equipment to the bedside and calling for the CPR team. This was a common strategy used from the late 1970s through the 1980s when a physician was aware of his or her legal duty to preserve a person's life, but did not believe such preservation to be appropriate. The physician therefore did not wish to expose the patient to the aggressive intervention of CPR. This type of order was most difficult for nurses.

3. In the U.S. case of Nancy Cruzan (Pence 1995), the courts would not accept the family's supposition that Nancy would not have wanted to live in a vegetative state. It was only when friends came forward to testify that they had heard her make such statements that the courts agreed to accept those statements as Nancy's wishes or will.

4. The majority ruled that the Criminal Code provisions did not violate section 7 (the right to life, liberty, and security of the person) or section 12 (no cruel or unusual treatment or punishment) of the Charter. The majority also ruled that it would be preferable not to decide the difficult and important issues raised by section 15 (equality), but rather to assume that any violation of section 15 would be saved by section 1 (which allows reasonable limits to be set on the guaranteed rights and freedoms) (Herbert 1996, 184). It should be noted that all of the judges of the Supreme Court of Canada strongly upheld the right to refuse treatment and that while the majority of the court distinguished this from any right to have assistance in committing suicide or access to euthanasia, four of the nine judges dissented and found that the criminal code provisions did violate the Charter of Rights and were not saved by the "reasonable limits" provisions in section 1. The majority questioned the distinguishing of withdrawal of treatment from an active step—they based the decision more on the basis that establishing a "fundamental right" to life, liberty, and security of the person cannot ignore the specific reference to "life" in the section and would also require some "general acceptance by reasonable people," and there was no evidence of this. As the majority stated, "Regardless of one's personal views as to whether the distinctions drawn between withdrawal of treatment and palliative care, on the one hand, and assisted suicide on the other are practically compelling, the fact remains that these distinctions are maintained and can persuasively defended. To the extent that there is a consensus, it is that human life must be respected and we must be careful not to undermine the institutions that protect it." (Source: An anonymous reviewer of this chapter).

5. This Ethics in Practice 13-4 account is written as a tribute to Sharon Nield, and it is printed with permission of her husband Jack Nield. At the time of her diagnosis, Sharon was Director of Nursing Policy at the Canadian Nurses Association, where she had previously served as a nursing policy consultant since 1990. In the latter position she was the CNA person responsible for ethics. Sharon was instrumental in developing the ethics program at CNA to maximize ethics education following the publication of the 1997 Code of Ethics, and she was instrumental in preparing for the 2002 Code of Ethics revision. Under her guidance the *Everyday Ethics* booklet to serve as companion to the 1997 Code of Ethics was developed, and five of a series of "Ethics in Practice" papers were commissioned. She was instrumental in facilitating breakfast or noon-hour sessions for nurses attending the Canadian Bioethics Society Annual Conferences and breakfast

meetings at the Canadian Nurses Association Conference for nurses involved and interested in ethics. At Sharon's funeral on December 30, 2002, one of her colleagues stated in her eulogy, "Although she was dying, Sharon gave us a gift—a lesson in living. Through the strength she showed, she reminded us of the power of love, the importance of family, and the depth and meaning that faith can give to life." (The eulogy was delivered by Barbara LaPerriere, December 30, 2002, at Glebe-St. James Church, Ottawa, Ontario.) We, the Editors of this book, will miss her leadership but know that she would want others to learn from her story.

REFERENCES

Alexander, M. 1980. The rigid embrace of the narrow house: premature burial and signs of death. *The Hastings Center Report, 12*(6), 25–31.

Ambrosio, E. 1994. Autonomy, oppression and "choice" in euthanasia. Unpublished doctoral dissertation. University of Toronto, Toronto.

Annas, G. 1980. Quinlan, Saikewicz, and now Brother Fox. *The Hastings Center Report, 10*(3), 20–21.

Bailey, Thomas. 2003. Personal communication. February 26. Victoria, BC.

Baker, C. 1980. The living will: The final expression. *Legal Medical Quarterly, 4*, 2–13.

Battin, M.P. 1995. A dozen caveats concerning the discussion of euthanasia in the Netherlands. In J.D. Moreno (Ed.), *Arguing Euthanasia* (pp. 88–93). New York: Touchstone.

Blondeau, D., Lavoie, M., Valois, P., Keyserlingk, E.W., Hebert, M. and Martineau, I. 2000. The attitude of Canadian nurses towards advance directives. *Nursing Ethics, 7*(5), 399–411.

Byock, I. 2003. Rediscovering community at the core of the human condition and social covenant. In B. Jennings, T. Ryndes, C. D'Onofrio and M.A. Baily (Eds.), *Access to Hospice Care: Expanding Boundaries, Overcoming Barriers.* Hastings Center Report, Special Supplement. (pp. S40–S41). New York: The Hastings Center.

Callahan, D. 1991. Medical futility, medical necessity: The problem-without-a-name. *Hastings Center Report, 21*(4), 30–35.

Canadian Healthcare Association, Canadian Medical Association, Canadian Nurses Association, and Catholic Health Association of Canada (in co-operation with the Canadian Bar Association). 1995. *Joint statement on resuscitative interventions.* Ottawa: Canadian Healthcare Association, Canadian Medical Association, Canadian Nurses Association, and the Catholic Health Association of Canada (in co-operation with the Canadian Bar Association).

Canadian Healthcare Association, Canadian Medical Association, Canadian Nurses Association, and Catholic Hospital Association. 1999. *Joint statement on preventing and resolving ethical conflicts involving health care providers and persons receiving care.* Ottawa: Canadian Healthcare Association, Canadian Medical Association, Canadian Nurses Association, Catholic Hospital Association.

Canadian Hospital Association, Canadian Medical Association, and Canadian Nurses Association. 1984. *Joint Statement on Terminal Illness.* Ottawa: Canadian Hospital Association, Canadian Medical Association, Canadian Nurses Association.

Canadian Nurses Association. 1998. *Advance directives: The nurse's role.* Ethics in Practice series paper. Ottawa: Canadian Nurses Association.

Canadian Nurses Association. 2001. *Futility presents many challenges for nurses.* Ethics in Practice series paper. Ottawa: Canadian Nurses Association.

Canadian Pedatric Society. 2000. *Treatment decisions for infants and children.* Ottawa: Bioethics Committee, Canadian Pediatric Society. Reference No. B8601. Available online: www.cps.ca/english/statements/B/b86-01.htm

Chambers-Evans, J. 2002. The family as window onto the world of the patient: Revising our approach to involving patients and families in the decision-making process. *Canadian Journal of Nursing Research, 34*(3), 15–32.

Commission on the Future of Health Care in Canada. 2002. *Building on values: The future of health care in Canada*. Ottawa: Commission on the Future of Health Care in Canada.

Corley, M.C. 2002. Nurse moral distress: A proposed theory and research agenda. *Nursing Ethics, 9*(6), 636–650.

Corley, M.C. 1995. Moral distress for critical care nurses. *American Journal of Critical Care, 4*(4), 280–285.

Davis, A.J., Phillips, L., Drought, T.S., Sellin, S., Ronsman, K. and Hershberger, A.K. 1995. Nurses' attitudes toward active euthanasia. *Nursing Outlook, 43*(4), 174–179.

De Wolf, G.D., Gregg, R.J., Harris, B.P. and Scargill, M.H. 1997. *Gage Canadian Dictionary*. Toronto: Gage Educational Publishing Company.

Doucet, H. 1992. *Someone I love is dying... euthanasia?* Ottawa: Novalis, St. Paul's University.

Ferris, F.D., Balfour, H.M., Bowen, K., Farley, J., Hardwick, M., Lamontagne, C., Lundy, M., Syme, A. and West, P.J. 2002. *A model to guide hospice palliative care: Based on national principles and norms of practice.* Toronto: Canadian Hospice Palliative Care Association.

Fisher, R., Ross, M.M. and MacLean, M.J. 2000. A guide to end-of-life care. Ottawa: University of Ottawa.

Foley, K. and Hendin, H. 1999. The Oregon report: Don't ask, don't tell. *Hastings Center Report, 29*(3), 37–42.

Glaser, B.G. and Strauss, A.L. 1965. *Awareness of dying*. Chicago: Aldine Publishing Co.

Godkin, M.D. 2002. *Apprehending death: The older adult's experience of preparing and advance directive.* Unpublished doctoral dissertation. University of Alberta, Edmonton.

Gramelspacher, G.P., Howell, M.D. and Young, M.J. 1986. Perceptions of ethical problems by nurses and doctors. *Archives of Internal Medicine, 146*, 577–578.

Georges, J.J. and Grypdonck, M. 2002. Moral problems experienced by nurses when caring for terminally ill people: A literature review. *Nursing Ethics, 9*(2), 155–178.

Hebert, P.C. 1996. *Doing right*. Toronto: Oxford University Press.

Hunter, S. 2000. Determination of moral negligence in the context of the undermedication of pain by nurses. *Nursing Ethics, 7*(5), 380–391.

Illich, I. 1975. *Medical nemesis: The expropriation of health*. London: Calder and Boyars.

Jameton, A. 1984. *Nursing practice: The ethical issues*. Englewood Cliffs, N.J.: Prentice Hall.

Justin, R.G. and Johnson, R.A. 1989. Recording end-of-life directives on hospital admission. *Nursing Management, 20*(3), 65–68.

Keenan, S.P., Mawdsley, C., Plotkin, D., Webster, G.K. and Priestap, F. 2000. Withdrawal of life support: How the family feels and why. *Journal of Palliative Care, 16* (Supplement/October), S40–S44.

Krisman-Scott, M.A. 2000. An historical analysis of disclosure of terminal status. *Journal of Nursing Scholarship,* First Quarter, 47–52.

Kubler-Ross, E. 1969. *On death and dying*. New York: Macmillan.

Kuhl, D. 2002. *What dying people want: Practical wisdom for the end of life*. Toronto: Doubleday Canada.

Kuhl, D. and Wilensky, P. 1999. Decision-making at the end of life: A model using an ethical grid and principles of group process. *Journal of Palliative Medicine, 2*(1), 75–86.

Kuhl, D. 1998. *Hospital bioethics committee: DNR Task Force*. Vancouver: St. Paul's Hospital.

Law Reform Commission of Canada. 1979. Criteria for the determination of death. Working Paper 23. Ottawa: Law Reform Commission of Canada.

Law Reform Commission of Canada. 1981. *Criteria for the determination of death*. Ottawa: Law Reform Commission of Canada.

Law Reform Commission of Canada. 1982. Euthanasia, aiding suicide and cessation of treatment. Working Paper 28. Ottawa: Law Reform Commission of Canada.

Mayo, D.J. and Gunderson, M. 2002. Vitalism revitalized. *Hastings Center Report, 32*(4), 14–21.

McPhail, A., Moore, S., O'Connor, J. and Woodward, C. 1981. One hospital's experience with a "do not resuscitate" policy. *Canadian Medical Association Journal, 15*, 830–836.

McTeer, M.A. 1999. *Tough choices: Living and dying in the 21st century.* Toronto: Irwin Law.

Molloy, D.W. 2002. *Let me decide.* Special British Columbia Edition. Troy, ON: Newgrange.

Moreno, J. (Ed.). 1995. *Arguing euthanasia.* Toronto: Simon and Schuster.

Morioka, M. 2001. Reconsidering brain death: A lesson from Japan's fifteen years of experience. *Hastings Center Report, 31*(4), 41–46.

National Health Forum. 1997. *Canada health action: Building on the legacy.* Final report of the National Health Forum. (Volumes 1 and 2). Ottawa: Minister of Public Works and Government Services.

Nelson-Martin, P., Braaten, J. and English, N. 2001. Promoting good end-of-life care in the intensive care unit. *Critical Care Nursing Clinics of North America, 13*(4), 577–585.

Parker, P. 2001. Sedation at the end of life: A challenging choice. *In Touch: The Provincial Health Ethics Network, 4*(1), 1–2.

Pence, G.E. 1995. *Classic cases in medical ethics.* 2nd edition. New York: McGraw-Hill.

Puopolo, A.L., Kennard, M.J., Mallatratt, L., Follen, M.A., Desbiens, N.A., Conners, A.F., Califf, R., Walzer, J., Soukup, J., Davis, R.B. and Phillips, R.S. 1997. Preferences for cardiopulmonary resuscitation. *Image: Journal of Nursing Scholarship, 29*(3), 229–235.

President's Commission for the Study of Ethical Problems in Medicine and Biomedical and Behavioural Research. 1981. *Defining death: Medical, legal and ethical issues in the determination of death.* Washington, DC: US Government Printing Office.

Raines, M.L. 2000. Ethical decision-making in nurses. *JONA's Healthcare Law, Ethics, and Regulation, 2*(1), 29–41.

Randal, J. 1983. Are ethics committees alive and well? *Hastings Center Report, 13*(6), 10–12.

Report of the Special Senate Subcommittee to update *Of Life and Death* of the Standing Committee on Social Affairs, Science and Technology. 2000. Chaired by S. Carstairs and G.A. Beaudoin. Ottawa: Supply and Services.

Report of the Special Senate Committee on Euthanasia and Assisted Suicide. 1995. *Of life and death.* Ottawa: Supply and Services.

Rocker, G. and Dunbar, S. 2000. Withholding or withdrawal of life support: The Canadian Critical Care Society position paper. *Journal of Palliative Care, 16* (Supplement/October), S53–S62.

Rodney, P., Dodek, P., Thompson, T., Kuhl, D., Calam, B., Chung, M., Jolliffe, C. and Nicholson, R. 1999. *Constructing bioethics policy through stakeholder participation and collaboration: Development of the St. Paul's hospital "do not resuscitate" protocol.* Unpublished manuscript. Vancouver: St. Paul's Hospital.

Rodney, P. and Howlett, J. In press. Elderly patients with cardiac disease: Quality of life, end of life, and ethics. In D. Fitchett (Ed.), *Canadian Cardiovascular Society Consensus Document on Care of the Elderly.*

Rodney, P.A., Thompson, T., Calam, B., Chung, M., Frost, L., Jolliffe, C., Murphy, K., McKenzie, L., Mulcahy, M., Dodek, P., Young, D., Mackinnon, M., Kuhl, D. and Budz, B. 2002a. *Constructing bioethics policy through consensus building and community participation: An evaluation of the St. Paul's Hospital DNR Protocol.* Unpublished research report sent to Providence Health Care and the Associated Medical Services Incorporated (Bioethics Division).

Rodney, P., Varcoe, C., Storch, J.L., McPherson, G., Mahoney, K., Brown, H., Pauly, B., Hartrick, G. and Starzomski, R. 2002b. Navigating towards a moral horizon: A multi-site qualitative study of nurses' enactment of ethical practice. *Canadian Journal of Nursing Research, 34*(3), 75–102.

Sahlberg-Blom, E., Ternestedt, B.M. and Johansson, J.E. 2000. Patient participation in decision-making at the end of life as seen by a close relative. *Nursing Ethics, 7*(4), 313.

Scanlon, C. 1996. Nurses as catalysts for improving end-of-life care. *Center for Ethics and Human Rights Communique.* Washington, DC: American Nurses Association, *5*(1), 1–2.

Schultz, L. 1997. Not for resuscitation: Two decades of challenge for nursing ethics and practice. *Nursing Ethics, 4*(3), 227-238.

Sharpe, V.A. 1997. The politics, economics, and ethics or "appropriateness." *Kennedy Institute of Ethics Journal, 7*(4), 337–343.

Singer, P.A. 1993. *Living will.* Toronto: University of Toronto Centre for Bioethics.

Singer, P.A. 1994. Advance directives in palliative care. *Journal of Palliative Care, 10*(3), 111–116.

Singer, P.A., Martin, D.K. and Kelner, M. 1999. Quality end-of-life care: Patient's perspectives. *Journal of the American Medical Association, 291*(2), 163.

Soderberg, A., Gilje, F. and Norberg, A. 1999. Transforming desolation into consolation: The meaning of being in situations of ethical difficulty in intensive care. *Nursing Ethics, 6*(5), 357–373.

Storch, J. 1983. *Medical legal issues: Ethical and legal issues of death and dying.* Calgary: ACCESS Alberta.

Storch, J. 1998. Advancing our thinking about advance directives: Ethics at the end of life. In E. Banister (Ed.), *Focus on Research: Mary Richmond Lecture Series* (pp. 73–91). Victoria: School of Nursing, University of Victoria.

Storch, J.L., Griener, G.G., Marshall, D.A. and Olineck, B.A. 1990. Ethics committees in Canadian hospitals: Report of the 1989 survey. *Healthcare Management Forum, 3*(4), 3–8.

Storch, J.L. and Griener, G.G. 1992. Ethics committees in Canadian hospitals: Report of the 1990 pilot study. *Healthcare Management Forum, 5*(1), 19–26.

Storch, J.L. and Dossetor, J. 1994/1998. Public attitudes towards end-of-life treatment decisions: Implications for nurse clinicians and nursing administrators. *Canadian Journal of Nursing Administration, 7*(3), 65–89. Reprinted in *CJNA, 11*(4), 8–33.

Storch, J., Rodney, P., Hartick, G., Varcoe, C. and Starzomski, R. 2000. *The ethics of practice: Context and curricular implications for nursing.* Victoria: University of Victoria.

Storch, J.L., Rodney, P. and Starzomski, R. 2002a. Ethics and health care in Canada. In B.S. Bolaria and H.D. Dickinson (Eds.), *Health, Illness and Health Care in Canada* (pp. 409–444). Toronto: Nelson Thomson Learning.

Storch, J.L., Rodney, P., Pauly, B., Brown, H. and Starzomski, R. 2002b. Listening to nurses' moral voices: Building a quality health care environment. *Canadian Journal of Nursing Leadership, 15*(4), 7–16.

Taylor, C. 1995. Medical futility and nursing. *Image: Journal of Nursing Scholarship, 27*(4), 301–306.

The SUPPORT Investigators. 1995. A controlled trial to improve care for the seriously ill hospitalized patients: The study to understand prognoses and preferences for outcomes and risk of treatment (SUPPORT). *Journal of the American Medical Association, 274*(20), 1591–1598.

Thomas, D. 1969. Do not go gentle into that good night. In C.M. Coffin (Ed.), *The Major Poets: English and American,* 2nd ed. (p. 553). New York: Harcourt Brace Jovanovich.

Truog, R.D. 1997. Is it time to abandon brain death? *Hastings Center Report, 27*(1), 29–37.

Truog, R.D., Cist, A.M., Brackett, S.E., Burns, J.P., Curley, M.A., Danis, M., DeVita, M.A., Rosenbaum, S.H., Rothenberg, D.M., Sprung, C.L., Webb, S.A., Wlody, G.S. and Hurford, W.E. 2001.

Recommendations for end-of-life care in the intensive care unit: The ethics committee of the Society of Critical Care Medicine. *Critical Care Medicine, 29*(12), 2332–2348.

Varcoe, C. and Rodney, P. 2003. Trends and new thinking. In G. Doane (Ed.), *Rethinking ethics education in nursing* (pp. 40–59). Unpublished manuscript. University of Victoria School of Nursing, Victoria, B.C.

Varcoe, C., Hartrick, G., Pauly, B., Rodney, P., Storch, J.L., Mahoney, K., McPherson, G., Brown, H. and Starzomski, R. In Review. Ethical practice in nursing—Working the in-betweens. *Journal of Advanced Nursing.*

Veatch, R.M. 1993. The impending collapse of the whole-brain definition of death. *Hastings Center Report, 23*(4), 18–24.

Veatch, R.M. 1977. Hospital ethics committees: Is there a role? *Hastings Center Report, 7*(3), 22–27.

White, K.R., Coyne, P.J. and Patel, U.B. 2001. Are nurses adequately prepared for end of life care? *Journal of Nursing Scholarship,* Second Quarter, 147–151.

Wilson, D.M. 2000. End of life care preferences of Canadian senior citizens with caregiving experience. *Journal of Advanced Nursing, 31*(6), 1416–1421.

Wilson, D.M., Smith, S.L., Anderson, M.C., Northcott, H.C., Fainsinger, R.L., Stingl, M.J. and Truman, C.D. 2002. Twentieth-century social and health-care influences on location of death in Canada. *Canadian Journal of Nursing Research, 34*(3), 141–161.

Zronek, S., Daly, B. and Lee, H. 1999. Elderly patients' understanding of advance directives. *JONA's Healthcare Law, Ethics and Regulation, 1*(2), 23–28.

chapter fourteen

Narrative Ethics in Health Care

Jeff Nisker

It is only with the heart that one can see truly, for what is essential is invisible to the eye.
—Antoine de Saint-Exupéry (1943): *The Little Prince*

My conversion from a theories-and-principles-based (Beauchamp and Childress 1994; Nisker 1995) to a **narrative**-based approach to moral exploration and ethics education occurred with the reading to my children of the above line in *The Little Prince* (de Saint-Exupéry 1943). With epiphanic clarity, this line opened the imperative to ask health care students and professionals to hear the hearts of the persons who come to our care. This line also encouraged me to explore ethical issues with the hearts of health care students and professionals, rather than just cognating moral issues or teaching the cognition of moral issues in the same manner health care students and professionals cognate symptoms and signs of disease (Nisker 1997a).

Hearing our patients' stories brings us to the inherent beauty of the persons too often confined within a diagnosis (Nisker 2001a). Hearing our patients' stories allows us to appreciate the position of the woman or man or child for whom the moral exploration is occurring; just as opening "Chalcedonies," the "lustreless rocks whose scabrous surface" conceals "crysoprase or agate or onyx" that can yield magnificent "jewelry, amulets, paperweights, bookends" (Nisker 2001a, 74) is required before we can appreciate their beauty within.

In this chapter, I will say more about the "beauty within"—but will start by suggesting the value of narratives and by supporting John Arras's contention that narrative is "an essential element in any and all ethical analysis [and] constitutes a powerful and necessary corrective to the narrowness and abstractness of some widespread versions of principle- and theory-based ethics" (Arras 1997, 84). I will describe the types of narrative used in health care ethics, which will lead me to a discussion of the advantages of "thick" narratives and how "thick" narratives improve traditional presentation of "cases."[1] I will continue by exploring the uses of narratives in health care ethics exploration, education, policy development, and research.

THE VALUE OF NARRATIVE

Exploring ethical issues through the narratives of a person at the centre of the issue helps us to better understand the person and the ethical issues involved in that person's care. Next to being a patient, or spending considerable time truly caring for the person who is our patient, hearing narratives is the best way a health care provider can experience what the persons who are in their care feel, how they want to be treated, and what they want to know. Narratives assist in clinical and moral decision-making because they bring us closer to understanding the uniqueness of the persons we serve.[2]

Story has provided moral footing for thousands of years. We experience moral learning when reading Greek mythologies, epic literary works like Homer's *Odysseus*, and religious texts like the Bhava Gita, Old Testament, and Quran, as well as Jesus' parables and the Gospels. Unfortunately, many great works, especially those created by women, as well as women and men from non-Western cultures, have been lost. Those that have survived the filter of time can, in a compelling manner, engage health care students and professionals, bringing us insight into the moral problems inherent in humanness. Over the centuries, poets and novelists have continued to surface ethical issues and help their readers explore right action. Telling our own stories[3] allows us to share our unique health care experiences with other caregivers, ethics explorers, policy-makers, and the general public.

Stories remain an engaging and memorable vehicle for moral learning, much more so than didactic, topic-based approaches. Stories may be fictional compilations of insights and feelings, or true stories of an illness experience. Anna Quindlen, former *New York Times* Op Ed columnist and author of the health-related novels *One True Thing* (1995) and *Black and Blue* (1998a), stated when she left journalism for novels that, "Facts sometimes need fiction to be told truly" (1998b). Nadine Gordimer, Nobel Laureate, goes further, stating, "There is always more truth in fiction" (1999).

For fictional works to significantly contribute to moral exploration in health care, it is not necessary that they describe medical moments, health care settings, or illness experiences. It *is* necessary, however, that they powerfully surface the feelings of the persons involved and explore humanness in a manner that can be absorbed for later understanding to assist other persons who are (or will be) confined beneath the medical microscope. "The universalizing tendency of the moral imagination is encouraged by the very activity of novel-reading of itself, with its alternations between identification and sympathy" (Nussbaum 1990, 166). This can be challenging to some health care students and providers for, as Philips suggests, to "engage with a narrative requires a leap of faith that suspends disbelief in order that what is told can be heard" (1994, 10). Although I find that this is true for some individuals in all health care disciplines, it is especially true for medical students and practitioners, culturally hardened to computer-like objectivization of data input.

Nonfiction stories and memoirs are also extremely valuable. In the writings of illness experience by Arthur Frank (1991; 1995), we have personal stories and personal reflections beautifully juxtaposed. They are at once self-reflective, compelling to the reader, and informative as to what can be learned from the author's personal experience. In scholarly texts, such as Howard Brody's *Stories of Sickness* (1987; 2003), the power of story as it relates to the provision of better health care is elegantly described.

Knowing as much as possible of the life stories of the persons for whom we care allows us to understand from where those persons' actions, hopes, and desires come and how we can best help those persons achieve their goals in relation to their illness experience. Let me say more about the various forms the stories may take.

Casuistry

Anne Hudson Jones describes **"casuistry"** as an ethical examination that "begins with the features of a particular 'case,'[4] then seeks to recall similar paradigm cases that may shed enlightenment about the best resolution for the case in hand" (Jones 1998, 222). As much of health care deliberation and learning (indeed law learning and business learning) is "case based," it is not surprising that cases have often been used in ethics deliberations and education. Jones refers to the "similarity of mental process in medical thinking and casuistical thinking" (222). Mark Kuczewski describes casuistry as case-based reasoning and claims "that comparing cases to a *paradigmatic case* in which the principle or common ethical maxim that should be predominant is clear, we can arrive at a sound moral judgment" (1997, 136).

Paradigm Cases

Paradigm cases are often used to stimulate ethics exploration of a specific topic. For end-of-life decision-making, the paradigm cases frequently used include Nancy B. or Sue Rodriguez (Hébert 1996). The presentation of such cases can vary from a thin half page, to a thick half page, to a book (Birnie and Rodriguez 1994), or even a film (Canadian Broadcasting Corporation 1998). I believe the "success" of a paradigm case is directly related to thickness of the story.

Thick and Thin Narratives

Thomas Murray (1997) argues that

> the "case" in bioethics is actually a collection of several different genres from telegraphically terse hypothetical use to illustrate a particular philosophical point, through the patient case— thick on numbers and thin on nuance—of the medical chart, to rich and complex narratives that weave together clinical facts with observations about human motivations, perceptions and relationships (7).[5]

We have had a tendency in health care to present "cases" that are of the **"thin"** variety on everything except medical data. These "thin" stories, by revealing only a smattering of family and social information, are rarely adequate to help us understand who the person *qua* patient is or what her desires for the present and future are—that is, the essentials in assisting with her health care. **"Thick"** stories, whether fictional, true, or fictional based on true, bring us to the deeper understanding we require as health care providers.

Arthur Frank's view that "narratives make the patient the ethicist" and "what is ethical is found in the story" (1995, 169) suggests that the narrative must be "thick" enough either to allow a person *qua* patient to tell her own story, or for someone else (such as her care provider) to express her story in an authentic fashion. This is not only imperative when the person *qua* patient is immersed in an ethical dilemma, but is important for the day-to-day assistance of all who come to our care.

Through "thick" narratives rather than the "thin" narratives in "cases," we are able to develop "empathetic imagining" (Halpern 2001) for each person we are hoping to help. "Thick" narratives do not have to be longer than "thin" narratives. Indeed, a poem, the densest form of narrative through its precision of words and the power of imagery per word, can concisely bring us to a person's condition. Short stories, short plays, and even novellas (and longer forms of each when there is sufficient time) are also very useful tools for imbuing insight in ethics exploration. Further, "thick" narratives can also be expressed in film, in song, and even in media where no words are used (such as paintings, photographs, other visual arts, and instrumental music).[6]

Let me provide an example to illustrate the differences. In our medical school, a "case-of-the-week," traditionally presented as "thin" on everything but medical data, is presented to the students each week and is referred to in all lectures and seminars. Adding a small but important amount of additional information regarding the person at the centre of the "case" and what the person feels about the "case," we convert "thin" cases to "thick" cases for ethics exploration. A "thick" case can deliver, through precision and compassion-imbued wording, much more about the person in the "case" without requiring much more ink or time. To illustrate, below is the "case-of-the-week" in the nephrology block of our second-year curriculum:

A 36-year-old male with end stage renal failure secondary to IgA nephropathy[7] has been on hemodialysis for 12 months. He comes to the hospital for four-hour dialysis treatments three times weekly, but intermittently does not show up. He has a history of depression, poor education, and poor social supports. He lives with his widowed mother and has been unemployed for the past 10 years. He has a history of alcohol abuse, but it has not been an issue in recent times. He is on erythropoietin, phosphate binders, Vitamin D, Vitamin B, and iron. He announces that dialysis is intolerable for him, that he has "nothing to live for" and that he is not going to come for further treatments. One of his dialysis nurses states that, while she is uncomfortable with his decision, she supports his right to make it. Another of his nurses, however, argues that he is too "unstable" to make a decision that will result in his death if he carries through with it.

I thickened the "case" by rewriting it as the poem "Tom" (below) to help bring the students to the person at the centre of the ethical issue being explored:

"Dialysis Patients Only" assigns Tom's place,
To park his 12-year-old car,
To live his 36-year-old life.
Tom's car has pulled up to this persecution
Three times a week, for a long year;
Except recently, more and more
His car chooses another way,
The way Tom wants to choose.
The car is transfixed by the sign
For the four hours Tom is fixed
To the dialysis machine

That cleans his body,
That contaminates his mind.
Alcohol once soothed the pain of Tom's uselessness,
But that was before IgA destroyed his kidneys.
IGA, like the supermarket
Where Tom bagged groceries ten years ago,
Demeaning himself before other adults.
So he quit and has not worked since.
Tom's mother takes care of him like when he was Tommy,
But Tom is not a child.
Tom's glad his father does not live
To see his latest incapacity,
His last incapacity.
The drugs to keep Tom's blood up are just another demean he suffers.
What's the point of living this helplessness, this hopelessness?
Tom proclaims he will break the chain
To the "Dialysis Patients Only" sign.

Lest the reader think I am singling out nephrologists for increased scrutiny, there is probably no more poignant example of thinning persons to cases than in my specialty of obstetrics, in which a woman (let's call her "Linda Smith") is reduced to "Mrs. S, 32, TPAL 3102,[8] having 3 normal vaginal deliveries (one at 22 weeks), presents at 32 weeks with a 3-hour history of RLQ[9] pain." How much more time would be required for "Mrs. S." to be "Linda, a 32-year-old woman, in the 32nd week of her fourth pregnancy, having given birth to three children through normal vaginal delivery, one of whom was 18 weeks premature and died shortly after birth, developed pain in the right lower quadrant of her abdomen gradually over the past three hours and is very worried that she will again deliver prematurely?"

TYPES OF NARRATIVE IN HEALTH CARE ETHICS

Narratives useful in ethics exploration, education, policy development, and research can be divided by their type or by their utility. Types of narrative can be categorized according to the form of presentation, such as a poem, play, short story, or film, or described in terms of content (see Exhibit 14-1).

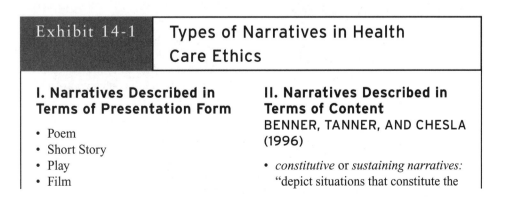

Exhibit 14-1	Types of Narratives in Health Care Ethics
I. Narratives Described in Terms of Presentation Form • Poem • Short Story • Play • Film	**II. Narratives Described in Terms of Content** BENNER, TANNER, AND CHESLA (1996) • *constitutive* or *sustaining narratives:* "depict situations that constitute the

person's understanding of what it is to be a nurse" and "capture the significance of the practice and demonstrate meaning-laden clinical episodes that convey the worth of the work" (237)

- *narratives of learning:* subdivided into "narratives about being open to experience" (241), "narratives of learning the skill of involvement" (242), "narratives of disillusionment" (245), "narratives about facing death and suffering" (248), and "liberation narratives" (249)

FRANK (1995)

- *restitution narratives:* dominate the stories of both those who are sick and are focusing on being healthy again, and how "contemporary culture treats health as the normal condition that people ought to have restored" (77)
- *chaos narratives:* the opposite of the restitution narrative, their plot imagines life never getting better (like a Holocaust story) (97)
- *quest narratives:* "stories meet suffering head on; they accept illness and seek to use it"
- *memoirs:* combines "telling the illness story with telling other events in the writer's life" (119)
- *manifestos:* "the truth that has been learned is prophetic, often carrying demands for social action" (120)
- *automythologies:* like the Phoenix myth, "where the protagonist reinvents herself from the ashes of the fire of [her] own body" (122)

NELSON (2001)

- *counter stories:* stories that resist an oppressive identity and attempt to replace it with one that commands respect
- *master narratives:* "stories found lying about in our culture that serve as summaries of socially shared understanding which over the years have 'exercised' a certain authority over our moral imaginations and play a role in informing our moral intuitions" (6)

SMYTHE AND MURRAY (2000)

- *personal narratives:* biographies, autobiographies, and works of fiction that are "centred on the individuality of a central main character or person... told from a consistent, personal perspective and is aimed at revealing the unique, idiosyncratic character and life circumstances of a particular individual" (327)
- *archetypal narratives:* stories "of mythological and religious texts" in which "the focus is not human individuality, as such, but... timeless human motifs that reflect fundamental spiritual, existential, and moral concerns" (327)
- *typal narratives:* based on "psychological and social" themes, in which the "principal aim is neither to capture the individuality of persons in detail nor to bring out archetypal human themes, but rather to concretely exemplify the theory-laden categories of contemporary social science" (327)

Presentation Forms

Poetry is the most concise **narrative form.** Each word, by itself or in phrases, is subconsciously calculated to convey maximum feeling—imagery created through similes and metaphors profoundly painting feeling through our hearts and minds. Many of my students prefer song to poetry, as it is more accessible to their generation and, for many students with talent in music, easier to present.

Short stories and poems are often best presented in a "readers' theatre" format in which each participant takes a turn reading a paragraph or stanza. These short stories or poems can be written by faculty members and/or students. Or they may be directed specifically toward a topic being discussed in the undergraduate clinical material, at a professional conference, or in a seminar. These literary works might be selected from anthologies, such as *Literature and Aging* (Kohn, Donley and Wear 1992). By involving the members of the class or conference participants in the narrative presentation, an ownership of the material and capacity to engage in moral exploration is achieved. The acting of plays similarly offers the opportunity to immerse many members of the class or conference in ethics exploration.

Film (video) is also a very valuable surfacing tool for narrative ethics exploration. Whether the central character is a nurse, as in *The English Patient*; a physician, as in *The Doctor*; another caregiver, as in *Passion Fish*; or a family member, as in *Marvin's Room* and *What's Eating Gilbert Grape?*, film engages participants. It is an attractive vehicle whether the film's importance lies in ethical issues for the person *qua* caregiver or person *qua* patient relationships (as in the films suggested above) or in the surfacing of specific ethical issues to be considered for later exploration by the group. Furthermore, scholarly analyses of films, such as Charles Weijer's (1997) work on Akiru Kurosawa's film *Ikiru* (translated as *To Live*), brings us to greater understanding of illness, healing, and moral behaviour—in this case, at the end of life.

A specific exploration of an ethical issue may use several narratives. For example, in exploring "end-of-life decision-making" I begin with a readers' theatre format of Earle Birney's poem, *David*. The poem brings participants to the position of David, not only as he is, lying quadriplegic on a rocky precipice after falling from a mountain, but, through the reflection of the narrator (David's friend), as he was throughout his life and while climbing the mountain. We are also placed in the position of the narrator as an unwilling substitute decision-maker. The issues surfaced by *David* are then explored using paradigm cases, including Sue Rodriguez and Nancy B. (from Philip Hébert's book *Doing Right* [1996, 174, 183]), that I "thickened" with permission of the author toward a "Tom"-like narrative.

Narrative-surfacing vehicles may vary in length from Rilke's three-stanza poem, *The Dwarf's Song*, to student-performed plays of varying length, to two-hour films (usually viewed in the week before the ethics exploration). Narratives allow learning through participation in the presentation, as well as in the discussion of the ethical issues surfaced.

USES OF NARRATIVE IN HEALTH CARE ETHICS

I believe that narrative is the place to begin **bioethics** exploration. Stories, whether true, fictional, or fictional based on truth, can help bring the reader or audience to the position of the person requiring health care, thus allowing a much deeper appreciation of that person's needs, rights, and desires than is possible in health care and philosophy tomes. By approximating empathy for the person at the centre of the decision-making, ethics explorers and educators can better contribute to moral resolution of the issue at hand, and provide better care.

Martha Montello tells us that "drawing on readers' own desires, memories, psychological defenses and imaginations enables readers to experience and understand things entirely unfamiliar, offering virtually limitless opportunities to engage their faculties in different ways of perceiving the world" (1997, 189). These different ways of perceiving the world should allow us "readers" to participate in more sensitive, and indeed informed, decision-making regarding the person and the issues affecting that person. This in turn enables more depth in our analysis and more empowerment of future persons *qua* patients to inform future decision-making. Further, these different perceptions could be used to promote public discussion of an ethical issue, national policy development, or specifically, for ethics education purposes.

Exhibit 14-2	**Purposes of Narratives in Health Care Ethics**

ARRAS (1997)

- To supplement principle-driven approaches
- To function as "the very ground of all moral justification" (73) (as described by MacIntyre and Hauerwas, e.g., MacIntyre 1981; 1988; Burrell and Hauerwas 1977)
- In a "postmodern ethical stance" in which "narrative and the authenticity of the narrator appear to play the role of substitutes for ethical justification" (68)[10]

MONTELLO (1997)

- To "reframe... the issues by focusing attention on the context of a patient's and family's life in all its moral complexity" (186)
- To "have long-term effects on the structure of the self by extending a reader's psychic map to include unfamiliar territory, taking in new values and knowledge and knowledge of other ways of seeing the world" (188–190)

NELSON (2001)

- "(1) to teach us our duties; (2) to guide morally good action; (3) to motivate morally good action; (4) to justify action on moral grounds; (5) to cultivate our moral sensibilities; (6) to enhance our moral perception; (7) to make actions or persons morally intelligible; and (8) to reinvent ourselves as better persons" (36)
- For compassionate health care decision-making
- For health care ethics education
- For health care policy development
- For health care ethics research

Narrative for Moral Exploration

Patricia Benner (1994) writes that "Narratives and narrative knowing allow us to examine practical moral reasoning and to get beyond abstractions" (59). Ann Hunsaker Hawkins

(1997) describes narratives as a "counter [to] the tendency in philosophy-based ethics to overemphasize moral principles and rules in considering a particular ethical situation" (154). Martha Nussbaum (1990) believes that "[t]he very difficulty of discovering a non-prejudicial description of the task of ethical inquiry will itself illuminate our problem: and the concealed prejudices in some prominent contemporary philosophical description of the task will begin to show us what moral philosophy has lost through the absence of dialogue with literary thought" (172).

Narratives can be written specifically for readers to use to begin their moral exploration of a particular issue or as stand-alone explorations in which authors use narratives as their argument. An example of the latter is my narrative exploration of the ethics of using economically disadvantaged women who request *in vitro* fertilization as "oocyte donors" for wealthier women who have delayed childbearing and have run out of eggs (Nisker 1997b). In this narrative exploration, I offered stories from multiple literary genres as analogies for what economically disadvantaged women (offered the opportunity to "share" their eggs in return for "free" IVF) have shared with me and others.

Another way to use narrative in moral exploration is that suggested by Rita Charon (1994; 1997) and other scholars (Jones 1998; Montello 1997; Nussbaum 1990) in which the principles of literary critical analysis are used to help health care providers better understand a patient's story and better practise medicine. As Martha Montello writes, "the same literary skills that critical readers use to interpret the meaning of events in a story allow clinicians to see the way ethical issues are embedded in the individual and continent nature of people's beliefs, cultures and biography" (1997, 186).[11]

Compassion Ethics

The utility of a narrative often works through its ability to approximate **empathy** for the person at the centre of the ethical issue, thus permitting us to better understand the ethical issue as it relates to that person. By developing a sensitivity to the position of the other, we are able to provide better care, not only for that person but for all those who come to our care. Indeed, though the purpose of using narrative in health care ethics can vary, the shared power of narratives lies in their link to **compassion:** "we see and hear and feel the same thing the characters do and from their perspective, so that when we close the book to render our own lives, that set of emotions and way of knowing is embedded in us, a part of us" (Montello 1997, 194). Defending the importance of compassion in ethics, David Thomasma argues that "not only rationality, but also emotional compassion, is an important teacher of bioethical decision making... our compassion can lead us to truths beyond reason and its analysis." (1994, 124).[12] Thomasma defines compassion as "more than pity or sympathy. It transcends social work, philanthropy, and government programs. It is the capacity to feel and suffer with the sick person—to experience something of the predicament of illness, its fears, anxieties, temptations, its insult on the whole person, the loss of freedom and dignity, the utter vulnerability, and the alienation every illness produces or portends... comprehension of the suffering experienced by another" (Thomasma 1994, 131–132).[13]

In the introduction to her book *From Detached Concern to Empathy* (2001), Jodi Halpern argues that by allowing patients to move us, we "gain access to a source of understanding illness and suffering that can make [us] more effective healers" (xi–xiii). The empathizer must be sufficiently affected by the patient "to be able to recognize and appreciate, in some quasi first-person way, how the rain and sun feel" (Halpern 2001, 67–68). Lois LaCivita Nixon, drawing on the work of Jones (1994), suggests that narratives function to "illuminat[e] ethical dilemmas with fictional materials that stretch the 'intuitive and imaginative faculties of mind'... [so that we] empathize with others, understand more fully what it means to be human, and develop moral wisdom" (Nixon 1997, 245).

Narratives teach us to integrate compassion with ethics. It is important to understand that this compassion applies to ourselves as health care providers and caregivers, as well as to patients. For example, the gift of being allowed to be a caregiver, which fuels our ability to help those we serve to the best of our potential, was beautifully presented in the film *Marvin's Room*. In this film, Bessie, a daughter caring for her bed-ridden father, defends her sacrifice as the gift of being able to care for her father, to be able to give love.

I believe, as does Frank (1995), that such stories are ends in themselves, but the writing of these stories is also a means to an end for the author—an exploration of self, of a relationship, of an issue. Indeed, the sharing of our stories with colleagues is a means to several ends: surfacing ethical issues for discussion, increasing awareness of an individual person's position (*qua* patient or *qua* health care provider), increasing sensitivity and compassion in members of a health care team, and even bringing the health care team closer together. For example, I wrote the play *Orchids: Not Necessarily a Gospel* (Nisker 2001b) as a narrative approach to the ethics exploration of issues in new genetic technology. The final line in the closing song of *Orchids* is "Help compassion happen every day" (Nisker 2001b). Those who viewed the original cast of health care students and professionals repeating this last refrain (as well as the cast themselves) not only explored what will be considered "normal" in "genetic technology's magic mirror" and how "disabled" people and "normal" people will see their reflections, but began to approximate empathy for women having to make decisions regarding genetic testing, for persons living with disabilities and for each other—indeed for all persons.

The term "compassion ethics" is frequently used to describe my narrative ethics courses because bringing the ethics explorer to the person's position imbues compassion for the person. Heath care students carry a "cargo" (Spiro 1996) of compassion into their chosen disciplines. It is important that the miles of medical ink and the consuming call schedules consistent with health care training not be allowed to evaporate any of this cargo (Nisker 1997a). Health care professionals ought to be adding to this cargo (Spiro 1996), even though the harried and hurried demands of too great a patient load too often discard compassion from our outward demeanor, and occasionally even from our inner feelings.

Narrative in Health Care Ethics Education

As I stated at the outset of this chapter, narrative helps us to hear the hearts of the persons who come to our care. As I also said earlier in the chapter, narrative helps us to better hear our own hearts. Given my convictions about the power of narrative, I strongly believe in using narrative in bioethics education. I have had the opportunity to use various narrative forms to teach (and learn from) medical students, students in other health care disciplines, and my colleagues in bioethics and health care communities. Here, I would like to describe some of what I have learned regarding the use of narrative in health care ethics education.

Overview

Ethics education is becoming an integral part of undergraduate and post-graduate health care curricula and continuing professional development. Thomasma (1994) worries that health care students, many of whom have a science background, are attracted to the principles-and-theories approach to ethics because the thought process is similar to clinical decision-making (123). This is true, but rather than committing to a principles-and-theories approach, ethics educators should take advantage of another characteristic of health care students and professionals. That is, they should take advantage of our most essential characteristic: a desire to care for others that brings us eagerly to stories of illness, of compassion, of others' needs, of caring for others. In a compassion-focused, narrative-based ethics curriculum, students eagerly come to class to share in an experience that might not only deepen their insight into ethical issues but also enhance their ability to understand their future patients' position so as to afford them compassionate care.

Scholars such as Charon (1994; 1997) validate the importance of narrative to help health care learners become better health care providers. Narrative fosters "empathetic imagining" (Halpern 2001, 185–190), whether as part of a narrative ethics or health care humanities curriculum, or indeed, in the form of the first-hand stories of the persons for whom we care. Empathetic imagining also helps us write narratives to help others experience empathy for the persons in our care. Martha Nussbaum (1990) suggests that "[b]y cultivating our ability to see vividly another person's distress, to picture ourselves in another person's place—we make ourselves more likely to respond with the morally illuminating and appropriate sort of response" (39). Narrative can help conserve compassion (Nisker 1997a) or even increase compassion through the years of undergraduate, post-graduate, and professional health care education. I have found that narrative is a powerful antidote for the "ethics-eyelid reflex" (Nisker 1995), and other non-verbal expressions of disinterest, that were contagious in many communities of students and professionals coming to traditional teaching templates.

Nixon (1997) explains that in her **medical humanities** classes "we search for understandings and interpretations of what humanness means by exploring literature, art, poetry, and film" (238). Medical humanities is a valuable part of any health care curriculum, whether listed separately from or combined with ethics explorations. The understandings and interpretations surfaced in literature, art, poetry, and film help keep open minds that may be gradually succumbing to the "tonnes of tutored words" (Nisker 1997a, 689) of most health care programs. Further, in undergraduate or post-graduate programs that find little time for curricula in both medical humanities and ethics (and often neither), combining the courses as a narrative ethics course can bring the importance of both to the student in the concise and attractive fashion demanded by "modern" programs and their students.

Writing "Thick" Narratives for Health Care Education

Just as health care education has evolved in the past 20 years from disease-based learning, to problem-based learning (PBL),[14] to patient-centred care (PCC) (Stewart et al. 1995), so too has the type of "case" evolved from cases consisting of diagnosis-driven facts, to relatively "thin cases" that include superficial reference to social circumstances and relationships, to "thick" narratives revealing the story of the person experiencing the health care issue through images that give deep insight into the social circumstances and relationships that surround the clinical condition. "Thick" narratives can assist in the evolution from PBL to PCC, forging a new person-centred learning. By keeping the story of the person for whom we are caring as the centre of our focus, we acknowledge the uniqueness of that person, as illustrated by the story of Tom provided earlier in the chapter. Moving from "a 36-year-old male" and a patient to "Tom," a person, meant that our action had to be much more than a decision to continue treatment or not. Our action also had to include attention to Tom's quality of life, including the meaning he found in his relationships and his day-to-day activities. Seeing Tom as a unique person, rather than as a "case" or a "patient," is essential for moral exploration of his dilemma.

It is not hard to convert "thin" stories to "thick" stories or, more accurately, to ensure that a person's story is not sliced down to its medical thread. In the workshops and seminars in which I suggest writing "thick" stories, I am always impressed with how quickly the participants are able to rewrite the "thin" cases I provide into "thick" narratives. Special talent or skill is not required, just a gentle reminder that there is a person inside that patient (Nisker 2001a). However, I also include the following suggestions:

1. Write from your heart, using "empathetic imagining" (Halpern 2001) to intuit what it is like to be in the person's position.

2. When possible, write in a first-person voice to more intimately bring to the reader what the person feels.

3. Use expressive adjectives, as well as similes and metaphors to create strong images.

4. Include tactile, auditory, and visual clues to imbue what the person is feeling, as in "I stopped the *coarseness* of the hospital's washcloth, as the *grating* sound of *yellowing* curtains opened me to the world."

5. Use a setting with which the participants can identify.

6. Make sure you include all necessary clinical information, but immerse it within the person's story.

7. When information from additional characters is necessary, reveal their words in the protagonist's recollection of a conversation that he or she had with them or that they had with others (i.e., an overheard conversation).[15]

Readers' Theatre

I find **readers' theatre** an extremely effective vehicle through which to bring poems and short stories to health care ethics explorers. Members of a class or participants in a conference are able to immerse themselves in the narrative and take mutual ownership in the discussion that follows the presentation. Ethics educators can write short stories specifically to be presented in a readers' theatre format. Dramatic phrasing, tending to purple (almost Shakespearean) prose seems particularly embracing. These short stories can be specifically written for subjects to be discussed in the classroom or conference auditorium. For example, to bring participants to the position of a 12-year-old boy suffering chemotherapy, I wrote the short story "Philip" (Nisker 2003a), which works well in my classroom as a readers' theatre but also required only minor modification by Danjiel Margetic, a University of Calgary theatre student, to be used as a short play at several Canadian pediatric conferences and rounds.

Victorian Parlour Game

Over the past seven years, I have been using a **Victorian parlour game** that I learned at a narrative bioethics course at Hiram College in August 1994. This game is a useful tool for both imbuing empathy and bringing together groups of students or professionals for moral exploration. Each Victorian guest (or seminar participant) is instructed to write one line in response to, "Imagine if you were in the position of a person in... [the ethical dilemma being explored]. How would you feel?" The first participant writes his or her line on the top of the page and folds the paper over the line (to conceal his or her response) and then passes the paper to the next person, who writes his or her line below the one already written and then folds the paper over again and passes it to the next person—and onward in succession until the last person (usually me) is charged to weave the lines into a group poem. In larger audiences, it may be necessary to have the paper passed down each row and (possibly) to construct a group poem for each row, or weave all the lines into one long poem. The poem constructor may change the order of the lines and, when necessary, the participants' words or phrases in order to achieve consistent tensing and rhythm and to avoid repetition, but may not introduce any new thoughts or images. This synthesis usually occurs after the class or on a break at a conference. The final poem is then presented to the group at the next session.

Let me provide an illustration. When exploring ethical issues of persons living with disabilities, I share with session participants Janice's story (Nisker 2001a). Janice is a woman who has been confined by multiple sclerosis to moving only her facial muscles. She is on a three-year waiting list to be allowed access to the technician and software to enable her to "go online." I then ask the participants to imagine themselves in Janice's position and to write one line each about how they would feel, after which these collections of lines are shaped into poems. Below are four of the twelve poems created at the 2000 Canadian Association of Critical Care Nurses (CACCN) Meeting in response to this question.[16]

CACCN Poem 1

I feel like an insect
Trapped in a glass jar.
It is warm,
I have air to breath,
But I am not free.
Time crawls incessantly.
I wait and wait and wait;
My day is filled with waiting
And I am running out of time.

How can I keep lowering my expectation
Without exploding with frustration,
As I stay segregated,
Needlessly silenced from cyberspace;
Placed in a dark tunnel
With no light at the end,
Just ghosts of a friend
That haunts with memories of monuments
Of my own?

Will you remember me
Or my medical nightmare?
Can you care for me
Without suffering yourself?
Please take my hand,
Make me feel real.

Empower me
By sharing my strength
With those who cannot see it.
For my mind is mighty;
Only my voice is small.
Be my microphone.

CACCN Poem 2

Let me in to laugh.
I would love another glass
With my love at sunset,
Wine like we first met;
Or somehow find a way
To feel my hands sculpt clay,
And tighten as they dry.
But I can only whisper why,
Why am I trapped in this tube
Of war-torn body
Screaming "hear me?"
Why am I an eagle
That can see the world so clearly
But cannot fly?

CACCN Poem 3

I watch an elastic raindrop
Struggle out of a puddle.
I watch an energetic fly
Struggle through a screen.
The fly is scared,
I am encouraged;
Give me a small opening
And I will soar.

CACCN Poem 4

I swim in strength
And patience and maturity.
I love life
Regardless of restriction.
I sink in isolation
And despair and futility.
I fear death
Even in exasperation.

The poem below is the result of the same narrative exploration with health care professionals (nurses, physicians), health law scholars, and graduate students in the 2001 Masters of Health Sciences in Ethics Program at the University of Toronto's Joint Centre for Bioethics:[17]

My chair's chain whines so slowly,
There is time to look in my eyes
And read my story:
I am locked in the prison cell of my body.
A place without physical feeling,
Even if someone wanted to touch me,
And allow me an intimate relationship.
I wish I could feel an itch
Just one more time,
But an itch is just another helpless aspiration
Waiting to erupt in a person incapable of eruption,
A volcano silent forever.
My world stands still though I still live,
Knowing all the me my silence has taught me.
How can I teach others what they need to know of me
When I can only smell what will become of me?
If only you would brush your cheek across my lips
So I could smell you instead.
Please keep talking to me
Even if I never respond.

"Yick Factor"

I encourage students to recognize their "gut feelings" as one of the important assessors of moral appropriateness (see also Chapter 21 and Chapter 22). Over the past eight years I have offered my students a "yick factor" (i.e., upsetting) scale (from 0 to 10, but as logarithmic as the Richter seismograph scale) as an impression of the appropriateness of a specific action, request, policy, or procedure. We also use the scale as a measure of the discomfort of participants when imagining themselves in the position of the person *qua* patient or person *qua* caregiver in the narrative. A high "yick factor" rating immediately draws the students to the need for ethics exploration. The use of this scale supports Nixon's view that ethics education has a role in helping students "gain practice in experiencing unsettling ideas and events" (1997, 247).

Evaluation

As can be seen from the power of the poems created through the Victorian parlour game above, the learning that occurs when narratives are used for health care ethics education can be profound. But how do we evaluate that learning, especially in formal professional education programs? Multiple-choice questions do not accurately or fairly assess moral competence or ethics learning at the best of times, they have no place in a narrative-based, ethics curriculum. Yet **evaluation** is necessary, not only to satisfy institutional requirements but to give students and professionals the impression that their ethics education is valued by universities, professional organizations, and licensing bodies, and, most importantly, that it is valuable to the persons for whom they will soon care.

As there is never one right way to evaluate, when I started an innovative program, it afforded me the opportunity for innovative evaluation. After experimenting with video vignettes followed by short answer questions, I became convinced that a narrative-based bioethics course should be evaluated through narratives. After consultation with students and faculty it was accepted that the student's bioethics "marks" over the first two years would be determined through a single major project to be presented and handed in at the end of the second year. Grades would be assigned in each semester (except for the first) for project development dates. The students take great pride in their achievements, as does the Dean. Several of these projects have been presented at national conferences and are in preparation for submission to scholarly journals. Further, this evaluation method was presented at the Association of Canadian Medical Colleges/Canadian Association of Medical Educators 2001 Annual Conference, where several students presented their poems and short stories, with encouraging acceptance of this as a valid evaluation method.

The third year in our medical school is clinical, and although narrative ethics seminars take place on some clinical rotations and ethics-related questions may be asked on the final clinical exam, no specific "grade" is afforded for ethics. However, the students are aware that in fourth year, their ethics "mark" will be based on an essay exploring an ethical dilemma they experienced in their hospital-based year. These essays are often very moving, and several of them are also on their way to publication. Knowing they will be writing this essay helps the students remain sensitive to ethical issues as they "rotate" through their clinical year. Writing the essay allows them to reflect on and through "student-centred" (Pendharkar 2001)[18] ethical issues in health care.

These methods of evaluation continue to evolve, and we have not yet undertaken a formal study of the evaluation of a narrative ethics curriculum in regard to its success in accomplishing the goals and objectives outlined in each module. Evaluation so far is limited to the comments of students and educators, which are useful as well as positive and have encouraged me to remain committed to this form of ethics education. Perhaps more objectively, our classroom is full of engaged students, whereas less than 20 percent of the class attended "compulsory" bioethics lectures and seminars in the previous traditional bioethics course. However, engagement remains but one factor in determining the appropriateness of a narrative-based approach to ethics education. In the future, specialists in evaluation will assist in obtaining a more accurate assessment of our narrative-based ethics curriculum.

On the Canadian Broadcasting Corporation (CBC) program "Daniel Richler Live" (1999), Richler asked medical students in my bioethics course whether I can teach compassion, and they answered (mistakenly in my opinion) "yes." Although I'm not sure that any of us can teach compassion, we *can*, through narrative, try to conserve the compassion our students already have and pave a softer path through the hard environment trodden by health care students and professionals (Nisker 1997a). Perhaps compassion ethics is "added value" to a bioethics curriculum, or moral awareness is "added value" to a compassion curriculum.

Narrative Ethics in Health Care Policy Development

Narratives, by surfacing ethical issues from the perspectives of a person central to the issue, can recruit the thoughts of the public, health care providers, ethicists, scholars, and policy-makers for their moral exploration. Stories from the heart thus have the potential to educate toward compassionate health care **policy development.** Narrative can engage the public in an open discussion of health care policy issues. Impressions gleaned from researchers and intellectual sources should be aired and debated, qualified and criticized, before public policy is made. This is in contrast to the current limited methods of public engagement and well-developed methods of "expert" engagement that currently exist (Buchanan et al. 2000, 305). Even in justice-based democracies such as ours, health care policy is largely developed by an oligarchy of "experts," including medical researchers, representatives of medical communities, government staff, as well as commercial interests (biotechnological, pharmaceutical, medical) and vested interest groups (health care funders and providers, disease focus groups, and politicians).

Any justice-based democracy requires the successful engagement of large numbers of participants for legitimate policy development. "As there are no obviously right or wrong answers in health care choices, it is therefore vital that decision makers get the process right, and that it has legitimacy in the eyes of both the public and professionals" (Lenaghan 1999, 60; see also Chapter 15). This is an urgent challenge for health care policy development. Rowe and Frewer (2000) contend that "[t]here is a growing call for greater public involvement in establishing science and technology policy, in line with democratic ideals" (p. 3), as a result of which we must consider which features of potential methods of engagement: (1) make it acceptable to the public and (2) ensure that the process is effective. In other words, the process by which we engage the public is crucial, yet we have a great deal to learn about *how*.

The idea that narrative may serve as a site of dialogical inquiry for policy has precedent in the seminal work of Augusto Boal, *Legislative Theatre: Using Performance to Make Politics* (1998). In this book, Boal describes theatre as a powerful tool for engaging the public to create a true form of democracy and effect social change and as a new and effective way to involve everyone in the democratic process. Boal's approach has primarily been used in North America in community-based educational settings, such as KYTES (The Kensington Youth Theatre Ensemble of St. Stephens) in Toronto, a program for street youth. A foundation for this kind of approach is Friere's formulation of a "pedagogy of the oppressed" (1993; 1994; 1995), which advocates critical consciousness of social-political systems through a dialogical and critical problematizing of the everyday experiences of the oppressed, leading to action for social change.

Similar initiatives have been suggested for health care policy. In their paper on ethics and genetics, Brunger and Cox (2002) suggest "a strategy for widening the space of public debate" (4) in a way that

1. provides the public with information about the production, distribution, and application of knowledge;
2. legitimizes lay knowledge;
3. attends to a multiplicity of voices;
4. welcomes dissent as a sign that all voices are being attended;
5. allows the debate to be transparent in public; and
6. promotes the accountability of government, industry, and science to the public.

There are obstacles to this list that are both macro and micro in nature. In Canada, health care providers face workplaces where the climate of compassion (and thus the moral climate) is deteriorating due to reduced resources for patient and family care. Staff shortages result in excessive workloads, loss of clinical leadership, and other efficiency-driven changes (see Chapter 10 and Chapter 11; for a fuller discussion, I also refer readers to Janice Stein's 2001 *Cult of Efficiency*).

Although most health care professionals are aware of their one-on-one obligation to those in their care, "out-of-the-box" moral obligations of health care professionals are less appreciated. As we will not be able to provide compassionate health care at the micro level if macro-level policy decisions are void of compassion, understanding our "out-of-the-box" moral imperatives is as important as our imperatives in the professional-patient relationship. In particular, we ought to challenge "efficiency"-based health policy (Nisker 2003b).

In macro health care policy-making, story may be an effective tool to bring a compassionate lens to policy-makers' scrutiny of the issues. Just as Solzhenitsyn shared what he observed and felt as a prisoner in the Soviet Gulag prison system in *Cancer Ward* (1969) and Boal (1998) and Friere (1993; 1994; 1995) shared what they observed and felt in totalitarian Brazil through their "street theatre" productions, health care providers can bring what we have observed and felt in order to effect social and political change. In our case, the change we are looking for is more compassionate health care policy, or perhaps a more compassionate society that will insist on more compassionate health care policy.

I wrote *Chalcedonies* (Nisker 2001a), Janice's story, upon her encouragement, to foster compassionate public policy development regarding accessibility issues for persons living with disabilities. All Janice wanted in life was to have the chin-operated joystick on her electric wheelchair hooked up to the Internet—technology that had been available for several years, but to which she was denied access because of the restrictions of our health care system. When I met Janice, her name still had approximately two years to languish on the "hook-up" waiting list. While neither Janice nor I deluded ourselves into thinking that the publishing of this story would cause an immediate compassionate response in health care policy development, we hoped, and I continue to hope (Janice died in 2000, shortly after the technician took her "measurements" for her Internet connection), that it might encourage others to write similar stories. And those who feel that they cannot write compassion-insisting stories might write their legislators compassion-insisting ballot box letters. Perhaps, eventually, legislators and other policy-makers will find themselves moved by narratives of both types.

Narratives in Health Care Ethics Research

In this section, I will reflect on both some of the promise that narrative holds for health sciences research and the problems particular to narrative research.

Narrative to Present Research

Narrative has been used by social scientists to present their research (Denzin 1997; McCall 2000), in scholarly journals (Cox 2003, Chapter 14) and books directed primarily to scholars (Frank 1991, 1995; Kuhl 2002) or primarily to the general public in books such as John Howard Griffin's *Black Like Me* (1961) and William H. White's *The Organization Man* (1956). The books of Frank (1991, 1995) and Kuhl (2002), drawing on personal experience, and patient interviews respectively, are extremely important to health care providers.

Theatre is also a useful way of presenting research (McCall, 2000). I had the privilege of collaborating with Vangie Bergum (Chapter 24) in bringing her research on "The experience of becoming mother through birthing, adopting, and placing a child" (Bergum, 1997). In the play titled *A Child On Her Mind,* my research and concerns regarding the use of economically disadvantaged women as surrogate mothers and as oocyte donors (Nisker 1996; Rodgers et al. 1997) was juxtaposed on Bergum's research to explore ethical issues common to both our areas of research. The play was originally performed for the Canadian Bioethics Society Conference in 1999 and the Social Sciences and Humanities Congress in 2000 with a cast of university students and staff. Since then the play has been performed with a professional cast, bringing the ethical issues inherent to large audiences of the general public and health care providers.

Most recently, Christina Sinding and Ross Gray have used theatre (Gray and Sinding 2002) to bring their research on women living with breast cancer (Gray et al. 2001) to audiences of health care providers, cancer patients and the general public.

Narrative for Research

Narrative can also be used as a powerful research tool. I believe narrative will be found useful to gather data, not only in social science fields, but also in ethics research. As an ethics **research** tool, narrative can not only bring the research of scholars to the public, but also engage the public to provide multiple and diverse thoughts and perspectives research as data.

For example, I have just completed the data collection on a study examining theatre for research in adult genetic testing. I melded the insights of ethicists, scientists and clinicians, as well as my own research and reflections on adult genetic testing into the one actor/one cellist play *Sarah's Daughters*. The communities involved were consulted, including participating in preliminary workshops of the script. The play was then performed for ten theatre audiences that included health care providers, vested interest groups, and policy makers as well as many members of the general public. The ensuing theatre discussions included from 20 to 150 audience members *qua* research participants and were audiotaped and transcribed. The transcribed tapes were then analyzed using a modified thematic approach (Strauss and Corbin 1994, 1998). Preliminary analysis of the data suggests that theatre is a very effective research tool to engage the public.

Should you choose to use theatre as a research tool, I believe it important to include in the invitations to participate in research (playbills, newspaper advertisements, posters, conference brochures, e-mail notices, etc.) and in the theatre lobby; the subject material of the play, that there will be an audience discussion following the performance, that the theatre experience is part of a research project, and that audience members choosing to share their perspectives into one of the microphones will be having their comments audiotaped and transcribed for research purposes. When the audience is seated, prior to each play's performance, I stress the importance of the reading of a formal (research ethics approved) invitation letter to participate in the research to explain the research in which they were invited to participate, the content of the play, and their choice to participate or not. I recommend the contents of the letter be reiterated prior to the audience discussion. I also recommend including a caution that it may not be possible to show the results of the research to the participants for their approval prior to publication. This was the case in the *Sarah's Daughters* research, as the participants were advised to remain anonymous and, indeed only if they were comfortable, indicate from where their perspective was offered (health care provider, patient, member of the general public, or policy maker). In the future this could be rectified by offering the opportunity for all participants to provide their name and contact information when entering the theatre so that they can be contacted with the results of the research and, if their comment is quoted, to verify their comments and provide permission for its publication.

Ethics of Using Narrative for Research, Education, and Policy Development

While using narrative for research is promising, it is not without its challenges. When using narrative as a research tool, "traditional **ethical principles governing research** with human participants offer insufficient guidance in dealing with our [qualitative research] unique dilemmas" (Smythe and Murray 2000, 312). Smythe and Murray draw our attention to the fact that "potential risks invoked by narrative research have to do with subtle and often unforeseen consequences of writing about other people's lives" (321) and that "extensive precautions often are necessary to protect the integrity of participants' reputations and their ongoing relationships with the others who figure in their stories" (321). This is an important warning as to how to go about achieving permission to tell a patient's story, or whether we should attempt to do so in a research or education or even moral exploration aegis.

Ethical guidelines for recruiting participants in narrative research, including narrative ethics research, are also different than other types of research. "[P]articipants in narrative research are asked to share more personal and identity laden data than in traditional, nomothetic research" (Smythe and Murray 2000, 339) and "[p]articipants might not always be the best judges of the potential consequences of their participation." Therefore the researcher (and, I would add, the educator) must use discretion in determining the suitability of specific persons as research participants (or sources of educational material).

I am especially concerned as to under what circumstance it is appropriate to present the narrative of a person we know, including persons who are (or have been) in our care or in the care of our colleagues. I am concerned not only when these stories are used for research or policy development purposes, but also when these narratives are used in classrooms, at rounds, at conferences, or other educational venues (Nisker and Daar 2003). In the clinician-patient relationship (Baylis 1990; Kenny 1994; Sherwin 1994), but also in other relationships such as in families, **power differentials** inexorably exist and exceed standard differentials in the researcher–research subject relationship. I have become increasingly concerned that stories in which the medical condition has a genetic basis—especially if the inheritance pattern is autosomal dominant or x-linked recessive, rather than an autosomal recessive or polygenic inheritance pattern that is less likely to identify family members—are quite different from other stories (Nisker and Daar 2003). This is because such stories may inadvertently violate not only the privacy of the person whose story is being told, but also family members' and that sacrifice of privacy may threaten the person's ability to access life insurance and employment opportunities. Striving for maximum camouflage of the persons kind (and brave) enough to allow us to tell their story not only requires changing names but also geographic locations and even at times factual material.

What is required to afford true choice in allowing an individual's story to be told if she is in the care of the storyteller or of a colleague of the storyteller? When compilations of patients' true stories create a fictional story, do we need the permission of all of these patients? How do we know which patients' (or friends') narratives subliminally contribute to our fictional narratives? If the patient is dead, do we need permission from his or her family?

IN CLOSING: THE BEAUTY WITHIN

While the questions above are troubling, they are not insoluble—they are places where we should seek further ethical inquiry. I remain committed to narrative because I believe narrative can help compassion happen. Hearing narratives of the persons who are in our care and their families is powerful. So is reflecting on these narratives as we write our narratives, exploring ourselves for our own narratives and sharing narratives with colleagues. And so is opening narratives to the scrutiny of health care students and providers, philosophers, scholars in other disciplines, health care policy advisors, writers, and the public.

Individual stories that promote compassion for the individual also promote compassion for society at large. In the end, we use narratives for the purpose of better serving those in our care or those who might come to our care. Ultimately, it is knowing that we have done our best each day (or night) for the persons in our care that allows us to be content with ourselves.[19]

FOR REFLECTION

1. How might "telling stories" of ethics problems assist practitioners working in direct care areas to improve their work environment?

2. How might educators better evaluate ethics learning involving narrative?

3. Think of ways in which you might use various forms of narrative to influence health care policy-makers. Provide specific examples.

4. What measures can be taken to preserve the confidentiality of persons when their stories are presented?

ENDNOTES

1. The use of the term "thick" narrative parallels Geertz's (1973) concept of "thick description."

2. Benner points out an interesting link to clinical reasoning here. Benner draws attention to Rubin's (1996) observation that "[p]ublic storytelling among practitioners allows for noticing distinctions and clinical learning. The forming of the story, where it begins, how it develops, what concerns shape the story, and how the story ends as well as the dialogue and perceptions of the storyteller present meaningful accounts of practical engaged reasoning" (Rubin's article cited as "in press" in Benner 1994, 58).

3. For the purposes of this chapter I am using the terms "story" and "narrative" interchangeably.

4. I believe the term "person" or "person *qua* patient" affords more dignity and respect than "case" or "patient" to the person at the centre of the ethical issue or moral exploration.

5. Childress (1997), an ethicist, gives a somewhat different perspective. He claims that "narrativists are inclined to make [cases] very thick to create a fuller picture, and this is often quite appropriate but not always necessary or unproblematic. There is also a place for thin cases" (259).

6. Note that some of these are not precisely qualified under the rubric of narrative.

7. IgA refers to immunoglobulin A, a protein that can build up inside the glomeruli of the kidney, usually as a response to a systemic bacterial infection. The buildup of IgA may cause a chronic glomerular nephritis, often resulting in renal failure.

8. TPAL refers to Term, Premature, Abortions, Living children. A TPAL of 2102 means the woman has had two pregnancies that went to term, 1 premature delivery, no abortions (spontaneous or therapeutic), and has 2 living children (thus assuming the premature child has died, which may not be the case, as indeed the premature child could have lived and one of the children born at term could have died).

9. RLQ refers to the right lower quadrant of the abdomen.

10. Arras (1997) warns, however, that in this last classification, the authenticity of the narrator might be mistaken for ethical truth. Also, he notes that narratives in his second classification risk either falling back into "a more principled version of ethics" or "sinking into a relativistic slough of incommensurable fundamental narratives" (85).

11. See also Charon and Montello (2002).

12. It is curious that compassion needs defending in the first place. Historically, Osler argued that distance from those for whom we care is required for the objectivity we need to be of assistance and to prevent our burnout caused by sharing too much of others' problems (Halpern 2001). But "[i]n unencumbering ourselves, we have shed much of our humanity. In our emphasis on legal ethics and rights, we have failed to meet our moral obligations of compassion and goodness" (Philips 1994, 4). In fact, if "[w]e are afraid that compassion will be excessive, ill-guided and expensive; we have overlooked the stories that tell us that compassion can be wise" (Benner 1994, 59).

13. Giving a contrary view, Arras states that "[i]t is an enduring temptation for Frank and the post-modernists in their single-minded embrace of creativity, empathy, and compassion uncritically to buy into the essentially romantic myth of the isolated individual or group, and thereby to ignore larger patterns and relationships that a more critical and socially attuned approach might recognize" (1997, 83). I must personally plead guilty to this temptation and propose that individual stories that promote empathy and compassion for the individual also promote empathy and compassion for society at large.

14. Credit for the development of problem-based learning goes in large part to the work done at McMaster University, Hamilton, Canada.

15. For a scholarly discussion on writing "thick" case-based narratives, I recommend Chambers (1997).

16. Used with permission of the conference organizer.

17. Used with permission of the course director.

18. The work on student-centred narrative ethics by Sachin Pendharkar was supported by an AMS/Wilson student fellowship (a fellowship that has supported several of my students over the past five years) for students to explore ethical issues in the summer and throughout the year.

19. I would like to acknowledge the assistance of Robyn Bluhm in the preparation of this chapter.

REFERENCES

Arras, J.D. 1997. Nice story, but so what? Narrative and justification in ethics. In H.L. Nelson (Ed.), *Stories and their limits: Narrative approaches to bioethics* (pp. 65–88). New York: Routledge.

Baylis, F. 1990. The ethics of ex utero research on spare "non-viable" IVF human embryos. *Bioethics, 4*, 311–329.

Beauchamp, T. and Childress, J.F. 1994. *Principles of bioethics*. New York: Oxford University Press.

Benner, P.A. 1994. Caring as a way of knowing and not knowing." In S. Philips and P.A. Benner (Eds.), *The crisis of care: Affirming and restoring caring practices in the helping professions* (pp. 42–62). Washington, D.C.: Georgetown University Press.

Benner, P.A., Tanner, C.A. and Chesla, C.A. 1996. *Expertise in nursing practice: Caring, clinical judgment and ethics*. New York: Springer.

Birnie, L.H. and Rodriguez, S. 1994. *Uncommon will: The death and life of Sue Rodriguez*. Toronto: Macmillan.

Boal, A. 1998. *Legislative theatre: Using performance to make politics*. London: Routledge.

Brody, H. 1987. *Stories of sickness*. New Haven, CT: Yale University Press.

Brody, H. 2003. *Stories of sickness*. 2nd edition. Oxford: Oxford University Press.

Brunger, F. and Cox, S.M. 2002. Ethics and genetics: The need for transparency. Available online: www.cwhn.ca/groups/biotech/availdocs/4-brun-cox.pdf

Buchanan, A., Brock, D.W., Daniels, N. and Wikler, D. 2000. *From chance to choice: Genetics and justice.* Cambridge, U.K.: Cambridge University Press.

Burrell, D. and Hauerwas, S. 1977. From system to story: An alternative pattern for rationality in ethics. In H.T. Engelhardt, Jr. and D. Callahan (Eds.), *Knowledge, value and belief.* Hastings-on-Hudson, NY: The Hastings Centre.

Canadian Broadcasting Corporation (CBC). 1998. *At the end of the day: The Sue Rodriguez story* (Film).

Chambers, T. 1994. The bioethicist as author: The medical ethics case as rhetorical device. *Literary Medicine, 13,* 60–78.

Chambers, T. 1997. What to expect from an ethics case (and what it expects from you). In H.L. Nelson (Ed.), *Stories and their limits: Narrative approaches to bioethics* (pp. 171–184). New York: Routledge.

Charon, R. 1994. Narrative contributions to medical ethics: Recognition, formulation, interpretation, and validation in the practice of the ethicist. In E.R. Dubose, R.P. Hamel and L.J. O'Connell (Eds.), *A matter of principles? Ferment in U.S. bioethics* (pp. 260–283). Valley Forge, PA: Trinity Press.

Charon, R. 1997. The ethical dimensions of literature: Henry James's *The Wings of the Dove.* In H.L. Nelson (Ed.), *Stories and their limits: Narrative approaches to bioethics* (pp. 91–112). New York: Routledge.

Charon, R. and Montello, M. (Eds.). 2002. *Stories matter: The role of narrative in medical ethics.* New York: Routledge.

Childress, J.F. 1997. Narrative(s) versus norm(s): A misplaced debate in bioethics. In H.L. Nelson (Ed.), *Stories and their limits: Narrative approaches to bioethics* (pp. 252–272). New York: Routledge.

Cox, S.M. 2003. Stories in decisions: How at-risk individuals decide to request predictive testing for Huntington Disease. *Qualitative Sociology, 26*(2), 257–280.

de Saint-Exupéry, A. 1943/1993. *The Little Prince.* San Diego: Harcourt Brace Jovanovich.

Denzin, N.K. 1997. *Interpretive ethnography: Ethnographic practices for the 21st century.* Thousand Oaks, CA: Sage.

Frank, A. 1991. *At the will of the body.* Boston: Houghton Mifflin.

Frank, A. 1995. *The wounded storyteller: Body, illness, and ethics.* Chicago: University of Chicago Press.

Freire, P. 1994. *Pedagogy of the oppressed.* New York: Continuum.

Freire, P. 1993. *Education for critical consciousness.* New York: Continuum.

Freire, P. 1995. *Pedagogy of hope: Reviving pedagogy of the oppressed.* New York: Continuum.

Geertz, C. 1973. *The interpretation of cultures.* New York: Basic.

Gordimer, N. 1999. Interview on CBC Radio.

Gray, R.E. and Sinding, C. 2003. *Standing ovation: Performing social science research about cancer.* Lanham, MD: AltaMira Press.

Gray, R.E., Sinding, C. and Fitch M. 2001. Navigating the social context of metastatic breast cancer: Reflections on a project linking research to drama. *Health, 5*(2), 233–248.

Griffin, J.H. 1961. *Black like me.* Boston: Houghton Mifflin.

Halpern, J. 2001. *From detached concern to empathy: Harmonizing medical practice.* New York: Oxford University Press.

Hawkins, A.H. 1997. Medical ethics and the epiphanic dimension of narrative. In H.L. Nelson (Ed.), *Stories and their limits: Narrative approaches to bioethics* (pp. 153–170). New York: Routledge.

Hébert, P.C. 1996. *Doing right: A practical guide to ethics for medical trainees and physicians.* Toronto: Oxford University Press.

Jones A.H. 1994. Literature as mirror or lamp? Commentary on literature, medical ethics, and "epiphanic knowledge." *Journal of Clinical Ethics, 5*(4), 340–341.

Jones, A.H. 1998. Narrative in medical ethics. In T. Greenhalgh and B. Hurwitz (Eds.), *Narrative-based medicine.*

Kenny, N.P. 1994. The ethics of care and the patient–physician relationship. *ANN RCPSC, 17*(6), 356–258.

Kohn, M., Donley, C. and Wear, D. 1992. *Literature and aging: An anthology.* Kent, OH: Kent State University Press.

Kuczewski, M. 1997. "Bioethics' consensus on method: Who could ask for anything more?" In H.L. Nelson (Ed.), *Stories and their limits: Narrative approaches to bioethics* (pp. 134–152). New York: Routledge.

Kuhl, D. 2002. *What dying people want: Lessons for living from people who are dying.* New York: Public Affairs.

Lenaghan, J. 1999. Involving the public in rationing decisions. The experience of citizens' juries. *Health Policy, 49*(1–2), 45–61.

MacIntyre, A.C. 1981. *After virtue: A study in moral theory.* Notre Dame, IN: Notre Dame University Press.

MacIntyre, A.C. 1988. *Whose justice? Which rationality?* Notre Dame, IN: Notre Dame University Press.

McCall, M.M. 2000. Performance ethnography: A brief history and some advice. In N.K. Denzin and Y. Lincoln (Eds.). *Handbook of Qualitative Research.* Second edition. Thousand Oaks, CA: Sage.

McLeod, C. 2002. *Self-trust and reproductive autonomy.* Cambridge, MA: MIT Press.

Montello, M. 1997. Narrative competence. In H.L. Nelson (Ed.), *Stories and their limits: Narrative approaches to bioethics* (pp. 185–197). New York: Routledge.

Murray, T.H. 1997. What do we mean by "narrative ethics?" In H.L. Nelson (Ed.), *Stories and their limits: Narrative approaches to bioethics* (pp. 3–17). New York: Routledge.

Nelson, H.L. 2001. *Damaged identities: Narrative repair.* New York: Cornell University Press.

Nisker, J.A. 1995. A user-friendly framework for exploration of ethical issues in reproductive medicine. *Association of Rep Rev, 5*(4), 272–279.

Nisker, J.A. 1997a. The yellow brick road of medical education. *Canadian Medical Association Journal, 156*(5), 689–691.

Nisker, J.A. 1997b. In quest of the perfect analogy for using in vitro fertilization patients as oocyte donors. *Womens Health Issues 7*(4), 241–247.

Nisker, J.A. 2001a. Chalcedonies. *Canadian Medical Association Journal, 164*(1), 74–75.

Nisker, J.A. 2001b. Orchids: Not necessarily a gospel. In *Mappa mundi: Mapping culture/mapping the world* (pp. 61–109).Windsor, ON: University of Windsor Press.

Nisker, J.A. 2003a. Philip. *Canadian Medical Association Journal, 168*, 746–747.

Nisker, J.A. 2003b. Rebuilding compassionate Canadian healthcare policy. *Journal of Obstet Gynaecol Can, 25*(1), 7–12.

Nisker, J.A. and Daar, A.S. 2003. Guiding principles for presentation of genetic-based narratives. *Submitted.*

Nixon, L.L. 1997. Medical humanities: Pyramids and rhomboids in the rationalist world of medicine. In H.L. Nelson (Ed.), *Stories and their limits* (pp. 238–272). New York: Routledge.

Nussbaum, M.C. 1990. *Love's knowledge: Essays on philosophy and literature.* New York: Oxford University Press.

Pendharkar, S. 2001. Seeking harmony: A medical student perspective on ethics education. Presented at the Royal College of Physicians and Surgeons of Canada Annual Meeting.

Phillips, S.S. 1994. Introduction. In S.S. Phillips and P. Benner (Eds.), *The crisis of care: Affirming and restoring caring practices in the helping professions.* Washington, D.C.: Georgetown University Press.

Quindlen, A. 1995. *One true thing.* New York: Dell.

Quindlen, A. 1998a. *Black and blue.* New York: Dell.

Quindlen, A. 1998b. Interview on *The Charlie Rose Show.*

Richler, D. 1999. The big life, with Daniel Richler. Canadian Broadcasting Corporation.

Rowe, G. and Frewer, L.J. 2000. Public participation methods: A framework for evaluation. *Science, Technology and Human Values, 25*(1), 3–29.

Rubin, J. 1996. Impediments to the development of clinical knowledge and ethical judgment in critical care nursing. In P.A Benner, C.A. Tanner and C.A. Chesla (Eds.), *Expertise in nursing practice: Caring, clinical judgment, and ethics* (pp. 170–192). New York: Springer.

Sherwin, S. 1994. Feminism, ethics, and cancer. *Humane Medicine, 10*(4), 282–290.

Smythe, W.E. and Murray, M.J. 2000. Owning the story: Ethical considerations in narrative research. *Ethics and Behavior, 10*(4), 311–336.

Solzhenitsyn, A. 1969. *Cancer ward.* New York: Bantam Books.

Spiro, H. 1996. *Empathy and the practice of medicine: Beyond pills and the scalpel.* New Haven, CT: Yale University Press.

Stein, J.G. 2001. *The cult of efficiency.* Toronto: Anansi.

Stewart, M.A., Weston, W.W., Brown, J.B., McWhinney, I.E., McWilliam C. and Freeman T.R. 1995. *Patient-centered medicine.* Thousand Oaks, CA: Sage.

Stewart, M.A. 2003 *Patient-centred medicine—Transforming the clinical method.* Second edition. Radcliffe Medical Press.

Strauss, A. and Corbin, J. 1994. Grounded theory methodology: An overview. In N.K. Denzin and Y.S. Lincoln (Eds.), *Handbook of qualitative research.* Thousand Oaks, CA: Sage.

Strauss, A. and Corbin, J. 1998. *Basics of qualitative research: Techniques and procedures of developing grounded theory.* Thousand Oaks, CA: Sage.

Thomasma, D.C. 1994. Beyond the ethics of rightness: The role of compassion in moral responsibility. In S.S. Philips and P.A. Benner (Eds.), *The crisis of care: Affirming and restoring caring practices in the helping professions* (pp. 123–143). Washington, D.C.: Georgetown University Press.

Weijer, C. 1997. Film and narrative in bioethics: Akira Kurosawa's *Ikuru.* In H.L. Nelson (Ed.), *Stories and their limits: Narrative approaches to bioethics* (pp. 113–122). New York: Routledge.

Whyte, W.H. 1956. *The organization man.* New York: Simon and Schuster.

Moral Horizons

Janet L. Storch
and Patricia Rodney

Almost every moment a nurse is confronted with the need to choose
between a greater or lesser good (Lanara 1981).

In Section III, we address areas that generate new and continuing challenges to our conceptions of health care ethics and nurs-
ing ethics. We also suggest ways in which nurses and other health providers can move
further forward in enhancing their enactment of ethical practice. We make no claim that
the chapters in this section encompass all the significant ethical concerns of present and
future. But we hope that they will stimulate more careful thinking about the many areas
in our lives to which we have not given sufficient attention in our scope of nursing
ethics, and, to some extent, in health care ethics in general. We believe that ethics provides "corrective vision"—in effect, a pair of new lenses—to help us see what we have
taken for granted and to prepare for what lies ahead.

In Chapter 15, Rosalie Starzomski leads off this section with her exploration of the
poorly charted course of biotechnology and nursing. Using xenotransplantation as her
exemplar, she shows us what nurses need to know to assist people to make difficult
choices and to be active and effective communicators in consultations with governments on public policy.

In Chapter 16, our often narrow thinking about ethics is exposed by Wendy Austin,
who draws our attention to global health challenges, including biotechnology. Austin
provides a "global picture" of health, uniting issues of poverty and conflict. She
reminds us about the importance of human rights—particularly a right to health care—
prior to her focus on the idea of a global ethic and a global moral community.

In Chapter 17, Kathleen Oberle and Janet Storch take up the issue of research ethics. Noting the marginalization of nurses in general research ethics literature and discourse, they recount the significant roles that *all* nurses have in the conduct of research involving human participants. From staff nurses who care for research subjects and carry out research protocols (e.g., by giving the required medications in a clinical trial); to nurses who serve as research assistants, co-ordinators, researchers, or research ethics board (REB) members; to nursing administrators who may be responsible for overseeing the REB, nurses play a vital role in health research. Oberle and Storch emphasize that nurses in all arenas need to be conversant with research ethics, and they lay out what knowledge is required.

In Chapter 18, using disability as an example, sociologist Susan Cox leads us through some of the "enduring moral questions" that must be addressed in genetic testing and screening. She suggests that nurses may not be prepared to deal with the ethical issues raised by genetics. Because nurses are well situated to play an important role, she urges us to become ethically fit to do so. She also challenges us to change our thinking about disability by seeing it as one form of diversity—that is, as one type among the many others that may be products of genetic makeup. She further urges us to distinguish between models of disability—the individual (medical) model and the social model.

The moral agency accorded to children is the substance of Franco Carnevale's Chapter 19, in which he offers rich narratives from his practice. Carnevale contrasts an "adult-centred" mode of construing the experiences of the child with a "child-centred" mode and shows the limitations of the former. Throughout the chapter he illustrates the clinical implications of a child's moral agency for nursing practice.

Writing on a topic largely excluded or marginalized by mainstream heath care ethics, in Chapter 20, Colleen Varcoe names violence against women as an ethical issue pertinent and central to health care. Her analysis of this particular issue is offered also with the intent to alert us to similar situations in which we might be involved in "othering" a person whom we perceive as different from us. By othering, we avoid dealing with an issue we believe could have nothing to do with us and our work. Varcoe implores us to strive to recognize our narrowness and to work to become more ethical in practice and more active in promoting ethical policy in the matter of violence against women and similar marginalized matters.

While the first six chapters in Moral Horizons point us to a diverse range of emerging challenges to ethical practice (and, hence, to inquiry in nursing ethics), the last four leave us with some promising new theoretical approaches. To return to the words of Joan Liaschenko that we cited in the introduction to the first section of the book, these last four chapters provide us with "a language that will enable us to sustain our patients and each other; that will serve as the vehicle for our ethical reflection; that will give voice to our ethical concerns" (Liaschenko 1993, 9).

In Chapter 21, Gweneth Doane calls for a more humanly involved ethics. Doane highlights the significance of nurses' moral identity and the embodied nature of ethics and ethical practice. She argues that since ethics is a deeply personal, embodied process, being and becoming a moral agent requires the cultivation of a mindful, critical awareness of and attunement to emotion and bodily experience. Per Nortvedt, a Norwegian nurse-philosopher, covers some related territory in Chapter 22. He elucidates how emotions overall are central to moral reasoning and moral behaviour in nursing. Nortvedt further suggests that moral sensitivity is highly essential to moral judgment and action in nursing and that this faculty in an important way is based on emotion. Finally, he explains how emotions play a significant role in moral judgments.

In Chapter 23, Jane Simington explores some interesting links between ethics and spirituality. She expands on present-day definitions of spirituality, calling for care providers to more courageously and effectively meet their ethical obligations. Overall, Simington's purpose in writing this chapter is to support the new ethic of an evolving spirituality.

Section III: Moral Horizons closes with Chapter 24, by Vangie Bergum. The focus of this chapter is relationship itself—which, Bergum argues, is the space where nurse and patient make connection. In this chapter, Bergum works from the assumption that all relationships as experienced are moral, for in each relationship we are enacting the question of what is the "right thing to do," both with ourselves and with others. With the use of a powerful narrative that threads through the chapter, Bergum focuses on a number of themes that she identifies as useful in increasing understanding and development of a relational ethic.

The location of Bergum's chapter at the end of Section III is purposeful on our (the Editors') part. We believe that it captures an important essence that has reverberated in different ways throughout the text. Nursing ethics can greatly benefit from—and has substantial contributions to make to—relational ethics.

REFERENCES

Lanara, V. 1981. *Heroism as a nursing value: A philosophical perspective.* Athens, GA: Sisterhood Evniki.

Liaschenko, J. 1993. *Faithful to the good: Morality and philosophy in nursing practice.* Unpublished doctoral dissertation. University of California, San Francisco.

chapter fifteen

The Biotechnology Revolution— A Brave New World? The Ethical Challenges of Xenotransplantation

Rosalie Starzomski

Men have become the tools of their tools.

—Henry David Thoreau[1]

The 21st century is developing into the century of **biotechnology,** the application of science and engineering to the use of living organisms or their constituent parts (Dhanda 2002; Rollin 2003). As the century unfolds, we find ourselves in the midst of a profound revolution in biotechnology—a revolution that is radically altering our view of who we are as human beings as well as our conceptions of health and health care. Banting and Best first discovered insulin for the treatment of diabetes in Canada in 1921, thereby launching the field of biotechnology.[2] However, it is only in the last few decades that we have seen the "biotech" industry emerge as the cutting-edge industry[3] of the new century. In 2003, we mark 50 years since Watson and Crick solved the mysteries of DNA (Lemonick 2003), a period during which remarkable strides have been made as a result of the historic discoveries in biotechnology. For instance, the identification of the human genome and the breakthroughs that have arisen in the world of genetics have resulted in significant changes regarding how we think about disease and disability (see Chapter 18; Sherwin 2000). In addition, we are faced with a myriad of new health care technologies emerging from research in such areas as human reproduction, stem cells, cloning, xenotransplantation, and nanotechnology.[4] The implications of this biotechnological reframing are vast. Today, developments are occurring at such a rapid rate that there is often insufficient discussion about the ethical and societal implications of the scientific advancements being made. Indeed, before the last half of the 20th century, few people paid much attention to these implications (Midgely 2000; Wiseman, Vanderkop and Nef 1991).

Sometimes it appears that, as a society, we are prepared "to boldly go where no one has gone before" (as described in the science fiction television program *Star Trek*), often with minimal critique of the direction in which we are moving. However, whereas each episode of *Star Trek* provided opportunities for the show's writers and actors to examine the moral dimensions of a featured technological "wonder," as a society, we have not always reviewed the social and ethical consequences of biotechnological developments prior to their implementation. Consequently, the diffusion of new technology into the health care system continues to be haphazard at best (Boyle and Callahan 1992; Deber 1992; Fox and Swazey 1992a; 1992b; Reiser 1992; Rettig 1989).

My goal in this chapter is to review the technology of xenotransplantation as an illustration of biotechnology development and to examine several of the ethical and societal challenges that are often pushed to the margins as we "boldly go where no one has gone before." **Xenotransplantation,** the transfer of living cells, tissues, or organs from one species to another for medical purposes, has arisen as one solution to increase the number of organs available for transplantation (Bloom et al. 1999; Canadian Public Health Association 2001; Platt 1997). Many of the issues, concerns, and troublesome questions that emerge in the debate about whether to allow xenotransplantation to become part of the therapeutic armamentarium to treat end-stage organ failure are also evident in other domains of biotechnology development. In what follows, I offer some approaches to advancing the dialogue and debate about the ethical and societal concerns that are emerging as part of the discussion about biotechnology, particularly strategies to enhance nursing leadership in the area. Although the focus of this chapter will be on reviewing developments in Canada, I also briefly examine several international issues and challenges.

BIOTECHNOLOGY—PROMISES AND PITFALLS

Biotechnology changes come in many forms (for example, the new developments in human genetics described in Chapter 18), and most share common features with respect to ethics. These include a rapid proliferation of the technology, corporate involvement in development and diffusion of the innovations, public pressure to make the biotechnology available, scientific progress with uncertainty, and inadequate attention to societal values.

Even though there may be little question that, generally, the capabilities and promises of biotechnology may be of benefit to society, there are concerns about the consequences of biotechnological innovation. For example, the serious worldwide public health crisis brought about by the outbreak of Severe Acute Respiratory Syndrome (SARS) and the recent news that a case of Bovine Spongiform Encephalopathy (BSE) (Mad Cow Disease) has been found in a cow in Canada[5] have fuelled fears about biotechnology and the crossover of viruses and other pathogens from animals and birds to humans (Health Canada 2003a; 2003b). These developments have resulted in more emphasis being placed on the need for extensive societal discussion about the use of new technologies prior to their implementation.

Technological development and decisions about how to use new technology have largely been under the control of so-called "experts," including researchers, governments, vested interest groups, as well as corporations, and have been highly politicized (Goodman 1992; Hadorn 1991; Rettig 1989; Yeo 1996). Today, there is widespread sentiment among a number of authors that societal input is required to debate the ethical issues that have surfaced in regard to biotechnology, not only to make decisions about what type of research ought to be pursued, but also to develop coherent public policy about the application of the innovations that emerge from the research. The call for public involvement about biotechnology policy and research comes from many sectors (Brunger and Cox 2000; Canadian Nurses Association 2002a; Health Canada 1997; Sherwin 2000; Sykes, d'Apice and Sandrin 2003) and has been a theme in health care system reviews as well as in meetings to discuss biotechnology (Canadian Public Health Association 2001; Commission on the Future of Health Care in Canada 2002; National Forum on Health 1997; "Proceed with care" 1993; Sherwin 2000). Interestingly, although support exists for the idea that decisions about the research, use, and outcomes of biotechnology have major implications for society, input from members of the public[6] has not always been sought. Further, in addition to the pivotal role members of the public could hold in determining the future direction for biotechnology, a substantial role is available for health care providers, such as nurses, not only to understand the ethical and societal concerns that surround the technology, but also to become involved in the ongoing debate about the manner in which to proceed with specific innovations (Barnard 1997; 2002; Broughton 2001; Canadian Nurses Association 1992; 1995; Marck 2000a; 2000b).

Public and health care provider involvement in decision-making about biotechnology is paramount in order to ensure that important societal values and expert knowledge are infused throughout the decision-making process. To illustrate how this can and should occur, I now turn to a discussion of the perplexing ethical and societal implications of biotechnology. Using xenotransplantation as an illustrative case, I first provide an Ethics in Practice narrative to contextualize the discussion. I then move on to review developments in the area and the benefits and concerns linked to the technology, especially as they apply to pathogen transmission and informed consent. Further, I elaborate on some of the challenges that arise in regard to corporate and regulatory issues related to xenotransplantation. I conclude with a discussion about public participation in biotechnology policy development and provide an example of a comprehensive approach used when attempting to obtain citizen input into whether Canada should proceed with xenotransplantation.

XENOTRANSPLANTATION: AN ILLUSTRATION OF THE BENEFITS AND CHALLENGES OF BIOTECHNOLOGY

Ethics in Practice 15-1	**Advice about Xenotransplantation**

Maria is an advanced practice nurse working within the transplant program in an urban quaternary care hospital. She, with other members of the trans-

plant team, is responsible for the assessment, education, and support of potential kidney transplant recipients. One of her patients, Paul, is a 47-year-old married teacher and father of two adult children. Paul has been receiving hemodialysis for five years and has been on the transplant waiting list for over three years. Maria has met with Paul and his family several times and has developed a trusting relationship with them. Unfortunately, Paul has developed a number of complications from his chronic renal failure, including a severe peripheral neuropathy. He has exhausted all possibility of receiving an organ from a living donor, as the friends and family members who have been tested are not compatible donors. He has been unsuccessful in obtaining an organ from a non-living donor, partly because he has a high level of panel-reactive antibodies, and with the waiting list growing and the number of organs available for transplantation decreasing, Paul realizes he could be waiting for some time to receive a kidney transplant. Paul's only daughter is being married in several months and he does not believe he will survive to attend her wedding and walk her down the aisle. He is quite despondent and is feeling absolutely desperate about obtaining a transplant. He has even considered going to a developing country to buy a kidney on the black market, but cannot afford the cost. Recently, he has heard that xenotransplant human clinical trials are being conducted in some countries, and he wants to be a volunteer. Paul's wife does not support the idea as she is concerned about what could happen to him, and she is also worried about the transmission of viruses to her and her children if he follows through with his idea. Paul's good friend and neighbour has also heard about the idea and believes that Paul is being irresponsible and putting his whole community at risk. Since Maria has been instrumental in helping Paul to make health care decisions in the past, he has approached her for advice about his idea. He also wants her to help him find a way to be a subject in a xenotransplant clinical trial in another country.

In this scenario, Maria is confronted with a variety of questions. How is she to advise Paul? How can she ensure that Paul has the information required to make an informed choice about xenotransplantation? What are the benefits and risks associated with xenotransplantation? What are her responsibilities as an advanced practice nurse in ensuring that patients and families in her care understand the risks, benefits, and implications of new technologies such as xenotransplantation? What are her responsibilities to the community regarding biotechnological innovations within the realm of her practice? In the sections that follow, I review several of the ethical and societal issues related to xenotransplantation emanating from Ethics in Practice 15-1. Further, by addressing the questions posed above, I will uncover ways in which Maria can demonstrate nursing leadership in the area of biotechnology.

Ethical and Societal Implications in the Development of Xenotransplantation

Organ, tissue, and cell transplantation have progressed from being impossible to becoming commonplace, with over one million people worldwide benefitting from organ transplants alone in the last 50 years (Alexander 1962; Bailey 1990; Murray 1992). With this success comes an increased demand for donor organs and a severe organ shortage, resulting in a growing number of individuals worldwide who die while waiting for suitable organs to become available[7] (Federal/Provincial Advisory Committee on Health Services 1996; House of Commons Standing Committee on Health 1999; Molzahn, Starzomski and McCormick 2003).

Xenotransplantation[8] has been proposed as one way to alleviate the shortage of organs, tissues, and cells available from non-living donors and to reduce the need for living humans to donate organs (a surgical process that is not without risk) (Land 1989). Significant ethical and societal implications of biotechnology are reflected in the debates that have surfaced around xenotransplant technology—debates that raise fundamental questions about social justice, informed consent, our relationships with one another as humans, our relationships with other species, the role of corporations, and the role of expert and public stakeholders in making decisions about biotechnology development and implementation (Caplan 1992; Canadian Public Health Association 2001; Daar and Phil 1997; National Kidney Foundation 1995; Nuffield Council on Bioethics 1996; Singer 1992).

The science of xenotransplantation has evolved over the past two decades, spurred on by major developments in genetics, and has transformed xenotransplantation from an area only being researched to one that is clinically feasible (Bach et al. 1998; Platt 1997; Reemtsma 1992). Other potential solutions to ameliorate the organ shortage, such as the use of organs and tissues engineered from stem cells, may be options to increase the number of organs, tissues, and cells for transplantation, but the solution closest to clinical application is likely to be xenotransplantation. Although xenotransplantation has the potential to supply cells to treat such disorders as Parkinson's disease and diabetes and to supply tissues such as skin and bone for transplant purposes (Canadian Public Health Association 2001; Council of Europe 2003), my emphasis in this chapter will be on the use of xenotransplantation in the field of **solid organ transplantation.** Further, while xenotransplantation can occur between animal species, I will be centering my review on transplantation of organs from animals to humans.

A major problem in the clinical application of xenotransplantation has been finding a suitable source animal from which to retrieve organs that will not be rejected by the human recipient (Platt 1997; Reemsta 1992). In the early days of xenotransplantation, the source animals were generally nonhuman primates. An example of such a case was that of newborn Baby Fae, one of the first humans to receive a **xenograft.** The case received much media attention in 1984 when Baby Fae received a heart transplant from a baboon to treat a condition often fatal in the first days of life called hypoplastic left heart syndrome—a condition in which her left atrium and ventricle were seriously underdeveloped. She died a few weeks post-transplant amid considerable controversy about the cause of her death since her heart did not show evidence of cellular rejection (McCormick 1985; National Institutes of Health 1985; Veatch 2000). Nonetheless, in the midst of the analysis and disputes after her death, xenotransplantation trials in humans were stalled because of the concerns related to possible organ rejection.

Currently, nonhuman primates have largely been removed from consideration as source animals for xenotransplantation, partly because of the high risk of unknown infections being transmitted from them to humans, as demonstrated by the HIV pandemic (Allan 1996). Major animal rights concerns exist regarding the use of nonhuman primates for research because of the close genetic link of these animals to humans (Singer 1992). Also, their long gestation period raises concern that insufficient numbers of animals would be bred to meet the need for organs (Allan 1996; Council of Europe 2003).

The current source animals of choice for xenotransplantation are transgenic pigs. Source animals, such as pigs, can be altered by genetic engineering to minimize rejection, thus optimizing organ function and providing potential advantages to the recipient. While some risks are reduced with the use of pigs as source animals (because of their greater phylogenetic distance from humans and the ability to breed them quickly in pathogen-free, closed environments), the risks associated with unknown infectious agents cannot be quantitatively assessed (Allan 1997; 1998; Fishman 1997). Most clinical developments in xenotransplantation have been in the area of cell transplantation, and there is growing emphasis on developing xenotransplant technology for solid organ transplantation. Because of the technological difficulties, few solid organ xenografts have been conducted worldwide. Most of the transplants done to date were for short-term bridging purposes—that is, while critically ill human recipients waited for human organs to become available (Council of Europe 2003).

This situation is rapidly changing, however, as scientific developments in the area of xenotransplantation are accelerating. It is now possible to clone pigs, and scientists are altering genetic systems in order to reproduce litters of piglets with organs that the human immune system will not reject. Recent developments—like the announcement by PPL Therapeutics that further to their cloning of the world's first piglets, they have now cloned a pig and "knocked out" a specific gene that has been implicated in transplant rejection—have moved the possibility of successful xenotransplantation closer to reality (Frankish 2002; "Xenotransplant news" 2003). As a result of the speed at which the science is moving, most countries in the world are embroiled in some way or another in attempting to develop an appropriate regulatory framework for xenotransplant human clinical trials and the therapeutic application of the technology, a topic I will take up later in this chapter.

Natural Law

Xenotransplantation, similar to other types of biotechnological innovation, is the focus of much controversy and debate, raising complex ethical, social, legal, and economic issues (Daar and Phil 1997; Health Canada 1997; Sykes, d'Apice and Sandrin 2003). The issues raised by xenotransplantation reflect the diversity of values, beliefs, and attitudes held by members of society about vital questions regarding who we are as humans and our role in the natural ecological order of our planet. Such questions are also important when discussing other forms of biotechnology such as genetics, stem cell research, cloning, and nanotechnology.

Societal beliefs, attitudes, and values about the nature of xenotransplantation are quite diverse. Some opponents of xenotransplantation suggest that the technology raises a problem of natural law because the intermixing of biological material from different species violates fundamental morality, impacting directly on who we are as humans (Canadian Public Health Association 2001; Veatch 2000). Some who support xenotransplantation propose that although the transplantation of organs from one species to another is cause for concern at first, it does not involve any more of a violation of natural law than does transplantation of an organ from one person to another, as long as the animal is treated with respect (Canadian Public Health Association 2001; Veatch 2000).

This diversity of societal opinion about the nature of xenotransplantation was clearly articulated by participants in a study I conducted, in which focus groups were held with 34 consumer and health care provider groups to determine their attitudes and beliefs about a number of ethical issues related to organ transplantation, including xenotransplantation (Starzomski 1997). One critical care nurse expressed her concern about xenotransplantation when she said,

> I'm a Christian, and I feel that death all along is natural; we are not immortal, and I see it as the final course of life, isn't it? And that's why, when you mentioned the pigs, I go no way! Because that is going to the mad scientist stage, and it's just beyond [imagination].

Providing a different view, an advanced practice nurse said,

> I would support it [xenotransplantation] as long as we are using, in real valued things, a lower-order animal like a pig (and I think there is still enough research done to know they already are lower-order animals) versus finding out later that they are actually smarter than we are, like the whales kind of thing. So, if there were some scientific assurances that that is the case then somehow I could bring myself to accept that.

One member of a group of reporters said,

> It sounds like a good idea, we eat them [animals] anyway, so we're not that sentimental about them. I wouldn't like to see them terribly exploited, but we exploit all over the place.

These opinions, generated by reflection on personal values, underscore several of the germane concerns related to xenotransplantation. In the next section, I will further explore many of the issues that have been raised in the discussion about biotechnology as I present a review of some of the benefits and concerns related to xenotransplantation.

Benefits and Challenges of Xenotransplantation

Although xenotransplantation has the potential to benefit many people, a number of societal and ethical concerns must be addressed if this technology is to move forward in a manner that optimizes its potential to benefit people while at the same time minimizing risk. In what follows, I will review the major benefits of xenotransplantation and discuss some of the potential problems that work against these benefits. Given the limited scope of this chapter, I will not address one of the concerns raised by xenotransplantation—that is, the rights of the animals who will be the donors if xenotransplantation becomes a reality (Canadian Public Health Association 2001; Singer 1992). For readers who wish more information about this topic, I include material in the endnotes that provides further background with respect to the animal rights challenges related to xenotransplantation.[9]

POTENTIAL BENEFITS OF XENOTRANSPLANTATION

Many potential benefits have been identified if xenotransplantation were to become a therapeutic treatment for end-stage organ failure. These include the following:

- The potential exists to eliminate the shortage of organs, tissues, and cells, as facilities would be established to produce pigs to serve as sources that would be available when required.
- In some jurisdictions where human organ donation has not been accepted because of ethical or ethnocultural concerns, xenotransplantation might provide an acceptable alternative.

- With ready access to organs, recipient selection criteria could be broadened, and the current ethical dilemma surrounding transplant allocation would disappear as, theoretically, everyone who needed an organ would be transplanted.
- Xenografts could be conducted in an early, controlled fashion before the ravages of disease affected patients.
- Xenografts could offer advantages similar to those associated with the use of human living donor organs. For example, the transplant surgery could be pre-scheduled; pretreatment of recipients would be possible; the quality of the organs would be known; the organs would be out of the body for a limited amount of time, thereby preventing rejection; and the effects of brain death on organ quality could be avoided.
- Finally, xenografts might not be susceptible to the human autoimmune diseases or viral infections that caused organ failure initially and which often limit the survival of organ transplants from human donors (Council of Europe 2003; Platt 1997; Sykes, d'Apice, and Sandrin 2003, 195).

This review of the possible benefits of xenotransplantation shows that biotechnology has the *potential* to provide therapeutic advantages in health care delivery. Similarities to the benefits described above exist for other biotechnologies. For instance, successful gene therapy and cloning technology could make available treatments that are tailored to an individual's genetic profile, thus preventing further disease and disability.

Although xenotransplantation offers benefits, a number of scientific and ethical barriers exist that must be addressed to ensure that advances in biotechnology are developed in a manner that optimizes potential to benefit society and minimizes risk (Daar and Phil 1997; Sykes, d'Apice and Sandrin 2003). In the sections that follow, I will review some of the risks and concerns as they relate to xenotransplantation, recognizing that comparable challenges are evident in other areas of biotechnology development.

RISK OF PATHOGEN TRANSMISSION

One of the significant societal and ethical concerns involved in xenotransplantation is the worry about the risk of transmission of animal pathogens to humans and the subsequent consequences for society. As with all mammals, pigs have viruses that are active, latent, or represented only by a partial genetic sequence embedded in the pig genome. It is difficult to assign exact numbers to the risk, but many experts agree that it is possible that pig endogenous retroviruses (PERVs) could be transmitted to human xenograft recipients (Bach and Ivinson 2002; Fishman 1997; Muir and Griffin 2001). The possibility has arisen that, under specific conditions, PERVs can infect human cells and be carried in tissue that is transplanted. Because PERVs could be transmitted to human xenograft recipients, it is further possible that such infections could be passed from recipients to other humans, and to society at large. Some authors have indicated that these fears are not unfounded by suggesting that current technology in antibody screening for potential xenozoonoses is fraught with problems and is in need of further study (Bach and Ivinson 2002; Dillner 1996; Michaels et al. 1994; Muir and Griffin 2001). Although investigators disagree about the magnitude of the risk, few dismiss it and many agree that it is sufficient to merit very serious concern (Dinsmore et al. 2000; Fishman 1997; Gunzburg and Salmons 2000; Muir and Griffin 2001).

Further complicating the issue of disease transmission is the reality that if researchers were aware of a particular virus or pathogen, they might be able to develop a test to determine if the pathogen was present. However, if it were a pathogen that had not yet been recognized, it would be impossible to determine if an animal were pathogen free (Sykes, d'Apice and Sandrin 2003). This is a very serious concern as precedents exist for the survival, replication, and spread of animal viruses to humans with subsequent human-to-human transmission. For example, some scientists believe that HIV may have originated in monkeys before spreading to humans (Allan 1996). And some epidemiologists believe that the Spanish Flu that killed close to 50 million people worldwide in the early part of the 20th century might have been triggered by swine flu. It is also thought that the influenza virus that struck Hong Kong in 1997 was spread from ducks to chickens to humans, killing 18 people. Experts indicate that if the outbreak had not been stopped in time, it would have caused a pandemic (Evanson 2000). Other situations linked to the jump of pathogens from animals to humans include the Ebola and Lassa fever outbreaks in Africa (Muir and Griffin 2001). Clearly, many gaps exist in our knowledge of the potential risks of disease transmission if xenotransplantation were to become a reality. Risks cannot be eliminated based on current evidence, and the uncertainty about the safety of xenotransplantation continues to be a significant obstacle to its implementation. Cloning and genetic modification techniques to address disease transmission are still in their early stages. Further scientific information may close the gap somewhat, but it will never be possible to say with absolute certainty that the risk is absent. Xenotransplantation falls into the category of experimental treatment. Although the risk is perhaps low and the benefits to humans substantial, the consequences for humanity could be catastrophic (Bach and Ivinson 2002; Fishman 1997; Muir and Griffin 2001). As one consumer in my 1997 study said:

> You know at this point, I think [xenografting is] a good idea, but where will it lead? I'm not sure, and I don't think any of us know where DNA manipulation is going to lead. It could be really scary stuff, and we need the answers to the questions, I suppose, to think about it at this point. I worry about the transmission of disease. What will happen to our world if we get another bug like HIV?

CONCERNS ABOUT INFORMED CONSENT

The tension between individual and societal rights is part of the difficult ethical debate about xenotransplantation. While subjects often accept risks arising from experimental treatment, believing them to be balanced by the potential benefits, one important distinction between xenotransplantation and other treatments is that xenotransplantation may put individuals other than the recipient at risk of contracting disease.

The concept of informed consent for individual patients is a central principle in Western health care delivery. When faced with health care decisions, the patient is informed of the various alternatives for treatment and the relative risks and benefits of each option. Given that the science in the area of xenotransplantation does not answer all the questions about possible risks, a potential patient would be put in a very difficult situation if he or she were considering being a participant in a clinical trial (Bach and Ivinson 2002).

As evident in Ethics in Practice 15-1, the risk is not restricted to the individual who is receiving the xenotransplant, but is also of concern to close contacts, family members, and indeed the community at large. Xenotransplantation raises the problematic challenge of applying the principle of informed consent to an entire community since the community as a whole would be potentially exposed to the risk (Bach and Ivinson 2002). In the situation in Ethics in Practice 15-1, Maria, the advanced practice nurse, will have to ensure that Paul has information about the risks of xenotransplantation and, as part of her responsibility, ensure that information is conveyed to Paul's family as well. To gain support in this work, Maria could access information about xenotransplantation, such as national standards and guidelines, and help to explain and interpret these to Paul and his family (Health Canada 1999; Sykes, d'Apice, and Sandrin 2003). Even though Paul is not currently enrolled in a clinical trial, Maria might find it useful to review information available about the role of the nurse in research (as described in Chapter 17) to help her determine what she could and should convey to Paul and his family.

But what of the larger community? What is Maria's responsibility to it? Viruses, and other infectious agents, do not respect national borders. The 2003 cases of SARS and BSE have made that evident. Along with other health care providers and health care researchers, nurses in leadership roles have a responsibility to ensure that information about issues such as xenotransplantation, genetics, cloning, and new reproductive technologies that are within the realm of their practice are discussed in the community. Further, it is essential that informed representatives of the public are given an opportunity to participate actively and meaningfully in the decisions about whether and under what conditions society is exposed to the risks associated with this and other biotechnological developments. If it is unethical to impose a health care risk on a patient, it is also unethical to expose the public to a risk without first considering societal opinion (Bach and Ivinson 2002). Strategies for nurses to become involved in the community at large in order to facilitate discussion about biotechnological advances will be discussed in more detail later in this chapter.

CORPORATE INFLUENCES

Xenotransplantation is big business, and it poses challenging problems from the perspective of business and corporate ethics. The economic implications are considerable, and many pressures are brought to bear by stakeholders for whom these considerations are at the forefront (Bach and Ivinson 2002; Nicholson 1996). For example, the U.S. organ and tissue transplant market will be worth 20 billion dollars by 2007, thus providing a huge potential market for biotechnology companies. Many companies have invested heavily in xenotransplantation and are eager to see their investment pay off ("Xenotransplant news" 2003).[10]

When considering the diffusion of new biotechnologies, it is important to ask questions about who is likely to benefit from the various types of biotechnology and who is likely to suffer from them (Sherwin 2000). When thinking about biotechnology, wealth can be seen as a benefit and poverty, a risk. It remains to be seen whether or not xenotransplantation and other technologies, such as gene therapies, will be accessible to the poor and disadvantaged. In the past, pharmaceutical and medical technologies have been readily available in the Western world but not accessible to the world's 50 poorest countries, which are inhabited by 75 percent of the world's population. Furthermore, issues regarding conflict of interest and research ethics have impacted on how companies choose to study new technologies and make them available globally (Baird 2003; Bodenheimer 2000; Neufeld et al. 2001).

Recently, because Western governments have been unwilling to approve xenotransplant clinical trials in their countries, corporations have moved to less regulated jurisdictions, such as Mexico and the Cook Islands, to pursue research and potential human clinical trials, raising the real concern of possible exploitation of research subjects in these less affluent countries. In addition, these jurisdictions do not have appropriate regulatory authorities to develop and maintain suitable guidelines to safeguard the patients and their contacts (BBC World 2002; Reuters Health 2002).

Moreover, it could be argued that in developing countries, biotechnology research is inappropriate when people are living without the basics of preventive care, maternal and child health services, and other fundamental health care needs (Veatch 2000). Although further discussion of resource allocation is beyond the scope of this chapter, see Chapter 4 for a review of the concept of justice and Chapter 16 for an in-depth discussion of globalization and health.

Another challenging problem that falls within the corporate realm is the lack of access to data from international clinical trials of xenotransplantation. Usually, such data, and any adverse reactions resulting from treatment, is confidential, and may only be made public at the discretion of the sponsor, something that generally only happens if positive outcomes are observed.

Corporate issues and concerns must be part of the public debate about biotechnology, and there is a need for members of the public and health care providers to work together with corporations to ensure that they are able to meet their ethical and social responsibilities (Dhanda 2002). Shareholders and society as a whole must hold corporations accountable in future work related to xenotransplantation as well as innovations coming from areas such as stem cells, cloning, nanotechnology, and genetic research.

REGULATORY CONCERNS

There are a variety of approaches used to regulate xenotransplantation research in different jurisdictions around the world (Council of Europe 2003). In Canada, xenotransplantation studies are currently being carried out using laboratory animals only. These pre-clinical or experimental trials do not involve human patients and are not regulated by Health Canada. Xenotransplants are considered therapeutic products and can only be used in clinical trials if authorized by Health Canada. A request to conduct clinical trials could be submitted to Health Canada at any time (Canadian Public Health Association 2001; Health Canada 1999). For Health Canada, one of the principles guiding the identification and evaluation of risks related to xenotransplantation has been the government of Canada's proposed precautionary approach or principle. This is an approach used to manage threats of serious or irreversible harm when there is scientific uncertainty, recognizing that full scientific certainty will not be used as a reason to postpone decisions when faced with the threat of serious or irreversible harm ("A Canadian perspective on the precautionary approach/principle" 2001).

In the United States, xenotransplant human clinical trials are approved and are tightly controlled. As a result, all experiments using animal tissues must be cleared through the Food and Drug Administration (FDA). The FDA has also banned xenotransplant recipients from donating blood because of the infection risk. As scientific knowledge about xenotransplantation increases, there is no consistency across the world about the status of xenotransplantation or how regulatory frameworks are developed and implemented. In January 1999, the Parliamentary Assembly of the Council of Europe called for a worldwide moratorium on xenotransplantation until the technology could be evaluated and guidelines could be established. However, countries worldwide have implemented a wide range of decisions about xenotransplantation research and clinical trials, including outright bans, moratoriums, and more relaxed safety rules (Council of Europe 2003; Dillner 1996). For example, clinical trials and folk treatments using xenotransplantation are being offered in Mexico under weak safety rules that could open the door for "international xenotourism," in which desperate patients bypass tight regulations in some developed countries by going to less developed ones for the surgeries, an option discussed in Ethics in Practice 15-1 (Council of Europe 2003; Reuters Health 2002).

The Ethics Committee of the International Xenotransplant Association has suggested that trials on humans should only be performed with oversight from a governmental regulatory agency with guidelines similar to those developed by the agencies in some Western countries. The committee proposes that the trials should include information about the source animals as well as monitoring procedures for xenotransplant research subjects and, where deemed appropriate, their close contacts. In addition, the group suggests the development of a national repository for holding specimens from human subjects in countries in which clinical trials are conducted and, if a repository is not possible, then specimens should be properly obtained, tracked, analyzed, and stored. The committee goes on to recommend that in the absence of such oversight and monitoring, clinical xenotransplantation should not occur. The committee proposes that the International Xenotransplant Association take leadership in facilitating the development of universally accepted procedures, standards, and guidelines about xenotransplantation since many countries around the world are beginning xenotransplant programs. Like others involved in xenotransplantation, the committee raises the concern that without such co-operation, efforts of countries to minimize the potential risks may be jeopardized as possible recipients travel from countries with regulation to those without for the purpose of undergoing xenotransplantation. In addition, the committee also raises concern about the potential entry of individuals (or their close contacts) who have received a xenotransplant in a country without regulatory guidelines into other countries (Sykes, d'Apice, and Sandrin 2003, 201–202).

Although the issues discussed here are focused on xenotransplantation, they are also applicable to other biotechnologies such as cloning, gene therapy, and stem cell research, in which similar regulations are required and are being discussed. Clearly, decisions about biotechnology require broad societal discussion and debate.

Opening Pandora's Box: Public Participation in Decisions about Xenotransplantation

I have previously made the argument that members of the public are often overlooked as participants in the discussions about biotechnology. And I suggested that in order to ensure that the required values and perspectives are represented, multiple voices are needed in the debate about biotechnology, with a prominent position for members of the public. The idea of public and health care provider involvement in decision-making is supported, but how can it happen in reality? Winner (1993), for example, supports broad involvement in decision-making about technology but points out that there is no moral community or public space in which technological issues are topics for deliberation and common action.

Brunger and Cox (2002), in their discussion about genetics and ethics, suggest strategies for widening the space of public debate about technology, including providing the public with information about the production, distribution, and application of knowledge; legitimizing lay knowledge; attending to a multiplicity of voices; welcoming dissent as a sign that all voices are being heard; allowing the debate to be transparent in public; and promoting the accountability of government, industry, and science to the public (4). Other authors have proposed several conditions that must be met for meaningful public participation to occur in health care decision-making, including assuring that consumers have adequate information; that there are a majority of consumers in the group; that there is a strong mandate from the community with formal and informal access to constituents; and that people selected to represent communities have strong personalities so that they will not be intimidated or dominated by the so-called experts within the group (Blue et al. 1999; Charles and DeMaio 1993; Eyles 1993; Jennings 1991; Lenaghan 1999; Lomas and Veenstra 1995; O'Neill 1992; Starzomski 1997, 2002). What follows is a description of a comprehensive public consultation process in which these strategies were evident in the discussion about whether Canada should proceed with xenotransplantation and, if so, under what conditions.

As part of efforts to hear the views and concerns of Canadians about xenotransplantation, Health Canada provided funding to the Canadian Public Health Association (CPHA) to strike a Public Advisory Group (PAG) to conduct an arm's length public consultation. The PAG was given the task of reporting back to the Minister of Health with recommendations about whether Canada should proceed with xenotransplantation. Members of the PAG represented a diversity of perspectives, regions, and interests. The process they designed included several options for Canadians to voice their opinions, including a telephone survey of 1519 randomly selected adults; opportunities to submit letters, faxes, and e-mails to the CPHA office and website; a "have your say" questionnaire (which was located on the CPHA website and also mailed to 3700 organizations); and regional citizen forums (sometimes also called citizen juries) of between 15–23 demographically representative citizens held in six cities across Canada. The forums were moderated by a professional facilitator and included opportunities for panelists to have discussions with experts and review resource material in the area of xenotransplantation. In addition, during each forum, prior to the private panelists meeting, time was allocated for members of the general public to participate (Canadian Public Health Association 2001).

Before the two-and-a-half-day forums were held, the members of the citizen juries were asked to complete a questionnaire to determine their attitudes and beliefs about xenotransplantation. Many participants held a positive view, but after discussing the risks and concerns during the forums, the majority changed their thinking, concluding that Canada should not proceed with xenotransplantation at this time: 34 percent said no, 19 percent said no with qualifications; and 46 percent said yes with qualifications. It appeared from these results that the more Canadians learned about xenotransplantation, the more concerned they became. Although not absolutely opposed to xenotransplantation, the forum participants favoured a precautionary approach, expressing concerns about uncertain health risks, an insufficient level of scientific knowledge in the area of xenotransplantation, and inadequate regulations (Canadian Public Health Association 2001; Wharry 2002).

In contrast to the citizen jury experience, in the telephone survey of 1519 Canadian adults, 70 percent were not very, or not at all, knowledgeable about xenotransplantation and yet, of this number, 65 percent supported clinical trials. These findings must be interpreted cautiously and illustrate some of the problems that occur when public opinion polls (where participants have little data about the issues) are used to solicit information about complex areas such as xenotransplantation. The final report of the PAG (Canadian Public Health Association 2001) describes the results of the complete public consultation process; it was delivered to the Minister of Health and subsequently released publicly in January 2002. The report does not close the door on xenotransplantation, but rather calls for more research into potential risks, suggesting that those who wish to proceed with xenotransplantation need to determine the level of risk and demonstrate how the benefits of the procedure would outweigh those risks. In addition, among the recommendations, the report suggests that pre-clinical research that does not involve humans, but which could provide more information about the viability of xenotransplantation, should occur. There is also a call for more stringent and transparent legislation and regulations covering all aspects of xenotransplant clinical trials. Further, it is recommended that Health Canada consider alternatives, such as disease prevention, the development of mechanical substitutes, and pursuit of stem cell research to expand the human donor pool. Finally, the report suggests that efforts should continue to further the knowledge and public discussion of xenotransplantation and that the citizen forum model be considered for future consultations on complex and not widely understood policy issues.

The consultation process described here for xenotransplantation is a model for other areas where innovations in biotechnology are occurring. Regardless of the particular approach taken, if public consultation of this sort is to be effective, it is crucial that participants be well informed. All sides of the issue must be presented without attempts to steer the dialogue, allowing the public participants to arrive at their own conclusions. There have been criticisms made about the CPHA process to solicit public opinion about xenotransplantation (Wright 2002). However, even with possible flaws, it stands as one of the only comprehensive experiments in Canada to engage the public in discussion about decisions regarding the diffusion of a new biotechnology into the health care system.

The practice of public consultation in biotechnology does not mean, however, that a few public representatives set policy. Such groups are not representative of the whole population and are not selected to represent the entire community (Bach and Ivinson 2002; Ivinson and Bach 2002). In the example described above, the PAG report was presented to the Minister of Health to inform the decisions that must be made by policy-makers and the political representatives to whom citizens delegate such authority. The CPHA experience has provided valuable information about including the values of the public in decision-making and engaging citizens in the debate about biotechnology development in Canada. At the writing of this chapter, Health Canada has not approved xenotransplant clinical trials in Canada, and the various expert groups involved in the issue are still studying the options.

The public must be involved in all facets of societal development (Morrison 1996). In particular, in developing policy about biotechnology, it is clear that public values are essential in making ethical choices that will benefit the community. Good health care decisions are not possible until the public supplies the value framework to be used. Value systems drawn from cultural, religious, and philosophical ideological systems are central to planning health care directions and act as the guides and justifications for choosing the goals, priorities, and means that guide policy development (Maxwell, Rosell and Forest 2003; Veatch 1985; 1991).

In this section I have made a case for public involvement in the decisions about biotechnology. In the following section, I discuss the implications for nurses in helping to open the moral space required for the discussion about the ethical and societal implications of biotechnology. As we have seen, the debate becomes all the more vital and complex with the introduction of ever more powerful biotechnologies that may offer potential benefits to individuals but that are counterbalanced by potential risks to society.

OPENING MORAL SPACE FOR DISCUSSION ABOUT BIOTECHNOLOGY: IMPLICATIONS FOR NURSES

In a rapidly changing world, we are inundated with material about biotechnology as well as information about the "good, the bad, and the ugly" of biotechnological innovations as we attempt to understand the vast amount of information that we are exposed to on a daily basis. Kingwell (2002) suggests that as conscientious citizens, we struggle to stay on top of what is happening in our technologically dominated and complex world and advises that we need to prepare ourselves for a "bumpy ride" as we try to determine where we are headed. Further, Saul (2001) points out that there are severe limitations to what we can understand in the face of constant technological change. He reminds us that

> In fact, with the explosion of technology over the last quarter-century, the percentage of what we understand versus what we know has probably slipped back to where it was a century ago (30).

As nurses, how do we sort through the information that is available, organize ourselves for the "bumpy ride," and ensure that we are prepared to deal with the societal and ethical implications of biotechnology? It is a difficult undertaking as the line between science and science fiction has become blurred, a plethora of information is available, and many conflicting points of view exist. We only have to review recent newspaper and magazine headlines to emerge with a sense of the complexity of the information provided for our perusal and the variety of perspectives and opinions that are presented to the public.[11]

In this book, and elsewhere, there has been a call to expand social, environmental, and political thinking in nursing, a call for a focus on the **common good,** a term used to describe the well-being of the community at large based on shared goals and common purposes (Fry 1985; Rodney and Starzomski 1993; Starzomski and Rodney 1997; Stevens 1989; 1992). For example, in the recent edition of the Canadian Nurses Association Code of Ethics (2002a) where a description of the challenges and opportunities for the ethical practice of nursing is presented, it is acknowledged that nurses need to be involved in understanding and facilitating broad societal discussion of issues related to biotechnology:

> The biological, genetic revolution, as well as other emerging technologies, raise profound changes in the human capacity to control diseases and human reproduction as well as to govern access to health information. Comparable philosophical development in considering the ethics of these advances is, as yet, limited. The public needs knowledge and ethical guidance to make well-informed choices about the appropriate use of many of these advances (4).

The Canadian Nurses Association (CNA) has made claims in other ways about the importance of the involvement of nurses and the public in making policy decisions about biotechnology. In various position statements, documents, and briefs developed by the CNA, support is expressed for including nurses in discussions about technology at all levels of the health care system. These documents suggest that nurses must be involved in all aspects of technology use, including identifying the need for such use, developing and implementing technology, and evaluating the impact on client care. CNA policy statements, such as those related to technology, primary care, and leadership, all include some reference to supporting a nursing role in discussions about technology development and implementation (Canadian Nurses Association 1992; 1995; 2002b). Further, CNA has shown national leadership in the area of biotechnology by ensuring that nurses are involved on committees and councils which make decisions about biotechnology.

The scope of understanding about biotechnology can be overwhelming. It is neither practical nor possible for every nurse to keep abreast of all the ethical and societal developments; nor is it possible to speak out on every issue as the issues are numerous and priorities vary. However, nurses could act as expert navigators of technology and become information brokers for their clients while ensuring that the core values of nursing are maintained. Further, there is a need for nursing leaders to examine the impact of biotech-nological changes on nursing recruitment, nursing work design, and the nursing workforce (Broughton 2001).

A solid understanding of nursing ethics can provide assistance to deal with the chal-lenges confronting us in health care and biotechnology and provide us with the ability to critically examine the issues and to devise solutions. In what follows, I suggest some strategies for continued nursing leadership in biotechnology at the micro, meso, and macro levels of the health care system. It is critical that nurses engage in this discussion with other health care providers and help to facilitate the involvement of members of the public. Many of the strategies that follow would be useful for Maria to consider (in Ethics in Practice 15-1) as she develops her plan about how to support Paul and his family.

Micro-Level Strategies

- Become educated about biotechnological developments and societal and ethical implications.
- Ensure that patients and families are informed about options, risks, and benefits when considering therapeutic biotechnological interventions.
- Help educate other nurses, health care providers, and members of the public.
- Ensure that ethical and societal issues about biotechnological developments are part of educational curricula, conferences, and symposia.
- Engage in advocacy to help patients and families have opportunities to express their views.

Meso-Level Strategies

- Participate in both clinical and research ethics committees where issues about biotech-nology are being discussed.
- Conduct research examining the ethical and societal implications of biotechnology.
- Ensure that ethical and societal issues about biotechnological developments are part of hospital, community, regional board, and health authority discussions.
- Work with provincial professional associations and groups to ensure that there is public dialogue about biotechnological concerns.

Macro-Level Strategies

- Participate in national committees, debates, and forums.
- Use methods such as citizens' juries, consensus conferences, town hall meetings, and the Internet to engage the public and health care providers in debates about issues.
- Participate with professional associations to ensure that nurses are represented in Parliament and provincial/territorial legislatures where laws are being made that govern biotechnology.

There is no doubt that, in the future, decisions about biotechnology will continue to demand the involvement of consumers and all health care providers, including nurses. These decisions will be complex and difficult, so that no one societal group or set of voices will be adequate to make the choices that are needed. Although, as a society, we may not always have the answers to questions related to choices about biotechnology, a collaborative effort will provide the best method to ensure that wise choices are made for future biotechnological developments.

FUTURE DIRECTIONS—THE TIP OF THE ICEBERG

Biotechnology raises major issues—issues of ethics, choice, trust, democracy, and globalization. Innovations in biotechnology come encumbered with intended and unintended social, political, and economic values (Barnard 1997; 2002; Marck 2000a; 2000b; Midgely 2000; Shenk 1999). I have argued throughout this chapter that policies surrounding xenotransplantation and other emerging biotechnological interventions must balance opportunity and risk. Further, I have advocated for an expansion in the debate about biotechnology that includes members of the public, nurses, and other health care providers in discussions about the societal and ethical issues facing us in the realm of biotechnology.

Public involvement in decisions about biotechnology is complex. There is no consensus on how to include the public in meaningful ways in the development of healthy public policy, although in this chapter I have presented several methods that I believe move us in the right direction. Clearly, we need to be sensitive to the contexts in which public participation is being asked to ensure that citizens are able to avail themselves of opportunities to be involved. This is an area where, definitely, "one size does not fit all" (Lomas and Veenstra 1995; Martin, Ableson and Singer 2002).

Although the future of dialogue and debate on issues of biotechnology is by no means assured, there are promising signs. As discussed throughout this chapter, researchers and governmental and non-governmental organizations are turning more of their attention to the issues. The xenotransplantation public consultation process in Canada is one example of the move in this direction. There is still time to seek meaningful societal participation regarding many of the issues facing us in biotechnology in order to make the best possible choices about future technological opportunities that are coming our way.

By its very nature, science alone will not give us answers with absolute certainty and can only tell us about the likelihood of the benefits and dangers posed by biotechnology. As citizens, we will need to continue to review the science and to make decisions based on our value systems, as what we currently see is just the tip of iceberg. The future possibilities in biotechnology are beyond many of our imaginations.[12]

Before us is a period of remarkable technological innovation. To our armamentarium of technological innovations we have added tools that have power over life and death. Will we use biotechnology to preserve our humanity and improve our quality of life, as exemplified in the optimistic future portrayed in *Star Trek*? Or will we choose a more pessimistic future such as that portrayed in Aldous Huxley's *Brave New World*, where humans have really become the tools of their tools. The manner in which we develop and use biotechnology today is a harbinger of what we can become as a society tomorrow (Starzomski 1994; 1997). We must use our tools wisely, keeping in mind that the wisdom we need for tomorrow comes from understanding the present and learning from the past.

FOR REFLECTION

1. Reflect on the situation described in Ethics in Practice 15-1. What actions do you think could support someone in Maria's position?

2. Think about your work setting and your role in your family and community. How can you facilitate discussion about the biotechnological innovations that affect you in those spheres of your life?

3. How can public input be obtained about biotechnology innovations like xenotransplantation, use of stem cells, cloning, and nanotechnology?

ENDNOTES

1. For these and other quotations about biotechnology see: www.brainyquote.com/quotes/quo; www.quoteworld.org

2. For more information about this historic discovery, see *Banting and Best isolate insulin.* Available online: www.pbs.org/wgbh/aso/databank/entries/dm22in.html

3. For further data about the growth of the biotechnology industry, see *Biotechnology: A hot career choice for the 21st century*. Available online: www.whybiotech.com/index.asp?id=2983

    It is expected that by 2011, 400,000 people will be employed by biotechnology companies and another 350,000 will be in related businesses (compared to 250,000 and 150,000 today). Biotechnology in Canada has grown to the level of being second only to the United States in its number of biotechnology companies. In 2002, Canada was home to more than 400 biotechnology firms, up from 282 in 1997. Biotechnology research-and-development spending has almost tripled from $494 million in 1997 to more than $1.5 billion in 2002. Ontario, one of the leaders of biotechnology in Canada, has approximately 120 biotechnology companies; in this province, almost $400 million was spent on research and development in 2002. Available online: www.biotech.ca/EN/nrMar2803.htm

4. For information about *new reproductive technologies* and recommendations for regulation, see *Proceed with care. Final report of the Royal Commission on New Reproductive Technologies* (1993). See also *Bill C-13—An Act respecting assisted human reproductive technologies and related research*. Available online: www.parl.gc.ca/37/2/parlbus/chambus/house/bills/government/C-13/C-13_2/90187bE.html

    For further discussion about *stem cell research,* see Baylis (2001); Holland, Lebacqz and Zoloth (2001); Meilander (2001); and Sanchez-Sweatman (2000).

    Stem cell research raises profound ethical issues. Human embryonic stem cells can divide indefinitely and have the potential to develop into a variety of different types of tissue. Research on these cells has brought about a new medical specialty: regenerative medicine. Because stem cells can be obtained from living embryos that are destroyed in the process, or from aborted fetuses, the discussion of stem cell research is linked with the debate on abortion. Work is occurring in many countries to develop ethical frameworks within which stem cell researchers can conduct research as well as guidelines for patents and informed consent for clinical trials. The Canadian Institutes of Health Research (CIHR) guidelines for human pluripotent stem cell research and a bill on assisted reproduction address the controversial issue of using human embryos in research. See Canadian Institutes of Health Research (2002). Human pluripotent stem cell research: Recommendations for CIHR-funded research (final report). Available online: www.cihr.ca/about_cihr/ethics/stem_cell/stem _cell_intro_e.shtml

    Some people are calling for a total ban on using stem cells collected from early embryos, arguing that because the embryo is destroyed in the process of extracting the cells, such research is unethical. However, scientific evidence suggests that embryonic stem cells may have the greatest versatility and potential to lead to therapies for a range of diseases. In the United States, publicly funded research is restricted to 60 existing stem cell lines. Although some countries have prohibited cloning, Canada is taking a cautious approach with Bill C-13 (in third reading in Parliament at the writing of this chapter), which will allow embryo and stem cell research under certain conditions, but without therapeutic cloning or reproductive cloning. Therapeutic cloning involves removing the nucleus from an egg and adding a nucleus from a somatic cell, or any adult body cell, from the person to be cloned. Recent research suggests that stem cells can be obtained from other body tissue (e.g., adipose tissue), thus potentially removing the need to use human embryos.

    See also Dekel et al. (2003), in which investigators discuss the potential of kidneys being developed from human or pig embryonic stem cells. Experiments from the Weizmann Institute in Israel indicate that primitive kidneys can be grown from human (if taken at 7–8 weeks) or pig (if taken at 4 weeks) embryonic stem cells, and that these kidneys, if transplanted, would need less immunosuppressive therapy for survival.

For a chilling work of fiction, see Atwood (2003), *Oryx and Crake* which describes a brave new world in which biotechnology takes over.

For information about the ownership of *genetically altered life forms,* see the Supreme Court of Canada judgment. Available online: www.scc-csc.gc.ca/Welcome/index_e.asp

On Dec. 5, 2002, the Supreme Court of Canada, in a 5–4 split, ruled that higher life forms, such as Harvard University's Onco Mouse, could not be patented. While some argue that the cellular changes in the mouse render it a composition of matter, the majority disagreed. Based on the esoteric language of Canada's 19th-century Patent Act, the Supreme Court judged the Harvard Mouse to be neither "a manufacture nor a composition of matter." The Court has asked Parliament to review the question. The Industry Minister says that Canadians will be consulted, as well the Canadian Biotechnology Advisory Committee, before a decision is made on rewriting the law. Canadian biotechnologists are concerned about the decision as this is contrary to laws in other places, such as Japan, the United States, and much of Europe, where patent rights to the Onco Mouse have long been extended (*Maclean's* 2002).

See Mnyusiwalla (2003) and Daar (2002) for further information about *nanotechnology*—the development of extremely small human-made machines that are measured in nanometers (billionths of a metre, and a thousand times smaller than the diameter of a human hair) and designed for use in disease treatment, surgery, and tissue repair. Nanotechnology is moving ahead with two billion dollars in research-and-development investment in 2002. Within the next decade, Daar predicts that human molecules will be able to stimulate repair and restoration of natural bodily functions. In greater than 10 years, there will be examples of developing tissues and organs outside of the body by treating stem cells with human signalling molecules. In the next 30 years, he says, there will be a resetting of the genetic clock, and in the next 50 years, nanotechnology.

For a disturbing view of nanotechnology, see *Prey,* a science fiction novel by Michael Crichton (2003), which portrays a future in which nanotechnology has caused a mechanical plague to roam the earth.

5. Beef that is ingested by some humans that comes from cows affected by bovine spongiform encephalopathy can lead to the neurological disorder new variant Creutzfeldt-Jakob disease. See, for example, Kluger (1997) and Health Canada (2003).

6. The terms "members of the public," "consumers," "society," "lay people," and "lay persons" will be used interchangeably in this chapter.

7. For information about the shortage of organs for transplantation see Molzahn, Starzomski and McCormick (2003). In the United States, 80,374 people were waiting for organ transplants in 2001. This is an increase from 21,914 in 1990. However, in 2001, there were only 6081 cadaveric donations and 6499 living donations. In the United States in 2001, 6124 people died waiting for transplants (United Network on Organ Sharing [2002]. Critical data: U.S. facts about organ donation. Available online: www.unos.org). A similar problem exists in Canada, where, over the five-year period from 1996 to 2000, the waiting list grew by 62 percent while the number of transplants increased by just 22 percent. By the end of 2002, there were almost 4,000 Canadians waiting for organ transplants, a 15.6 percent increase in three years (Canadian Organ Replacement Registry [CORR] [2002] Available online: http://secure.cihi.ca/cihiweb).

8. For more information about xenotransplantation, see: The Xenotransplantation Discussion Scenario. Available online: http://strategis.ic.gc.ca/SSG/bb00009e.html; See also Health Canada (2002), Xenotransplantation facts. Available online: www.hc-sc.gc.ca/hpfb-dgpsa/bgtd-dpbtg/xeno_fact_e.html. See also Nicholson (1996), where he suggests that successful xenografting would increase transplantation tenfold worldwide, thus producing a profit of more than three billion U.S. dollars annually for just one pharmaceutical company involved in the process.

9. Opponents of using animals as sources for xenotransplantation vehemently state that the use of animals for food or research does not automatically justify their use in transplantation. They question whether scientists will be able to meet the social and behavioural needs of animals in a respectful manner. Further, there have been major concerns raised about the use of nonhuman primates in research. Some countries, such as New Zealand, have banned all research using nonhuman primates. See, for example, Nuffield Council on Bioethics (1996); Singer (1975, 1992).

10. For updated information about how Canada is dealing with these issues, see material available from the CBAC (Canadian Biotechnology Advisory Committee). The CBAC is an expert, arm's-length committee created under the renewed Canadian Biotechnology Strategy (CBS) to advise Ministers, raise public awareness, and engage Canadians in an open and transparent dialogue on biotechnology matters. The CBAC

advises government on broad policy issues associated with the ethical, social, regulatory, economic, scientific, environmental, and health aspects of biotechnology (CBAC 1999). Available online: http://cbac.gc.ca

See also Dr. Chris McDonald's website: www.biotechethics.ca. The site includes descriptions about a program of research focused on corporate governance, ethics, and the biotechnology industry, with links to several other organizations such as BIOTE Canada and the U.S Biotechnology Industry Organization. The site also includes a decision-making guide to recognizing, evaluating, and resolving key ethical issues in the biotechnology industry, by MacDonald and Dharma, titled Ethics in Biotechnology— An Executive Guide.

11. Just in the last few weeks, several headlines that have been noted are: Skepticism Greets New Cloning Claim; Why Not Clone a Human? Ethical Challenges of Biotechnology; Cloned Sheep Dolly Put Down; Rejection Free Pigs Cloned; Law on Human Cloning Shouldn't Pass As It Stands; Genetic Patenting Ruling Hurt Canadian Biotechs; Scientists Find Reason Humans Can't Be Cloned; Human, Pig Cells Make Mice; Creation: The Promise of Stem Cells; Big Danger Seen in Tiny Machines; Could Tiny Machines Rule the World? and Face Transplant Technology Something To Be Envisaged.

12. For several future technologies that are being developed, see www.business2.com/articles/mag/0,1640,49104,00. html. This site provides a description of "God's Ink-Jet," a device that could build human organs and tissues from scratch. Assistant professor of bioengineering, Thomas Boland, at Clemson University, has modified surplus ink-jet printers to squirt out a "bio ink" of cells, growth factors, and degradable gel to form three-dimensional tubes of living tissue. The gel acts as a scaffold for the cells to rest on as they naturally fuse together into the desired form. Funding comes from NASA. Hewlett-Packard (HPQ) and Canon (CAJ) have both expressed interest in the novel ink-jet application. The investigators propose that organ printing will be a great contribution to personalized medical care since it might be possible to build every single fiber of a human being. They suggest that "It's a huge step toward the eternity of mankind."

Marcikic et al. (2003) report that they "beamed" information that organized tiny bits of matter (smaller than an atom, called qubits) more than a mile away, the furthest instance of teleportation yet reported. Although "beaming" human beings may be a far off reality, if it ever is in fact possible, the stuff of science fiction is now becoming a reality.

REFERENCES

Alexander, S. 1962. They decide who lives, who dies: Medical miracle puts a burden on a small committee. *Life,* November 9, 102–104, 106, 108, 110, 115, 117–118, 123–125.

Allan, J. 1996. Xenotransplantation at a crossroads: Prevention versus progress. *Nature Medicine, 2*, 18–21.

Allan, J. 1997. Silk purse or sow's ear. *Nature Medicine, 3*, 275–276.

Allan, J. 1998. Cross-species infection: No news is good news? *Nature Medicine, 4*, 644–645.

Atwood, M. 2003. *Oryx and Crake.* Toronto: McClelland and Stewart.

Bach, F. and Ivinson, A. 2002. A shrewd and ethical approach to xenotransplantation. *Trends in Biotechnology, 20*(3), 129–131.

Bach, F., Fishman, J., Daniels, N., Proimos, J., Anderson, B., Carpenter, C., Forrow, L., Robson, S. and Fineberg, H. 1998. Uncertainty in xenotransplantation: Individual benefit versus collective risk. *Nature Medicine, 4*(2), 141–144.

Bailey, L. 1990. Organ transplantation: A paradigm of medical progress. *Hastings Center Report, 20*(1), 24–28.

Baird, P. 2003. Getting it right: Industry sponsorship and medical research. *Canadian Medical Association Journal, 168*(10), 1267–1269.

BBC World. 2002. *Cook Islands plans xenotransplant trials*, March 5.

Barnard, A. 1997. A critical review of the belief that technology is a neutral object and nurses are its master. *Journal of Advanced Nursing, 26*, 126–131.

Barnard, A. 2002. Philosophy of technology and nursing. *Nursing Philosophy, 3*, 15–26.

Baylis, F. 2001. The Canadian stem cell debate: Stuck in the '80s. *Journal of the Society of Obstetricians and Gynaecologists of Canada, 23*(3), 248–252.

Bloom, E., Moulton, A., McCoy, J., Chapman, L. and Patterson, A. 1999. Xenotransplantation: The potential and the challenges. *Critical Care Nurse, 19*(2), 76–82.

Blue, A., Keyserlingk, T., Rodney, P. and Starzomski, R. 1999. A critical review of North American health policy. In H. Coward and P. Ratanakul (Eds.), *An intercultural dialogue on health care ethics* (pp. 215–225). Waterloo, ON: Wilfred Laurier University Press.

Bodenheimer, T. 2000. Uneasy alliance—Clinical investigators and the pharmaceutical industry. *New England Journal of Medicine, 342*(20), 1539–1544.

Boyle, P. and Callahan, D. 1992. Technology assessment: The missing human dimension. *Hastings Center Report, 22*(3), 38–39.

Broughton, H. 2001. *Nursing leadership: Unleashing the power*. Ottawa: Canadian Nurses Association.

Brunger, F. and Cox, S. 2000. Ethics and genetics: The need for transparency. In F. Miller, L. Weir, R. Mykitiuk et al. (Eds.), *The gender of genetic futures: The Canadian biotechnology strategy, women and health* (pp. 27–31). Proceedings of the National Strategic Workshop, York University, Toronto, February 11–12, 2000.

Canadian Nurses Association. 1992. *The role of the nurse in the use of health care technology.* Ottawa: Canadian Nurses Association.

Canadian Nurses Association. 1995. *The role of the nurse in primary health care.* Ottawa: Canadian Nurses Association.

Canadian Nurses Association. 2002a. *Code of ethics for registered nurses.* Ottawa: Canadian Nurses Association.

Canadian Nurses Association. 2002b. *Position statement: Nursing leadership.* Ottawa: Canadian Nurses Association.

Canadian perspective on the precautionary approach/principle, A. 2001. Available online: www.hc.sc.gc.ca/english/protection/precaution.html

Canadian Public Health Association. 2001. *Animal-to-human transplantation: Should Canada proceed? A public consultation on xenotransplantation.* Ottawa: Canadian Public Health Association.

Caplan, A. 1992. Is xenografting morally wrong? *Transplantation Proceedings, 24*(2), 722–727.

Charles, C. and DeMaio, S. 1993. Lay participation in health care decision making: A conceptual framework. *Journal of Health Politics, Policy and Law, 18*(4), 883–904.

Commission on the Future of Health Care in Canada. 2002. *Building on values: The future of health care in Canada - Final report.* Ottawa: Government of Canada.

Council of Europe. 2003. Report on xenotransplantation. Available online: www.coe.int/T/E/Legal_Affairs/Legal_co-operation/Bioethics/Activities/XenotransplantationXENO(2003)1E_state_of_art_final_website.asp#TopOfPage

Crichton, M. 2003. *Prey.* Toronto: Harper Collins.

Daar, A. and Phil, D. 1997. Ethics of xenotransplantation: Animal issues, consent, and likely transformation of transplant ethics. *World Journal of Surgery, 21*, 975–982.

Daar, A. 2002. Aspects of regenerative medicine today. *Proceedings of the International Congress on Ethics in Organ Transplantation,* Munich, Germany, Dec. 10–13, 2002.

Deber, R. 1992. Translating technology assessment into policy: Conceptual choices and tough issues. *International Journal of Technology Assessment in Health Care, 8*(1), 131–137.

Dekel, B., Burakova, T., Arditti, F., Reich-Zeliger, S., Milstein, O., Aviel-Ronen, S., Gideon Rechavi, G., Friedman, N., Kaminski, N., Passwell, J. and Reisner, Y. 2003. Human and porcine early kidney precursors as a new source for transplantation. *Nature Medicine, 9*(1), 53–60.

Dhanda, R. 2002. *Guiding Icarus: Merging bioethics with corporate interests.* Toronto: Wiley.

Dillner, L. 1996. Pig organs approved for human transplants. *British Medical Journal, 312*(7032), 657.

Dinsmore, J., Manhart, C., Raineri, R., Jacoby, D. and Moore, A. 2000. No evidence for infection of human cells with porcine endogenous retrovirus (PERV) after exposure to porcine fetal neuronal cells. *Transplantation, 70,* 1382–1389.

Evanson, B. 2000. What if there's a virus hiding in a pig organ? *National Post*, Aug. 17, A16.

Eyles, J. 1993. *The role of the citizen in health care decision making.* McMaster University Centre for Health Economics and Policy Analysis. (Policy Commentary C93-1).

Federal/Provincial Advisory Committee on Health Services. 1996. *Organ and tissue distribution in Canada: A discussion document.* Ottawa: Health Canada.

Fishman, J. 1997. Xenosis and xenotransplantation: Addressing the infectious risks posed by an emerging technology. *Kidney International, 51*(58), S41–S45.

Fox, R. and Swazey, J. 1992a. Leaving the field. *Hastings Center Report, 22*(5), 9–15.

Fox, R. and Swazey, J. 1992b. *Spare parts: Organ replacement in American society.* New York: Oxford University Press.

Frankish, H. 2002. Pig organ transplantation brought one step closer. *Lancet, 359*(9301), 137.

Fry, S. 1985. Individual vs. aggregate good: Ethical tension in nursing practice. *International Journal of Nursing Studies, 22,* 303–310.

Goodman, C. 1992. It's time to rethink health care technology assessment. *International Journal of Technology Assessment in Health Care, 8*(2), 335–358.

Gunzburg, W. and Salmons, B. 2000. Xenotransplantation: Is the risk of viral infection as great as we thought? *Molecular Medicine Today, 6*(5), 199–208.

Hadorn, D. 1991. The role of public values in setting health care priorities. *Social Science & Medicine, 32*(7), 773–781.

Health Canada. 1997. *National forum on xenotransplantation—Clinical, ethical and regulatory issues.* Ottawa: Health Canada.

Health Canada. 1999. *Proposed Canadian standard for xenotransplantation.* Ottawa: Health Canada.

Health Canada. 2003a. *Summary of severe acute respiratory syndrome (SARS) cases: Canada and international.* Available online: www.hc-sc.gc.ca/pphb-dgspsp/sars-sras/eu-ae/sars20030602_e.html

Health Canada. 2003b. *Mad cow disease-Frequently asked questions.* Available online: www.hc-sc.gc.ca/english/diseases/bse/faq.html

Holland, S., Lebacqz, K. and Zoloth, L. 2001. *The human embryonic stem cell debate: Science, ethics and public policy.* Cambridge, MA: MIT Press.

House of Commons Standing Committee on Health. 1999. *Report on organ and tissue donation and transplantation: A Canadian approach.* Available online: www.parl.gc.ca

Ivinson, A. and Bach, F. 2002. The xenotransplantation question: Public consultation is an important part of the answer. *Canadian Medical Association Journal, 167*(1), 42–43.

Jennings, B. 1991. Possibilities of consensus: Toward democratic moral discourse. *Journal of Medicine and Philosophy, 16*(4), 447–463.

Kingwell, M. 2002. *Practical judgments: Essays in culture, politics and interpretation.* Toronto: University of Toronto Press.

Kluger, J. 1997. Where now mad cow? *Time, 149*(4), 44–45.

Land, W. 1989. The problem of living organ donation: Facts, thoughts, and reflections. *Transplant International, 2,* 168–179.

Lemonick, M. 2003. The DNA revolution: A twist of fate. *Time, 161*(6), 31–40.

Lenaghan, J. 1999. Involving the public in rationing decisions. The experience of citizens' juries. *Health Policy, 49*(1–2), 45–61.

Lomas, J. and Veenstra, G. 1995. If you build it, who will come? Governments, consultation and biased publics. *Policy Options, 16*(9), 37–40.

Maclean's. 2002. The week: Law: Patents and rodents. *Maclean's,* December 16, 15.

Marcikic, I., de Riedmatten, H., Tittel, W., Zbinde, H. and Gisin, N. 2003. Long-distance teleportation of qubits at telecommunication wavelengths. *Nature, 421*, 509–513.

Marck, P. 2000a. Recovering ethics after "technics": Developing critical text on technology. *Nursing Ethics, 7*(1), 5–14.

Marck, P. 2000b. Nursing in a technological world: Searching for healing communities. *Advances in Nursing Science, 23*, 63–81.

Martin, D., Abelson, J. and Singer, P. 2002. Participation in health care priority-setting through the eyes of the participants. *Journal of Health Service Research Policy, 7*(4), 222–228.

Maxwell, J., Rosell, S. and Forest, P. 2003. Giving citizens a voice in healthcare policy in Canada. *British Medical Journal, 326*, 1031–1033.

McCormick, R. 1985. Was there any real hope for Baby Fae? *Hastings Center Report, 15*, 12–13.

Meilander, G. 2001. The point of a ban: Or, how to think about stem cell research. *Hastings Centre Report, 31*(1), 9–16.

Michaels, M., McMichael, J., Brasky, K., Kalter, S., Peters, R., Starzl, T. and Simmons R. 1994. Screening donors for xenotransplantation: The potential for xenozoonoses. *Transplantation, 57*, 1462–1465.

Midgely, M. 2000. Biotechnology and monstrosity: Why we should pay attention to the "yuk factor." *Hastings Centre Report, 30*(5), 7–15.

Mnyusiwalla, A. 2003. Mind the gap: Science and ethics in nanotechnology. *Nanotechnology, 14*, R9–R13.

Molzahn, A., Starzomski, R. and McCormick, J. 2003. The supply of organs for transplantation: Issues and challenges. *Nephrology Nursing Journal, 30*(1), 17–28.

Morrison, I. 1996. *The second curve: How to command new technologies, new consumers and new markets.* New York: Ballantine Books.

Muir, D. and Griffin, G. 2001. *Infection risks in xenotransplantation.* Prepared for U.K. Department of Health. Available online: www.doh.gov.uk/pub/docs/doh/76035_doh_infection_risks.pdf

Murray, J. 1992. Human organ transplantation: Background and consequences. *Science, 256*, 1411–1416.

National Forum on Health. 1997. *Canada health action: Building on the legacy* (Volumes 1 and 2). Ottawa: National Forum on Health.

National Institutes of Health. 1985. *Report of the National Institutes of Health: The report of the NIH team investigating Baby Fae.* Washington, D.C: National Institutes of Health.

National Kidney Foundation. 1995. *Survey on xenotransplantation.* Unpublished report. New York: National Kidney Foundation.

Neufeld, V., MacLeod, S., Tugwell, P., Zakus, D. and Zarowsky, C. 2001. The rich–poor gap in global health research: Challenges for Canada. *Canadian Medical Association Journal, 164*(8), 1158–1159.

Nicholson, R. 1996. This little pig went to market. *Hastings Center Report, 26*(4), 3.

Nuffield Council on Bioethics. 1996. *Animal-to-human transplants: The ethics of xenotransplantation*: London: Nuffield Council on Bioethics.

O'Neill, M. 1992. Community participation in Quebec's health system: A strategy to curtail community empowerment. *International Journal of Health Services, 22*(2), 287–301.

Platt, J. 1997. Xenotransplantation: A potential solution to the shortage of donor organs. *Transplantation Proceedings, 29*, 3324–3326.

Proceed with care. 1993. *Final report of the Royal Commission on New Reproductive Technologies.* Canada: Minister of Government Services.

Reemtsma, K. 1992. Xenografts. *Transplantation Proceedings, 24*(5), 2225–2227.

Reiser, S. 1992. Out of chaos: A rational approach to assessing technology. *Hospitals, 66*(15), 22–23.

Rettig, R. 1989. The politics of organ transplantation: A parable of our time. *Journal of Health Politics, Policy and Law, 14*(1), 191–227.

Reuters Health. 2002. *Panel worried about "xenotourism" for animal organ transplants*, March 12.

Rodney, P. and Starzomski, R. 1993. Constraints on the moral agency of nurses. *The Canadian Nurse, 89*(9), 23–26.

Rollin, B. 2003. *The Frankenstein syndrome: Ethical and social issues in the genetic engineering of animals.* New York: Cambridge University Press.

Sanchez-Sweatman, L. 2000. Reproductive cloning and human health: An ethical, international, and nursing perspective. *International Nursing Review, 47*(1), 28–37.

Saul, J. 2001. *The unconscious civilization.* Toronto: Penguin.

Shenk, D. 1999. *The end of patience: Cautionary notes on the information revolution.* Bloomington, IN: Indiana University Press.

Sherwin, S. 2000. Placing values at the center of biotechnology policy: The Canadian biotechnology strategy and women's health. Opening remarks. In F. Miller, L. Weir, R. Mykitiuk et al. (Eds.), *The gender of genetic futures: The Canadian biotechnology strategy, women and health* (pp. 1–8). Proceedings of the National Strategic Workshop, York University, Toronto, February 11–12, 2000.

Singer, P. 1975. *Animal liberation.* New York: Random House.

Singer, P. 1992. Xenotransplantation and speciesism. *Transplantation Proceedings, 24*(2), 728–732.

Starzomski, R. 1994. Ethical issues in palliative care: The case of dialysis and organ transplantation. *Journal of Palliative Care, 10*(3), 27–33.

Starzomski, R. 1997. *Resource allocation for solid organ transplantation: Toward public and health care provider dialogue.* Unpublished doctoral dissertation. University of British Columbia, Vancouver.

Starzomski, R. 2002. Listening to multiple voices: Consumer involvement in health promotion. In L. Young and V. Hayes (Eds.), *Transforming health promotion practice: Concepts, issues and applications* (pp. 71–86). Philadelphia: F.A. Davis.

Starzomski, R. and Rodney, P. 1997. Nursing inquiry for the common good. In S. Thorne and V. Hayes (Eds.), *Nursing praxis: Knowledge and action* (pp. 219–236). Thousand Oaks: Sage Publications.

Stevens, P. 1989. A critical reconceptualization of environment in nursing: Implications for methodology. *Advances in Nursing Science, 114*, 56–68.

Stevens, P. 1992. Who gets care? Access to health care as an arena for nursing action. *Scholarly Inquiry for Nursing Practice, 6*, 185–200.

Sykes, M., d'Apice, A. and Sandrin, M. 2003. Position paper of the Ethics Committee of the International Xenotransplantation Association. *Xenotransplantation, 10*, 194–2003.

Veatch, R. 1985. Lay medical ethics. *Journal of Medicine & Philosophy, 10*(1), 1–5.

Veatch, R. 1991. Consensus of expertise: The role of consensus of experts in formulating public policy and estimating facts. *Journal of Medicine and Philosophy, 16(*4), 429–445.

Veatch, R. 2000. Transplantation ethics. Washington, D.C.: Georgetown University Press.

Wharry, S. 2002. Canadians not ready for animal-to-human transplants. *Canadian Medical Association Journal, 166*(4), 493.

Winner, L. 1993. Citizen virtues in a technological order. In E. Winkler and J. Coombs (Eds.), *Applied ethics—A reader* (pp. 46–69). Cambridge: Blackwell.

Wiseman, H., Vanderkop, J. and Nef, J. 1991. Ethics and technology: Across the great divide. In H. Wiseman, J. Vanderkop and J. Nef (Eds.), *Critical choices! Ethics, science and technology* (pp. x–xiv). Toronto: Thompson Educational Publishing Inc.

Wright, J. 2002. Alternative interpretations of the same data: Flaws in the process of consulting the Canadian public about xenotransplantation issues. *Canadian Medical Association Journal, 167*(1), 40–42.

Xenotransplant news. 2003. *Xenotransplantation, 10*(3), 191–193.

Yeo, M. 1996. The ethics of public participation. In M. Stingl and D. Wilson (Eds.), *Efficiency vs. equality: Health reform in Canada* (pp. 39–54). Lethbridge, Alberta: Fernwood Publishing.

chapter sixteen

Global Health Challenges, Human Rights, and Nursing Ethics[1]

Wendy Austin

Globalization... refers to a process by which the economic, political, social, technological, and ecological forces are creating a new supranational world order.

It is increasingly apparent that the lives of all beings on the planet are essentially intertwined and that the moral question "How should we live together?" must be addressed. What role can nurses play in searching for answers to this question? What are the challenges that we face in striving to bring health to all? From a global perspective, what should be the ethical concerns of nurses (Austin 2001a)? In this chapter, these questions are considered. Overall, it is argued that the time has come for Canadian nurses to reflect and act upon their responsibilities as professional health practitioners in a global community. The chapter begins with a brief overview of the meaning of globalization and with the identification of some global health issues. It continues with four themes that are important to a global view of nursing ethics: poverty, biotechnology, conflict, and health as a human right. The chapter concludes with a discussion of the quest for a universal or macro-level ethic to guide moral actions in our small world.

GLOBALIZATION

That it is a *small* world is becoming more obvious every day (Robertson 1992; Waters 1995). Journeys that would have taken months a century ago can now be concluded in a matter of hours. Communication technologies (telephone, fax, and electronic mail) allow us to converse with others whether they reside in Accra, Moscow, Sydney, or Kathmandu. Television permits us to watch events as they happen even though they are occurring thousands of miles away. The geographical constraints that once shaped our social connections and defined our individual worlds are significantly diminishing. In the 21st century, we find ourselves living in a global village (McLuhan 1964).

Globalization is a term sometimes used to indicate economic globalization, but more accurately it refers to a process by which economic, political, social, technological, and ecological forces are creating a new supranational world order. In this new world, lines between international and domestic issues are not easily drawn, and political borders are increasingly irrelevant (Jowitt 1992). The balance of power in the world is shifting as the locus of economic power moves from the nation-state to the multinational corporation (Freidman 1999). Our most pressing problems, although locally experienced, are now global in magnitude: the effects of human activities on the environment; weapons of mass destruction; chemical and biological terrorism; emerging and resurgent infectious diseases (Albrow 1996; Beck 1992; Howson, Fineberg and Bloom 1998; Ignatieff 1998). Our technological powers are affecting the very nature of existence—not just human existence but that of other forms of life and of the earth itself. Just as the wheel, the printing press, the clock, and currency altered human life in extraordinary ways, electronics has, in a sense, changed our very experience of time and space (Waters 1995). Today, we are taken beyond our family, neighbourhood, and nation in such an immediate way that the scope of our moral community is changing.

The process and substance of this change remains open. A globalized world may become a single society, but it will not necessarily be a harmonious one (Waters 1995). Globalization will not necessarily fulfill hopes of a universal order in which life chances become more equable for every newborn child. Bauman (1998), in *Globalization: The Human Consequences*, argues that the process of globalization divides even as it unites. Those with resources may become "global" and literally or virtually mobile, but those without resources are fixed in their localities and thus separated and excluded. Separation is a strategy of the new global order, according to Bauman. One does not love or hate one's neighbours; one just keeps them at a distance, with economic globalization and free market ideology promoting the idea that no one is responsible for any one else. At a time when the solidarity of our interests with one another should bring us responsibly together, we may, paradoxically, be increasingly separated.

Making globalization an inclusive and positive force may be the central challenge of this millennium (Annan 2000). Kofi Annan, Secretary-General of the United Nations (UN), argues that a new global partnership is required among all countries, rich and poor. It is in this spirit that a UN Millennium Declaration (2000) was made. The Declaration outlines eight goals that the world community needs to achieve if the lives of its citizens are to be improved:

1. eradicate extreme poverty and hunger;
2. achieve universal primary education;

3. promote gender equality and empower women;

4. reduce child mortality;

5. improve maternal health;

6. combat HIV/AIDS, malaria, and other diseases;

7. ensure environmental sustainability; and

8. develop a global partnership for development.

It is readily apparent from the nature and substance of these goals that the knowledge, skills, imagination, and commitment of nurses throughout the world will be necessary to meet them. Do nurses recognize and accept such a responsibility? Are we able to accept it? In order to thoughtfully consider these questions, nurses will need to understand the extent of the challenges involved.

Ethics in Practice 16-1	A Personal Struggle toward a Global Perspective

In 2001, I was a Visiting Professor in the Department of Nursing at the University of Ghana. Among other activities, I taught an advanced practice course. This role gave me an opportunity to see at first hand the health situation of many Ghanaians. The students whom I supervised nursed persons living with mental illness and persons living with HIV/AIDS. At the hospitals, and especially during home visits to patients and their families, I was faced with the enormous differences between the resources available to Ghanaians and the resources that would be available to Canadians with similar illnesses. For instance, the persons with HIV/AIDS that I met not only lacked access to antiretroviral medication, but could not afford vitamins or sometimes even food. They could not afford many critical things, such as schooling for their children. On returning home, I learned that my brother-in-law's sister had just received a lung transplant. This was a happy moment for the family—Ivy lived to meet two new grandchildren. She lived for a further ten months before she died of a cancer that recurred, possibly because of her immunosuppressant chemotherapy.

The theoretical arguments about taking "a global perspective on health" became real for me in 2001. Questions of resource allocation, such as "Is it ethical to spend thousands of dollars to extend one Canadian life when the same amount might extend or transform the lives of many elsewhere,?" became associated with the faces of actual people. I see Ivy's face and recognize the priceless gift of a transplant. I see the faces of a dying Ghanaian woman and her small children and recognize the great need elsewhere. How am I to understand and respond to such profound and competing moral claims? Moving toward a true global perspective is an unsettling experience. There are no easy answers to the complex questions that must arise. In this chapter, I can only aspire to raise some of the questions and issues that we must face as members of a truly global community.

HEALTH FROM A GLOBAL PERSPECTIVE

It can be difficult to grasp health issues at a world level, especially when one's viewpoint is situated in an affluent, democratic society in which sophisticated biotechnical and pharmaceutical interventions are readily available. Can we take hold of the reality that on this day more than 30,000 children will die of a preventable disease (UN Development Programme 2002)? When obesity is one of our prominent local health concerns—obesity-related diseases cause the death of about 500,000 North American and Western European adults annually, with more than one billion adults overweight and 300 million clinically obese (World Health Organization [WHO] 2002a)—can we truly comprehend that some of the children dying today will do so from starvation, that being underweight accounts for the death of over three million children a year?

For many of the children, the disease that causes their death today will be an Acute Respiratory Infection (ARI). Although selective use of antibiotics could save a majority of them, ARIs kill approximately two million children under the age of five every year in developing countries.[2] Malaria will kill some of the children on this day, especially those already suffering from malnutrition and respiratory disease. Malaria killed 906,000 children under the age of five in 2000 (WHO 2002b, 14). It is disheartening that only five per cent of "at-risk" children sleep under the insecticide-treated nets that could protect them. Last year the number of persons succumbing to malaria and the other two major infectious diseases, tuberculosis and Human Immunodeficiency Virus/Acquired Immunodeficiency Syndrome (HIV/AIDS), was 5.7 million. It is estimated that two billion people are carriers of the tuberculosis bacillus, with about 8.8 million developing active tuberculosis (TB) and 1.7 million dying of it every year. HIV/AIDS is the fourth leading cause of death in the world and has already killed over 21 million people, including 4.3 million children.

The life chances of many children are reduced by the fact that they are made orphans by these diseases: HIV/AIDS alone has orphaned 13 million children.[3] Complications of pregnancy and childbirth are also orphaning children: today approximately 1,600 women will die from such complications (WHO 1996). It is in this statistic that the disparity between have and have not nations is most evident. Maternal mortality rates are 18 percent higher in poor nations than in rich ones.

Nurses who take a global view of health will realize that the global burden of disease is accounted for by a relatively few risk factors (WHO 2002a). **Risk** is defined as "a probability of an adverse outcome, or a factor that raises this probability" (WHO 2002a, 1). What is more, these risk factors are strongly related to patterns of living and particularly to consumption. WHO identifies the top ten risks as underweight, unsafe sex, high blood pressure, tobacco consumption, alcohol consumption, unsafe water, sanitation and hygiene, iron deficiency, indoor smoke from solid fuels, high cholesterol, and obesity. Nursing knowledge and skills can make an enormous impact on the reduction of such risks. It is preventive strategies, rather than high-tech medical interventions (so central to health care in industrialized nations) that are necessary to combat them. Simply put, reducing tobacco and alcohol consumption, unsafe sex, and unhealthy diets will save many lives and vastly improve others. The application of nurses' current knowledge of risk reduction and of population health measures can produce substantial, positive change in the health of the world.

Nursing research that focuses on health promotion, health policy, and the prevention of disease could augment existing knowledge and further strengthen its impact. Unfortunately, there exists an imbalance in the funding of health research. It has been estimated that less than 10 percent of health research dollars go to addressing 90 percent of the global disease burden (UNDP/World Bank/WHO 2003, 7). The poor and disadvantaged persons in all societies bear the greatest burden of health risks, but their interests do not guide the health care "industry" or the health research agenda.

Poverty

Do the great inequities revealed in WHO's statistics on disease, disability, and death constitute an ethical issue for nurses? Canadian nurse ethicist Smith (2002), in an article in *The Globe and Mail* titled "Medicare for us, malaria for millions," argues that as we are perfecting our own health care system, we must not forget those without health care. She notes, "there's something awfully wrong with spending all our money on ourselves while most of the world goes health-care hungry, and if we don't find a way to bridge the widening health gap between rich and poor, there will be a day of reckoning" (A19).

The correlation between poverty and poor health is readily apparent. Persons in the least developed countries can expect, on average, to live to 49 years, although 1 in 10 will never make it to their first birthday. Contrast this to the situation in high-income countries, where the average life span is 77 years and the infant mortality rate is 6 per 1,000 live births (UN Population Fund 2002). **Poverty** is want of the necessities of life. From a capability perspective, poverty means the absence of basic capabilities to function, like being well nourished, adequately clothed and sheltered, and able to avoid preventable morbidity, as well as being able to participate in community life. The World Bank defines poverty as consumption expenditure under U.S. $1 per day (World Bank 2002). In 1997 the UN Development Programme introduced a measure, the Human Poverty Index (HPI), which has three elements: longevity (life expectancy), knowledge (literacy), and standard of living (access to safe water and health services, and percentage of malnourished children under five). The HPI highlights the presence of poverty within every country, as a high income per capita does not mean poverty does not exist in a nation. For instance, the United Nations Human Development Report (HDR) for 2002 indicates that the United States has the second highest level of income per person in 17 industrial countries, but also has the highest rate of poverty.

Just as world health statistics can be difficult to grasp in an immediate, real-life sense, so can those describing wealth and poverty in the world. For instance, in 1996, the HDR indicated that 358 people had more wealth than the combined incomes of 45 percent of the world's population—that is, 358 rich people owned more than 2.3 billion poor people. In 2002, the richest 1 percent had a yearly income equivalent to the poorest 57 percent. Despite the wealth generated by global markets, 2.8 billion people live on less than U.S. $2 a day (UN Development Programme 2002). This appalling gap between rich and poor (between and within nations) is widening with the forces of globalization. At the beginning of the 20th century the wealthiest 20 percent of the world was nine times richer than the poorest 20 percent. At the end of the century, the ratio had grown to over 70 times (Benatar 2002).

Benatar (2002), a South African physician and health ethicist, eloquently argues that the social and economic forces producing such disparity must be addressed. He uses the HIV/AIDS pandemic as an example of the instability that exists in the world in terms of health burdens and resources. It is a good example. Sub-Saharan Africa is the poorest area of the world and bears over 70 percent of the global burden of HIV/AIDS. Extreme poverty helps proliferate and encourage HIV illness as it brings malnourishment, lack of safe water and sanitation, compromised immune systems, high exposure to other infectious diseases, illiteracy, pressures encouraging high-risk behaviour (e.g., labour migration, substance abuse, gender violence), and lack of hope (UN Population Fund 2002). Obviously, the pandemic must be understood and responded to in ways that encompass more than a biomedical perspective (Benatar 2002).[4]

The moral understanding of the pandemic must be broader than a medical ethics perspective as well. Benatar notes that the ethical debates in regard to HIV/AIDS have, for the most part, been situated at the micro (interpersonal) level, dealing with such issues as confidentiality. While the meso level of ethics (civic morality) has drawn some attention (for example, stigmatization), we have yet to respond to the complexity of the ethical issues at the macro level (international relations). Economic, military, cultural, and political dimensions need to be addressed and the roles of health professionals broadened to include commitment to global professional ideals.

As the HIV pandemic is teaching us, global health problems require mobilization of an integrated global response. For that to be possible, a genuine sense of **solidarity** among the citizens of the world will be necessary. Solidarity is a unity of feeling or action along with a sense of mutual support among individuals with a common interest. We must come to recognize that humanity has a common interest—that of human survival and flourishing. Can we find a way to be responsive to the powerful forces that are impacting the health of the world, to deal with the glaring disparities in wealth and health? Benatar believes that self-interest, if nothing else, should impel us to try (173). Like Smith, Benatar suggests that if we don't try—if we don't succeed—there will be dire consequences. On this small planet, our physical and moral interdependence is too great for the result to be otherwise.

Biotechnology

Advances in biotechnology, and the business that is arising from those advances, are changing our world in significant ways. These changes will impact our lives as radically as communication and transportation technology have, but in ways that are difficult to foresee. Biotechnology is the application of science and engineering to the use of living organisms (or their parts) in the provision of goods or services. Examples of biotechnology include medically assisted reproduction, organ transplantation, human gene therapy, and the creation of transgenic organisms. Biotechnology has incredible, if unpredictable, possibilities for the quality of human and nonhuman life. The mapping of the human genome, for instance, will have ramifications that we cannot fully imagine; human evolution may be fundamentally changed. We know that this science will bring enormous opportunities to promote human health and extend human longevity in such ways as identifying predispositions to inheritable diseases (for example, diabetes and Alzheimer's disease); developing genetically oriented disease strategies (for example, the breast cancer suppressor gene); and creating biological therapeutics and vaccines (Austin 2001a). There is, however, enormous potential for abuse of this new knowledge. Our fears about the dark side of biotechnology are as old as Mary Shelley's story of Frankenstein and as new as contemporary cinema stories like *Jurassic Park* and *Gattaca*. It should give us pause that the reality of our new technological powers actually rivals that portrayed in such science fiction. We are creating new beings, like the "Frankencell" (Mooney 2002), and recreating extinct ones, like the Tasmanian tiger (Holloway 2002). Astoundingly, human cloning may be a reality (Galloway 2002). What danger does this type of knowledge open to the world? How can such activities be regulated?

Because biotechnology and nursing ethics are the focus of Chapter 15, I will not explore the issues here. I do want to emphasize, however, that their relevance lies at a global level. Gadamer (1996) warns, in *The Enigma of Health*, that "the progress of technology encounters an unprepared humanity" (24). He argues that our sociopolitical consciousness has not evolved at a pace with our scientific and technological progress. There is good evidence that he is right. Our efforts to gain control of emerging scientific and technological advances (or to simply give ourselves time to consider and address the social, political, and moral issues) seem to be failing.

Like other forms of technology, biotechnology is big business. New developments are patented, and this can have negative effects when only those with sufficient monetary resources can gain access to new treatments and equipment. Whether or not biotechnologies will be used to help the disadvantaged and poor of the world remains to be seen. Research seems focused on the most lucrative markets. Applications of new biotechnologies in food and agriculture could allow for enormous strides in feeding the world and bringing health to all. There are great possibilities for genetically modified (GM) plants, made drought resistant or more nutritious or modified to act as vaccines for diseases like Hepatitis B (Dawson 1998). There is, however, "a definite lack of a pro-poor bias in most agricultural biotechnology research" (Spillane 1999, 49).

Vaccines and pharmaceuticals are other components of biotechnology business in which profit severely limits availability. Although tropical infections like tuberculosis, malaria, sleeping sickness, Chagas' disease, and leishmaniasis affect 14 million people a year, less than 1 percent of the drugs approved between 1975 and 1999 (i.e., 13 of the 1,393 new drugs) were treatments for tropical disease[5] (Médecins Sans Frontières 2002). Creating drugs to combat baldness and erectile dysfunction is far better business. A case in point, Eflornithine, the cure for trypanosomiasis (a fatal sleeping sickness infecting about 300,000 Africans a year) was not readily available until it became more marketable as a means to remove female facial hair (McMaster 2001). Lack of affordability is a major barrier to using biotechnologies to improve health in developing countries, even though appropriate application of technology could make a real difference (Daar et al. 2002).[6]

As discussed by Starzomski, nurses must ensure that, where biotechnology is concerned, they are neither low in knowledge or engagement. The public obviously expects health professionals to be on top of the issues. We need to be informed about new initiatives and the tensions and conflicts that surround them. There are questions of regulation (e.g., Should governments control the development and use of biotechnology? If so, how?), of access (e.g., Who owns genetic information?), of informed consent (e.g., Should consumers know that the food they are purchasing has been genetically modified?), of risk (e.g., What will happen if a new organism escapes into the local ecosystem?), of respect for nature (e.g., Should we be creating transgenic organisms?), of business (e.g., Should life forms be patented?), and of moral constraint (e.g., Are there limits to the kinds of research that may be conducted with living things?). We need to ask questions and to be involved in informed dialogue and debate. We need, perhaps most importantly, to ensure that there *is* dialogue and debate.

Conflict

The human ingenuity that makes biotechnology possible has also created atomic, biological, and chemical weapons with the capability to destroy all life on earth (Galtung 1997). Global terrorism has made the threat of such weapons a very real health issue. For instance, smallpox, a disease eradicated 25 years ago, has become a biological weapon. This fact has resulted in the United States implementing plans for the vaccination of up to 10.5 million medical personnel and emergency response workers, who are being encouraged to get the vaccine (despite potential negative consequences) as a patriotic duty. The cost of the vaccination program is estimated between 600 million and 1 billion U.S. dollars—money now unavailable for other health initiatives (Connolly 2002; Foege 2002). Conflict is a major public health problem in our global community.

Many people struggle daily to avoid being killed, maimed, tortured, or displaced by war or conflicts. Even though wars between countries have declined, civil conflicts within states have killed over 3.6 million people in the past decade (WHO 2002c). Although in World War I only 10 percent of the dead were civilians, since WWII, civilians comprise 90 percent of those killed in war (Galtung 1997). Conflict affects health in a myriad of ways. For example, recently, fighting in Kisangani disrupted planned immunization days and over 180,000 doses of polio vaccine were wasted (WHO 2002c). Despite the Mine Ban Treaty of 1997 (which China, Russia, and the United States have yet to sign), 15,000 to 20,000 people are victims of landmines each year (UN Development Programme 2002). Children in some conflict areas are recruited and used as soldiers, resulting in serious physical and psychological damage to them.[7] The UN High Commissioner for Refugees is currently caring for nearly 20 million people who are unable to go home.[8] Even attempts to maintain global order and reduce the chance of war have negative health consequences. UN economic sanctions (used 14 times since 1945, 12 times since 1990) were imposed on Iraq following its invasion of Kuwait. Despite an "oil-for-food" program begun in December 1996, the health conditions in Iraq continued to deteriorate because of the sanctions (Gordon 2002). It is estimated that 25 percent of children in south and central Iraq (750,000 children) suffer from chronic malnutrition. Child mortality doubled during the sanctions,[9] posing a serious moral dilemma for the UN. Clearly, since these statistics were made available, the people of Iraq have experienced even further devastation.

The skills of nurses and other health practitioners are vital in dealing with the terrible results of conflict, but they are also recognized as vital for the preservation and promotion of peace. In fact, the World Health Assembly has declared the peace-builder role of health workers to be the most significant factor in the attainment of health for all (1981 Resolution 34.38). In 1997, WHO developed the concept of "Health as a Bridge for Peace (HBP)," which integrated peace-building concerns, concepts, principles, strategies, and practices into health relief and health sector development.[10] The HBP concept is based on values of human rights, humanitarian principles, and medical ethics. It is an acknowledgment that health personnel are positioned well to contribute to peace building.

The motivations and capabilities of health practitioners also transfer well to the role of peacemaker (Galtung 1997; Garber 2001). Health practitioners are on the ground, prepared to alleviate suffering and save lives. Their humanitarian ethos and the explicit demands of professional ethics mean that all persons receive care (even an enemy) according to their health needs, not their status or politics. Health professionals are trained to take responsibility, to be accountable, and to do so with an attitude of service, not domination. The ability to be empathic and skilled at communication is key to their role and they inspire trust and respect in others. Health problems can be a basis for collaboration across lines of conflict, and there is much precedence for practitioners working together. Health professionals have networks of contacts and belong to professional associations organized at the international level.

Within the HBP program, specific peace-building roles have been suggested for nurses and other practitioners. They can promote security as a health determinant and manage health information in times of conflict, including giving early warning of conflict (Garber 2001). They can be dialogue partners with parties in conflict, organize such dialogues, and help broker agreements, as well as play a role in reconstruction and reconciliation (Galtung 1997). The most important peace role for nurses, including nurses outside of conflict areas, may be as an exemplar of human solidarity. Nurses who recognize that the quality of life in our global community, perhaps its very survival, depends upon our success at creating a safe, peaceful, and just world for everyone can enact this common interest in their everyday lives and practice. This enactment may simply mean living in a more environmentally friendly way or becoming involved in a project to help a struggling community or being politically active in promoting solutions to global problems.

If we live with a conscious awareness of the fundamental rights of all humans and accept some responsibility for helping to protect and support those rights, we can do much to improve the world.

HUMAN RIGHTS

As I write this chapter, Russian security troops are forcing thousands of refugees to leave a UN-supplied border camp in −10°C weather to return to an active war zone. Russia's human rights commissioner, Oleg Mironov, is decrying this action, calling it one of the worst human rights disasters in Russian history (Weir 2002). Naming this action as a violation of human rights is a way to capture the attention of the international community and to secure protection for persons experiencing inhumane treatment. Human rights, possibly our most common global value (Austin 2001b; Wilson 1997), can be thought of as a kind of language that we may use to engage one another across our diversities (cultures, religions, and politics) when fundamental human issues are at stake (Ignatieff 2001).

Human rights were formalized by the UN in the aftermath of WWII and the Holocaust as part of an attempt by the world to create "firewalls against barbarism" (Ignatieff 2001, 5). The Universal Declaration of Human Rights (UDHR) was adopted by the General Assembly of the UN on December 10, 1948. It made the protection and fulfillment of human rights the responsibility of national governments. Since 1948 other rights instruments have been developed: including national charters of rights; international treatises on civil and political rights; economic, social, and cultural rights; and rights of protection against racial discrimination. The concept of **peoples' rights** (the collective rights of specific groups, such as women, children, gays, indigenous peoples, minorities) is a new, if highly controversial, way of addressing group oppression (Felice 1996). Peoples' rights is a controversial concept because certain groups are given special attention, and human rights are based on the idea that, when it comes to rights, we are all the same. This criticism is countered by the argument that some groups are particularly vulnerable and need protection as a group. A rights approach was used to address concerns regarding interventions on human genes when the United Nations Educational, Scientific and Cultural Organization (UNESCO) adopted The Universal Declaration on the Human Genome and Human Rights in 1997, and the United Nations General Assembly endorsed it the following year.[11]

Based on the assumption that every member of the human species has certain entitlements simply because of being human, a human rights perspective explicitly recognizes the dignity and worth of every person. Despite its intuitive and political appeal, the human rights paradigm has been severely criticized on several accounts:

- as lacking a sound theoretical basis (i.e., it is nonsense to assert that humans are born with inherent rights);
- as being too legalistic (i.e., legislation enacts human rights, but infrastructures to support legal solutions to rights violations are often not in place);
- as being too Western and individualistic (i.e., Eastern cultures value family and community above the individual); and
- as essentialist (i.e., based on a false idea of universal humanness).

Rights, nevertheless, have rhetorical force and the power of shame over violators, and they are understood and accepted by ordinary people around the world (Austin 2001b).

One serious problem for the human rights approach is, hopefully, being overcome. Prosecuting rights violators has been difficult (or impossible) in the past. On July 1, 2002, however, the world's first permanent, independent International Criminal Court (ICC) came into existence. The ICC is an effort to ensure that no one (even dictators, politicians, and military leaders) can perpetrate human rights abuse with impunity.

Within the rights paradigm, health is conceived as an entitlement. Having a "right to health" means that everyone, regardless of gender, race, religion, ethnicity, social status, or political identity has the "right to a standard of living adequate for the health and well-being of him [or her]self and his [or her] family, including food, clothing, housing, and medical care and necessary social services, and the right to security in the event of unemployment, sickness, disability, widowhood, old age, or other lack of livelihood in circumstances beyond his [or her] control" (Article 25 of the UDHR). Governments who have ratified UN agreements with articles pertaining to health must indicate the ways they are working to improve the health of their people.

It is important that nurses understand and are attentive to the interaction of human rights and health. For instance, human rights violations can have substantial consequences for health. Individuals being tortured or discriminated against or being denied access to safe water or to health information will suffer negative consequences to their health and well-being. As well, health policies and practices can violate human rights. Acts of discrimination can range from the extreme, such as *apartheid* or ethnic cleansing, to the subtle, such as social barriers that curtail access of marginalized groups to health services. The creation of environmental health hazards, the utilization of unethical research practices, and disrespectful treatment of persons with disabilities are other examples of health rights violations. Some health policies may inherently constrict rights, such as policies for infectious disease control, which often involve mandatory testing, reporting, and quarantine. Awareness of rights, however, can lessen the negative impact of such policies, as when WHO integrated human rights concerns with health care strategies in its Global AIDS response and explicitly addressed the protection of persons with HIV/AIDS from discrimination (Gruskin, Mann and Tarantola 1997).

Nurses need to actively ensure the right to health. Rights violations must be identified and documented, and nurses need to testify about those rights; health rights must be promoted by the provision of scientific information about public health problems; the public must be helped to monitor and question health systems; and policy development must be informed by individual practitioners and their professional associations (Hannibal and Lawrence 1996; Mann et al. 1999; Moore et al. 1997).

For nurses in some parts of the world, protecting the right to health may be a dangerous activity. International rights documents[12] and the International Council of Nurses' (ICN) position validate nurses' efforts in their statements on nurses' role in the protection of human rights and in the care/protection of prisoners/detainees.[13] There are organizations, in addition to ICN, such as Physicians for Human Rights, Global Lawyers and Physicians, and Amnesty International to look to for help and guidance. Although it has been unsuccessful to date, ICN has been requesting that the UN assign a Special Rapporteur to monitor and protect the independence and integrity of health professionals (ICN 2000). Despite the struggles it often entails, the human rights approach remains a powerful way of addressing some of the barriers encountered in achieving health for all. Nurses need to become skilled in the language of rights so that their voices may be heard to greater effect.

A UNIVERSAL ETHIC FOR A GLOBAL COMMUNITY

How do we find answers to our global health problems? How do we determine the answers to the fundamental ethical questions: How should we live? How should we live together? Given the great diversity of a global community, is it possible to conceive of common moral values and basic ethical principles that can serve as a foundation for every person's ethical life? Is it possible to form a meaningful moral community to which every human belongs (Rorty 1996)?

Optimists argue that we already have shared values. Some point to human rights documents as evidence of that. Others, uneasy regarding anything "universal" in these postmodern times, note that values and norms are embedded in context and history, and no common system of ethics can have validity. Cultures and societies that have been colonized and/or oppressed are particularly wary of any hegemonic ethic. Despite these concerns, the need to secure some foundation for addressing our global problems and for understanding responsibility and moral obligations beyond national borders is moving many to try to articulate a global ethics (or what Apel [1997] calls a "planetary macroethic" [5]) for 21st-century society, as daunting as that task may be.

International groups have taken up the challenge. The Commission on Global Governance[14] in its 1995 report, *Our Global Neighbourhood,* calls for a "global civic ethic." The principle of reciprocity (or the "golden rule") is identified as a value for all, with respect for life, liberty, justice and equity, mutual respect, caring, and integrity given as basic values, along with their accompanying rights and responsibilities. These rights are seen as the right to a secure life, equitable treatment, an opportunity to earn a fair living, participation in governance at all levels, equal access to information, and equal access to the global commons. Responsibilities include gender equity, protecting the interests of future generations, safeguarding the global commons, preserving humanity's cultural and intellectual heritage, participating actively in governance, and working to eliminate corruption. The Commission also proposes that new ways be found to establish funds for global purposes, suggesting such methods as a tax on foreign currency movements or charges for using flight lanes, sea lanes, and other common global resources.

Other groups working to balance rights with duties and responsibilities are the InterAction Council,[15] which in 1997 produced a Declaration of Responsibilities in which rights are balanced with responsibilities (e.g., to behave with integrity, honesty, and fairness) and the Valencia Third Millennium Foundation (1999) which created a Declaration of Human Duties and Responsibilities.[16] In 1993, at the Parliament of the World's Religions, a "global ethic" was declared based on principles said to be found in all major religious and ethical traditions. Two principles were stipulated as representing the fundamental demand of all religions: that every human should be treated humanely and that we should treat others as we would have others treat us. These principles are seen as giving rise to certain moral commitments: to a culture of peace; to a culture of solidarity and a just economic order; to a culture of tolerance and a life of truthfulness; and to a culture of equal rights and partnership between men and women (Kung 1993). Rushworth Kidder, founder of the Institute for Global Ethics, has used a more empirical approach to explore universal values.[17] Using a Delphic method, he asked leading thinkers, artists, educators, scientists, and business, political, and religious leaders for their vision of a global code of ethics (Kidder 1989, 1994). Values identified by Kidder include compassion, truth, responsibility, fairness, freedom, tolerance, and reverence for life (Loges and Kidder 1996). UNESCO has been integrating the efforts of these various groups and proceeding with its own mandate to derive a global civic ethic. UNESCO launched the Universal Ethics Project in 1997 (Kim 1999).

Those contributing to the Universal Ethics Project learned early on that, when describing moral universals discernible beyond cultural differences, a major issue becomes whether a maximalist or a minimalist approach should be taken. Should a thick description of an ethical foundation be derived even if some principles might not be accepted by all cultures? Or should a thin, basic ethic and a common moral language be secured (Kim 1999)? Bok (1995), for instance, suggests that we start with minimal "down to earth values" recognized by all human groups as preconditions of their survival and delineates three categories of global values: duties of mutual support and loyalty, constraints on violence and dishonesty, and ideas of procedural justice.

The common framework for ethics ultimately developed in the UNESCO project, however, is a maximalist one, founded on an inclusive idea of universality that can accommodate cultural differences. "Such a conception is based on two concrete facts: the commonality of ethical practice in the daily life of different cultures, and the commonality of the tasks which humanity faces" (Kim 1999, 40). The framework focuses on four areas in which ethical values and principles related to global problems seem to cluster: sustainability for the earth, human fulfillment in the exercise of rights and responsibilities, complementarity between the individual and the community, and peace through justice (Kim 1999, 41).

Other efforts to create what amounts to a planetary code of conduct for humans have led to the Earth Charter, accepted formally by UNESCO in the year 2000.[18] The Charter declares that, as peoples of the planet Earth, we recognize our responsibility to one another, to the greater community of life, and to future generations. It commits us to the goal of achieving a sustainable global society founded on respect for nature, universal human rights, economic justice, and a culture of peace. It now awaits UN endorsement.

Toward the development of a global health ethic, a working group of the International Bioethics Committee (IBC) recently met to explore the possibility of elaborating a universal instrument on bioethics (UNESCO 2002). **Bioethics** is the study of moral issues in biological and medical research and practice. Its evolution overlaps that of nursing ethics, and a universal instrument on bioethics will have relevance for the 11 million nurses in the world. In the preliminary work on the instrument, some fields for consideration have been identified. These include practices that have implications beyond national borders (e.g., international research, import of embryos, tissue collections, genetic data), access to health care (inequality between rich and poor), human reproduction issues, end-of-life issues, biomedical research with humans, personal health care data (e.g., genetic data), intellectual property protection (e.g., patents, benefit sharing), organ and tissue transplantation, use of embryonic stem cells in therapeutic research, and genetically modified organisms. It is intended that the instrument will be used to promote the basic principles of bioethics across the global community. Like the other efforts to make universal values and principles explicit, it is a document for raising awareness and stimulating debate.

Nurses need to participate in such debate and to initiate their own. This can be accomplished in ways such as supporting the Canadian Nurses Association's efforts to describe and address ethical practice, participating in bioethics discourse in arenas like the Canadian Bioethics Society's conferences, and contributing ideas to local and international bioethics journals. As nurses gain a global, as well as local, perspective, some of our assumptions regarding the values and virtues of nursing itself may need to change. Davis (1999) suggests that one such assumption might be the Western view of the self-reliant individual as the human ideal. She asks the question about whether there are ethical notions of caring, principles, and virtues that all nurses could endorse. Nurses in Canada— a multicultural and plural society—should have much to offer to the discourse evolving from this question.

Reflection upon the themes that arise from efforts to capture a global ethic reveal that one principle, at least, seems fundamental to human ethical life—that of reciprocity. It seems that we need to aspire to live by the golden rule. Our basic challenge, then, is to be willing to create conditions under which we truly do treat our neighbours as we would want to be treated. Can we do this in a global neighbourhood? Can the suffering of distant humans come to have the same moral claim as the suffering of proximate ones (Laquer 2001)? Is our moral imagination strong enough for us to see ourselves in the place of the poor, the war-torn, the sick, and the dying though they live thousands of miles away?

Ethics in Practice 16-2	**Moral Community**

The British nurse was picking her way through the mass of women and children squatting in the dust at the entrance of the field hospital of the refugee camp in Korem, Ethiopia. She was selecting which children could still be helped. She was choosing who would live and who would die. A television crew trailed behind her, moving its way among the starving. A television reporter approached with a mike and asked her how she felt about what she was doing. It was not a question she felt capable of answering (Ignatieff 1998, 9).

The scene in Ethics in Practice 16-2 is a real one, and it is not difficult to imagine watching the nurse, the dying children, and their mothers on our home television set. What is difficult, perhaps, is to carefully imagine and honestly consider our reactions to it. Would we move to quickly change the channel? Are we tired of seeing such terrible suffering in far-off places? Do we feel we have too many troubles on the home front to be opening ourselves to more? Are we annoyed at the TV reporter for being there, for going for the heartstrings, as if a silent image of dying children is not enough? Or are we relieved that someone is there to get the story out, to allow us to know what is happening? Would our response be different if the camera was recording a camp in Canada rather than in Ethiopia? Does this scene make us feel appalled, frustrated, and at a loss for what to do? Can we imagine ourselves as this nurse, making the decisions she is making? Do we feel a bond, a connection with her, or is she and her role so remote from our own practice that she seems entirely foreign, a saint or a fool? Are we able to put ourselves in the place of the mothers, to imagine watching our own child starve before our eyes? Can we imagine being one of the children? Are we able to see ourselves in such a vulnerable state that a nurse's nod means the difference between life and death? This latter is likely the most difficult image of all. The profound silence of the nurse may best capture our response to this scene.

A precondition of moral performance is a receptivity to situations that require a moral response (Vetlesen 1997). In this era of globalization, our moral space is changing and we need to develop an openness, an attentiveness to persons and other living things outside our immediate geographical community or nation-state. Our moral perspectives must encompass the global, as well as the local, as we become more cognizant of the economic, political, military, historical, and cultural issues that impact human health. Our moral space can no longer be readily divided into those for whom we have responsibility and those for whom we do not (Ignatieff 1999). Our conception of professional accountability must be expanded to include the world community when, as nurses, we decide: How should I act? What is the right thing to do? (Austin 2001a). Nurses can take action to address their professional accountability at various levels (micro, meso, and macro) according to their situation. As individual nurses and as individual citizens, they can maintain an awareness of world events, knowing that because of globalization most of these events will impact their life and their work. They need to think globally and act locally. For example, at the local level they can promote recycling in hospitals and/or take actions to promote the conservation of water. Through collective actions via their professional associations (for example, the Canadian Nurses Association, the International Council of Nurses), nurses can be involved in addressing issues of world health, poverty, advances in biotechnology, conflict, and human rights. For example, they can promote discussion and action on homelessness and the effects of industrialization, and they can participate in councils or committees to prevent the buying and selling of organs and/or to create position statements about the prevention of torture. A few nurses may also be able to contribute their nursing expertise to international aide. Whatever their level of participation, nurses can be effective in building a global moral community.

FOR REFLECTION

1. Do you believe that, as a nurse, you have responsibilities to persons outside your local community? If so, what are those responsibilities and how do you act upon them?

2. Do you believe that nursing education should include the study of political science and economics?

3. What leadership activities do you want from ICN and/or the WHO Collaborating Centres for Nursing and Midwifery in relation to nurses' role in the global community?

ENDNOTES

1. Features of this chapter are closely related to aspects of two of my papers that have been previously published: Austin, W. 2001. Nursing ethics in an era of globalization. *Advances in Nursing Science, 24*(2), 1–18; and Austin, W. 2001. Using the human rights paradigm in health ethics: The problems and the possibilities. *Nursing Ethics, 8*(3), 183–195.

2. A UNICEF and WHO statistic for the year 2000.

3. See www.unchr.ch/children/covero1.html

4. A new field has been proposed by the Gates Foundation—that of "global health sciences." It would merge economics and political science with public health (Brumfiel 2002).

5. See MSF campaign for access to essential medicines: www.accessmed-msf.org

6. Daar, Thorsteinsdottir, Martin, Smith, Nast and Singer (2002) asked eminent scientists with expertise in global health to identify the top 10 biotechnologies that could make a difference in developing countries. These made the list:
   - modified molecular technologies for affordable, simple diagnosis of infectious diseases
   - recombinant technologies to develop vaccines against infectious diseases
   - technologies for more efficient drug and vaccine delivery systems
   - technologies for environmental improvement (sanitation, clean water, bioremediation)
   - sequencing pathogen genomes to understand their biology and to identify new antimicrobials
   - female-controlled protection against sexually transmitted diseases, both with and without contraceptives
   - bioinfomatics to identify drug targets and to examine pathogen-host interactions
   - genetically modified crops with increased nutrients to counter specific deficiencies
   - recombinant technology to make therapeutic products (e.g., insulin) more affordable
   - combinatorial chemistry for drug discovery (230)

7. UN Secretary-General Kofi Annan has submitted a report to the Security Council, listing parties to conflicts on the Council's agenda that continue to recruit and use child soldiers: Afghanistan, Burundi, the Democratic Republic of Congo, Liberia, and Somalia (UN Press release, December 16, 2002). See: www.un.org/special-rep/children-armed-conflict/index.html

8. See UNCHR: www.unhcr.ch/cgi-bin/texis/vtx/home

9. See UNICEF: www.unicef.org/newsline/prgva11.htm

10. See WHO's program, "Health as a Bridge for Peace": www.who.int/disasters/bridge.cfm

11. See: www.unesco.org/opi/29gencon

12. International human rights instruments can be found at the website of the United Nations Office of the High Commissioner for Human Rights: www.unhchr.ch/html/intlinst.htm

13. See: www.icn.ch/policy.htm

14. Formed in 1992, the Commission evolved from earlier efforts of West German Chancellor, Willy Brandt. Its work is based on hopes of global co-operation in securing peace, sustainable development, and universal democracy. The members are 28 independent distinguished public figures. See: www.cgg.ch

15. This is an independent international organization created in 1983 to offer recommendations and practical solutions for humanity's problems in three principle areas: peace and security; world economy; development, population, and environment. Members are statesmen who have held highest office in their own countries.

16. See: http://globalization.icaap.org/content/v2.2/declare.html

17. See: www.globalethics.org/default.html

18. See: www.earthcharter.org/earthcharter/charter.htm

REFERENCES

Albrow, M. 1996. *The global age: State and society beyond modernity.* Cambridge: Polity Press.

Annan, K. 2000. *We the peoples: The role of the UN in the 21st century.* New York: United Nations.

Apel, K.O. 1997. *Globalization and the need for universal ethics: The problem in light of a transcendental-pragmatic and proceduralistic conception of discourse ethics.* Paper presented at the Challenges of the Third Millennium Congress of the Valencia Third Millennium UNESCO Project, February, 1997. Available online: www.valenciatercermilenio.org/ingles/ingles.html

Austin, W. 2001a. Nursing ethics in an era of globalization. *Advances in Nursing Science, 24*(2), 1–18.

Austin, W. 2001b. Using the human rights paradigm in health ethics: The problems and the possibilities. *Nursing Ethics, 8*(3), 183–195.

Bauman, Z. 1998. *Globalization: The human consequences.* Cambridge: Polity Press.

Beck, U. 1992. *Risk society: Towards a new modernity.* Translator: M. Ritter. London: Sage. Original work published 1986.

Benatar, S. 2002. The HIV/AIDS pandemic: A sign of instability in a complex global system. *Journal of Medicine and Philosophy, 27*(2), 163–177.

Bok, S. 1995. *Common values.* Missouri: University of Missouri Press.

Brumfiel, G. 2002. Health initiative gets warm welcome. *Nature, 420,* 5.

Commission on Global Governance. 1995. *Our global neighbourhood.* Oxford: Oxford University Press.

Connolly, C. 2002. Smallpox plan may force other health cuts. *Washington Post*, December 24, A01.

Daar, A., Thorsteinsdottir, H., Martin, D., Smith, A., Nast, S. and Singer, P. 2002. Top ten biotechnologies for improving health in developing countries: Commentary. *Nature Genetics, 32*, 229–232.

Davis, A. 1999. Global influence of American nursing: Some ethical issues. *Nursing Ethics, 6(*2), 118–125.

Dawson, C. 1998. Vaccines growing on trees will take the sting out of immunizations—scientists. *The Edmonton Journal*, December 7, A.

Felice, W. 1996. *"Taking suffering seriously." The importance of collective human rights.* Albany, NY: State University of New York Press.

Foege, W. 2002. Can smallpox be as simple as 1-2-3? *Washington Post*, December 29, B05.

Freidman, F. 1999. *The Lexus and the olive tree: Understanding globalization.* New York: Farrar, Straus and Giroux.

Gadamer, H.-G. 1996. *The enigma of health: The art of healing in a scientific age.* Translators: J. Gaiger and N. Walker. California: Stanford University Press. Original work published 1993.

Galloway, G. 2002. Cult set to present first clone of human. *The Globe and Mail*, December 27, A1.

Galtung, J. 1997. *"Health as a bridge for peace" in the context of humanitarian action in complex emergency situations.* Paper for WHO, Geneva, Division of Emergency and Humanitarian Action. Available online: www.who.int/disasters/hbp/case_studies/health_as_bridge.htm

Garber, R. 2001. Professional to professional: A methodology for health professionals working together in conflict areas. Paper presented at *Health without Borders*, Annual Meeting of The Israel National Institute for Health Policy and Health Services. December 18, Jerusalem, Israel.

Gordon, J. 2002. Cool war: Economic sanctions as a weapon of mass destruction. *Harper's Magazine,* November, 43–49.

Gruskin, S., Mann, J. and Tarantola, D. 1997. Past, present and future: AIDS and human rights. *Health and Human Rights, 2*(4), 1–3.

Hannibal, K. and Lawrence, R. 1996. The health professional as human rights promoter: Ten years of physicians for human rights. *Health and Humans Rights, 2*(1), 111–127.

Holloway, G. 2002. Cloning to revive extinct species. *CNN*, Sydney, Australia, May 28.

Howson, C., Fineberg, H. and Bloom, B. 1998. The pursuit of global health: The relevance of engagement for developed countries. *Lancet, 351*, 586–590.

International Council of Nurses. 2000. *Nurses, pharmacists and doctors call for a UN Special Rapporteur to monitor the protection and independence of health professionals.* ICN Press Release, April, 10. Geneva, Switzerland.

Ignatieff, M. 1998. *The warrior's honour: Ethnic war and the modern conscience.* Toronto: Penguin.

Ignatieff, M. 2001. *Human rights as politics and idolatry.* Princeton, NJ: Princeton University Press.

Jowitt, K. 1992. *The new world disorder.* Berkeley: University of California Press.

Kidder, R. 1989. *Reinventing the future: Goals for the 21st century.* San Francisco: Institute for Global Ethics.

Kidder, R. 1994. *Shared values for a troubled world.* San Francisco: Institute for Global Ethics.

Kim, Y. 1999. *A common framework for the ethics of the 21st century.* Geneva: UNESCO.

Kung, H. 1993. *A global ethic: The declaration of the Parliament of the World's Religions.* Chicago: Continuum Publishing Group.

Laquer, T. 2001. The moral imagination and human rights. In M. Ignatieff (Ed.), *Human rights as politics and idolatry* (pp. 127–139). Princeton, NJ: Princeton University Press.

Loges, W. and Kidder, R. 1996. *Global values, moral boundaries: A pilot survey.* San Francisco: Institute for Global Ethics. Summary available online: www.globalethics.org/gvs/summary.html

Mann, J., Grostin, L., Gruskin, S., Brennan, T., Lazzarini, Z. and Fineberg, H. 1999. Health and human rights. In J. Mann, S. Gruskin, M. Grodin and G. Annas (Eds.), *Health and human rights: A reader* (pp. 7 –20). New York: Routledge.

McLuhan, M. 1964. *Understanding media.* London: Routledge.

McMaster, G. 2001 (March 9). Confronting the drug dilemma: Will the Third World get the drugs it needs? *University of Alberta Folio, 38*, 13. Available online: www.ualberta.ca/folio

Médecins Sans Frontières. 2002. *Lancet: Brundtland sets out priorities at annual World Health Assembly.* Available online: www.accessmed-msf.org/prod/publications

Mooney, C. 2002. Nothing wrong with a little Frankenstein. *Washington Post*, December 1, B01.

Moore, K., Randolph, K., Toubia, N. and Kirberger, E. 1997. The synergistic relationship between health and human rights: A case study using female genital mutilation. *Health and Human Rights, 2*(2), 137–146.

Robertson, R. 1992. *Globalization.* London: Sage.

Rorty, R. 1996. *Moral universalism and economic triage.* Paper presented at "WHO are we?" The Second UNESCO Philosophy Forum. March, Paris, France. Available online: www.unesco.org/p7

Smith, J. 2002. Medicare for us, malaria for millions. *The Globe and Mail,* November 26, A19.

Spillane, C. 1999 (April). *Recent developments in biotechnology as they relate to plant genetic resources for food and agriculture.* Background Study Paper 9. Commission on Genetic Resources for Food and Agriculture. Rome, Italy: Food and Agricultural Organization of the UN.

United Nations Economic, Social and Cultural Organization. 2002. *Preliminary report on the possibility of elaborating a universal instrument on bioethics.* Paris: Division of the Ethics of Science and Technology, UNESCO.

United Nations. 2002. *Secretary-General says Security Council should seek every opportunity to alleviate suffering of people of Iraq.* Press Release SG/SM/7338 IK/292 SC/6834, March 24.

United Nations Development Programme (UNDP). 2002. *Human Development Report: Deepening democracy in a fragmented world.* Oxford: Oxford University Press. Available online: http://hdr.undp.org/reports/global/2002

UNDP/World Bank/WHO. 2003. *Investing in health and development: Research capacity building in developing countries.* Available online: www.who.int/tdr/publications/publications/pdf/rcs_grantee.pdf

United Nations Millennium Declaration. 2000. Available online: www.un.org/millennium/declaration See also: www.un.org/millennium/sg/report

United Nations Population Fund. 2002. *State of the World Population 2002.* Available online: www.unfpa.org

Universal Declaration of Human Rights (United Nations) (UDHR). 1948. Available online: http://www.unhchr.ch/udhr

Vetlesen, A.J. 1994. *Perception, empathy and judgment: An inquiry into the preconditions of moral performance.* Philadelphia: Pennsylvania State University Press.

Waters, M. 1995. *Globalization.* London: Routledge.

Weir, F. 2002. Chechens forced out of refugee camp. *Christian Science Monitor*, December 7. [Online] Available: http://www.hrvc.net/news/07b-12-2002.html.

Wilson, R. (Ed.). 1997. *Human rights, culture and context.* London: Pluto Press.

World Health Assembly. 1981. Resolution 34.38. Available online: http://www.who.int/disasters/bridge.cfm

World Health Organization. 1996. *Revised 1990 estimates of maternal mortality: A new approach by WHO & UNICEF.* Geneva: WHO.

World Health Organization. 2002a. *World health report 2002: Reducing risks, promoting life.* Available online: www.who.int/whr/2002/overview/3n/print.html

World Health Organization. 2002b. *Report on infectious diseases.* Geneva: WHO.

World Health Organization. 2002c. *Health as a bridge for peace.* Available online: www.who.int/disasters/bridge.cfm

World Bank. 2002. *World development indicators.* Washington, DC: World Bank.

chapter seventeen

Nursing Ethics
and Research

Kathleen Oberle
and Janet L. Storch

... [N]urses are always expected to uphold ethical values in patient care, [but] their obligation takes on different nuances when research is involved.

We live in a research-intensive age, with health care research escalating at a rapid pace in Canada. Not only has federal funding for research increased steadily over the past decade, but the effects of globalization on clinical research (e.g., multinational clinical trials and international research guidelines)[1] have also been felt in Canada. Accompanying this increased activity is a concomitant growth of interest in the ethics of research. Historically, the horrors of the Nazi experiments, purportedly conducted in the interests of science, and such projects as the Willowbrook and Tuskegee studies, which are well described in most basic nursing research textbooks (see, for example, Gillis and Jackson 2002; LoBiondo-Wood and Haber 2002; Polit, Beck and Hungler 2001), have clearly pointed to the need for formalized approaches to protect human research subjects. In Canada, protections are afforded through the Tri-Council Policy Statement, *Ethical Conduct for Research Involving Humans* (TCPS 1998), designed to serve as a comprehensive guide for medical and socio-behavioural research, as well as through several national bodies and committees focusing on research ethics.[2] The impact at the local level of this interest in protecting human subjects is staggering. **Research Ethics Boards (REBs),** created specifically to review research proposals in institutions, and called

Institutional Ethics Boards (IRBs) in the United States, have multiplied at an astonishing rate, concurrent with the rise in the number of clinical studies. Yet only some of the growing need for vigilance can be met through formal mechanisms (such as REBs). Ensuring that people are informed about the research they are being asked to participate in, guarding against exploitation of vulnerable people, and ensuring that risks are minimized are some of the ongoing challenges of research ethics. Nurses, because of their privileged position of ongoing contact with people in hospitals, nursing homes, community health clinics, educational institutions, workplace sites, patients' homes, and a multitude of other places, have unique roles to play in the protection of human research participants.

In this chapter, a brief account of the background to Canadian research ethics will be provided and the local effects discussed. Emerging issues in research and research ethics will also be considered to emphasize the critical role nurses must play in safeguarding human participants. Following this background, a more detailed analysis of the various roles nurses must take in research ethics will be provided.

BACKGROUND TO RESEARCH ETHICS IN CANADA

Until the late 1980s the primary guides for research ethics in Canada included the Medical Research Council's *Ethical Considerations in Research Involving Human Subjects* (1978) and *Guidelines on Research Involving Human Subjects* (1987), which had been based upon international guidelines for medical research,[3] the Social Science and Humanities' *Guidelines for Research with Human Subjects* (n.d.), and various other guidelines for social and psychological research, as well as the research ethics or general ethics guidelines of various professional associations (Law Reform Commission of Canada 1990; Storch 2001). In 1989, at the request of the Medical Research Council, the National Council on Ethics in Human Research (NCEHR) was formed as an arms-length body. It was established by the Royal College of Physicians and Surgeons and was initially funded by Health Canada and the Medical Research Council. NCEHR's purpose was to advance the protection and promotion of the well-being of human participants in research and to foster high ethical standards for the conduct of research involving humans (NCEHR 1998). This mission NCEHR accomplished through education, print materials to support education, and educational site visits to local REBs.

In the early 1990s a Tri-Council Policy committee was formed, with a mandate to develop a set of guidelines that would guide researchers and research ethics committees in evaluating the ethics of proposed studies. Membership included representatives of each of the three major research funding agencies in Canada (Social Sciences and Humanities Research Council [SSHRC], Natural Sciences and Engineering Research Council [NSERC], and the Medical Research Council [MRC], which in 2000 was transformed into the Canadian Institutes of Health Research [CIHR]).[4] When the Tri-Council Policy guidelines were released in 1998, the three granting councils immediately announced that every institution receiving funding from one of the three agencies must be in compliance with the policy statement or funding would no longer be forthcoming. "Compliance" in this case meant that every protocol (whether funded by a Tri-Council agency or not) must be approved by an REB constituted according to the TCPS and that all studies must adhere to the policy in every aspect. This led to major changes in procedure in some institutions and increased the general interest in research ethics within and outside universities.

In 2002, for example, the health-related REB at the University of Calgary reviewed and approved about 600 new research protocols. Because many studies were also continuing from the previous year, it is safe to say that at any point in time there were over 1000 studies being conducted in the Calgary Health Region. The vast majority of these were randomized controlled clinical trials, most sponsored by pharmaceutical agencies seeking to test the safety and efficacy of new drugs. However, many were nursing studies, most of which were non-experimental in design. This plethora of research applications for ethics review is by no means unique. In fact, every major academic centre in Canada is experiencing a similar growth in research activity. Even at universities without medical schools or without significant clinical trial research, the volume of research ethics reviews and approvals (or denials) continues to grow. At the University of Victoria, for example, where health research is largely focused on socio-behavioural research, upwards of 500 applications for ethics review were submitted in 2002, and an estimated 700 studies were ongoing. Thus, whether applications emanate from a medical school or from a university with no medical school, the increase in health research and in research involving human participants is unprecedented.[5]

Gaps and Challenges in Ethics Review

All research involving human participants should be reviewed for attention to research ethics. Indeed, a recent statement from an international coalition of editors of medical journals indicates that they will not publish research articles in which evidence of ethics review is lacking. Yet many research projects involving human subjects are not reviewed because there is no logical place for them to be reviewed. This applies particularly to projects conducted outside the umbrella of a university REB. Universities are not anxious to take on the task of research ethics reviews outside of their own research community for at least two reasons: the REBs are already overloaded with university researchers' applications for review, and liability issues are too difficult to manage. In some cases, private REBs are engaged to conduct the research ethics review, in other cases the research may not be reviewed at all, and in yet other cases the clinical ethics committee in an agency may conduct the review. Few provinces have found a solution to these gaps in coverage, although Alberta has set an important standard in this regard. In Alberta, for example, the College of Physicians and Surgeons recently struck an REB to review medical research protocols that fall outside the domain of university-affiliated institutions, such as those in private clinics. For those researchers who are neither physicians nor affiliated with a university, the Alberta Heritage Foundation for Medical Research has also developed an REB. Thus, Albertans can have much greater confidence that all health research will have received careful scrutiny for possible ethical concerns.

Despite the assurance that a study has received an ethics review, concerns still arise as studies are being carried out (Law Commission of Canada 2000). The mechanisms for follow-up by REBs are poorly developed across Canada. Most REBs rely on researchers to provide annual reports on the progress of the research but do not undertake active monitoring of studies in progress. Instead, the institution depends on the researcher to follow the approved protocol exactly and rests its confidence on the thoroughness of the REB review. As Michael McDonald indicated in his report for the Law Commission, "institutions and sponsors have a far better idea of what happens to research funds than what happens to research [participants]" (Law Commission of Canada 2000).

Clearly, with a large volume of studies to be reviewed, almost always by volunteer board members, it is possible that some ethical dimensions of studies might be missed. It is also possible that interpretation of procedures might differ between REBs and researchers and that researchers might not always act in compliance with ethical standards. Because recognition, prestige, merit, and promotion in a university system are significant rewards for researchers, they might be tempted to overlook the impact of their research on human participants. This may have been the case, for example, in the continued conduct of the "sleep room" experiments at the Allan Memorial Institute in Montreal, where in the late 1950s and 1960s mind-altering drugs and electroshock therapy were used experimentally (Collins 1988). Thus, the role of others in maintaining vigilance for protection of participants is critical. This means that all those who are in contact with research participants must be mindful of their direct and indirect involvement in research and attentive to potential needs for advocacy or for risk minimization. Nurses have major roles to play in human research participant protection.

ROLES FOR NURSES IN RESEARCH ETHICS

In the rapidly growing literature on health research ethics—outside the nursing literature—nurses' roles and obligations in research ethics are seldom mentioned. This is despite the fact that nurses are almost always the direct care providers for patients who are research subjects, are most often the research co-ordinators for medical research, are frequently principal investigators or co-investigators, and are often members of REBs. In any of these roles (caregiver, research assistant/co-ordinator, principal investigator, or REB member), nurses' obligations to patients or clients, particularly with respect to advocacy, may make them especially sensitive to ethical dimensions of situations and may place them in distinct conflict positions. The lack of attention to nurses' ethical concerns around research is perhaps not surprising, for as Johnstone (1999) has pointed out, "the moral concerns of nurses generally continue in varying ways to be marginalized, invalidated and/or even ignored altogether" (10).

Within the nursing literature, however, attention is increasingly being paid to research ethics as it becomes clear that nurses have important obligations regarding protection of research participants (see, for example, Benhamou-Jantelet 2001; Foster 2000; Holloway and Wheeler 1995; Latvala, Janhonen and Moring 1998; Milton 2000; Pallikkathayil, Crighton and Aaronson 1998; Platzer and James 1997; Robley 1995; Usher and Holmes 1997; Williamson 2001; Working Group 2003; Wysoker 2000).

In 2002, in an effort to direct nurses' attention to the growing issues involved in research ethics, and to provide a practical guide for action, the Canadian Nurses Association released its revised document, *Ethical Research Guidelines for Registered Nurses* (CNA 2002a, see Appendix B). It contains a clear statement about the breadth of research ethics roles nurses should take by stating that the guidelines apply to staff nurses and to nurses who serve as research assistants, as clinical research co-ordinators, as principal or co-principal investigators, as members or chairs of REBs, as nurse administrators who may be responsible for the provision of research ethics review, and as nurse educators. These guidelines also provide details about problems and cases, an in-depth analysis of typical ethical conflicts around research, and ways for nurses to approach these conflicts. Although this is a valuable resource, nurses need a more detailed account of ethics in research if they are to act in an advocacy role.

Whereas nurses are always expected to uphold ethical values in patient care, their obligation takes on different nuances when research is involved. In many research studies there may be little or no direct benefit to the patient, and in fact, the potential for harm might be much greater than in standard practice. An inherent distinction exists between researcher-participant and nurse-patient relationships, since, in research, ethical justification can be made for the participant's best interests not being the *sole* purpose of the relationship. However, that is not meant to indicate that deliberately causing serious harm is ever ethical. Nurses need to be aware of that difference and to learn to develop sensitivity to ethical issues in research. They also need to understand that considerable **moral courage**—that is, the courage to do what ought to be done—may be required in challenging the activities of researchers who fail to pay attention to research ethics. Some of the unique research-related concerns experienced by nurses will be described below.

Nurse as Care Provider

What kinds of issues arise for nurses when they care for patients who are research subjects? Close examination of clinical research studies reveals an interesting phenomenon. As caregivers of patients involved in a clinical study, nurses are, in some sense, participants in the study, particularly when they are expected to administer experimental treatments. Staff nurses are, however, seldom asked whether they wish to participate in the trial—that is, their consent is rarely, if ever, sought. Nor are they considered co-investigators. Yet their participation in a trial may cause them extreme distress, a fact that is seldom acknowledged and has not been discussed in the literature to date.

Conversations with nurses indicate that the most worrying situation is the blinded placebo-controlled trial. When neither patient nor caregiver knows whether the patient is on placebo or experimental treatment, a particular set of problems arises, as illustrated in Ethics in Practice 17-1.

Ethics in Practice 17-1	**Withdrawing from a Clinical Trial**

Mr. Peters was a 52-year-old man with acute myelocytic leukemia. I was looking after him the day his doctor came to ask him if he would consent to being in a clinical trial. The doctor explained that they wanted to try a combination of drugs that might have a better chance of putting him into full remission. A new, experimental drug was to be added to the usual medications. The study was a placebo-controlled trial, so he would have a 50-50 chance of getting the experimental drug. He would not know whether he was in the experimental arm of the study because either way he would be getting an extra pill once a day, and it could be either the placebo or the experimental drug. The doctor explained all the side effects of the usual chemotherapy protocol and added a list of side effects that were possible from the new drug. Mr. Peters said he would give it a try—anything that might help him and others get better. The next morning Mr. Peters started on his treatment regimen. He experienced terrible side effects—severe nausea, vomiting and diarrhea, a blinding headache, and awful itching. He was so weak he could hardly lift his head from the pillow except to vomit. It seemed like he suffered more with side effects than any patient I had cared for, and I was surprised that they came on so fast. Each day when I gave him his meds he asked me if I thought it was worth it. On the fifth day he told me that he was pretty sure the worst of the side effects were from the new drug and that he wouldn't take the new pill. He said it wasn't worth it to him to be in the trial any more—he wanted to drop out. I tried to get hold of his doctor, but she was unavailable. I didn't know what to do because it was stressed that the drugs had to be given together and at the same time every day. Should I honour Mr. Peters' choice or try to talk him into taking the pill?

In this scenario the nurse experiences distress in administering an unknown drug for which she is unable to predict usual side effects or to determine when the side effects are unusually toxic. Nurses see this treatment situation as contrary to professional standards. They have a moral obligation to help prevent patient suffering, but if they are unable to establish whether suffering is intensified by the experimental treatment, it is difficult to determine what would be in the patient's best interests. They report that it is sometimes obvious when a patient is on the experimental drug rather than placebo, either because of the drug's effects or its side effects, and they question what recourse they have if they believe the treatment is harming the patient in some way. A related problem occurs when the patient is receiving a drug or a placebo that clearly does not offer as much benefit as what they are certain is offered by the experimental treatment. They then have difficulty administering the placebo if they feel that patients are being denied effective treatment by its continued use.

Blinded clinical trials are not the only source of concern for nurses. Important issues arise for all kinds of studies around the consent process. Nurses' concerns seem to centre around two things: their perception that patients frequently fail to understand the nature of the study, despite having signed a consent form, and their belief that patients are sometimes coerced into taking part in studies. Nurses report that patients frequently remain ignorant of the details of their participation despite having signed a consent form. For example, many patients involved in placebo-controlled trials appear not to understand that they may be receiving an inactive substance. Many of these patients may be under a **therapeutic misconception**—that is, they may believe that the medications they are taking are all therapeutic and to their advantage (Miller and Brody 2003). Often patients do not understand that their participation in research is entirely voluntary, that the medication may not benefit them in any way, and that their care will not be adversely affected if they choose not to participate. When they believe that consent was not informed, free, or voluntary, nurses feel distressed by being required to administer experimental treatments, particularly if the patient begins to express doubt about participation.

A problem may also arise when researchers provide direct care as part of a research protocol. Staff nurses are accountable for the care provided to their assigned patients, but they are often unsure as to their responsibility for interventions provided by researchers. Should they chart the nature of the intervention and the patient's response? Should they stand by and supervise the researcher? What if the nurse observes an intervention that appears to be below standard or with which he or she disagrees? Does the fact that a study has been approved by an REB mean that the nurse should quietly accept whatever is being done to the patient? At what point should the nurse speak up? If the requirements of the research project are impacting on workload to the extent that other patients are not receiving adequate care, what is the nurse's responsibility?

What should nurses do when they experience such concerns? Even today, many administrators and physicians believe that nurses should do what they are ordered to do (Ahern and McDonald 2002). However, in the 21st century, nurses are expected to be critical thinkers and to take an active advocacy role on behalf of their patients (Johnstone 1999). It is no longer acceptable to expect nurses, as primary caregivers, to be passive about their participation in research studies as to do so may contravene the Code of Ethics for Registered Nurses (CNA 2002b). Nurses hold a **fiduciary obligation**—that is, a relationship based upon trust and confidence—to patients in their care. They are expected to uphold a principle of **nonmaleficence,** or "do no harm," and to be vigilant in ensuring that patients' rights and safety are protected. This extends to the research context.

It is worth noting that, despite the many issues raised above, nurses should not automatically assume that participation in a research protocol is harmful to a patient. Indeed, according to the CNA Code, "Nurses should continue to contribute to and support procedurally and ethically rigorous research" (2002b, 11). It is a nurse's obligation as caregiver to understand the nature of the study and to support it whenever possible. However, this does not imply that nurses should accept without question any research project they encounter.

Given their obligations to patients, nurses are justified in questioning patients' participation in research studies. In clinical research this would include, for example, questioning the whole matter of **clinical equipoise,** which is defined as "a genuine uncertainty on the part of the expert medical community about the comparative merits of each arm of a clinical trial" (Freedman 1987; TCPS 1998). To elaborate, clinical equipoise suggests that a study of a new treatment is justified if it is genuinely unclear as to whether the new treatment is as good as or better than either a placebo or the usual standard of care. McCleary (2002) notes that "as long as the nurse accepts that there is disagreement among the expert community about what is best, the nurse can, in good conscience, enroll participants in a clinical trial.... [But] the problem is that while clinical equipoise may mean that a trial is ethical, it may not be ethical for particular clinicians... to recommend the trial to a particular patient" (52). Thus, nurses may experience moral distress when they believe either that the experimental treatment is inferior to the standard of care or that the experimental treatment is inferior for a particular patient (Olsen 2000). If such is the case, they are not only justified, but morally obligated, to question the research.

Patients, by definition, are considered to be a vulnerable population because they are in need of care, and some patient groups are even more vulnerable than others. For instance, people experiencing mental illness (Koivisto, Janhonen, Latvala and Vasanen 2001; Tillson and Zbogar 2002; Usher and Holmes 1997), pediatric patients (Kankkunen, Vehvilainen-Jukunen and Pietila 2002), and palliative patient populations (Wilkie 1997) may be considered at particular risk. Their capacity to give free and informed consent might be in question, as, due to their own lack of understanding and/or due to power imbalances in health care, they might be especially subject to coercion. The nurse's role as patient advocate is salient here. A nurse who perceives that a patient is lacking comprehension about his or her involvement in a research study (whether because of limited cognitive capacity or merely because he or she has received an insufficient explanation) has a moral obligation to ensure that the patient's participation is, indeed, fully informed and voluntary. This involves assurance that the patient understands the relative risks and benefits of the study, is able to weigh them in making a decision about participation, and in no way feels pressured to participate. If the patient lacks cognitive capacity, consent from an appropriate proxy must be sought, and the proxy must, likewise, be fully informed of risks and benefits and be equally free from pressure. If a nurse believes that a patient (or proxy) does not have full comprehension, yet is being asked to consent for research, the issue must be addressed with the investigator. Failing that, the REB must be informed.

The CNA Code of Ethics emphasizes informed choice as a fundamental value and indicates that "Nurses should provide the desired information and support required so people are enabled to act on their own behalf in meeting their health and health care needs to the greatest extent possible" (2002b, 11). However, if nurses are not provided with such information, they are not able to comply with that requirement. They should therefore expect to be apprised of details of every study in which their patients are involved—that is, the researchers must see themselves as responsible for keeping nurses apprised of their studies. Nurses should also expect that contingency plans around patients' expressions of desire to withdraw from studies would be discussed with them (the nurses) before the study commences. Researchers and research co-ordinators should make all necessary information available to staff nurses, including contact numbers where the researcher can be reached around the clock. If such information is not ready-at-hand, nurses have every right to contact the REB to report their concerns.

At the institutional level, nurses should also be prepared to agitate for policies to cover their participation in research. These policies should include clear statements of nurses' rights. In many institutions, the signature of the nurse manager is required before a researcher is permitted to bring a research protocol onto a nursing unit. Before providing that signature, a nurse manager must become familiar with the protocol and ask those difficult questions. Until satisfactory answers are provided by the researcher, the manager should not sign the permission form. If research within an institution does not require a signature, nurses should again be prepared to agitate for a change in institutional policy. Once such a policy is in place, nurses can feel more comfortable demanding that responsibilities of staff nurses vis-à-vis research be outlined. Institutions should not be silent on such matters, as both patients and nurses may be placed at unnecessary risk or put under undue stress by clinical protocols (Johnson 1998).

In summary, nursing staff may be reluctant or enthusiastic participants in research protocols and/or may have important moral questions about their rights and responsibilities in studies being carried out with their patients. Certainly it is part of good clinical practice to support the advancement of knowledge through research, and nurses should have a working understanding of the research process. When patients are recruited into clinical studies, the nurse is responsible for being familiar with the basic elements of the protocol such that he or she can interpret appropriately to patients and contribute positively to the study. That said, it should be noted that a nurse's first obligation is to the patient, and any nurse who believes that a patient is being harmed through participation in a study has a duty to address the issue with the investigators and managers and, if necessary, with the REB. To the extent possible, issues should be discussed with the researcher in advance in order to enable support of the project. However, if issues are not addressed, nurses have an obligation to take an active advocacy role. Failing to take action is no longer an option.

Nurses as Research Assistant or Co-ordinator

The role of the nurse as research assistant or project co-ordinator (research nurse) and the ethical challenges that such a role entails are subjects that have been conspicuously absent from published literature to date, although almost all clinical trial co-ordinators are nurses. Conversations with trial co-ordinators indicate that, for them, the primary issue occurs when they are caught between the demands of the research project and the demands of their nursing ethic of obligation to the patient. As has been pointed out in other parts of this book, nursing ethics is unique in that it is founded in personal relationships and caring (Bishop and Scudder 2001). The ethics of nursing tends to be highly autonomy oriented and focused on the individual good of the patient (Elder, Price and Williams 2003; Robertson 1996). By contrast, the goal of science is, essentially, to further the greater good of humanity on a larger scale. Thus, when a research nurse encounters a situation in which the goals of science appear to be at odds with the individual good, the nurse feels conflicted, as illustrated in Ethics in Practice 17-2.

Ethics in Practice 17-2	**Recruitment to a Study**

Roger is a research assistant for an intervention study of an exercise and diet program designed to enhance well-being after surgery for breast cancer. Mrs. Smith is a potential subject as she meets all the inclusion criteria. However, she is quite elderly, is very frail, and lives alone. Follow-up for the study includes frequent visits to the clinic for extensive testing. Roger feels reluctant to invite Mrs. Smith to participate, recognizing that her participation in the study will likely expose her to significant inconvenience, possibly for minimal or no direct benefit. At the same time, Roger has a commitment to the study, which he believes to be important.

Ethics concerns of nurses as research assistants or trial co-ordinators are not unique, and in fact, are similar to those expressed by staff nurses as caregivers of research subjects. However, the research nurse may feel a dual obligation to his or her employer (the researcher or research organization) and to the patient. The professional caring commitment may make such problems more distressing than they would be for a non-nurse. For example, issues around consent may exist, which are made more salient to nurses because of the emphasis on choice as a core value in the Code of Ethics. The Code states, "Nurses respect and promote the autonomy of persons and help them... obtain desired information and services so they can make informed decisions" (2002b, 11). If, while obtaining consent, the nurse feels obligated to recruit subjects even when sensing that that they are not fully competent, a feeling of moral distress or **moral blurring** (the inability to distinguish clear demarcations between right and wrong) may occur (Ray 1998). Here, despite a belief that potential benefits outweigh risks to the subject, the nurse may still feel uneasy at the possible breach of patient autonomy. Similarly, if the employer encourages increased recruitment numbers, the nurse may experience some unease about whether recruitment activities involve persuasion or coercion. The same concern might arise when a patient expresses a desire to withdraw from a study. The nurse must question at what point explaining or reinterpreting the study to the patient becomes a form of harassment or coercion.

Another ethical issue related to recruitment has to do with inclusion/exclusion criteria and who gets into the study. Although the criteria in research protocols appear to be quite precise, personal communication with research co-ordinators indicates that they require, in fact, a certain degree of interpretation. If the nurse, who is morally obligated to act in the patient's best interests, has strong feelings about whether the patient would be harmed, or conversely, would benefit, from being in the protocol, it is possible to interpret the selection criteria in such a way that the nurse's beliefs are supported. This could conceivably introduce a selection bias into the study.

Significantly, as front-line research workers, nurses may be the first to observe, or may even be requested to participate in, breaches of ethical conduct. Although most researchers will behave in an ethical manner, recent evidence suggests that this is not always the case (Pharmasource Information Services 2000). Unethical situations can be extremely difficult for the nurse, who may find him- or herself in the position of **whistle-blower**—the person who reports a perceived wrongdoing. When one's employment is threatened, or when one feels obligated to "betray" an employer for whom one has had respect, considerable moral courage will be required to act according to one's conscience (Ahern and McDonald 2002). Nurses should take responsibility to follow appropriate lines of communication in reporting a perceived wrongdoing, carefully document concerns and processes followed, call for a meeting of like-minded people, and refer back to the REB or even clinical ethics committees for assistance.

In summary, nurses as research assistants or project co-ordinators may experience a variety of moral problems in the conduct of the research. The nurse must always keep in mind that his or her first obligation is to the patient, and, that despite difficulties, the nurse as professional is required to act in accordance with the professional Code of Ethics. When the nature of the obligation is not made clear during recruitment, these problems should be discussed with the principal investigator. The nurse will have to be aware, however, that some conflicts may remain unresolved. Here again, a cultivated ethical awareness and active reflection on practice are necessary to ensure that nurses have a clear sense of how they ought to act. They then must find the moral courage to follow through on that obligation.

Nurses as Researchers

Guidance for nurses in the ethical conduct of research is discussed to some extent in every basic textbook on nursing research (Gillis and Jackson 2002; LoBiondo-Wood and Haber 2002; Polit, Beck and Hungler 2001), but for the most part this coverage centres on issues of informed consent and protection of confidentiality. In Canada, nurses as researchers will be guided by the Code of Ethics for Registered Nurses (CNA 2002b), but this code does not speak directly to research involvement. As was mentioned earlier in this chapter, the CNA document *Ethical Research Guidelines for Registered Nurses* (CNA 2002a) is an excellent resource for research-related issues. In addition, ethical guidelines for research with human subjects are carefully spelled out in a number of non-nursing documents, of which the most important for Canadian researchers are the *Tri-Council Policy Statement*

(TCPS 1998), the Declaration of Helsinki (World Medical Association 2002), and the International Conference on Harmonization guidelines (2002), which articulate international standards. Finally, each university will have specific guidelines that must be followed when developing research proposals. It should be noted, however, that the documents speak in generalities, and the specifics of cases may be open to interpretation.

Nurses as researchers are subject to the same constraints as any other researcher—that is, they have an obligation to ensure that their studies are methodologically strong, that issues of risk and benefit are appropriately weighed and justified, that consent is fully informed and voluntary, that confidentiality is maintained, and that the benefits (and burdens) of the research are distributed equally. Nurses, however, may experience some rather unique problems because of the nature of their research and their relationship with patients. In fact, the nurse planning to undertake a clinical research study might find him- or herself in something of an ethics minefield. It is important that these potential problems be anticipated and avoided to the greatest extent possible at the proposal development stage. Some issues, however, may be difficult to predict, and nurse researchers need to work hard to develop sensitivity to ethical issues in research.

First, it should be noted that ethical constraints imposed by the REB may present nurse researchers with difficulties in accessing research subjects in clinical settings. To uphold the principle of respect for persons and to protect confidentiality, most REBs require participant recruitment to follow one of two pathways: self-selection, in which the participant responds to advertisements or word-of-mouth contacts by approaching the researcher directly; or face-to-face recruitment, in which the initial approach is made by a direct caregiver or a third party on behalf of the caregiver. If the researcher and the caregiver are the same person, the process is simplified (although the potential for coercion is much greater). With concerns about coercion in mind, even if the organization's ethics review allows nurses to assume a **dual role** as caregiver and as researcher, nurses should recognize the importance of third party assistance in recruitment. This is important to assure that no patient is agreeing to be part of the study to please his or her caregiver. Some, but not all, REBs require that any researcher who is a direct caregiver must rely on others to make the first contact. For example, the individual might ask staff nurses to identify potential participants and ask them for permission to have the researcher approach them if they appear to meet study criteria. Thus, nurses and other researchers may be required to place much of the onus for recruitment on staff nurses, which may increase the nurses' workload. This possibility may in itself be an ethical concern for nurse researchers who may be reluctant to do anything to make their colleagues' work more difficult. Recruitment may also become more laborious because of the need to explain the study, remind nurses to identify patients, and to be present when patients are available for recruitment. This same constraint applies if a nurse or other researcher wishes to collect identifiable data from charts and databases. Another constraint might be an organizational requirement that nurses seek permission from the physician before a patient is contacted. Although nurses might well disagree with the right of doctors to control nursing research and to prevent their patients from enrolling in studies, the fact is that it remains standard practice in some institutions. Therefore, nurses considering recruitment of a clinical population would be well advised to seek advice from the local REB before proceeding.

Such practical considerations aside, nurse researchers may encounter ethical issues related to the nature of the research design. In particular, nurse researchers often use qualitative methods, which are accompanied by a number of particular ethical considerations (de Laine 2000; Oberle 2002; Orb, Eisenhauer and Wynaden 2001). One of the most important of these is a function of the relationship that a qualitative researcher develops with the participant and the possible blurring of roles between researcher and caregiver (Holloway and Wheeler 1995; Siebold 2000). For example, a doctoral student, who is an expert practitioner, was interviewing patients about barriers to care. It soon become clear to her that the patients had agreed to participate in the study because they needed help that they thought she could provide. They asked her many questions about what they should do. Her caring response, experienced as a moral obligation, was to provide what assistance she could, but her role as researcher was not intended to involve caregiving. She felt that respect for her participants demanded that she repay them for their time by offering her expertise, so she resolved this dilemma by indicating to participants that she would attend to their questions after data collection was completed—that is, after she had turned off the tape recorder. Still, she was concerned that the promise of care could affect the interviews in some way and influence the information that participants were interested in sharing with her. The flip side of this situation is represented in Ethics in Practice 17-3. Here, the nurse has expertise to offer and is surprised when patients are reluctant to participate. She believes that taking part in the study would be of benefit to patients but is reluctant to press the point because she thinks that it borders on coercion. Clearly, she is aware of ethical issues in recruitment and is determined to uphold ethical standards despite suggestions to the contrary. Such conflicts should be anticipated when the study involves a population with health problems in the nurse's area of expertise. Moreover, the case makes it clear that the nurse researcher requires great strength of purpose if she is to act ethically in such difficult situations, and it underscores the importance of having a plan in place for dealing with such problems.

Ethics in Practice 17-3	**Recruiting Participants Who Need Care**

As a Master's student undertaking thesis research, Millie went to her supervisor with a problem. She was having some difficulty recruiting participants for her study. What she wanted to do was go to their homes after they were discharged from surgery to provide a kind of supportive care that she believed would enhance their healing, reduce the number of visits to the emergency and/or the physician after surgery, reduce complications such as infection, and enhance well-being. First, she had trouble getting the nurses to remember that they were to ask patients if she could come in and talk to them. Secondly, the nurses kept suggesting that she simply look over the OR slate each day and find the patients herself, which would make it much easier for them. Also, when she did talk to patients, they seemed very reluctant to sign the consent. Many indicated that they wanted to ask their doctor if he thought it was a good idea. Others said they didn't think they wanted to be bothered at home. Millie was quite convinced that patients would do better if they had her support, but she was reluctant to try to talk them into being in the study because she was afraid that she was pressuring them too much.

In this situation, the nurse researcher might have enlisted the assistance of the manager or supervisor to give tangible support to the study by encouraging recruitment of suitable participants. Other important issues arise in the context of informed consent. In a qualitative study, it may be difficult to anticipate risks, and one must question just how informed a consent can be if risks cannot be disclosed *a priori*. For example, an interview might open sensitive wounds (Holloway and Wheeler 1995), the location of the interview might make the participant feel vulnerable (Elwood and Martin 2000), and observational studies might result in unflattering descriptions of groups or communities (Bosk 2001; Ellis 1995; Herdman 2000). In-depth interviews and the reporting of data also raise special concerns about engagement and confidentiality. Nurses' skills in relational communication make them especially effective interviewers. Individuals may reveal far more than they expected and may feel exploited in some way by having disclosed highly personal information. Although they have agreed to the interview, they may regret it later. In reporting data, qualitative researchers often use verbatim portions of interviews to illustrate key points, and recognizing themselves in the report might cause participants even more distress. Verbatim reports, combined with detailed demographic data, may make participants identifiable to those who know them, which make promises of confidentiality suspect. Purposefully masking biographical details and letting the reader know that this is being done is one way of protecting confidentiality.

How can researchers minimize other harm they cause to participants? Part of the answer is to approach informed consent as **process consent,** in which the researcher frequently seeks permission to proceed as the study progresses. However, process consent does not avoid the problem of damage caused by the raising of unexpected emotions or memories. It is important that the nurse researcher "expect the unexpected" and have a plan in place for such eventualities, including the provision of counselling support if necessary (Milton 2000). Researchers should also consider carefully whether demographic data are really necessary to the integrity of the project, particularly when findings are reported, and whether the quotations they use are too revealing. Perhaps process consent should extend not just to the data collection phase of the study, but also to the reporting phase. Further to this last point is the issue of "who owns the story." Qualitative research is often portrayed as an egalitarian endeavour designed to present the participant's viewpoint—the so-called "emic perspective." What happens, then, when the researcher and participant disagree with the findings? Whose interpretation is to be respected? Smythe and Murray (2000) suggest that these and related questions must be discussed with participants as part of the process of obtaining informed consent. This kind of discussion requires that the researcher has thought the issues through before seeking consent, and by extension, that he or she has examined the philosophical premises on which the research is based.

Similarly, ethical considerations for international nursing research, as outlined by the Working Group (2003), emphasize a collaborative approach to research in the researcher-participant relationship. These researchers suggest that participant recruitment should be considered as a set of "conditions for ethical entry into a protocol and [as] continuation of the person's participation in research" (129). They remind us that it is ethnocentric to assume that informed consent, which is based upon individualism (a Western concept), is meaningful or appropriate to people in all cultures. Further, Western researchers must recognize the dynamic nature of culture and understand that common ethical principles in Western cultures (such as confidentiality, privacy, and benefit and risk) are based on different values.

The research ethics issues outlined in this chapter are just the "tip of the iceberg;" as mentioned earlier, the TCPS and ICH provide more detailed guidance for nurse researchers. The focus in those documents is primarily on quantitative studies, but as awareness grows, interest in the ethics of qualitative research is also increasing (see, for example, Boman and Jevne 2000; de Laine 2000; Eysenbach 2001; Fitzgerald and Hamilton 1997; Herdman 2000; Herndl and Nahrwold 2000; Holloway and Wheeler 1995; Ramcharan and Cutliffe 2001; Rowan 2000; Thorne 1998; Van Den Hoonard 2001). The key point is that nurses undertaking any kind of research should reflect carefully on how their research might impact negatively on those being studied. Nurses occupy a special position of trust with people in their care, and, while research is essential to the improvement of care, nurses should never allow their enthusiasm for a study to overshadow their obligation to fulfill that trust. An awareness of the kinds of issues that can arise is an essential part of the research process, and the CNA document on ethics in research can be invaluable in helping the nurse to gain the necessary sensitivity (CNA 2002a).

Nurses as Members of Review Boards

A research role that is growing in importance for nurses is membership on review boards, including REBs. Nurses are accustomed to acting in an advocacy role, and their perspectives on how studies might affect patients are generally informed by previous experience. Therefore, their voice is exceptionally important. For example, in one study being reviewed by an REB, it was a nurse who identified the potentially coercive nature of the recruitment process. She was basing her concerns on having talked to patients who admitted that they had felt coerced in a similar situation. Nurses are often more aware than other health care providers of the kinds of worries patients have because patients say things to nurses that they do not share with anyone else. As patients themselves are seldom consulted in developing research proposals, the nurse has a greater obligation to reflect the patient's viewpoint.

It is important that nurses be present at the table when decisions are being made about which studies may proceed. REBs generally consider the scientific merit of the study in their deliberations based on the premise that conducting scientifically unsound research is inherently unethical. A problem may arise if the REB does not have sufficient knowledge of the kinds of methods nurses use to make an accurate assessment of the scientific merit of a study. For example, researchers schooled in experimental design may have difficulty seeing the worth of a qualitative study that has no control group, no hypotheses, and no calculation of sample size. Such a lack of knowledge on the part of an REB raises a danger that valuable qualitative nursing studies could be blocked unreasonably on the basis of perceived inadequate methods; this could translate into inappropriate controls on the development of nursing knowledge (Dolan 1999). Nursing membership on the REB can provide the necessary expertise, but this is only valuable if the nurse is prepared to speak out and champion well-developed nursing proposals. Since the preponderance of members on most clinical REBs are physicians, with perhaps one nurse member, this may be a daunting task for some. At the same time, interest in qualitative research is growing among some physicians, which means that nurses can encourage and support colleagues in other disciplines who are trying to break into new methodologies. But the importance of nurses speaking up about research ethics concerns cannot be underestimated.

It should be remembered that, despite recent advances, the possibility still exists that some areas do not have REBs for the review of research protocols. This could be the case, for instance, in rural settings or private clinics. Nursing expertise may then be required to review protocols and to assess their merits, as in remote Northern communities where the nurse may be the only person with advanced education. Community leaders might request the nurse's advice regarding the impact of the study and whether the researcher should be allowed to collect data. Clearly it is incumbent on the nurse to have a good working understanding of research methods, sensitivity to ethics issues, and a defined route for seeking further advice. Ethics in Practice 17-4 illustrates how such a situation might arise and be handled. Nurses working in remote areas should be prepared for such eventualities.

Ethics in Practice 17-4	**Voicing Concerns about a Protocol**

Heather was a nurse manager of a public health unit in a remote rural area. She contacted me because she knew I chaired the research ethics board of a large city hospital. She told me that a research protocol had been submitted to her Chief Medical Officer (CMO) by a psychiatrist who was also the CMO's close friend. The CMO read the proposal, approved it, and forwarded it to Heather for nursing approval. When Heather reviewed the proposal, she became concerned that the study would create problems for the nurses and the community. The topic was elder abuse, and the nurses were expected to collect the data using a questionnaire that they would fill in after visiting homes in which there were dependent elders. Unfortunately, in Heather's view, the questionnaire was badly designed, and the questions decidedly biased. In fact, Heather felt that if the nurses were to fill out the questions, it was almost guaranteed that the community would be revealed as having a high incidence of elder abuse, even though she believed that to be incorrect. Her worry was that the community could be harmed by faulty study results and that the trust relationship between the nurses and the community would be badly damaged. Consequently, she informed her CMO that she would not sign off on the protocol until it had been reviewed by an ethics board and made a written request to me as REB chair. Her CMO was annoyed, but had little choice but to accept her decision. When our REB reviewed the protocol we agreed with Heather's assessment and sent her a written statement that the study would not have received approval from our REB. When faced with this response, the CMO rescinded his approval and the study was stopped.

NURSES AS LEADERS IN ETHICS AND ETHICS RESEARCH

To this point in the chapter, discussion has focused on "ethics in research." We will now turn our attention briefly to another area in which nurses have an important role: "research in ethics"—that is, research about ethics. Until recently, little nursing research had been done in this area. In fact, most undergraduate nursing research textbooks suggested that questions of ethics, as value questions, were inherently "unresearchable." However, that view has changed. Nurses are now turning to research to help them define nursing ethics and the kinds of ethical issues nurses encounter in their practice. Canadian nurses have begun to explore and explicate the nature of relational ethics (Bergum 1994; 2002); ethics of trust (Peter and Morgan 2001; Peter 2000); ethics in home care, community, and public health (MacPhail 1996; Oberle and Tenove 2000; Peter 2002); ethics in acute care (Oberle and Hughes 2001; Rodney 1997); the meaning of ethics in practice (Rodney et al. 2002; Storch et al. 2002); and ethics and technology (Marck 2000a; 2000b). These kinds of studies are shaping our understanding of nursing ethics and ethical practice. The journal *Nursing Ethics,* established in 1994, is an important forum for dissemination and discussion of international nursing ethics scholarship.

Nurses also conduct studies on research ethics, although the numbers of studies are relatively small to date. This is unsurprising given that few researchers from any discipline have undertaken research in this area. Recent nursing examples include a study to examine, from within a nursing conceptual framework, women's decision-making about taking part in a cancer clinical trial (Ehrenberger, Alligood, Wallace and Licavoli 2002) and another study to explore the kinds of ethical issues identified in nursing studies by a research ethics board (Olsen and Mahrenholz 2002). Nurses are also making contributions to the field of research ethics by writing philosophical papers in which they discuss the issues (see, for example, Jeffers [2001], who discusses the use of biological materials in research, and Olsen [2001], who presents a nurse's view on equipoise).

Clearly, nurses have a unique perspective and something important to say about research ethics. It is essential that this viewpoint be brought to light through research and scholarly writing, as the nurse's voice must be heard. Nurses are at the front line of care and, as such, have an obligation to support research and knowledge development for clinical practice. At the same time, nurses' role as patient advocate places them in a position to ensure that participants in health research are protected from harm. The obligations are clear; what is needed now is the moral courage and commitment to fulfill those obligations. Nurses, as caregivers and researchers, are ideally situated to be leaders in this area; they have a moral obligation to strive for growing ethical sensitivity regarding research and its conduct.

In this chapter, the important roles nurses play in health research are underscored. These roles include those involving direct and indirect involvement in research. Despite the lack of attention in the literature, at current research ethics conferences and in the popular press, to the nurses' varied roles and responsibilities in the ethics of research, there is no question that nurses are vital to the protection of human participants in health research and to fostering good research.

This chapter has also focused on key documents and structures in research ethics in Canada as a reminder to nurses (and others) of the guidance that is available and that continues to be developed. Nurses are and can continue to be key contributors to research ethics through their own practice and research, their participation on REBs, and their leadership in developing structures for research ethics review where none currently exist. All these moves will take significant energy and moral courage, but they are tasks nurses are well positioned to carry out.

FOR REFLECTION

1. What kinds of guidelines are in place in your institution to guide nurses' involvement in research?

2. Why might a gap exist between what nurses believe they ought to do in research-related situations involving another's research and what they actually do?

3. What kinds of research-related issues have you encountered in your practice, and what action have you taken?

ENDNOTES

1. Other research guidelines pertinent to Canadian researchers conducting clinical research are: *Good Clinical Practice: Consolidated Guidelines,* published by Health Canada as an ICH harmonized Tripartite Guideline (International Conference on Harmonization of Technical Requirements for the Registration of Pharmaceuticals for Human Use); *Canada Gazette, Part II*, June 20, 2001, Statutory Instruments, which paved the way for phase 1 trials; and *Operational Guidelines for Ethics Committees That Review Biomedical Research*, World Health Organization, 2000.

2. For example: the National Council on Ethics in Human Research (NCEHR), the Tri-Council Advisory Group (TACG), which was replaced by the Interagency Advisory Panel on Research Ethics (PRE), the Canadian Institutes of Health Research Ethics Committee, the Canadian Association of Research Ethics Boards (CAREB).

3. The Nuremburg Trials following World War II (1949) set the stage for the development of research ethics to right the wrongs of the Nazi experiments conducted on subjects who were involuntarily conscripted for research. In 1964, the World Medical Assembly meeting in Helsinki, Finland adopted the Declaration of Helsinki as a further guideline for research involving human subjects. (This Code has been revised regularly, the latest revision published in 2002.) These two events and the documents developed from them have had a major impact on national codes of research ethics worldwide.

4. Throughout the development and implementation of the Tri-Council Policy Statement, the Medical Research Council was undergoing its own transformation to become the Canadian Institutes of Health Research (CIHR), the intention of which was to broaden its focus on research funding from medical research to health research through a series of institutes with specific health research foci integrating institutions and disciplines. (*A new approach to health research for the 21st century: The Canadian Institutes of Health Research.* n.d. Ottawa: Government of Canada).

5. The Canadian Institutes of Health Research's (CIHR) mandate opened the door for increased funding to socio-behavioral research.

REFERENCES

Ahern, K. and McDonald, M. 2002. The beliefs of nurses who were involved in a whistleblowing event. *Journal of Advanced Nursing, 38*, 303–309.

Benhamou-Jantelet, G. 2001. Nurses' ethical perceptions of health care and of medical clinical research: An audit in a French university teaching hospital. *Nursing Ethics, 8*(2), 114–122.

Bergum, V. 1994. Knowledge for ethical care. *Nursing Ethics, 1*, 71–79.

Bergum, V. 2002. Discourse: Ethical challenges of the 21st century: Attending to relations. *Canadian Journal of Nursing Research, 34*(2), 9–15.

Bishop, A. and Scudder, J. 2001. *Nursing ethics: Holistic caring practice.* 2nd edition. Boston: Jones and Bartlett.

Boman, J. and Jevne, R. 2000. Pearls, pith and provocation: Ethical evaluation in qualitative research. *Qualitative Health Research, 10*, 547–554.

Bosk, C.L. 2001. Irony, ethnography and informed consent. In B. Hoffmaster (Ed.), *Bioethics in social context* (pp. 199–200). Philadelphia: Temple Press.

Canadian Nurses Association. 2002a. *Ethical research guidelines for Registered Nurses.* Ottawa: Canadian Nurses Association.

Canadian Nurses Association. 2002b. *Code of ethics for Registered Nurses.* Ottawa: Canadian Nurses Association.

Collins, A. 1988. *In the sleep room: The story of the CIA brainwashing experiments in Canada.* Toronto: Lester and Orpen Dennys.

de Laine, M. 2000. *Fieldwork, participation and practice.* Thousand Oaks: Sage.

Dolan, B. 1999. The impact of local research ethics committees on the development of nursing knowledge. *Journal of Advanced Nursing, 30*(5), 1009–1010.

Ehrenberger, H.E., Alligood, M.R., Wallace, D.C. and Licavoli, C.M. 2002. Testing a theory of decision-making derived from King's systems framework in women eligible for a cancer clinical trial. *Nursing Science Quarterly, 15*, 156–163.

Elder, R., Price, J. and Williams, C. 2003. Difference in ethical attitudes between registered nurses and medical students. *Nursing Ethics*, *10*(2), 149–164.

Ellis, C. 1995. Emotional and ethical quagmires in returning to the field. *Journal of Contemporary Ethnography, 24*(1), 68–98.

Elwood, S.A. and Martin, D.G. 2000. "Placing" interviews: Location and scales of power in qualitative research. *Professional Geographer*, *52*, 649–657.

Eysenbach, G. and Till, J.E. 2001. Ethical issues in qualitative research on internet communities. *BMJ, 323*, 1103–1105.

Fitzgerald, J.L. and Hamilton, M. 1997. Confidentiality, disseminated regulation and ethico-legal liabilities in research with hidden populations of illicit drug users. *Addiction, 92*, 1099–1107.

Foster, R.L. 2000. Building the ethics of nursing inquiry as we build the science. *Journal of the Society of Pediatric Nurses, 5*(3), 107–109.

Freedman, B. 1997. Equipoise and the ethics of clinical research. *New England Journal of Medicine, 317*(3), 141–145.

Gillis, A. and Jackson, W. 2002. *Research for nurses: Methods and interpretation.* Philadelphia: F.A. Davis.

Herdman, E. 2000. Pearls, pith and provocation: Reflections on "making somebody angry." *Qualitative Health Research, 10*, 691–702.

Herndl, C.G. and Nahrwold, C.A. 2000. Research as social practice. *Written Communication, 17*, 258–297.

Holloway, I. and Wheeler, S. 1995. Ethical issues in qualitative nursing research. *Nursing Ethics, 2*, 223–232.

International Conference on Harmonization of Technical Requirements for Registration of Pharmaceuticals for Human Use. 2002. *ICH guidelines.* Geneva: ICH Secretariat. Available online: www.ich.org

Jeffers, B.R. 2001. Human biological materials in research: Ethical issues and the role of stewardship in minimizing research risks. *Advances in Nursing Science, 24*, 32–46.

Johnson, M. 1998. Researcher, clinician, advocate—What happens when ethics and clinical practice collide? *Prairie Rose, 66*(1), 13–15.

Johnstone, M.J. 1999. *Bioethics: A nursing perspective.* 3rd edition. Sydney: Harcourt Saunders.

Kankkunen, P., Vehvilainen-Julkunen, K. and Pietilia, A.M. 2002. Ethical issues in paediatric nontherapeutic pain research. *Nursing Ethics, 9*(1), 80–91.

Koivosto, K., Janhonen, S., Latvala, E. and Vaisanen, L. 2001. Applying ethical guidelines in nursing research on people with mental illness. *Nursing Ethics, 8*(4), 328–339.

Latvala, E., Janhonen, S. and Moring, J. 1998. Ethical dilemmas in a psychiatric nursing study. *Nursing Ethics, 5*(1), 27–35.

Law Commission of Canada. 2000. *The governance of health research involving human subjects (HRIHS).* McDonald M., principal investigator. Ottawa: Law Commission of Canada.

Law Reform Commission of Canada. 1990. *Toward a Canadian advisory council on biomedical ethics.* Protection of Life series study paper. Ottawa: Law Reform Commission of Canada.

Levine, R. 1986. *Ethics and regulation of clinical research.* 2nd edition. New Haven, CT: Yale University Press.

LoBiondo-Wood, G. and Haber, J. 2002. *Nursing research: Methods, critical appraisal and utilization.* 5th edition. St. Louis: Mosby.

MacPhail, S. 1996. Ethical issues in community nursing. Unpublished Master's thesis. University of Alberta, Edmonton.

Marck, P. 2000a. Recovering ethics after "technics": Developing critical text on technology. *Nursing Ethics, 7,* 5–14.

Marck, P. 2000b. Nursing in a technological world: Searching for healing communities. *Advances in Nursing Science, 23,* 63–81.

McCleary, L. 2002. Equipoise in clinical nursing research. *Canadian Journal of Nursing Research, 34*(3), 49–60.

Medical Research Council. 1978. *Ethical considerations in research involving human subjects.* Working Group on Human Experimentation. Ottawa: Health Canada.

Medical Research Council. 1987. *Guidelines on research involving human subjects 1987.* Ottawa: Medical Research Council.

Milton, C.L. 2000. Informed consent: Process or outcome? *Nursing Science Quarterly, 13,* 291–292.

Miller, F.G. and Brody, H. 2003. A critique of clinical equipoise: Therapeutic misconception in the ethics of clinical trials. *Hastings Center Report, 33*(3), 19–28.

National Council on Ethics in Human Research. 1998. Information booklet, 5th edition. Ottawa: National Council on Ethics in Human Research.

Oberle, K. 2002. Ethics in qualitative health research. *Annals of the Royal College of Physicians and Surgeons of Canada, 35*(December supplement), 563–566.

Oberle, K. and Hughes, D. 2001. Doctors' and nurses' perceptions of end-of-life decisions. *Journal of Advanced Nursing, 33,* 707–715.

Oberle, K. and Tenove, S. 2000. Ethical issues in public health nursing. *Nursing Ethics, 7*(5), 425–438.

Olsen, D.P. 2000. Equipoise: An appropriate standard for ethical review of nursing research? *Journal of Advanced Nursing, 31,* 267–273.

Olsen, D.P. and Mahrenholz, D. 2002. IRB-identified ethical issues in nursing research. *Journal of Professional Nursing, 16*(3), 140–148.

Orb, A., Eisenhauer, L. and Wynaden, D. 2001. Ethics in qualitative research. *Journal of Nursing Scholarship, 33,* 93–96.

Pallikkathayil, L., Crighton, F. and Aaronson, L.S. 2001. Balancing ethical quandaries with scientific rigor: Part 1. *Western Journal of Nursing Research, 20,* 388–393.

Peter, E. 2002. The history of nursing in the home: Revealing the significance of place in the expression of moral agency. *Nursing Inquiry, 9*(2), 65–72.

Peter, E. 2000. Politicization of ethical knowledge: Feminist ethics as a basis for home care nursing research. *Canadian Journal of Nursing Research, 32*, 103–118.

Peter, E. and Morgan, K.P. 2001. Explorations of a trust approach for nursing ethics. *Nursing Inquiry, 8*(1), 3–10.

PharmaSource Information Services Inc. 2000. OHPR issues first MPA suspension letter; calls for new IRB chair, research head. *Clinical Trials Advisor, 5*(14), 1–4.

Platzer, J. and James, T. 1997. Methodological issues conducting sensitive research on lesbian and gay men's experience of nursing care. *Journal of Advanced Nursing, 25*, 626–633.

Polit, D.F., Beck, C.T. and Hungler, B.P. 2001. *Essentials of nursing research: Essentials, appraisal and utilization.* 5th edition. Philadelphia: Lippincott.

Ramcharan, P. and Cutliff, J.R. 2001. Judging the ethics of qualitative research: Considering "ethics as process" model. *Health and Social Care in the Community, 9*, 358–366.

Ray, M.A. 1998. A phenomenologic study of the interface of caring and technology in intermediate care: Toward a reflexive ethics for clinical practice. *Holistic Nurse Practitioner, 12*(4), 69–77.

Robertson, D.W. 1996. Ethical theory, ethnography, and differences between doctors and nurses in approaches to patient care. *Journal of Medical Ethics, 22*, 292–299.

Robley, L.R. 1995. The ethics of qualitative nursing research. *Journal of Professional Nursing, 11*(1), 45–48.

Rodney, P. 1998. Towards ethical decision-making in nursing practice. *Canadian Journal of Nursing Administration, 11*(4), 34–45.

Rodney, P., Varcoe, C., Storch, J.L., McPherson, G., Mahoney, K., Brown, H., Pauly, B., Hartrick, G. and Starzomski, R. 2002. Navigating towards a moral horizon: A multisite qualitative study of ethical practice in nursing. *Canadian Journal of Nursing Research, 34*(3), 75–102.

Rowan, J. 2000. Research ethics. *International Journal of Psychotherapy, 5*, 103–111.

Siebold, C. 2000. Qualitative research from a feminist perspective in the postmodern era: Methodological, ethical and reflexive concerns. *Nursing Inquiry, 7*, 147–155.

Smythe, W.E. and Murray, M.J. 2000. Owning the story: Ethical considerations in narrative research. *Ethics and Behavior, 10*, 311–336.

Storch, J.L. 2001. Current status of human participant protection in research in Canada. *Annals RCPSC, 34*(4), 201–204.

Storch, J.L., Rodney, P., Pauly, B., Brown, H. and Starzomski, R. 2002. Listening to nurses moral voices: Building a quality health care environment. *Canadian Journal of Nursing Leadership, 15*(4), 7–16.

Thorne, S. 1998. Pearls, pith and provocation: Ethical and representational issues in qualitative secondary analysis. *Qualitative Health Research, 8*, 547–555.

Tillson, T. and Zbogar, H. 2002. Putting human research on trial. Research with vulnerable populations raises ethical issues. *The Journal of Addiction and Mental Health, 6*(1), 12–13.

Tri-Council Policy Statement. 1998. *Ethical conduct for research involving humans.* Ottawa: Public Works and Government Services of Canada. Available online: www.nserc.ca/program/ethics/english/policy.htm

Usher, K. and Holmes, C. 1997. Ethical aspects of phenomenological research with mentally ill people. *Nursing Ethics, 4*, 49–56.

Van Den Hoonard, W.C. 2001. Is research ethics review a moral panic? *Canadian Review of Sociology and Anthropology, 38*, 19–36.

Wilkie, P. 1997. Ethical issues in qualitative research in palliative care. *Palliative Medicine, 11*, 321–324.

Williamson, G. R. 2001. Does nursing need an ethical code for research? *Nursing Research, 6*, 785–790.

Working Group for the Study of Ethical Issues in International Nursing Research, Chair Douglas P. Olsen. 2003. Ethical considerations in international nursing research: A report from the International Centre for Nursing Ethics. *Nursing Ethics*, *10*(2), 122–137.

World Medical Association. 2002. Declaration of Helsinki. Available online: www.wma.net/e/policy/ 17-c_e.html

Wysoker, A. 2000. Legal and ethical consideration. Informed consent: The ultimate right. *Journal of the American Psychiatric Nurses Association, 6*(3), 100–102.

chapter eighteen

Human Genetics, Ethics, and Disability

Susan M. Cox

Nurses are well situated to play an important role in genetics within clinical and community, as well as research and educational, settings. Nurses can also do a lot to shift predominantly negative stereotypes of persons with disabilities and to question the potentially eugenic uses of new genetic knowledge and techniques.

Genetics is "an area that nursing can no longer ignore or consider superficially, or it will find itself wholly unprepared to deal with tomorrow's health-care requirements" (Gottlieb 1998, 4). Recent advances in human genetics are reshaping contemporary understandings of health and illness and transforming the practice of medicine. A map of the human genome has been completed, and there is now a plethora of potential uses for genetic information in the prediction, diagnosis, treatment, and prevention of disease. The demand for genetic services is placing an increasing emphasis on the need to integrate genetics with the provision of primary health care (Guttmacher et al. 2001), and there is mounting pressure from commercial interests to accelerate the introduction of predictive, diagnostic, and therapeutic interventions. Nonetheless, scientists, experts in population health, and policy analysts warn about the dangers of over-emphasizing genetics (Caulfield et al. 2001; Lewontin 2000). The role of genetics in human health is complex, and, when packaged in simplistic terms, the message that "genes cause disease" overlooks other important socio-economic and environmental determinants of health (Baird 2002).

In this chapter, I focus on current applications of genetics in the area of human health. In the first section, I describe the Human Genome Project and some of its implications for the prediction, diagnosis, and treatment of adult onset hereditary conditions. Though prenatal and other routinized forms of genetic testing raise many significant ethical issues, I focus on predictive testing because it creates a whole new subpopulation—that is, the "worried well" (Kenen 1996). In the second section, I explore the relationship between genetics and disability, looking at how an increasingly geneticized view of health compels a re-examination of taken-for-granted views of normality and abnormality, difference and disability (Lippman 1998). In the third section, I identify challenges and opportunities for ethical practice from the standpoint of nurses and other health professionals seeking to assist patients, families, colleagues, and society in responding to recent advances in human genetics.

Throughout the chapter, I introduce Ethics in Practice examples drawn from research and teaching I have been engaged in over the last few years. The stories featured exemplify ethical practice issues identified by nurses and other health professionals. My perspective, however, is that of a sociologist working within applied ethics. I am especially interested in everyday morality and narrative; thus, I emphasize the value of listening to people's stories in order to identify enduring moral questions. **Enduring moral questions** are questions that we must live with (Burgess et al. 1998). They defy easy answers but teach us much about our moral commitments and the meaning of being human.

SOCIAL, FAMILIAL, AND ETHICAL IMPLICATIONS OF THE NEW GENETICS

The Human Genome Project

In 1990, the Human Genome Organization launched a multibillion dollar international effort to map and sequence the human genome.[1] Proponents of the Human Genome Project (HGP) promised that unlocking the secrets of the "book of life" would result in cures for common as well as rare diseases and that genome mapping would resolve long-standing puzzles of human development and cellular function (Kevles and Hood 1992). Critics argued that the HGP advanced an overly deterministic view of the relationship between genes, human health, and behaviour, and, moreover, that the project would siphon attention and resources away from other important health issues (Lippman 1992). Many also raised concerns about the consequences of an increasingly geneticized approach to health. These consequences include an overemphasis on individual risk, social stigmatization and discrimination, lack of respect for human diversity, commercialization and lack of regulation of genetic services, and eugenic applications of genetic knowledge and techniques[2] (Duster 1990; Hubbard and Wald 1993).

In recognition of these implications, the United States arm of the project established an Ethical, Legal and Social Implications (ELSI) program to prospectively evaluate the various impacts of new genetic knowledge and techniques. In 1992, the Canadian Genome and Technology (CGAT) Program also included an ELSI program. Critics perceived these programs as a necessary and positive step, yet many remained concerned that the eugenic potential of the new genetics was not being taken seriously enough (Garver and Garver 1994).

Now that a draft of the human genome is complete, it is important to ask what this new knowledge and its application means for human health and well-being, as well as for social justice. Does possession of a computerized catalogue containing the biochemical "recipes" for life enhance our ability to detect and treat common as well as rare forms of disease? Or do the predictive powers of the new genetics engender new anxieties around health and "normalcy" and contribute to new forms of discrimination and stigmatization?

Answers to these questions are not straightforward. The genetic basis for many single-gene disorders was known before completion of the HGP. Genome mapping has, however, had a dramatic impact in stepping up the pace of gene discovery and the range of available DNA-based tests. Genomic medicine is, perhaps, also qualitatively different in that it now emphasizes the importance of understanding the interplay between genes and the environment in the causation of many common etiologically complex diseases. These are diseases such as heart disease, breast and ovarian cancer, colorectal cancer, prostate cancer, diabetes, Alzheimer disease, and asthma (Guttmacher et al. 2001). Some believe that this shift in thinking is ushering in a new medical paradigm—pharmacogenomics—in which therapeutic interventions will be tailored to each individual's genetic characteristics and disease (Guttmacher et al. 2001). For the time being, however, medicine's growing ability to detect harmful genetic traits continues to outstrip the ability to offer treatment or cure for the resulting diseases.

Genetic Testing and Screening

There are now many types of testing and screening used in the prediction and diagnosis of hereditary and/or genetic disease.[3] The decision to proceed with individual testing is typically made within the context of the individual physician-patient or genetic counsellor–client relationship; at other times, decisions are made on a population basis. The purpose of all genetic testing and screening is, however, to learn something about an individual's genotype (Clayton 2002).[4]

Some types of testing and screening have been in use in Canada's health system for many years. A common example is newborn screening for phenylketonuria, a rare but treatable genetic metabolic disease that has been tested for since the 1960s. Another example is prenatal testing for detection of chromosomal anomalies such as Down syndrome. Pregnant women considered at high risk have been offered amniocentesis since the 1970s, and it is now considered a routine part of prenatal care. Predictive or presymptomatic genetic testing for adult onset conditions is a more recent phenomenon. The first predictive test for an adult onset condition became available in the late 1980s, when scientists located genetic markers for **Huntington Disease (HD)**[5] (Bloch et al. 1989). Since then, predictive and/or susceptibility tests have become available for many other adult onset conditions.

Early or presymptomatic detection of mutations that predispose at-risk individuals to particular conditions may lead to interventions that delay onset of disease or avert its most serious consequences. For instance, some women found to carry one of the mutations strongly associated with hereditary breast cancer may undergo radical mastectomy to reduce their chances of developing breast cancer (Hallowell et al. 1997). Alternately, the 1–2 percent of the population found to have a single-gene form of hyperlipidemia may, through diet and medication, avoid early heart disease (Baird 2002). There are, however, a great many cases in which there is no effective intervention available.

In the absence of effective treatment or cure, genetic testing and the provision of information about risk and disease susceptibility have emerged as new types of medical interventions. The paradigmatic example of this is Huntington Disease. As psychologist Nancy Wexler (1990)—who is herself at risk for HD—points out, predictive genetic testing differs from other more routine forms of testing in several important ways.

First, predictive testing creates the novel situation in which some asymptomatic individuals learn, with a high degree of certainty, of impending illness while others learn they have escaped such a fate. As I indicated earlier, this creates a new health status, that of the "worried well" (Kenen 1996). When there is no effective treatment available for the resulting disease, as is the case with HD, great care must be taken to ensure that there is adequate pre- and post-test counselling and support. In contrast with HD, mutations conferring susceptibility to other dominant disorders may demonstrate incomplete penetrance;[6] thus, genetic testing will not confer the same degree of certainty that the person will develop onset of the disease. For instance, women with BRCA1 mutations (associated with familial breast cancer) have an 80 to 85 percent lifetime risk of developing breast cancer, and some of these women will not develop symptoms at all (Clayton 2002). Those who are not found to have a known mutation are not, however, free of risk, as the vast majority of breast cancer is non-hereditary.

The second aspect that distinguishes predictive genetic information from other types of medical information is that it does not "belong" to just one person. Given that we inherit DNA from both parents and share an average of 50 percent of the same genes as our siblings, predictive and/or susceptibility testing reveals information that is both individual and familial in orientation. The modification of risk that accompanies an informative test result may, therefore, have implications not only for the individual being tested but also for his or her offspring and other family members. This creates ethical dilemmas for at-risk individuals and families as well as genetic service providers because there is an inherent tension between upholding the confidentiality of the person being tested and discerning where there may be a duty to warn other family members of potential harms related to an altered risk status. Further, since it is often necessary to obtain DNA samples from multiple family members, there is always the potential for discovery of misattributed paternity.[7] Though it is difficult to accurately assess the incidence of misattributed paternity, those who work in genetics estimate that it is a factor for approximately 10 percent of the population. As such, genetic counsellors emphasize the importance of discussing the implications of misattributed paternity with clients well in advance of any genetic testing (Smith et al. 1998).

Third, genetic information has an intimate connection with our individual (as well as collective) need to define ourselves in relation to others and, in so doing, to recognize both our similarity to, and difference from, others. Genetic information is, therefore, intertwined with ongoing existential processes of self-identity and perception—that is, one's sense of physical, intellectual, emotional, and spiritual "beingness" in the world. It is also deeply connected to our notions of uniqueness and personhood, agency, and self-determination (Brock 1994).

These aspects of genetic information (that is, predictive power, familial orientation, and existential quality) are central to understanding the social and ethical implications of hereditary risk and genetic testing for a range of adult onset conditions. The decision to undergo testing is highly personal, although it must be emphasized that many at-risk individuals feel responsible to other family members in making this decision (Burgess and Canning 2001; Cox 2003). For instance, some of the most common reasons given for testing for HD include relief of uncertainty; general planning for the future; specific planning in marital, reproductive, career, or financial areas; and the perceived responsibility to provide information to children (Bloch et al. 1989). Reasons for choosing not to be tested for HD include the burden of having knowledge of the increased risk of one's children, the absence of an effective cure, the potential loss of health insurance and other related financial implications, and the inability to "undo" the knowledge offered by predictive testing (Quaid and Morris 1993).

Whether or not genetic testing is employed, the implications of hereditary risk ripple through families, surfacing a welter of feelings about responsibilities to self and others (Burgess and Canning 2001). In Ethics in Practice 18-1, a nurse educator tells a story about a woman who has autosomal dominant polycystic kidney disease (ADPKD).[8] Through spending time at the woman's bedside, the nurse comes to understand that parental responsibility is often a significant source of moral distress for persons diagnosed with hereditary disease. The nurse in this example participated in a recent qualitative study on the social construction and clinical management of ADPKD.[9]

Ethics in Practice 18-1	**Feeling Guilt-Ridden**

There was one family that I spoke with and I remember how the woman was feeling quite guilt-ridden about knowing that one of her children was going to be experiencing what she was experiencing—having to come to the dialysis unit three times a week. It was very difficult for her. The whole issue around dialysis would have been easier for her to cope with if it was just her. But knowing that one of her children was actually in the process of realizing that their kidneys were starting to decline in function, I think it was becoming quite a difficult situation for her. We talked about it. This was a number of years ago, when I was working with her at the bedside and during the time when I was taking her off dialysis. I remember talking about her family and she went over the facts... her children all live back in Ontario. She didn't even have the opportunity to be close to them to support them because they were out of province. So I think there were a number of issues there for her, and you could see it was very painful for her. I mean her husband had passed away, she was in her late sixties, and it was so difficult. I think she had this huge feeling of responsibility on her shoulders.

As this example indicates, autosomal dominant[10] conditions (such as ADPKD and HD) impose a double burden. Patients must contend not only with their own symptoms and gradual loss of function, but also with the knowledge that their children may one day experience the same disease. Such knowledge may evoke profound feelings of responsibility, guilt, and shame (Cox and McKellin 1999).[11]

Knowing that one may develop the onset of a hereditary disease also raises many everyday dilemmas around the management of personal information. In Ethics in Practice 18-2, Jocelyn talks with Dan (note: these are pseudonyms) about how being at risk for HD shaped her career and sense of professional responsibility as a nurse. Both of these individuals participated in a focus group conducted during a recent qualitative study on moral aspects of HD.[12]

Ethics in Practice 18-2	**Being at Risk, Being Responsible**

Jocelyn: Being at risk (for HD) pushed me to go back to school and get my RN. I was a practical nurse for years, but being at risk stopped me from getting my nursing degree. I did start, I took three courses for my degree, and then I thought this isn't fair, it's a waste of time and money for me to do this, in case I do have Huntington's, to put in another two years at school. So I stopped that and I don't regret it, but being at risk did push me to hurry up and get my RN diploma before it was too late. So that was okay, it was a positive thing for me. And I've told people at work, you know, "If I start acting a little strange, if you think I've had a nip [an alcoholic drink], let me know because you guys might be the ones [to first notice symptoms]. Because I work

closest with you guys." So I'm very up front with them.

Dan: Well that's good that you can do that because in a lot of jobs you wouldn't want your fellow employees to know that you had any defects, especially the way things are going in this world. I mean everybody's out to get somebody else's job sort of thing. In the private sector anyway, I mean it's dog-eat-dog. It's not like working in a seniority system or like it used to be in the past, right?

Jocelyn: But I guess my job makes it different. Like being a nurse and being responsible for life-and-death situations at times, I want my co-workers to be aware that I might start having some short-term memory (problems) or something; they need to know that and I need them to know that.

In Ethics in Practice 18-2, Jocelyn describes the impact her risk status has in making significant life decisions. Uncertain about whether she might develop HD, she pursues a diploma in nursing but decides not to earn her degree. Though she elects not to pursue predictive testing, she still confronts the difficult issue of whether she should disclose her risk status to co-workers. As a nurse, she believes that it is her moral responsibility to reveal that she could experience symptoms affecting her work. Dan suggests that not everyone will be comfortable with such disclosures. There is still a great deal of misunderstanding, and persons at risk for hereditary conditions may be seen as "defective." There is also the possibility of employment- or insurance-related discrimination (Lemmens 1998).

In Ethics in Practice 18-3, Jocelyn describes how some of her co-workers mistakenly assumed that a man with HD was a drunk.[13] This occurred before Jocelyn knew that she was at risk, but it made a lasting impression.

Ethics in Practice 18-3	**Stereotypes and Assumptions**

Before I really knew anything about Huntington's, and about two years before

my mother was diagnosed, I was working in the back room in the emergency

> department and the girls from the front came into the back and they were talking about "this drunk" that was in the social service room. Before the end of the night it came out that he was actually end-stage or mid-stage with HD. And that's just never left my mind because those nurses all assumed something that just wasn't so. Then, when my mother ended up being diagnosed with HD, that was the first flash that went through my head. That's affected me, whereas I used to have social drinks with ease, I don't any more.... I don't ever want anyone to assume I'm an alcoholic. But it's interesting, one of my sisters, she doesn't drink, but she said, "Well I might as well start drinking," because she is gene positive, and she said, "They're going to assume I'm a drunk anyway."

In Ethics in Practice 18-3, Jocelyn compares her response to social stigmatization with that of her sister, who has had predictive testing and knows she inherited the mutation associated with HD. Though Jocelyn's sister does not drink alcohol, she anticipates that people will assume she is drunk once she develops onset of HD. Hence, she feels that her own moral agency is diminished and that there is no escaping the social stigmatization that surrounds HD.

Social responses to disability have a profound influence in the lives of persons with disabilities. Negative stereotypes of persons with disabilities permeate the practice of health care and the policies guiding medical uses of genetic knowledge (Silvers 2001). In the next section, I reflect on some of the links between genetics and disability, emphasizing in particular the need to re-think and positively value disability as a form of human diversity.

DISABILITY AND DIVERSITY

As it becomes possible to test for an increasingly wide array of genetic conditions at all stages of life, we are confronted in an especially acute way with the need to question predominant beliefs about disability, think critically about the social construction of "normality" and "abnormality," and evaluate criteria used to define quality of life. Such issues arise in many practical settings—from assisting patients in decision-making to evaluating the benefits and harms of new social policies on genetics and disability.

Here, it is necessary to clarify the relationship between genetics and disability. Although there are many substantive areas of overlap, genetics involves more than disability, and disability involves more than genetics. Further, disability is not synonymous with disease. If we focus on biological aspects only, some forms of disability are congenital or hereditary while others are the result of an accident, trauma, chronic illness, surgery, or the natural process of aging. Time of onset and duration are other factors that differentiate experiences of disability. Some persons with disabilities are disabled from birth, while others become disabled later in life. Likewise, some forms of disability are episodic, others are progressive, and still others are static and permanent (Mahowald 1998).

To distinguish too sharply between genetic and nongenetic causes of disability is, however, to miss the critical issue—that is, our ways of thinking about disability. Why is it that we acknowledge and celebrate some forms of diversity and yet ignore or even disparage others? There are many examples of how we positively value other forms of diversity. I am, for instance, fortunate to live in Vancouver, one of the most ethnically diverse cities in Canada.

I chat with a woman from Somalia about world history over morning coffee. I learn about the symbolism of honey in traditional Persian wedding ceremonies from the woman who cuts my hair. I learn to speak a little Italian when I shop for groceries. The people I interact with and the cultures I participate in enhance my appreciation of life and what it means to be human.

Why is disability not seen as another form of difference or as an inevitable aspect of being human? Why is there so much emphasis on instrumental issues such as "how to prevent disability, how to cure it, and what to do with it when it cannot be either" (Michalko 2002, 167)? Disability rights activist Morris (1992) argues that ableism and the depreciation of the lives of persons with disabilities are grounded in profound fears about the body and vulnerability. People are afraid of becoming dependent on others and thus dissociate themselves from anything or anyone that is not "normal." This is also the case within medicine, as disability is viewed as "extremely different from—and worse than—other forms of human variation" (Asch 2002, 125–126).

The exclusion of disabled people is particularly striking within the context of recent debates about genetic diversity and the application of research on hereditary conditions. Nondisabled experts define both the problem and the solution with little reflection on the ableist assumptions informing their judgments about quality of life. Yet there are experts available from within the community of persons with disabilities.

Established in 1981, Disabled Peoples' International (DPI) is a human rights organization committed to the protection of disabled people's rights and the promotion of their full and equal participation in society. In 2000, DPI Europe developed a position statement emphasizing the need to strictly regulate the uses of new genetic discoveries, techniques, and practices in order to avoid discrimination, protect the human rights of disabled people, and positively value human diversity:

> We want to see research directed at improving the quality of our lives, not denying us the opportunity to live... Human genetics poses a threat to us because while cures and palliatives are promised, what is actually being offered are genetic tests for characteristics perceived as undesirable... These technologies are, therefore, opening the door to a new eugenics which directly threatens our human rights (Disabled Peoples' International Europe 2002).

There is perhaps no more cogent reminder of the moral issues at stake than the atrocities committed by Nazi Germany during the Holocaust. The campaign against all so-called "undesirable and useless" people included those with psychological illnesses and mental disabilities, schizophrenia, epilepsy, paralysis, Huntington Disease and other neurological conditions, as well as those who were physically disabled, deaf, blind, elderly, or ill.The Nazis were, however, not alone in pursuing eugenic goals. Many U.S. states adopted mandatory sterilization programs. Moreover, the dubious "results" of family studies of feeble-mindedness and other heritable "defects" were exhibited at state fairs and expositions (Paul 1995). Nor did Canada escape unsullied. In 1933, British Columbia followed Alberta's lead in adopting legislation that sanctioned forced sterilization of the mentally ill and retarded. These programs remained in effect until the 1970s. Manitoba and Ontario rejected such legislation, but "eugenically based racial concerns were all-pervasive in interwar Canadian society and the most extreme policies tended to be advanced, not by conservatives, but by progressives and medical scientists" (McLaren 1990, 91). Indeed, social activists such as suffragist Nellie McClung and magistrate Emily Murphy were active supporters of sterilization and the eugenics campaign in Alberta and British Columbia (McLaren 1990).

Ways of Thinking about Disability

For health care professionals contemplating the eugenic implications of new genetic technologies, there is perhaps no more important task than reflecting on the way that disability is constructed and experienced. Disabilities vary according to many factors, and two approaches to thinking about disability emphasize these factors in different ways.

The **individual (or medical) model of disability** emphasizes the type and severity of biological impairment the individual experiences. Impairments may involve appearance, mobility, ability to perform physical functions, cognitive ability and psychological capacity, ability to communicate, or ability to function without pain. In this model, impairment is seen as abnormality, pathology, defect, or loss. Suffering is the "natural" result, but this is largely seen as a personal tragedy rather than a social problem. Its remedy lies in assisting the disabled individual to adopt the appropriate attitude so that he or she can effectively adapt to his or her disability.

Many people with disabilities feel as if they are seen as little more than their disabilities. When the medical labels that describe various impairments become descriptors totalizing the personhood and identity of disabled persons—as in "the deaf" or "the blind"—we commit the fallacy of allowing the part to stand for the whole. We also fail to account for the social and economic context within which disability is experienced. As the Union of the Physically Impaired Against Segregation stated in one of the first articulations of an alternative model of disability:

> In our view, it is society which disables physically impaired people. Disability is something imposed on top of our impairments by the way we are unnecessarily isolated and excluded from full participation in society (Oliver 1996).

In contrast to the individual model, the **social model of disability** reframes the emphasis on individual impairment, focusing instead on social deficits. This model thus directs attention to the social and physical obstacles that prevent people with disabilities from participating fully in society. These obstacles include everything from discriminatory employment practices to inaccessible public buildings. Suffering, according to this model, is therefore the unjust result of socially created disadvantage. The social model also recognizes the importance of nondisabled persons' perceptions of impairment. Some disabilities arise from the perceptions of others: obesity and stuttering are good examples since each may become a disability if it is perceived as such and evokes discriminatory practices from others (Mahowald 1998). Here, the history of discrimination against nonsymptomatic carriers of sickle cell disease[14] also offers a warning that is germane to thinking about discrimination associated with susceptibility for late onset hereditary conditions. As we test more widely for various mutations, persons who test positive may find they are socially disabled by depression, psychological trauma, stigmatization, and/or discrimination.

In contrast to the individual model, the experience of people with disabilities suggests that it is through collective identification with the social experience and causes of disability that meaningful change occurs. The remedy is not to be found in using prenatal or other forms of testing to prevent the existence of biologically anomalous people. Rather, it lies in challenging predominant views of disability as pathology and promoting respect for difference and human genetic diversity. Within the context of prenatal testing, this means that prospective mothers must be provided with an appropriate range of information as well as support from competent counselling professionals (Roeher Institute 2002).

Making a Difference

Although the differences underlying these models of disability are fundamental, supporters of each can agree on the commitment to social support for people with disabilities, and supporters of both share the desire to eliminate discriminatory practices. These commonalities are significant. Progress can be made if the question of how to best respect "persons of difference" is disentangled from the question of how to respond to concerns raised by disability rights activists about the ableist assumptions informing the use of prenatal and other forms of genetic testing (Koch 2001).

From the standpoint of many persons with disabilities, issues of respect for difference and the ableist uses of prenatal testing are inextricably linked since the practice of preventing the existence of future persons with disabilities is seen as inherently devaluing existing persons with disabilities (Asch 2002). Here one's standpoint and life experience matter greatly. Though I cannot speak from the experience of parenting a child with a disability or having a disability myself, I have struggled with the question of when difference should make a difference and, moreover, what nondisabled persons can do to support persons of difference.

Ethics in Practice 18-4 focuses on "interactional ethics." It balances the individual and social models of disability to show how quality of life can be improved for persons with disabilities when difference is appropriately acknowledged and persons of difference participate in both defining the problem and creating a workable solution. This example is based on the author's firsthand observations.

Ethics in Practice 18-4	**Interactional Ethics**

When I (the author) was working as a volunteer staff person at a week-long retreat for people with Huntington Disease (HD), we held a group discussion about what it means to lose one's independence. Several people with mid-stage HD talked about their frustration with social situations where they were mistaken for being drunk or were simply not treated with respect. This occurred in banks or grocery stores when cashiers or tellers became impatient with the amount of time it took for people with HD to complete a routine transaction. People with HD said they would become so angry at being treated disrespectfully that they simply could not find words or the will to respond. The problem was not their inability to carry out independent activities; it was the lack of patience and understanding that characterized the social response. Thus the solution lay in creating a card with a short message clarifying the situation for cashiers or tellers. Assisting people with HD in creating this card was an intensely rewarding experience. They identified the most relevant aspects of their lived experience of HD and everyone then worked collectively to formulate an appropriate message. It was important to avoid negative biomedical language that reinforces HD as pathology, defect, or inevitable loss. The message was printed on business cards and a pilot version was distributed by the Huntington Society of Canada. According to anecdotal reports, it worked well in a variety of situations, easing social interactions for persons with HD and increasing awareness of the disease within the community. The card has now been re-printed and is in use across the country.

> *I have Huntington disease... but I am very aware of what is going on around me. Sometimes I may be forgetful, have slurred speech, or difficulty with my balance. It may take me some time to express my thoughts. Thank you for your patience and understanding. For further information, please contact:* Huntington Society of Canada

A second example of valuing difference comes from the educational context. Curriculum revision is a vital way of encouraging students and faculty to think about how disability is socially constructed. In Ethics in Practice 18-5, a general nursing student talks about the personal and pedagogic impact of working at the annual Huntington Disease retreat. Her comments derive from a conversation I had with her.

Ethics in Practice 18-5	**Valuing Disability**

As nurses in training, we don't have much training or teaching about genetic disorders, so when I first went to the Huntington's camp I was very apprehensive. I didn't know what to expect. I had never met anyone with HD before the camp. Also, being one of the youngest people at the camp added to my anxiety. So, the first day of camp it was really overwhelming for me to meet all of these people coping with a huge disability. But once you get past that and start to talk with them, not only about their disease but about them as individuals, you start to realize how strong they are and how much they have to teach you. When I went back to school after the camp, other student nurses were really interested in what I had to say. And because we have a class that is based on reflections, I had a good opportunity to talk with all of the other student nurses. Because I've had the opportunity to experience the camp, it has helped me to bring a more holistic view in helping people deal with not just HD but other chronic illnesses as well. It is an opportunity that everyone should have a chance to experience. It is somewhat included in our curriculum because we do community visits with acute and chronic illness patients, but it would be interesting to do that with people with hereditary conditions too. Especially with HD, this is something that is often unexpected. Also, some chronic illnesses are not life threatening, and there is an opportunity for cure or medical intervention. HD has no cure and it is all the more devastating. Personally, though, I've learned through camp to appreciate what I have in my life. Even though I am there helping people with HD, I feel that I am taking more out of it than I am giving.

The nursing student in this example recognizes the moral value of listening closely to what people have to say about their experiences. Frank (1995) describes this type of empathetic listening as "witnessing" people's illness narratives. Through witnessing, the nursing student learns that people with disabilities have a lot to teach health care professionals. When she returns to the classroom, she reflects on her experiences with other nursing students and discovers that she has enlarged their understanding.

The experience of working and socializing with persons with disabilities also leads to greater reflexivity in research and practice. As nursing student Tracie Culp Harrison (2002) discovered, disability researchers are ultimately dependent upon persons with disabilities, not because their perspectives are more valid than dominant perspectives, but because non-dominant perspectives are often missing from the dominant discourse. Simply adding people with disabilities as subjects in research is, however, not enough. It is important to ask the questions that people with disabilities believe to be important in their lives and to structure the research so that people with disabilities can participate meaningfully. As the Disabled Peoples' International (2002) statement on genetics states, "Our experience as disabled people places us in a unique position to contribute to comprehensive ethical discourse leading to scientific development which respects and affirms the essential diversity of humankind."

PRACTICAL CHALLENGES AND OPPORTUNITIES FOR NURSING

The Canadian Nurses Association's Code of Ethics for Registered Nurses recognizes that genetic and other emergent technologies pose new challenges and opportunities for the ethical practice of medicine. A lack of basic knowledge about genetics and hereditary aspects of disease and disability is one challenge that nurses face. Other significant challenges include uncertainty about the most effective methods to convey complex information about genetic risk to patients and assist in promoting client-driven, ethically informed decision-making (Jansen 2001). How can nurses begin to address these challenges and opportunities?

In assessing possible nursing roles in genetics, it is vital to distinguish between what is appropriate to expect of most nurses and what requires specific genetics training and education. This means that there is both good and bad news in relation to nursing roles in genetics:

> The good news is that many of the things that nurses should be prepared to do in relation to genetics they are already doing generally in relation to non-genetic conditions. The bad news is that they may not realize it and [may] represent themselves as inadequate in this knowledge (Lashley 2000, 798).

A national survey conducted by the Health Canada Working Group on Public and Professional Educational Requirements Related to Genetic Testing of Late Onset Disease confirms that both nurses and physicians experience a lack of confidence with the provision of genetic services and, moreover, that this is often tied to a lack of knowledge about genetics (Bottorff et al. 2003).

In Ethics in Practice 18-6, a nephrology nurse reflects on her feelings of inadequacy when she imagines how she would respond if a patient asked about hereditary aspects of his or her condition.[15]

Ethics in Practice 18-6	The Limits to Our Knowledge

We (nurses) would be of very little help to patients because we don't know much about hereditary aspects of disease. We don't know anything about genetic counselling so we would just be able to empathize. All we would be able to do is say "Oh" and "I know" and maybe send them back to their doctor. That is really all that we would be able to do. So other than just listening and trying to be supportive, we wouldn't be able to offer anything in particular, anything concrete if they were looking for that. We might talk about exercise, diet, those kinds of things. We can help them with lifestyle things but there is a limit to our knowl- edge, and certainly [to] our knowledge of genetic counselling! I remember in nursing school, twenty years ago, they would say "Huntington's is a genetic disease, so if you have it then chances are that your children will have it too." You know that's about as far as that went.... [B]ut for us to delve into counselling about what that means for the child to grow up knowing their parent has Huntington's? Or maybe the grand-parents died young, maybe nobody knew it was in the family, and now here it is, you have Huntington's at forty-three AND you've got two little kids?

The nurse in this example feels overwhelmed by the prospect of mastering a new and specialized area of knowledge. Although she is willing to empathize with patients' concerns and offer practical advice on lifestyle modifications, she is aware that she lacks basic knowledge about genetics. Recalling that her education about genetics was minimal, she recognizes that patients and families may need in-depth counselling to help them deal with the significant psychosocial and familial implications of hereditary risk. She also implies that because she is not equipped to offer this type of counselling, she has little to contribute to the delivery of genetic services. She may, however, be wrong in arriving at this conclusion.

Nurses already have many of the skills and abilities required to assist patients and families at risk for hereditary conditions. Nurses spend more hours interacting with patients than do most other health care providers. Further, nurses are often adept at deciphering complex medical information and communicating with patients in understandable language (Wright 2001). As such, nurses' "constant presence" (Weeks 1994)—whether at the bedside, in a community health clinic, or in the home—is an important contextual feature that must be factored into deliberations about how to integrate nursing with genetic services.

The nurse in Ethics in Practice 18-6 is an empathetic listener and clearly exercises moral sensitivity in imagining what it is like to grow up in a family affected by HD. She is aware of the limits of her own professional knowledge and recognizes that it might be appropriate to refer patients for specialized genetic counselling. Although there remains a need to provide nurses with specific genetics training and education, the skills and abilities she has already are important contributions to the delivery of genetic services.[16]

In Ethics in Practice 18-7, a social worker talks about her experiences in working with families with hereditary kidney disease. Like the nephrology nurse in Ethics in Practice

18-6, she acknowledges feelings of professional inadequacy in knowing how to respond to patients' fears.[17]

Ethics in Practice 18-7	**Being There**

I don't know how to put this. Where sometimes I feel at a little bit of a loss is with people who are having to deal with these major issues arising from genetic components of the disease and, you know, all the fears. Because the fears are real! Obviously you can't give false reassurance. But again it's like many other things in this job, you can't solve the problems, what you can do is be with the person as they're going through them and be as supportive as you can... I think social workers and many health care professionals feel inadequate in the face of the kinds of problems that patients have to deal with. You have to realize that you can't make it all better... But you can be there for people. I found again and again that you may think that you're doing nothing for a person, but you'll find later on that it's very important that you were there.

The social worker in this example does not want to offer false reassurance, nor does she want her clients to feel overwhelmed. She recognizes how important it is to be there *for* people, even if it is not possible to solve all of their problems. Providing accurate information and appropriate support is, in this sense, vital. As another social worker emphasized, families often operate on the basis of information that is out of date. Hence, their fears are sometimes based on unfounded concerns, and knowledgeable health care providers may be able to lay some worries to rest.

Nurses must not practise beyond their own level of competence, but when aspects of care demand the acquisition of new knowledge and skills, there is an ethical responsibility to seek out and employ such knowledge in their area of practice. Further, given that nurses have an ethical commitment to building trusting relations with patients and families, nurses also need to identify and respond to the range of issues that create moral distress for families affected by hereditary conditions (Canadian Nurses Association 2002).[18]

Effective integration of nursing with genetic services will, therefore, have curricular implications. There is a need for basic as well as more specialized education about genetics. The International Society of Nurses in Genetics (ISONG), in conjunction with the American Nurses Association, produced a Statement on the Scope and Standards of Genetics Clinical Nursing Practice (1998) that reviews theories and ethical frameworks used in genetics nursing practice, the scope of basic and advanced genetics clinical nursing, and appropriate standards for professional performance.

There is also a need to develop a vision for how best to integrate genetic services within the existing health care system. To this end, in Canada, a study funded by the Canadian Institutes of Health Research will be the first to document and describe nursing practice roles and expertise related to genetic services. The study will also propose a set of recommendations that will support the development and expansion of genetic nursing practice in Canada (Bottorff et al. 2002).

Nurses are well situated to play an important role in genetics within clinical and community, as well as research and educational, settings. Nurses can also do a lot to shift predominantly negative stereotypes of persons with disabilities and to question the potentially eugenic uses of new genetic knowledge and techniques. Although there are many practical and theoretical challenges confronting nurses in these developing roles, there is also great potential for nurses to contribute to the humane and sensitive delivery of genetic services.

FOR REFLECTION

1. What aspects of your nursing education and practice best equip you to assist patients and families coping with hereditary and/or genetic conditions? In what areas do you feel least equipped?

2. Would you want to take a genetic test revealing which diseases you are likely to develop later in life? If so, why? If not, why not? Are there some diseases that you would want to know about and others you would not? Are there some diseases that you have a responsibility to know about? Why or why not?

3. Williams syndrome is a hereditary condition that causes intellectual deficits (such as developmental delay and attention deficit) and a range of physical differences (including broad forehead and/or flattened midface). People with Willams syndrome may, however, also be gifted with special abilities such as expressive language skills, an extremely social personality, and/or exceptional musical ability (Milunksy 2001). Do you think Williams syndrome challenges common assumptions about disability? If so, how?

ENDNOTES

1. Mapping involves compilation of genetic linkage and physical maps indicating where an estimated 30,000 genes reside on each of the 23 pairs of human chromosomes. Sequencing, a separate but related activity, involves working out the precise order of nucleotide bases.

2. Eugenics is based on notions of racial purity and superiority and presumes that human attributes such as personality and intelligence are determined by heredity. Although eugenic thinking is most often associated with Adolf Hitler, the goals of eugenics derive from Francis Galton's view that the governing classes should strive to control and improve the human gene pool.

3. Currently, there are tests for at least 960 genetic diseases. See the GeneTests website (www.genetests.org) for a listing of laboratories, clinics, genetics information, and educational materials.

4. Not all types of testing for hereditary or genetic conditions involve DNA analysis. For example, ultrasound is routinely used to diagnose autosomal dominant polycystic kidney disease.

5. Huntington Disease (HD) is an autosomal dominant neuropsychiatric disorder. There is currently no effective prevention or cure. Onset typically occurs in mid-life, causing loss of control over voluntary movements and gradual but inexorable physical and cognitive decline (Hayden 1981).

6. Incomplete penetrance occurs where there is inconsistent phenotypic expression of a gene, even though the gene is present.

7. Misattributed paternity occurs when a child of any age incorrectly believes that a male, other than the true biological father, is his or her biological father.

8. Autosomal dominant polycystic kidney disease (ADPKD) is one of the most common single-gene hereditary diseases. It typically presents in mid-life, causing progressive enlargement of the kidneys as normal tissue is replaced by fluid-filled cysts. In the absence of restorative treatment (i.e., dialysis or kidney transplant) the disease may cause renal failure and death (Qian et al. 2001).

9. The Social Construction and Clinical Management of the Hereditary Aspects of ADPKD (Principal Investigator: Rosalie C. Starzomski). Funded by the Kidney Foundation of Canada.

10. With autosomal dominant inheritance, all affected individuals have a 50 percent chance of passing the trait to each of their offspring. This is because only one copy of the variant allele is required for expression of the trait. Autosomal dominant conditions affect both women and men.

11. Autosomal recessive conditions, such as sickle cell disease, are experienced differently since gene carriers are usually unaffected by the condition.

12. The Ethical and Moral Dimensions of Genetic Risk: Huntington Disease and Breast Cancer (Principal Investigator: Michael M. Burgess). Funded by the Huntington Society of Canada, the Earl and Jennie Lohn Foundation, and the Canadian Breast Cancer Foundation.

13. Example is drawn from the study cited in endnote 12.

14. Sickle cell disease is a recessive disorder linked to a mutation in the hemoglobin gene. It results in red blood cells becoming sickle shaped, causing anemia and blood vessel blockages (Milunksy 2001).

15. Example is drawn from the study cited in endnote 9.

16. The National Coalition for Health Professional Education in Genetics is a non-profit organization that offers health professionals a range of educational resources on genetics. See the NCHPEG website: www.nchpeg.org

17. Example is drawn from the study cited in endnote 9.

18. See also the position papers and fact sheets available through the Canadian Nurses Association website: www.cna-nurses.ca/pages/ethics/ethicsframe.htm

REFERENCES

Asch, A. 2002. Prenatal diagnosis and selective abortion: A challenge to practice and policy. In J.S. Alper, C. Ard, A. Asch, J. Beckwith, P. Conrad and L.N. Geller (Eds.), *The double-edged helix: Social implications of genetics in a diverse society* (pp. 123–150). Baltimore: The Johns Hopkins University Press.

Baird, P.A. 2002. Identification of genetic susceptibility to common diseases: The case for regulation. *Perspectives in Biology and Medicine, 45*(4), 516–528.

Bloch, M., Fahy, M., Fox, S. and Hayden, M. 1989. Predictive testing for Huntington disease: Demographic characteristics, life-style patterns, attitudes, and psychological assessments of the first fifty-one test candidates. *American Journal of Medical Genetics, 32*, 217–224.

Bottorff, J.L., Blaine, S., Carroll, J.C., Esplen, M.J., Evans, J., Nicolson Klimek, M.L., Meschino, W. and Ritvo, P. 2003. *The educational needs and professional roles of Canadian physicians and nurses regarding genetic testing and adult onset hereditary disease.* Unpublished report.

Bottorff, J.L., McCullum, M., Balneaves, L., Esplen, M.J. and Carroll, J. 2002. *Genetic services and adult onset hereditary diseases: Current and future nursing roles.* Ottawa: Canadian Institutes of Health Research.

Brock, D. 1994. The genome project and human identity. In R. Weir, S. Lawrence and E. Fales (Eds.), *Genes and human self-knowledge: Historical and philosophical reflections on modern genetics* (pp. 18–33). Iowa City: University of Iowa Press.

Burgess, M.M. and d'Agincourt Canning, L. 2001. Genetic testing for hereditary disease: Attending to relational responsibility. *The Journal of Clinical Ethics, 12*(4), 361–372.

Burgess, M.M., Rodney, P., Coward, H., Ratanakul, P. and Suwonnakote, K. 1998. Pediatric care: Judgements about best interests at the onset of life. In H. Coward and P. Ratanakul (Eds.), *A cross-cultural dialogue on health care ethics* (pp. 160–175). Waterloo: Wilfrid Laurier University Press.

Canadian Nurses Association. 2002. *Code of ethics for registered nurses.* Ottawa: Canadian Nurses Association.

Caulfield, T.A., Burgess, M.M., Williams-Jones, B., Baily, M.A., Chadwick, R., Cho, M., Deber, R., Fleising, U., Flood, C., Friedman, J., Lank, R., Owen, T. and Sproule, J. 2001. Providing genetic testing through the private sector: A view from Canada. *Isuma, 2*(3), 72–81.

Clayton, E.W. 2002. Bioethics of genetic testing. In *Encyclopedia of Life Sciences* (pp. 1–7). London: Macmillan Publishers Ltd.

Cox, S.M. 2003. Stories in decisions: How at-risk individuals decide to request predictive testing for Huntington disease. *Qualitative Sociology, 26*(2), 257–280.

Cox, S.M. and McKellin, W.H. 1999. "There's this thing in our family": Predictive testing and the social construction of risk for Huntington disease. *Sociology of Health and Illness, 21*(5), 622–646.

Culp Harrison, T. 2002. *Socializing and working with persons with disabilities: A student autoethnography*. 8th Annual Qualitative Health Research Conference, Banff.

Disabled Peoples' International Europe. 2002. *Disabled people speak on the new genetics*. London, UK: DPI Europe. Available online: www.dpieurope.org

Duster, T. 1990. *Backdoor to eugenics*. New York: Routledge.

Frank, A.W. 1995. *The wounded storyteller: Body, illness, and ethics*. Chicago: University of Chicago Press.

Garver, K.L. and Garver, B. 1994. The human genome project and eugenic concerns. *American Journal of Human Genetics, 54*, 148–158.

Gottlieb, L.N. 1998. The human genome project: Nursing must get on board. *Canadian Journal of Nursing Research, 30*(3), 3–4.

Guttmacher, A.E., Jenkins, J. and Uhlmann, W.R. 2001. Genomic medicine: Who will practice it? *American Journal of Medical Genetics, 106*, 216–222.

Hallowell, N., Statham, H., Murton, F., Green, J. and Richards, M. 1997. "Talking about chance": The presentation of risk information during genetic counseling for breast and ovarian cancer. *Journal of Genetic Counseling, 6*(3), 269–286.

Hayden, M. 1981. *Huntington's chorea*. Berlin: Springer-Verlag.

Hubbard, R. and Wald, E. 1993. *Exploding the gene myth: How genetic information is produced and manipulated by scientists, physicians, employers, insurance companies, educators, and law enforcers*. Boston: Beacon Press.

International Society of Nurses in Genetics. 1998. *Statement on the scope and standards of genetics clinical nursing practice*. Washington, DC: American Nurses Publishing.

Jansen, L.A. 2001. Role of the nurse in clinical genetics. In M.B. Mahowald, V.A. McKusick, A.S. Scheuerle and T.J. Aspinwall (Eds.), *Genetics in the clinic: Clinical, ethical, and social implications for primary care* (pp. 133–141). St. Louis: Mosby.

Kenen, R. 1996. The at-risk health status and technology: A diagnostic invitation and the "gift" of knowing. *Social Science and Medicine, 42*(11), 1545–1553.

Kevles, D.J. and Hood, L. (Eds.). 1992. *The code of codes: Scientific and social issues in the human genome project*. Cambridge: Harvard University Press.

Koch, T. 2001. Disability and difference: Balancing social and physical constructions. *Journal of Medical Ethics, 27*, 370–376.

Lashley, F.R. 2000. Genetics in nursing education. *Nursing Clinics of North America, 35*(3), 795–805.

Lemmens, T. and Bahamin, P. 1998. Genetics in life, disability and additional health insurance in Canada: A comparative ethical and legal analysis. In B.M. Knoppers (Ed.), *Socio-ethical issues in human genetics* (pp. 120–275). Cowansville, Quebec: Les Editions Yvon Blais.

Lewontin, R.C. 2000. *It ain't necessarily so: The dream of the human genome and other illusions*. New York: New York Review of Books.

Lippman, A. 1992. Led (astray) by genetic maps: The cartography of the human genome and health care. *Social Science and Medicine, 35*(12), 1469–1476.

Lippman, A. 1998. The politics of health: Geneticization versus health promotion. In S. Sherwin (Ed.), *The politics of women's health: Exploring agency and autonomy* (pp. 64–82). Philadelphia: Temple University Press.

Mahowald, M.B. 1998. A feminist standpoint. In A. Silvers, D. Wasserman, and M.B. Mahowald (Eds.), *Disability, difference, discrimination: Perspectives on justice in bioethics and public policy* (pp. 209–251). Lanham, MD: Rowman & Littlefield.

McLaren, A. 1990. *Our own master race: Eugenics in Canada, 1885–1945*. Toronto: McClelland & Stewart.

Michalko, R. 2002. *The difference that disability makes*. Philadelphia: Temple University Press.

Milunsky, A. 2001. *Your genetic destiny*. Cambridge, MA: Perseus Publishing.

Morris, J. 1992. Tyrannies of perfection. *New Internationalist,* July, 16–17.

Oliver, M. 1996. *Understanding disability: From theory to practice*. Houndmills: Basingstoke, Hampshire, Macmillan.

Paul, D.B. 1995. *Controlling human heredity: 1865 to the present*. New Jersey: Humanities Press.

Qian, Q., Harris, P.C. and Torres, V.E. 2001. Treatment prospects for autosomal-dominant polycystic kidney disease. *Kidney International, 59*, 2005–2022.

Quaid, K.A. and Morris, M. 1993. Reluctance to undergo predictive testing: The case of Huntington Disease. *American Journal of Medical Genetics, 45*, 41–45.

Roeher Institute. 2002. *The construction of disability and risk in genetic counselling discourse*. North York, Ontario: L'Institute Roeher Institute.

Silvers, A. 2001. Normality and functionality: A disability perspective. In M.B. Mahowald, V.A. McKusick, A.S. Scheuerle and T.J. Aspinwall (Eds.), *Genetics in the clinic: Clinical, ethical, and social implications for primary care* (pp. 89–100). St. Louis: Mosby.

Smith, D.H., Quaid, K.A., Dworkin, R.B., Gramelspacher, G.P., Granbois, J.A. and Vance, G.H. 1998. *Early warning: Cases and ethical guidance for presymptomatic testing in genetic diseases*. Bloomington: Indiana University Press.

Weeks, S.L. 1994. From high-touch to high-tech: Hospital nursing and technological change. *Technology Studies, 1/2*(2), 153–174.

Wexler, N. 1990. *Presymptomatic testing for Huntington's disease: Harbinger of the new genetics*. Paper presented at Genetics, Ethics and Human Values: Human Genome Mapping, Genetic Screening and Gene Therapy, XXIVth Conference of CIOMS, Japan.

Wright, L. 2001. Documenting nursing expertise in genetics: Where are we going? *American Journal of Medical Genetics, 98*, 13–14.

chapter nineteen

Listening Authentically
to Youthful Voices:
A Conception of the Moral
Agency of Children

Franco A. Carnevale

... [W]e ought to listen to the moral voices of children in a deeply engaged manner, and not trivialize them.

In opening this chapter, I present six narratives drawn from my clinical experience. These narratives express a range of encounters lived by children that are commonly under-recognized as moral experiences.[1] These give rise to profound feelings and concerns among children, families, and health professionals.

In biomedicine today, such stories are frequently interpreted within adult-centred psychological frameworks that marginalize the moral lives of children. The prevalent psychological models commonly minimize the moral experiences of children as expressions of immaturity. For example, children like William, in Ethics in Practice 19-1, may be regarded as cognitively incapable of understanding their care requirements. Therefore, common practice calls for rapid persuasive (frequently forceful) intervention. In Ethics in Practice 19-2 and 19-4, the practice of withholding meaningful information from a minor in order to "protect" him or her is "justified" because it is thought that such information would overwhelm the child's limited capacities.

My aim in this chapter is to (1) highlight the limitations of the prevalent adult-centred modes of construing the experiences of children, (2) outline a child-centered conception of moral agency (that is, how children enact their moral capabilities), and (3) briefly discuss some of the implications for the clinical care of children that can be derived from this analysis. I will refer to the Ethics in Practice cases below throughout the remainder of the chapter.

NARRATIVES OF MORAL EXPERIENCE

Ethics in Practice 19-1	"Good boy, William..."

William is a five-and-a-half-year-old boy who has come in for day treatment requiring the administration of an intravenous antibiotic. His parents have indicated that he has been seriously dreading coming to the hospital to have this needle put into him. He has shed a lot of tears in the couple of days leading up to this treatment. As the nurse very gently approaches him to start the intra-venous, he becomes very pale and silent. He readily cooperates with every instruction that the nurse gives him, holding out his arm, making a fist, and taking a deep breath as the needle goes in. Every step of the way, each time little William cooperates with an instruction, the nurse very warmly tells him, "Good boy, William—you're such a good boy—what a big boy you are."

Ethics in Practice 19-2	Unspoken Diagnosis

Benjamin is a twelve-and-a-half-year-old boy with a metastasized inoperable abdominal tumour. His parents have been asking for help because he has been frequently crying at home—seem-ing to be discouraged about all the time he has to spend at the hospital, while missing his friends so much. His par-ents have also indicated that they do not want Benjamin to know his diagnosis because that would discourage him too much. They have been telling him that the intravenous chemotherapy he was receiving was actually antibiotics to help fight an infection.

Ethics in Practice 19-3	Anticipating Suffering

Gloria is a six-year-old girl with a degenerative neuromuscular disorder. She has been admitted to hospital with respiratory failure that has been judged to be an end-stage manifestation of her neuromuscular disorder. She will require long-term mechanical ventila-tion. Her parents, who have always been by Gloria's side providing her exceptional care and love, are devastated by the fact that she will never be able to breathe on her own again. They have decided that they would like to have her life-support terminated in order to let Gloria die and prevent the long life of suffering that they foresee for her.

Meanwhile, when most of the health care professionals look at Gloria, they see a playful girl who loves loud music and celebrities and frequently laughs out loud as she watches videos with her parents or her favourite nurses. She seems to enjoy life.

Ethics in Practice 19-4	Protective Secrets?

Nine-year-old Marianne has been in the intensive care unit for two days for the care of severe injuries following a major car accident that took her father's life. Following two days of unconsciousness, she is awakening rapidly despite her ongoing need for support of numerous vital functions (such as mechanical ventilation). She is clearly very agitated and is mouthing many questions about the accident and asking for her father. Her mother and the clinicians caring for her are torn over whether it is better to immediately tell her the truth about her father's death or invent a less painful account to tell her for now, and wait to tell her the truth at a later time.

Ethics in Practice 19-5	Hurt in the Crossfire

David is an eight-year-old boy who frequently comes to hospital for the management of recurrent back pain. One day he discloses that he is very upset inside over how much his divorced mom and dad fight over him. He feels that "they're so busy fighting all the time that they don't think that maybe it hurts me so much to see my mom and dad fighting about me. Sometimes I wish I wasn't there so they wouldn't have to fight so much. What good am I? I wish that some days they would just play with me or just think about *me*."

Ethics in Practice 19-6	Struggling to Escape

Robbie is a fourteen-year-old boy who has recently survived a four-week stay in an intensive care unit for the care of severe burns that he sustained through a supposed accident while manipulating a heating stove. He has just been weaned off the ventilator and had his endotracheal tube removed so that he can once again use his voice. During a particularly intense conversation, talking about the painful ordeal he has just been through, he says that the incident that caused his burns was not an accident. He tried to kill himself. He wanted to die because he could no longer bear to see his father physically beat his mother every evening after he got drunk.

EXAMINING THE CONVENTIONAL FRAMEWORK

The prevalent bioethical and legal framework for examining medical treatment decisions involving children—that is legal minors—is centred on the best-interests standard (American Academy of Pediatrics 1994; 1995; Buchanan and Brock 1990; Carnevale 1996; Koocher and Keith-Spiegel 1990; Macklin 1995). This requires a weighing of the burdens and benefits associated with each treatment option. However, many cases present a complex scenario whereby the benefits and burdens are difficult to judge because they relate to goods that cannot be ranked according to any universally agreed upon criteria. For example, in Ethics in Practice 19-3, the various adults in Gloria's life cannot agree on whether the burdens in her life render it unworthy of ongoing support. Furthermore, how can the significance of quality of life be ranked in relation to the sanctity of life as a good in itself? Some cultural communities argue that the preservation of life is mandatory regardless of the quality of that life; whereas, others argue that life is only valuable in terms of the quality of life that can be achieved.

In light of the difficulties inherent in trying to reconcile such dilemmas, the most widely accepted view is to recognize parents as the surrogate decision-makers for the child (American Academy of Pediatrics 1994; 1995; Blustein 1993; Buchanan and Brock 1990; Carnevale 1996; Koocher and Keith-Spiegel 1990; Kopelman 1995; Macklin 1995). This can be traced to a modern Western valuation assigned to the autonomy of families. It is largely held that families should be enabled to establish their own respective moral norms because such judgments should be based on the loving intimacy that is commonly inherent in familial relationships (Nelson and Nelson 1995).[2]

It is also recognized that the cultural and religious freedom of families should be respected (Canadian Charter of Rights and Freedoms 1982). Here too, the state imposes some limitations in situations where such freedoms conflict with some more fundamental rights. For example, in cases where a minor has a life-threatening medical condition that can be effectively corrected with a blood transfusion, the courts have commonly overruled the objection to such transfusions by Jehovah's Witnesses families, declaring that the child's right to have his or her life preserved overrides the family's religious freedom.[3]

FROM MORAL SUBJECT TO MORAL OBJECT

Throughout this chapter, I will argue that children should be regarded as moral subjects—agents who are highly capable of moral experience. However, a significant body of literature has demonstrated that children are frequently exploited as moral objects; that is, they are regarded as means to the moral pursuits of the more powerful adults in their lives.

It is remarkable that the moral worthiness of the lives of individual children has not consistently held a universal value. Wright's (1988) historical analysis of the medicalization of infant mortality in turn-of-the-century England (from 19th to 20th century) highlights a particular constellation of social phenomena that shaped the valuation of these lives. The historical period during which there was a turn to medicine to combat the high prevalence of infant death corresponded with a period of urbanization and diminution of family size. Consequently, each child's worth within his or her own family and society as a future source of labour and revenue increased.[4]

The moral objectification of children is particularly highlighted within the series of papers edited by Nancy Scheper-Hughes and Carolyn Sargent (1988) in *Small Wars: The Cultural Politics of Childhood*. Children are construed on the one hand as material possessions and on the other hand as "selfish" burdens on their surrounding adults. They are regarded as helpless consumers in need of protection.[5]

Elements of the moral objectification of children can be traced within the contemporary North American clinical encounter. In my work with critically ill children, parents commonly speak of the enormous burden they feel toward doing right by their children, ensuring that they get the kind of care they deserve (Alexander et al. 2002; Carnevale 1998; 2002). Parents are often overwhelmed by the weight of their sense of duty toward being a good parent.[6] Concurrently, they struggle with profound apprehensions about the possibility that their child may no longer live. Although parents are commonly the most appropriate advocates for a child's interests, the child's interests are intertwined with the parents' self-interests.

Further, health care professionals attempt to judge if parents are genuinely serving a child's best interests, with the knowledge that some parents clearly neglect or harm their children. A conscientious professional may be authentically concerned about a child-patient's interests. However, these interests are difficult to clearly distinguish from the professional's own interests in having a reasonable quality of work life (e.g., a manageable workload, some opportunities for breaks, and so on) while pursuing interesting opportunities for clinical innovation that may be beneficial for the child but that could also yield some professional recognition. Similarly, health care institutions (e.g., hospitals) may be interested in ensuring that patients get the care they require while balancing such care with their interests in containing costs or pursuing politically meaningful projects.

Thus, although an ill child is surrounded by a variety of adult moral agents claiming to advocate for the child's best interests, these adults are also involved in pursuing their own interests. Given the significant power imbalance between these adult-centred agents and the largely silent, morally subordinated children, the latter run a significant risk of moral objectification. As moral subjects navigating within an adult-centred moral universe, children can readily come to serve as objects of the moral interests of the surrounding adults. This risk justifies a move toward a more genuine recognition of the moral agency of children to ensure that the moral voice of children is centred in discourses regarding their child-centred interests.

WHAT ABOUT THE VOICE OF THE CHILD?

The "best-interests model" for examining ethical issues related to children casts the child in a highly passive role as a moral agent. The voice of the child is essentially muted. I would attribute this problem to two phenomena: (1) an underestimation of the "maturity" of moral reasoning children are capable of, and (2) the "adult-centredness" of the "best-interests model." I will discuss these separately.

Recognizing the "Maturity" of Moral Reasoning in Children

I have placed the term "maturity" within quotation marks to set it off as a contestable expression, primarily because it is commonly construed within an adult-centred viewpoint, an issue that will be taken up in the next section. Despite this problem, children (or legal minors) are more capable of engaging in what is regarded as mature adult moral reasoning than is typically recognized. To illustrate, in a 1990 brief submitted by the American Psychological Association (APA) in the *Hodgson v. Minnesota* case, the APA stated:

> [By] middle adolescence (age 14–15) young people develop abilities similar to adults in reasoning about moral dilemmas, understanding social rules and laws, reasoning about interpersonal relationships and interpersonal problems, and reasoning about custody preference during parental divorce.... Thus, by age 14 most adolescents have developed adult-like intellectual and social capacities including specific abilities outlined in the law as necessary for understanding treatment alternatives, considering risks and benefits, and legally competent consent (Schnieder et al. 1989, 8–20, cited in Melton 1999).

Christine Harrison and colleagues (1997) outlined three groups of children with respect to their decisional capacities: (1) preschool children who cannot provide their own consent because they have no significant decision-making capacity; (2) primary-school children who do not have full decision-making capacity, so parents should authorize or refuse treatments although the child's assent should be sought and sustained dissent should be taken seriously; and (3) adolescents who can have the decision-making capacity of an adult although this capacity will need to be assessed specifically for each child.[7]

In other words, this conventional framework limits the extent to which children should participate in decisions regarding their care in terms of their decision-making capacities. An inference that can be drawn from this view is that it is wrong to tell Benjamin, the adolescent boy in Ethics in Practice 19-2, that his chemotherapy is an antibiotic.

Despite the work of the APA and experts such as Harrison and her colleagues, there does not exist any universally accepted standard for determining when the child's voice is to be regarded as a sufficiently competent expression of an autonomous will. The child's voice matters, but when and how it matters is subject to a case-by-case interpretation of the child's "maturity." This framework implies that six-year-old Gloria in Ethics in Practice 19-3 is too immature to express meaningful preferences regarding life-support decisions. Perhaps this view can be extended further, to the withholding of a grave prognosis from Benjamin in Ethics in Practice 19-2 on the basis of his parents' belief that he would be unable to deal with such news.

Confronting the Adult-Centredness of the "Best-Interests Model"

The "best-interests model" is mistakenly premised on an adult-centred conception of moral agency. This model corresponds with the doctrine underlying ethical decision-making in adults—the doctrine of self-determination. This regards adults as self-determining agents capable of independently judging their respective moral interests. Furthermore, persons should not be impeded in their pursuit of these interests.[8]

This ideal of autonomy is further expressed through the leading psychological frameworks "explaining" moral development (Erikson 1950; Levinson 1978). These establish a moral norm for mature adults as highly rational and autonomous. Children are consequently regarded as less mature—or immature—and therefore as not worthy of a comparable recognition as moral agents.[9] Consequently, these immature agents, construed as incapable of rationally discerning their own moral interests, are classed as moral minors who are dependent upon adult custodians for the care of their interests. However, the cases of David and Robbie in Ethics in Practice 19-5 and 19-6, wherein both boys conceal their diminished sense of self-worth, demonstrate how adult custodians can be highly mistaken in their understanding of their children's moral lives.

Jean Piaget, a pioneer in the formulation of such psychological frameworks, characterized moral development in terms of three stages (Piaget 1932/1965): constraint, co-operation, and generosity. Lawrence Kohlberg (1981) drew on this Piagetian model to develop his own three-level framework for moral judgment in adolescents and adults: preconventional, conventional, and postconventional levels. The preconventional level is self-centred; the individual formulates moral norms in terms of his or her own needs and is essentially incapable of construing socially shared views. Conventional morality (associated with the preadolescence-adolescence juncture) relates the "good or right thing to do" with the surrounding social values and moral norms that serve to sustain relationships, communities, and societies. The postconventional level involves a reflective view that transcends the conventional, seeking to discover—through a process of personal enlightenment—a universal construal of morality.

Kohlberg's framework is differentiated along a six-stage (three-level) model of moral development. The child is characterized by Kohlberg as developing from an egocentric and individualistic view of rightness based on avoidance of punishment and individual need (stages one and two), to an understanding based on "The Golden Rule" (putting oneself in the shoes of the other person) and shared conventions of societal agreement (stages three and four). Finally, the child develops a principled understanding of morality that upholds the basic rights and values of a society and a free-standing logic of universal principles that all humanity should follow (stages five and six) (Kohlberg 1981). For Kohlberg, the ultimate morally mature person is capable of engaging in rational reasoning (drawing on a highly deductive logic) to arrive at an ethically principled conception of justice.

The conceptual soundness of these leading theories of moral development is challenged by Carol Gilligan (1982) through her study of moral experience among girls and women. She argues that the Piaget and Kohlberg models are based on studies of boys and men and consequently give rise to a male-centred conception of moral development.[10] Whereas Piaget and Kohlberg argue that humans (meaning, that is, men) strive to become independent moral agents, Gilligan reported that girls and women strive to be interdependent. Her research findings suggested that females speak of moral matters "in a different voice" (1).

Gilligan's moral orientation toward care and responsibility distinguishes the moral agency of women from men; the latter are primarily concerned about justice and the preservation of the rights of individuals with an entitlement to freedom from interference in their pursuit of self-fulfillment. This feminist challenge to the conventional (male-centred) view of human morality suggests that women employ a "different" moral framework and raises the plausibility that additional distinctive moral frameworks can exist. In the next section, I will argue that although children may not reason according to the prevailing adult, male-centred Kohlbergian morality, there exists a significant body of evidence indicating that children are capable of a rich degree of moral awareness. The moral viewpoints of children should not be judged in terms of how they might resemble or approximate adult moral reasoning, but instead warrant recognition on their own merits.

The Moral Awareness of Children

Numerous works have highlighted that children have a greater awareness of morally significant matters than is commonly granted. Psychiatrist Irwin Yalom (1980) has asserted that children's first awareness of death can emerge as early as three years of age. Anthropologist Myra Bluebond-Langner (1978) conducted a highly respected ethnographic study of three- to nine-year-old children's encounters with leukemia. She poignantly voiced the silent experiences of children's struggles with sickness and dying, demonstrating a depth and richness in the children's comprehension that far surpassed the understandings attributed to them by the adults in their lives. Particularly remarkable was how these children willfully complied with social taboos and respected the silence that the adults seemed to prefer in relation to the children's foreseen mortality. This finding corresponds with Benjamin's case in Ethics in Practice 19-2. This invites us to scrutinize that which is unheard from children. Their silence may be expressive of their motivation to conform to socially desired behavioural norms for children, rather than a simple demonstration of moral immaturity.

Psychologist Barbara Sourkes (1996) has reported accounts of anticipatory grief among children facing their own deaths. Examples from her work follow:

> One seven-year-old told her parents that she was too tired to fight anymore and she wanted to give up. She added, "If I have to continue suffering, I would rather be in heaven" (57).

> A three-year-old child played the same game with a stuffed duck and a toy ambulance each time he was hospitalized. The duck would be sick, and need to go to the hospital by ambulance. The boy would move the ambulance making siren noises.
>
> **Therapist:** How is the duck? **Child:** Sick.
>
> **Therapist:** Where is he going? **Child:** To the hospital.
>
> **Therapist:** What are they going to do? **Child:** Make him better.
>
> **Therapist:** Is he going to get better? **Child:** Yes, better.
>
> During what turned out to be the child's terminal admission, he played the same game with the duck. However, the ritual changed dramatically in its outcome.
>
> **Therapist:** How is the duck? **Child:** Sick.
>
> **Therapist:** Is he going to get better? **Child:** (Shook head slowly) Ducky not get better. Ducky die (57).

Sourkes (1995) has also highlighted that children can have a significant awareness of temporality, an awareness that is particularly related to morality. Moral awareness is enriched by an ability to construe a temporal account of actions, with a comprehension of ensuing consequences and contributory causes. An eight-year-old boy reported, "The doctors think my bone marrow is fine for now—and *for now* is *for now*" (119; italics in original text). An eight-year-old girl stated, "I like being myself. It is nice being myself. I like being myself forever" (122).

In the cases of Benjamin and Gloria (Ethics in Practice 19-2 and 19-3), both appear to have a highly limited moral awareness of their situation. This can be partially attributable to restrictions in the amount of information about their condition that was available to them. In light of Bluebond-Langner's (1978) findings, they may have also realized that the adults in their lives prefer that they inhibit particular expressions of their moral experience.

Sourkes (1995) has further illustrated children's capabilities to reflect on matters pertaining to a broad moral order:

> An eight-year-old boy who had just relapsed worked on his picture in the playroom. In response to the child life specialist's query about all the "eyes" that he had so carefully glued onto the paper, he explained: "It's God watching over me" (133).

Similarly, philosopher Thomas Attig (1996) has argued that children are able to anguish existentially, wondering about how they view their "finite existence, the nature and purpose of life, God, punishment, fate, what is fair, and the meanings of suffering and death" (21). David, in Ethics in Practice 19-5, describes himself as a cause of his parents' fighting while also expressing moral outrage toward the unfairness of their spending insufficient "quality time" with him.

Psychiatrist Robert Coles (1986) has examined the moral experiences of children in detail in his acclaimed text *The Moral Life of Children*. He argues that children strive to maintain a sense of moral dignity despite highly trying circumstances. He relates accounts from poor families in the American South to convey that children do not simply express parental views, but are capable of formulating and asserting their own independent sense of how the world should be. In one of the accounts relayed by Coles, Ruby, a black ten-year-old,

> ... walked past hostile mobs at age six to enter a once all-white school in New Orleans.... "I knew I was just Ruby... just Ruby trying to go to school, and worrying that I couldn't be helping my momma with the kids younger than me, like I did on weekends and in the summer. But I guess I also knew I was the Ruby who had to do it—go into that school and stay there, no matter what those people said (10).

Coles further explains that the moral life of children can be characterized as charitable but also "by extended stretches of moral stinginess, amoral self-absorption, even a persistent immorality that takes the form of spitefulness, rudeness, assaultiveness" (44).

In my own work with critically ill children and their siblings, I have witnessed rich expressions of children's moral agency (Carnevale 1997; 1998). Bereaved siblings, ranging from 5 to 19 years of age have expressed feelings of guilt about the "rude" or "mean" ways they may have acted toward their deceased brother or sister. Six-year-old Joseph, whose younger sister died as a result of septic shock, said, "Maybe this is God's way of punishing me for being so mean to my sister." Despite the apparent self-centredness of this remark (I would however add that many grieving adults can also exhibit a significant "inward turn"), Joseph demonstrated a capacity for moral contemplation. That is, he searched for a meaningful order in his world that would help explain his tragic loss. Many siblings of critically ill children, as well as bereaved siblings, commonly express an outrage toward the amount of attention accorded to the seriously ill child. Although their parents may regard such sentiments as amoral, they nonetheless express the child's sense of right and wrong.

Eight-year-old Melissa, who had battled acute leukemia over a number of years, expressed a sense of malaise about the impact her illness had on her parents:

> I feel bad that I'm always asking them to be with me. I know that I should be a big girl and leave them alone sometimes. But I don't feel good when I'm alone, so I know they try to make sure one of them is always with me. But I feel bad for being so selfish.

David, in Ethics in Practice 19-5, expressed outrage toward his father because he frequently did not follow through on his promises to make time for him:

> He thinks only about himself. He's selfish! I feel like I'm useless to him—just a bother for him.

Here, David condemns what he perceives as morally wrong parenting.

In short, although the apparently selfish moral demeanour of children may frequently fall short of what adults might consider virtuous, it nonetheless expresses a moral stance toward their world. Children are morally aware, sometimes with rich sophistication, at other times with a simplistic matter-of-factness. Although the moral values children subscribe to may sometimes correspond with those commonly held by adults, their moral awareness should not be judged according to such an adult-centred standard. Given their unique perspectives on the world, it ought to be understandable that children will hold some distinctive moral outlooks on the world. Rather than construing these as immature forms of what is to follow later in their developing lives, according to adult-centred moral development models, the moral views of children ought to merit recognition in their own right. The works outlined above justify a call for the recognition of the moral voice of children—a further "different voice."[11]

WHAT ABOUT MORAL RESPONSIBILITY?

Some may argue that it is mistaken to speak of moral agency in children without a direct implication of moral responsibility. That is, it can be argued that the moral agency of children should be construed narrowly because of the limitations in which formal responsibility can be assigned to their actions, given the limits of their understanding of the moral world that surrounds them. On the other hand, it could be conversely argued that if we want to grant children a broad measure of moral agency in light of the depth of their moral awareness, then we ought to correspondingly assign them a proportional degree of responsibility.

This "inherent" relating of responsibility with moral agency can be traced to Aristotle's *Nichomachean Ethics* (350 BCE/1985).[12] Aristotle rooted moral responsibility in the voluntariness of human action. He further elaborated two conditions that excuse the voluntariness of an act: ignorance or compulsion.[13] Perhaps some children's actions could be considered morally involuntary in light of their variable degrees of ignorance with regard to the morally significant particulars in their surrounding world and their compulsive urges to seek immediate gratification of emerging needs—which may both be manifested, for example, in an act of running across a highly dangerous street to chase after a ball.

Following Aristotle's framework, it can be argued that the degree of moral responsibility that ought to be assigned to children's actions should vary according to the genuine "voluntariness" of their actions. Although there may be grounds for limiting their responsibility for the consequences of their actions, this should not imply a diminution of their moral agency. Considering the depth of the moral awareness that children are capable of, they can experience moral distress, guilt, remorse, indignation, and pride—a full range of conscientious sentiments. Therefore, they should be accorded significant recognition as moral agents. That is, children's voices should merit genuine attention—not curious "listening to" the perspective of an immature moral inferior. Such listening ought not to be neglected by adults who might wish to do to the child whatever they consider required through the use of coercion that they judge necessary.

Toward a Broad Conception of Assent

Such a position raises questions about how we ought to enact such a recognition within the clinical encounter. How do we genuinely attend to the moral voices of children, while also recognizing potential limits to the degree of responsibility that can be assigned to their acts?

The genuine attention I am implying here could resemble the "authentic listening" advocated by Carl Rogers (1951) within his client-centred therapy framework, wherein the clinician seeks a profoundly empathic attunement to the experiential perspective of the patient.[14] This kind of approach could fairly readily be managed by interpreting the current standard of child assent more broadly. Assent implies seeking the child's willingness to accept the proposed care based on a developmentally appropriate understanding of his or her condition and the proposed tests and treatments. The American Academy of Pediatrics (AAP) recommends that for children who cannot give consent themselves, parents should be responsible for giving permission for treatment while giving great weight to the clearly expressed views of the child. Situations involving older children and adolescents should also include the assent of the child, to the greatest extent possible (AAP 1995).

The foregoing discussion of the moral awareness of children implies that this AAP recommendation ought to be applied with an *a priori* valuation of the richness of the moral lives of children. What children say should be regarded as morally meaningful, and the adults in their lives (e.g., parents and/or health care professionals) should genuinely seek to reconcile any matters that seem to be causing the child moral distress. This would involve attending meaningfully to their questions, objections, contestations, and possible protests.

Some clinical situations can involve a complexity of phenomena—clearly oriented toward the child's long-term good—that a child may not be able to grasp (such as emergency surgery for a four-year-old with appendicitis). Although the responsible adults in such a situation (typically the parents) might authorize surgery despite the child's objections, such an authorization should follow the adults' best efforts to recruit the child's acceptance of such an intervention. In the end, if it is judged that some interventions may be warranted despite the child's objections, such a coercive overriding of the child's moral voice should still be regarded as a source of moral distress. Although such a situation may be considered excusable, it should still carry the moral significance of a harm—a consequence that should be prevented and ameliorated as much as possible.[15] This scenario can be distinguished from the approach used by Benjamin's parents in Ethics in Practice 19-2. Here, morally significant information that would help Benjamin to understand what is happening to his body and enable him to express his own preferences toward his care is withheld by his parents, requiring him to undergo chemotherapy without his consent or his assent. In light of the arguments presented in this chapter outlining (1) the depth of children's moral capacities and (2) the moral harms that can be attributed to a neglect of their moral agency, the withholding of morally significant information from Benjamin is difficult to justify.

AGENCY WITHIN A MORAL WORLD

I have argued throughout this analysis for a maximization of our attentiveness to the moral voices of children. I should add that attending to the moral lives of children consists of more than solely recognizing their individual moral experiences. In light of their relative position of disempowerment, consideration should also be given to the fragility of their "moral worlds." Given their limited capacities to shape their own particular worlds, children rely on the significant adults in their lives (who model enactments of "right and wrong" ethical comportment) to help build and sustain the moral order of their world. Children also form their own moral outlooks, in the manner outlined in this chapter. They forge modes of coexistence, continually negotiating co-operation with their significant adults. Co-operation enables children to develop their particular moral character that they can express and cultivate within their adult-powered moral order.

Some traumatic experiences for children can be morally distressing in that they may rupture their moral order (Carnevale 1997; 1998; Carnevale and Rafman 1998; Rafman et al. 1997). For example, for Robbie, in Ethics in Practice 19-6, life seemed meaningless in light of his repeated experiences of witnessing his mother's beating by his father. This distress can be traced to disruptions in children's socio-moral order. Such disruptions can cause profound discontinuities in the everyday webs of relationships that constitute the children's social worlds. These webs of relationships also constitute the children's moral order. Such profound experiences can disrupt the children's socially mediated moral order: their ability to rely on significant adults as (1) sources of comfort and security that can protect them from the multitude of threats perceived within the everyday lives of children, as well as (2) significant sources of moral inspiration and support for the constitution and maintenance of the children's own idiosyncratic moral systems. Significant disruptions in children's socio-moral orders can give rise to profound distress. In turn, preservation or restoration of such socio-moral orders can serve as vital sources of comfort.

Therefore, attending meaningfully to the moral lives of children ought to consist of not only authentic listening but also devoting genuine consideration toward securing children's socio-moral order—their moral world. Within the clinical context, this implies the enactment of strategies that optimize the stable maintenance of relationships that are morally significant for the afflicted children.

Implications for Clinical Care

The narratives presented at the beginning of this chapter highlight a diversity of moral dilemmas that can be experienced by children in clinical settings. The occurrence of such dilemmas suggests the potential for children's moral experience to be under-recognized by the adults in their lives, including their families and health care professionals. Some implications for clinical care can be inferred from this analysis of moral agency.

First, this discussion calls for an authentic recognition of the moral voices of children. The views and sentiments of children have moral worth and ought to be treated as such. For example, there exists a significant body of evidence justifying the requirement of consent for treatment decisions from young adolescence onward (AAP 1995; Harrison et al. 1997; Melton 1999; Schneider et al. 1989). Second, health care professionals should seek to maximally apply the standard of assent, with a genuine stance toward the (spoken and bodily) voices of children. Health care professionals should regard children's views as worthy in their own right and not just as immature expressions requiring attention and pacification (the latter being a stance arising from an adult-centred conception of moral agency).

Finally, health care professionals should also attend to childrens' socio-moral order, predominantly constituted and sustained by the web of significant relationships in their social world. This would require (1) identifying the persons who matter (morally) in each child-patient's life, (2) seeking to understand how these persons matter, and (3) striving to find ways to help preserve the continuity of such relationships within the context of clinical care. To illustrate, hospital policies should facilitate the presence of significant adults for children (Brinchmann, Forde and Nortvedt 2002; Hayes and McElheran 2002). In addition to serving the psychological needs of these adults, these policies can be fundamentally important toward minimizing the traumatization of children. So-called hospital "visiting policies" imply a subordination of the significance of families (Carnevale 1998). When parents tend to their hospitalized children, they are "parenting" not "visiting." Characterizing significant family members as visitors serves to marginalize their importance, helping to justify limiting their presence through restrictive policies.

REVISITING THE ETHICS IN PRACTICE NARRATIVES

I will end this chapter by returning to the Ethics in Practice narratives at the beginning of the chapter to discuss corresponding implications for clinical care. Space constraints permit only a brief treatment of each situation. An authentic approach to these would require a commitment to examining the particularities of each narrative in order to uncover the specific moral phenomena and the corresponding circumstances at issue within each case. It should also be noted that the actual discovery of the moral angst reported in each narrative demonstrates a child-centred attunement to moral experience in itself.

One of the most profound messages that runs through every one of the Ethics in Practice narratives (taken from my experiences within my practice) is that we ought to listen to the moral voices of children in a deeply engaged manner, and not trivialize them. In Ethics in Practice 19-1, for instance, this meant sitting with William to listen to what he was afraid of rather than only rewarding the behaviour we wanted.

In a more extreme situation, for Robbie in Ethics in Practice 19-6, engagement meant ensuring that Robbie was able to continue to express his psychological as well as his physical pain. In fact, after expressing my dismay over the possibility of losing him in my life, by which I aimed to emphasize his moral significance, Robbie told me that my relationship with him helped him to talk about all his pain and lighten the meaninglessness he felt in his life.[16]

The promotion of authentic listening is particularly important for fostering a deepened awareness of the moral lives of children among the significant adults in their world. Parents are commonly moved by their children's expressed wishes, especially when these are articulated with a demonstration of the richness of their moral awareness. In Ethics in Practice 19-3, in which six-year-old Gloria's parents wanted to end her life support, we were able to engage her in a dialogue through which she was able to explicitly express that she enjoyed many aspects of her life. Although she was frustrated by her dependence on technology, she clearly indicated that it was better to be alive in this manner than to not be alive at all.

In Ethics in Practice 19-5, David was so distraught over his parents' fighting that he was unable to speak with them about the pain this was causing him (and for Robbie in Ethics in Practice 19-6, this gave rise to suicidal feelings). Children in such situations can benefit from advocacy that facilitates the revealing of their masked sentiments. For example, when I arranged a family conference to help David express his feelings, he said that he felt safe in knowing that I would be there as an adult who would help ensure that he was heard. David's parents were very upset with themselves after hearing their child's despair. They promised him that they would do everything they could to stop fighting.

In Ethics in Practice 19-2 and 19-4, the cases of Benjamin and Marianne each involve situations in which some of the adults in the children's lives were withholding significant information from them. Although keeping such secrets may be intended to protect children from emotional pain, they in fact distance the children from the significant moral matters at hand. This impedes the children's ability to understand what is happening, as well as their ability to express how this matters to them morally. In such situations, I have found that parents themselves appear morally distressed about such secrets. Commonly, parents demonstrate a form of relief once the secret is broken (because they feel that on some level it is wrong to not tell the truth), and a deeper intimacy between the parents and the child is fostered. It is also important to recognize that parents commonly strive to protect their children from harm, which can give rise to a profound sense of burden when they acquire emotionally painful information about their children's lives.

The promotion of authentic listening is also important for enhancing health professionals' awareness of children's moral worlds. In caring for children like William in Ethics in Practice 19-1, this can involve discussing how the use of normative terms such as "good boy" can significantly limit the range of feelings that children will openly express while privately experiencing fear, pain, and distress.

Much has been written regarding ethical issues surrounding treatment decisions for children. This literature has predominantly focused on which adults are most suited to decide on behalf of children and the normative standards that should be employed for such decisions. In this chapter, I strive to give voice to the silent agents that are the objects of these decisions: morally aware youthful subjects living their own moral experiences.

FOR REFLECTION

1. How does this chapter affect your understanding of the role of parents?

2. Identify a situation from your practice where a child's moral agency was under-recognized.

3. How would you approach a child differently after reading this chapter?

ENDNOTES

1. Portions of these narratives, which are not fundamentally relevant to the arguments that follow, have been modified in an attempt to preserve the anonymity of the persons involved. For example, all of the names presented are pseudonyms.

2. Although the family is generally viewed as the most suitable unit for creating the moral milieu conducive for fostering the healthy development of children, it is also recognized that, on occasion, some families can neglect or abuse children. In such cases, there is some acceptance of state interference in family life.

3. See *B.(R.) v. Children's Aid Society of Metropolitan Toronto* (1995) 1 S.C.R. 315.

4. For a broader socio-historical analysis of turn-of-the-century childhood in England, see Walwin (1982). See Field (1995) and Lock (1990) for an analysis of adult coercion of contemporary Japanese children. Finally, see Foucault (1972/1984) for his analysis of medicalization patterns in 18th-century France.

5. In another context, Scheper-Hughes (1992) has reported that poor mothers in the shantytowns of Brazil systematically suppress their maternal compassion toward their weaker and sicker children and allow them to die of neglect, while turning their attention to the healthier, more "viable" children. Children are accorded attention in relation to their estimated outlook. They are not regarded as moral ends in themselves.

6. This resembles a central argument outlined by Benjamin Freedman (1999) in his study of Jewish traditions among adult children of incompetent parents. He argued that family members dreaded, rather than welcomed, their involvement in life-support decisions. Although family members demanded

decision-making authority, this claim was grounded on a felt duty of the family to care for its members that cannot care for themselves.

7. Decision-making capacity should be judged on the basis of an ability to understand relevant information, think and choose with some degree of independence, and assess the potential for benefit as well as harm, as well as the achievement of a fairly stable set of values (Harrison et al. 1997). The decisional sophistication of adolescents has been further discussed by Weir and Peters (1997).

8. This view can be traced to a fundamental ethos of individualism in modern Western societies, wherein each human ought to become an independent or autonomous agent capable of judging morally significant matters through a developed faculty of rational discernment (Carnevale 1999; Taylor 1989).

9. This highlights a fundamental tension whereby cognitive "maturity" is presumed as a necessary condition for moral agency. Moral development is related to the development of general skills of rational reasoning (Kohlberg 1981; Piaget 1932/1965). This presumption is valid for an adult-centred conception of moral agency. However, I will argue for a recognition of children's moral agency, regardless of their level of cognitive development.

10. Kohlberg subsequently put forth a reformulated theory that attempted to address criticisms of his earlier work (Kohlberg, Levine and Hewer 1983). This was regarded as complex and unclear, such that his earlier work persisted as his most influential (Shweder, Mahapatra and Miller 1987).

11. Although I am employing the metaphor of voice in this discussion, drawing on Gilligan's (1982) acclaimed work, "listening" to the moral experiences of children should not be limited to attending to their *verbal* expressions. Children commonly express outrage and protest or comfort and acceptance through various modes of *bodily* expression, as well as through the verbal realm (Carnevale 1997; 1998). Also, see Kagan and Lamb (1987) for a discussion of the relation of culture to moral development in children.

12. My discussion of moral responsibility is deeply indebted to Carl Elliott (1996) for his insightful philosophical analysis of responsibility in his study of mentally ill offenders.

13. According to Aristotle, the type of *ignorance* that can make an action involuntary refers to an ignorance of the particular circumstances of an action (e.g., injuring someone in response to a suspected yet false threat, an ignorance-based involuntary injury). *Compulsion* refers to an act where the drive resides outside the person. This essentially refers to acts committed out of necessity or duress, wherein many would agree that they could not really have done otherwise under those particular circumstances. For example, your family is taken hostage and you are instructed to set a neighbour's home on fire in order to salvage your family—an intentional yet formally involuntary act.

14. This is further related to the clinical care of children in Schultz and Carnevale (1996).

15. This acknowledges the importance of (1) retaining some form of the best-interests standard (balancing benefits and burdens) for a preliminary discernment of which treatment options might be most appropriate for a particular child, and (2) continuing to recognize the significance of parents as "surrogate" decision-makers because the common intimacy of their relationship predisposes them (more than most other adults) to think in terms of the child's interests. However, a corresponding recognition of the moral views of children problematizes objections or exclusions they experience toward treatment decisions made by their parents. This can foster a greater consideration of the child's voice as well as enrich the parents' understanding of the benefits and harms attributed to various treatments by better recognizing that certain courses of action are *morally* distressing for their child. It is noteworthy that in the context of *research* it is widely held that a child's expression of dissent should be respected (Medical Research Council 1998). "Children can be seriously harmed by having something done to them without their knowledge or understanding" (Baylis et al. 1999, 8).

16. Similar to how suicide ideation might be managed with adults, it is important to immediately direct (verbal and nonverbal) attention toward demonstrating a deep valuation of the significance of such a self-disclosure. It is essential to establish an engaged relationship with the child that aims to highlight ways in which the child's life is morally meaningful. In Robbie's case, I encouraged him to tell me about the specific aspects of his life that demoralized him, while expressing my commitment to help him find ways to significantly improve these conditions. This aimed to diminish his sense of isolation and alienation while demonstrating under-recognized resources that were available to him, to help him feel less overwhelmed by the enormity of his situation. I promised to help him mobilize specific strategies (in particular, specific relationships) that could comfort him. I explicitly attempted to demonstrate that, regardless of his youthful age, his malaise was deeply significant and legitimate.

REFERENCES

American Academy of Pediatrics (AAP). 1994. Guidelines on forgoing life-sustaining medical treatment. *Pediatrics*, *93*(3), 532–536.

American Academy of Pediatrics (AAP). 1995. Informed consent, parental permission, and assent in pediatric practice. *Pediatrics*, *95*(2), 314–317.

Alexander, E., Rennick, J.E., Carnevale, F.A. and Davis, M. 2002. Daily struggles: The experience of families with children requiring assisted ventilation at home. *Canadian Journal of Nursing Research*, *34*(4), 7–14.

Aristotle. 350 BCE/1985. *Nichomachean ethics*. Translator: D. Ross. Oxford: Oxford University Press.

Attig, T. 1996. Beyond pain: The existential suffering of children. *Journal of Palliative Care*, *12*(3), 20–23.

Baylis, F., Downie, J. and Kenny, M. 1999. Children and decision making in health research. *IRB: A Review of Human Subjects Research*, *21*(4), 5–10.

Bluebond-Langner, M. 1978. *The private worlds of dying children*. Princeton: Princeton University Press.

Blustein, J. 1993. The family in medical decisionmaking. *Hastings Center Report*, *23*(3), 6–13.

B.(R.) v. Children's Aid Society of Metropolitan Toronto. 1995. 1 S.C.R. 315.

Brinchmann, B.S., Forde, R. and Nortvedt, P. 2002. What matters to the parents? A qualitative study of parents' experiences with life-and-death decisions concerning their premature infants. *Nursing Ethics*, *9*(4), 388–404.

Buchanan, A.E. and Brock, D.W. 1990. *Deciding for others: The ethics of surrogate decision making*. Cambridge, U.K.: Cambridge University Press.

Canadian Charter of Rights and Freedoms, Canada Act 1982 (U.K.), c. 11.

Carnevale, F.A. 1996. "Good" medicine: Ethics and pediatric critical care. In D. Tibboel and E. van der Voort (Eds.), *Intensive care in childhood: A challenge to the future* (pp. 491–503). Berline: Springer-Verlag.

Carnevale, F.A. 1997. The experience of critically ill children: Narratives of unmaking. *Intensive and Critical Care Nursing*, *13*, 49–52.

Carnevale, F.A. 1998. "Striving to recapture our previous life"—The experience of families of critically ill children. *Dynamics—Official Journal of The Canadian Association of Critical Care Nurses*, *9*(4), 16–22.

Carnevale, F.A. 1999. Toward a cultural conception of the self. *Journal of Psychosocial Nursing and Mental Health Services*, *37*(8), 26–31.

Carnevale, F.A. 2002. Moral binds and conflicts of interests: Ethical considerations for innovative therapies. *Pediatric Intensive Care Nursing*, *3*(2), 4–6.

Carnevale, F.A. and Rafman, S. 1998. *Socio-moral transformations in childhood trauma*. Proceedings of the XXII International Congress of Pediatrics, Amsterdam, August, 407.

Coles, R. 1986. *The moral life of children*. New York: Atlantic Monthly Press.

Elliott, C. 1996. *The rules of insanity: Moral responsibility and the mentally ill offender*. Albany: State University of New York Press.

Erikson, E.H. 1950. *Childhood and society*. New York: W.W. Norton.

Field, N. 1995. The child as laborer and consumer. In S. Stephens (Ed.), *Children and the politics of culture* (pp. 51–78). Princeton: Princeton University Press.

Foucault, M. 1972/1984. The politics of health in the eighteenth century (from *Power/Knowledge*). In P. Rabinow (Ed.), *The Foucault reader* (pp. 273–289). New York: Pantheon Books.

Freedman, B.1999. *Duty and healing: Foundations of a Jewish bioethic*. New York: Routledge.

Gilligan, C. 1982. *In a different voice: Psychological theory and woman's development.* Cambridge, MA: Harvard University Press.

Harrison, C., Kenny, N.P., Sidarous, M. and Rowell, M. 1997. Bioethics for clinicians: Involving children in medical decisions. *Canadian Medical Association Journal, 156*(6), 825–828.

Hayes, V.E. and McElheran, P.J. 2002. Family health promotion within the demands of pediatric home care and nursing respite. In L.E. Young and V. Hayes (Eds.), *Transforming health promotion: Concepts, issues, and applications* (pp. 265–283). Philadelphia: F.A. Davis Company.

Kagan, J. and Lamb, S. (Eds.). 1987. *The emergence of morality in young children.* Chicago: University of Chicago Press.

Kohlberg, L. 1981. *The philosophy of moral development.* San Francisco: Harper and Row.

Kohlberg, L., Levine, C. and Hewer, A. 1983. *Moral stages: a current formulation and a response to critics.* New York: Karger.

Koocher, G.P. and Keith-Spiegel, P.C. 1990. *Children, ethics, and the law: Professional issues and cases.* Lincoln, Nebraska: University of Nebraska Press.

Kopelman, L.M. 1995. Children: Health-care and research issues. In W.T. Reich (Ed.), *Encyclopedia of bioethics* (pp. 357–367). New York: Simon & Schuster Macmillan.

Levinson, D.J. 1978. *The seasons of a man's life.* New York: Alfred A. Knopf.

Lock, M. 1990. Flawed jewels and national dis/order: Narratives of adolescent dissent in Japan. *Journal of Psychohistory, 18*(4), 507–531.

Macklin, R. 1995. Deciding for others. In F. Baylis, J. Downie, B. Freedman, B. Hoffmaster and S. Sherwin (Eds.), *Health care ethics in Canada* (pp. 282–289). Toronto: Harcourt Brace.

Medical Research Council of Canada, Natural Sciences and Engineering Research Council of Canada, and Social Sciences and Humanities Research Council of Canada. 1998. *Tri-Council Policy Statement: Ethical Conduct for Research Involving Humans.* Ottawa: Public Works and Government Services Canada.

Melton, G.B. 1999. Parents and children: Legal reform to facilitate children's participation. *American Psychologist, 54*(11), 935–944.

Nelson, H.L. and Nelson, J.L. 1995. *The patient in the family: An ethics of medicine and families.* New York: Routledge.

Piaget, J. 1932/1965. *The moral judgment of the child.* New York: The Free Press.

Rafman, S., Canfield, J., Barbas, J. and Kaczorowski, J. 1997. Children's representations of parental loss due to war. *International Journal of Behavioral Development, 20*(1), 163–177.

Rogers, C. 1951. *Client-centered therapy.* Boston: Houghton Mifflin.

Scheper-Hughes, N. 1992. *Death without weeping: The violence of everyday life in Brazil.* Berkeley: University of California Press.

Scheper-Hughes, N. and Sargent, C. 1998. Introduction: The cultural politics of childhood. In N. Scheper-Hughes and C. Sargent (Eds.), *Small wars: The cultural politics of childhood* (pp. 1–33). Berkeley: University of California Press.

Schneider, M.D., Bersoff, D.N. and Podolsky, S.R. 1989. Brief for *amici curiae* American Psychological Association, National Association of Social Workers, and the American Jewish Committee in *Ohio v. Akron Center for Reproductive Health* and *Hidgson v. Minnesota.* Washington, D.C.: Jenner and Block.

Schultz, D.S. and Carnevale, F.A. 1996. Engagement and suffering in responsible caregiving: On overcoming maleficence in health care. *Theoretical Medicine, 17*(3), 189–207.

Shweder, R.A., Mahapatra, M. and Miller, J.G. 1987. Culture and moral development. In J. Kagan and S. Lamb (Eds.), *The emergence of morality in young children* (pp. 1–83). Chicago: University of Chicago Press.

Sourkes, B.M. 1995. *Armfuls of time: The psychological experience of the child with a life-threatening illness*. Pittsburgh: University of Pittsburgh Press.

Sourkes, B.M. 1996. The broken heart: Anticipatory grief in the child facing death. *Journal of Palliative Care, 12*(3), 56–59.

Taylor, C. 1989. *Sources of the self: The making of the modern identity*. Cambridge, MA: Harvard University Press.

Walwin, J. 1982. *A child's world: A social history of English childhood 1800–1914*. Harmondsworth, U.K.: Penguin.

Weir, R.F. and Peters, C. 1997. Affirming the decisions adolescents make about life and death. *Hastings Center Report, 27*(6), 29–40.

Wright, P.W.G. 1988. Babyhood: The social construction of infant care as a medical problem in England in the years around 1900. In M. Lock and D. Gordon (Eds.), *Biomedicine examined* (pp. 299–329). Dordrecht: Kluwer Academic Press.

Yalom, I.D. 1980. *Existential psychotherapy*. New York: Basic Books.

chapter twenty

Widening the Scope of Ethical Theory, Practice, and Policy: Violence against Women as an Illustration

Colleen Varcoe

Often self-questioning and redefinition have come from outside what is considered philosophy proper (Nye 2000, 102).

As earlier chapters have argued, the nature and scope of what is considered relevant in nursing ethics is widening. This chapter contributes to that trend by considering **violence against women**[1] and health care responses to violence as ethical issues. In contributing this chapter to this ethics text, I hope to point out the usefulness of an ethical analysis of violence against women for movement toward more ethical practice. I also draw attention to how such an analysis raises questions about nursing practices in general, particularly practices that involve certain forms of "othering." Finally, I point to the importance of incorporating post-colonial theory and contextual ethical theory (including feminist and relational theory) with nursing ethical theory.[2] Thus, in this chapter, violence against women is used as an exemplary illustration that both requires and contributes to current movement and debates in ethics.

VIOLENCE AGAINST WOMEN AS AN ETHICAL ISSUE IN HEALTH CARE

Over the past several decades, Western society has become increasingly aware of the epidemic nature of violence against women. Yet little progress has been made in terms of women's lives. Women in most countries around the world continue to be terrorized in their homes, beaten, sexually assaulted, and murdered. Despite increasing awareness of the problem, the social response has made little impact on the problem. In particular, the health care response to violence against women has been shown to be at best inadequate and, at worst, damaging to women. Women who are abused are often not identified as such, leading researchers and health care providers to advocate widely for routine screening for abuse in all health care settings (e.g., Fishwick 1998; Humphreys, Parker and Campbell 2001). Despite these calls, persistently low rates of screening for abuse by health professionals have been documented (e.g., Erickson, Hill and Siegel 2001; Groth, Chelmowski and Batson 2001; Grunfeld, Ritmiller, MacKay, Cowan and Hotch 1994; Willson et al. 2001). Research has found that the attitudes of health care providers are often unsympathetic or negative toward women who have been abused (e.g., Cochrane 1987; Garimella, Plichta, Houseman and Garzon 2000; McCauley, Yurk, Jenckes and Ford 1998; Moore, Zaccaro and Parsons 1998; Sugg, Thompson, Thompson, Maiuro and Rivara 1999). Attitudes vary by gender and position, with women and nurses generally having more positive attitudes when compared with men and other health care workers (Cann, Withnell, Shakespeare, Doll and Thomas 2001; Rose and Saunders 1986). Attitudes have a profound influence on care (Corbally 2001; Woodtli 2001). When abuse is recognized, treatment is often inappropriate and/or accompanied by disbelief, blame, and negative judgments (e.g., Gerbert et al. 1996; Loring and Smith 1994; Shields, Baer, Leininger, Marlow and Dekeyser 1998; Warshaw 1998). Intervention is often based on what Ewing (1987) called an *impositional ethic*—that is, the intentions of health care providers are imposed on the woman. As a result, women experience loss of control, stigma, isolation, humiliation, and lack of respect (McMurray and Moore 1994), which may deter disclosure (McCauley et al. 1998) and further diminish their health. Analyzing national data in Canada, Ratner (1995) found that women who came into contact with health care providers in relation to abuse they experienced had slightly poorer outcomes than women who did not, even when severity of abuse was taken into account.

Ethics in Practice 20-1	**"Hey, she's had the choices..."**

... [S]he was a [Muslim][3] lady, complaining of a migraine and... when the nurse interacted with the lady and her husband, the nurse was suspicious that there might have been some kind of abuse going on. So she was in one of the regular stretcher bays where all the curtains are normally opened and [the nurse] got the social worker involved and it was confirmed that it was, in fact, abuse and the nurse [let] the Charge Nurse know that we shouldn't let the husband in for now until the social worker was finished talking to the lady.

They pulled the curtains around the lady, turned off the lights in the space that she was in.... [T]hey left the next bed empty, and when they talked about her there was no question of addressing the pain of her headache or what might be causing her migraines or any kind of physiological basis for her complaint, she immediately became the abused patient. Everybody spoke in very hushed tones and the only conversation about her became the conversation about the abuse. She didn't fit the victim model that we like to construct. We like people who maybe haven't accessed services before, have never been offered help, have been violently abused etc., but she didn't fit it because it had been taking place over a long period of time, she had been offered help before and returned. She had resources to leave [her husband] but wasn't leaving, and so because she wasn't doing what we wanted her to do she didn't get the—I wouldn't use empathy, I would actually use sympathy—that the people tend to get if they fit the mold that we want them to fit, and she didn't fit it. So not only was her physical problem not dealt with but she wasn't given any empathy or respect because people said, "Hey, she's had the choices, she's had the opportunity, there she is behind the curtain, social work is dealing with it" and nothing further was done or said.... [B]ecause I have had a lot to do with [Muslim] people in the last three years, I would say overall that, as a group of nurses, [here] people are more suspicious of abuse in a multicultural type of patient situation than they are in an actually Caucasian situation.[4]

As Ethics in Practice 20-1 suggests, and as research on the health care response to violence illustrates, there are multiple ethical issues embedded in the problem of violence against women in general and, more specifically, in the failure of health care providers to respond in a meaningful way to abuse. Because gender-based violence is grounded in gender inequity, it is by definition an ethical issue if one operates from a morality that values equity and justice. However, violence against women is a neglected topic in **bioethics** (Wilkerson 1998). Ethical analyses of issues related to violence against women and health care are few and have tended to focus on the issue of confidentiality and the conflict between autonomy and beneficence that arises when a woman requests that health care providers not report abuse to others (Larkin, Moskop, Sanders and Derse 1994; Limandri and Tilden 1993; Tilden and Schmidt 1994). Even from a traditional bioethical perspective, the failure to identify abuse, blaming women for the abuse they experience, and treating women in ways that deter help-seeking can be seen as problematic. Clearly, such practices do not "do good" and can be seen as harmful. And such practices do not respect the persons who experience them. In this chapter, I will posit that violence against women serves as a case-in-point for contemporary critiques of ethical theory and illustrates the promise of new trends in ethical theory that move us toward deeper analyses.

Stories like the one in Ethics in Practice 20-1 make most people uncomfortable. The story offers an illustration of what is known from research about the health care response to violence against women: the woman is blamed for not changing her situation and is judged negatively for not complying with health care providers' directions. The practices can be seen as isolating and disrespectful, with little likelihood of a meaningful outcome for the woman. But what exactly is *wrong* with the practices described? Surely there are limits to what health care providers can do? If the woman has been offered services to help leave her husband and she has "chosen" not to, surely her autonomy should be respected, and the health care providers' abandonment is justified? Is there a reason to be more suspicious of abuse with racialized people than with those from dominant groups?

I argue that part of what is problematic in Ethics in Practice 20-1 is the failure to account for the social conditions of **health care access.** Although the woman was deemed to have "resources," the health care response does not seem to be informed by an understanding of the ways that gender, ethnicity, the dynamics of abuse, and the responses of health care providers might shape the woman's decisions. Bourdieu (2000) identifies various forms of scholastic fallacy, all of which he claims are based on the same principle— that of universalizing a particular case and failing to account for the social conditions that make that case possible. A particular form of fallacy, he claims, is expressed in some types of ethical universalism that overlook the economic and social conditions of access, and therefore overlook those who are deprived of such access. Overcoming such fallacies is central to contemporary trends in ethical theorizing and will facilitate recognition of the social nature of violence against women, which Wilkerson (1998) argues is necessary for prevention and treatment.

One of the central social conditions that recent ethical theorizing has taken into account is that of **gender. Feminist ethics** draws attention to inequality in power relations (based on gender, race, class, ability, and so on) and repeatedly calls into question the idea that the "role of ethics is to clarify obligations among individuals who are viewed as paradigmatically equal, independent, rational and autonomous" (Sherwin 1992, 21). Re-reading the above excerpt through the lens of gender would require asking how the social expectations of women and gender economics might shape this woman's apparent choices. Understanding that women are still held largely responsible for family and for maintaining relationships might lead the health care providers to ask how this woman's relationship values might shape her willingness to "leave" in accordance with their wishes. Taking into account the static gender gap in most economic indicators, and the specific knowledge that economic independence is the single most important factor in determining whether women enter or leave abusive relationships (Barnett 2000; Gurr, Mailloux and Kinnon 1996; Lambert and Firestone 2000), might lead health care providers to re-think their judgment that "she had the resources for leaving." Taking into account the dynamics of abuse would raise awareness that abusive partners often escalate violence when separation is threatened or attempted (Campbell, Rose, Kub and Nedd 1998; McFarlane et al. 1999; Tjaden and Thoennes 1998). Such thinking might then lead to questioning the extent to which this woman, or indeed any woman who is being abused, is an independent, autonomous actor.

Ethics in Practice 20-1 illustrates many of the features of the response to violence against women that I observed in an ethnographic study of emergency units (Varcoe 2001). Nurses and other health care providers were concerned about violence and abuse but were frustrated by their inability to affect change in women's lives and tended to blame the women. They particularly blamed the women for failing to leave an abusive partner. In subsequent research with women who had been battered by their partners[5], I found that women were deterred from help-seeking in general by disbelief and negative responses that they experienced themselves or anticipated based on the experiences of others (Varcoe, Jaffer and Kelln 2002). By responding to women in ways that might deter further help-seeking, health care providers thus inadvertently compound gender-based violence and create gender-based barriers to access to health care.

It is also evident, though, that gender alone is not the sole social condition under consideration in Ethics in Practice 20-1. The question of resources points to the intersection between gender and **class** as a condition of health and access to health care. And the **racialization** of the patient as well as the suggestion that health care providers are more suspicious about violence in certain groups point to the intersection between race and gender in the case of violence against women. Indeed, similar to what was described in the United States by Richie and Kanuha (1993), in the Canadian context I found that nurses and other health care providers routinely associated violence with poor and racialized people (Varcoe 2001; 2002). This association did not mean that racialized and poor people were more likely to receive meaningful and helpful responses from health care providers in relation to violence. Rather, poverty and race played a role in explaining abuse in a stereotypical manner; racialized and poor men were thought to be more likely to be violent, and racialized and poor women were thought to be more vulnerable to abuse.

In both Canada and the United States, poverty is associated with higher levels of interpersonal violence (Canadian Centre for Justice Statistics 1993; Tjaden and Thoennes 1998). In the United States, researchers found that higher rates of domestic violence among black populations compared to white populations were fully explained by socioeconomic status (Centerwall 1995). There is evidence that poverty and racialization do make women more vulnerable to violence in that fewer social and economic resources and more limited access to support systems fundamentally shape the experience of violence and women's life options (Crenshaw 1994; Richie and Kanuha 1993; Walker 1995). Further, the former authors and other authors (e.g., Agnew 1998; Mosher 1998) argue that women of colour must weigh their interests in protecting their communities from further racism against the need to deal with abuse. That is, women from racialized groups may find it difficult to disclose violence in a society that tends to treat members of those groups harshly (such as with imprisonment) and where such disclosure will feed racist stereotypes. *However, there is a vast difference between understanding that the complex of racism and poverty may make women vulnerable to violence and making stereotypical assumptions that poor and racialized people have a propensity to violence.*

Ethics in Practice 20-2 shares many features with Ethics in Practice 20-1 but is more explicit in the treatment of race. In this second example, the nurse is seeking to place responsibility for violence on women who are abused. Rather than seeing violence against women as a gender-based social problem, the nurse sees it as an individual's problem, which leaves her struggling with questions regarding what role women play in exacerbating their partners' violence. Further, she explicitly associates violence with particular racialized groups, in this case "Native Indian" women. She sees such women as "particularly vulnerable," but it is not clear whether she associates this vulnerability with the social conditions of Aboriginal people in Canada, or with "race" as a biologically determined set of traits.[6]

"OTHERING" AS AN ETHICAL ISSUE

Ethics in Practice 20-2 amplifies the process of **"othering"** evident in the first excerpt and highlights the utility of post-colonial theory for ethical analysis. Mary Canales (2000)

Ethics in Practice 20-2	**"What is it about women's personalities?"**

I would have to say from my practice that the case[s of violence] that come to mind most easily would be with Native Indian women. [In this hospital] we see quite a few of them, so that is really what I can remember dealing with. Native Indian women are very vulnerable to that sort of thing, and I think they come to us for help and when I have seen them they have been fairly significantly battered and it is usually not something where you are wondering about the woman having had some abuse. She is either telling you or she's not telling you, but if you questioned her she will reveal it. I think in some ways they are a little more open than some other segments of our society. These women are the ones that I can talk to you about really only.

I have found that they are usually physically battered to the point where there is open bruising and sometimes significant abdominal injuries and we have dealt with that. But to speak to the woman and ask her whether or not she wants... to press charges or move along with counselling, it is very, very often something that she is not prepared to do. My experience with them has been fairly brief. I've never followed a case through to find out how the woman is doing in the community, but I have seen repeat offenders and repeat women

coming through, so have seen their injuries that way.

I have found Native women very open really, about the fact, maybe because they are often under the influence of alcohol, so that they themselves are somewhat more vocal just because they are not as defensive, so they will speak about him hitting them and relate to it in a way that seems a very normal part of their relationship with this man, or person, but it doesn't necessarily mean that they recognize it as being something they don't.... [T]hey speak about it very openly, not in a way that they are accusing and blaming [their partners], whatever.

The other issue that I find that they deal with, or don't deal with actually, is if, in fact, there is any part that they played in either exacerbating or stimulating this scenario to occur in the first place. It is a part of the whole violence against women issue that I have a bit of difficulty with, and that is how do women, what do women do, now though I feel, I don't want to get into a difficult scenario here, I feel very strongly about women and violence and that women should not have to put up with it, but I keep wondering what is it about women's personalities that allows us to get to a point where violence is an issue?[7]

defines "othering" as the way we engage with others—those perceived as different from ourselves. She further defines exclusionary othering as a process that utilizes the power within relationships for domination and subordination. In Ethics in Practice 20-1 and 20-2, women who are battered by their partners are seen as different from the speakers who are telling the stories, and, further, the women are "othered" on the basis of race. In these

[handwritten in margin: experience this at home. / I am different than you + I will not experience]

excerpts, the nurses are seen to view certain racialized people as more likely to engage in or be vulnerable to violence. In Ethics in Practice 20-2, the speaker draws upon the racial stereotypes about alcohol and Canadian Aboriginal people as a component of the process of othering.

While feminist ethics often purports also to draw attention to forms of inequality beyond gender, **post-colonial theory** brings specific attention to the social conditions occasioned by colonialism and its constant companion, **racism**.[8] Post-colonial theory draws attention to the historicity of social conditions and draws attention to the voices of those who have been, and continue to be, marginalized (see also Chapter 7). Therefore, taking a post-colonial approach to the ethical issues embedded in the health care response to violence against women draws attention to the process of othering as one of achieving social distance and justifying limits to the obligations of health care providers to certain patients. *Associating race (or gender) with a tendency to or vulnerability to violence naturalizes violence and, in the process, absolves health care providers of an obligation to act: "Hey, she's had the choices, she's had the opportunity...."*

Taking socio-historical conditions into account would lead to an analysis of why and how some health care providers come to see themselves as "different" on the basis of race,[9] how racial stereotypes are used in the process, and then to question how this process of othering operates. Such analysis could lead to the understanding that racialization and stereotyping might predispose health care providers to identify abuse more readily in some groups, thus reinforcing their previously held biases. A perceived preponderance of abused women among certain groups may therefore be at least partially a product of anticipation and intensified scrutiny on the part of health care providers. As Canales (2000) notes, stereotypes dramatize separation: stereotypical representation of those stigmatized as other often defines their identity for dominant group members.

An ethical analysis from a post-colonial perspective might lead to the understanding that stereotypes shape perspective in ways that devalue certain persons. For example, an Aboriginal person who is under the influence of alcohol may be seen as a "drunken Indian," a naturalized state for which there is no remedy, whereas a white person under the influence of alcohol may be seen as merely drunk, a temporary and reversible situation that does not alter the person's social worth. An ethical analysis from a post-colonial perspective would also bring into view the particular ways in which racism and classism "unmindfully" influence clinical judgment in predicting abuse (Limandri and Sheridan 1995, 15). Finally, such analysis would call into question the effects of othering on help-seeking and access to health care and the influence of racism on health care provision in general (e.g., Anderson and Kirkham 1998; Henry, Tator, Mattis and Rees 2000b; Whaley 1998)—and specifically on women who experience abuse (e.g., Richie and Kanuha 1993; Walker 1995; Williams and Becker 1994). *As Browne and her colleagues (Browne, Johnson, Bottorff, Grewal and Hilton 2002) illustrate, patients who encounter racism and other forms of discrimination are less likely to re-enter the health care system to seek appropriate care.*

Such analysis is also useful in helping to understand how othering might work despite an apparent lack of difference between health care providers and clients. In my research in emergency units, health care providers, who were predominantly white professionals, saw women who were abused as different from themselves based on race or class if the women were non-white or poor. However, because health care providers found abused women who were like themselves in terms of race/ethnicity and class difficult to understand, they searched for differences between themselves and such women in terms of personality, strength of character, and so on.

Othering as a process of exclusion and as a basis for limiting the ethical obligations of health care providers toward their clients can be seen as a contentious ethical issue. Othering as a dynamic in the enactment of social judgments is incongruent with the ethical obligations of nurses as outlined in national and international codes of ethics (Pauly and Varcoe In review; Shaha 1998). Shaha argues that in maintaining an ethnocentric attitude towards clients, nurses may violate the client's dignity and autonomy, fail to respect clients, and fail to develop a therapeutic nurse-client relationship necessary to adequate care.

SCREENING FOR ABUSE AS AN ETHICAL ISSUE

In the past two decades, health care providers and researchers have drawn attention to the extent to which abuse is not recognized or is overlooked, have described the deficiencies in practice when violence is recognized, and have advocated for effective responses (e.g., Bell and Mosher 1998; Cann et al. 2001; Gerbert et al. 1996; McLeer and Anwar 1989). Because the lack of recognition of abuse is so marked, recommendations for improvement usually begin with strategies for increasing recognition, primarily through the practice of **"screening"** (e.g., Ellis 1999; Lazzaro and McFarlane 1991; Tilden and Shepherd 1987; Waalen, Goodwin, Spitz, Petersen and Saltzman 2000; Wiebe and Janssen 2001). In brief, all health care providers are advised to inquire of all women, or in some cases, all clients, whether they have experienced abuse. However, given the complexity of the issue of violence against women, and its entanglement within interlocking forms of oppression, improving the health care response is no simple matter. This practice of screening serves as a further illustration of the utility of an ethical analysis in relation to violence against women and of the importance of expanding ethical theory, particularly in the direction of anti-oppressive analyses.

Screening protocols are typically a brief series of questions designed to identify whether a person has been the victim of various forms of interpersonal violence. The recommended screening tools range from single to multiple items, some of which distinguish between current, recent, or historical abuse. The tools typically contain a question such as, "Have you ever been hit, slapped, kicked or otherwise hurt by your male partner?" to focus on physical abuse and other questions to examine other forms of abuse (McFarlane, Greenberg, Weltge and Watson 1995, 392). For example, in recent research, D'Avolio and colleagues used the Abuse Assessment Screen (AAS), a five-item tool that asks pregnant women about frequency and type of current and past domestic violence that includes physical, sexual, and emotional abuse and that "can be completed in less than a minute" (D'Avolio et al. 2001, 356).

The practice of screening women for abuse rests on several assumptions that are congruent with the notion of moral actors who are equal, independent, rational, and autonomous individuals. First, screening presumes the main reason that violence is not recognized is that women do not disclose abuse by choice. A second assumption is that if health care providers ask, women will disclose. Third, advocating screening presumes that the health care provider must know that the woman has experienced abuse in order to provide a meaningful response. Finally, screening presumes that the health care provider understands the dynamics of abuse and will make a meaningful response when abuse is disclosed.

If, however, the idea of moral agents as relational, gendered, and embedded in particular and power-laden contexts is taken into account, a number of questions must be raised. First, given the economic and social position of women, what are the factors that a woman must take into account when deciding whether or not to disclose abuse? Might fear of loss of her children, partner, or means of economic support figure in her response? Might fear of racial stereotypes or fear that her partner might be mistreated by the judicial system deter her from disclosure? Second, given the problematic attitudes of health care providers toward women who have experienced violence and the evidence of blaming and judgmental responses, what is the likelihood that a woman could anticipate a helpful response? Given that women claim that they are deterred from help-seeking by their anticipation of disbelief or blame, what is the likelihood that they will disclose abuse, particularly when questioned in "less than a minute?" Given the mounting acuity in health care, the limited resources of health care providers, and the attitudes of health care providers toward women and abuse, what is the likelihood that health care providers will provide meaningful support if and when abuse is recognized?

The *application* of the practice of screening is also likely to be problematic. If health care providers tend to associate violence with certain groups, and if they are more comfortable questioning certain groups of people than others (for which there is evidence) (Varcoe 2001; 2002), then is screening more likely to be implemented along the lines of race, class, and stereotypical thinking? Despite training and protocols, persistently low rates of screening have been documented. With few exceptions (e.g., Grunfeld et al. 1994), the question of who is and is not being screened in terms of race, class, and so on has not been addressed.

Finally, given the complexities of this issue, what is the likelihood that women will experience a meaningful outcome as a consequence of screening? Chalk and King (1998) reviewed all available evaluative studies on all forms of abuse in the United States. They did not find any studies examining the potential benefits of screening programs against the potential risks, and they expressed concern that risks include false negatives and false positives in "programs characterized by inadequate staff training and responses" (306). They also cited a lack of follow-up services, the inability of other services to manage the increased case loads generated by screening, and the risk of labelling women and exposure to negative attitudes (Chalk and King 1998). Ramsey et al. (2002) conducted a systematic review of quantitative research regarding screening and concluded that

> other than increased referral to outside agencies, little evidence exists for changes in important outcomes such as decreased exposure to violence. No studies measured quality of life, mental health outcomes, or potential harm to women from screening programmes.... Although domestic violence is a common problem with major health consequences for women, implementation of screening programmes in healthcare settings cannot be justified. Evidence of the benefit of specific interventions and lack of harm from screening is needed (314).

As this conclusion clearly indicates, an ethical analysis of potential harm must be undertaken in designing practice. And to do so requires more robust ethical theory.

WIDENING THE SCOPE OF ETHICAL THEORY

Feminist and anti-racist scholars argue that feminism and anti-racism are inherently and explicitly ethical projects as they challenge **oppression.** Valdivia (2002) argues that race, like gender, accords value and worth in our social structure. Valdivia further argues that by rendering some people superior and others inferior, such differentiation contradicts a morality of mutual respect. Nye (2000) contends that some philosophers "discard feminist and multicultural thought as mere 'politics'" (102). However, authors such as Nye argue that philosophy and ethics require feminist and post-colonial theory to address contemporary ethical issues. For example, Valdivia argues that a minority[10] politics of ethics ought to "inform, change and revolutionize the mainstream" (430). These calls complement critiques charging that traditional ethical theory (dominated by rational-analytic approaches that presuppose independent, context-free actors) is inadequate for contemporary health care practice (Rodney et al. 2002; Sherwin 1992; 1998; Taylor 1992).

An adequate analysis of the potential harm or good that might be derived from policy and practice in relation to violence against women requires attention to the dynamics of intersecting forms of oppression, including gender, race, class, ability, age, and sexual orientation. Such attention might in turn highlight the ways in which ethical theory is shaped by race, class, gender, and other biases (see Saunders 1996; Warren 1989; Yeo 1994). For example, traditional theory regarding informed consent implies that if women are competent, un-coerced, and informed, they will make the "right choices," as is reflected in Ethics in Practice 20-1 and 20-2. Yet traditional analysis of informed consent misses the multiple ways that power runs through the lives of women who have experienced abuse and the relationships that are intertwined in their decision-making. Developing an understanding of informed consent that takes interlocking forms of oppression into account in relation to violence against women may offer a broader understanding of informed consent.

TOWARD MORE ETHICAL PRACTICE

If countering oppression is inherently an ethical project, then ethical practice for nurses and other health care providers demands countering oppression. As Shaha (1998) has observed regarding nursing in general, Browne et al. (2002) note that Canadian nursing literature has tended to ignore issues of discrimination, racism, and inequities in health care. Employing an ethical analysis of violence against women underscores the importance of attention to such issues. And it opens up a world of possibilities for the enhancement of ethical practice offered by feminist and post-colonial theorists who have struggled with how to work together in overcoming oppression.

Most authors note that **anti-oppressive practice** begins with the practitioner and with an examination of the practitioner's motives (e.g., Lugones and Spelman 1983; Nye 2000). Browne and her colleagues (2002) suggest beginning with working toward the development of a critical consciousness of one's own power, knowledge, and privilege. They continue by advising explicit naming of discrimination, attention to the language we use to refer to "others," active reflection upon generalizations and biases that may inform action, and attending to patients' claims of discrimination. Canales (2000) suggests engaging with others perceived as different from ourselves in an actively inclusionary manner. She conceptualizes this "inclusionary othering" as a process that attempts to utilize power within relationships for transformation and coalition building. In concert with post-colonial and feminist authors such as Collins (e.g., 1990; 1993) and Lugones and Spelman (1983), Canales advises nurses to work to know the other's world, to reconceptualize meanings and understandings, and to connect with "others" as allies and in friendship.

In relation to violence against women, such strategies would direct nurses to seek to understand the experience of women who are abused and to attempt to understand the way in which their social and economic circumstances shape their lives and options. Consider the example in Ethics in Practice 20-3. In this excerpt, the nurse describes imagining what she "can't imagine." She engages in "moral imagination" (Babbitt 1996) to work toward a different stance in her relationship with patients.

Ethics in Practice 20-3	**Bulldozer**

I had one woman in tears one night. She came in with a broken arm. Her husband had slammed her arm in the door and broken her arm, and it was intentional. I terrified her, I absolutely terrified her. I said, "You've got to leave now. You can't stay with him. You have got to believe him if he says he is going to hurt you, he could kill you, he could buy a gun, he could [pause]".... I mean I can't imagine what I did to this poor woman, because obviously that wasn't helpful.... So I think I probably didn't do a good job of helping women... because I was just this bulldozer—bulldozer is a good word for it. I had blinders on and I couldn't see anything.

I have come full circle from that now, I believe... in that I can really understand women and why they stay in relationships and what is at stake for them and all of the variables, instead of just the one variable [of violence]. I think that makes a big difference to them. I can't imagine what it would be like to be alone, without a job, maybe with kids, or without kids, maybe in a city where you don't know anybody else, versus being with somebody who is actually supporting you, even though he is hurting you at times, he is still bringing in money and feeding you and the kids. So it would be a horrible, horrible situation to be in.[4]

Seeking to understand women's experiences and circumstances, working across difference in friendship, and connecting with women as allies are likely to decrease blame and negative judgment and increase the likelihood of a meaningful and supportive experience for women. With such a perspective, nurses would examine racializing language, such as "Native Indian," would explore how stereotypes might work with their thinking about Muslim women, and would reflect on how traditional ideas about the role of women might shape practice. *Nurses would consider a woman's access to resources as gendered and raced, and would strive to offer respect rather than judgment, and support rather than blame.*

TOWARD MORE ETHICAL POLICY

The practices of individual health care providers will not end discrimination or violence. Rather, as argued in Chapter 1, policy that supports ethical practice is required. An ethical analysis of the issue of violence against women provides the basis for such policy at the level of client care, at the level of programs and organizations, and at the level of governments and other societal structures. So, at the level of client care, rather than a policy that requires all health care providers to "screen" women for a past or current history of abuse, policy might be established that requires all health care providers to learn about the dynamics of gender-based violence and to develop **culturally safe**[11] practices (see Agnew 1998; Austin et al. 1999; Browne and Fiske 2001; Lee, Sanders Thompson and Mechanic 2002; Polaschek 1998; Smye and Browne 2002). The concept of cultural safety not only turns attention to the attitudes and practices of individuals, but also directs attention to examining how dominant organizational, institutional, and structural contexts shape health and social relations and practices. The concept of cultural safety also prompts the unmasking of the ways policies and practices may be perpetuating neo-colonial approaches to health care (Smye and Brown).

Program policy might be developed that provides for comprehensive responses to the issue of violence against women. As economic independence is the greatest determinant of whether women leave or stay in abusive relationships, and as it influences the extent to which women are exposed to sexual assault and other forms of gender-based violence such as sexual harassment, health care responses must be integrated with programs to foster the economic independence of women. Such integration is required both to assist women to leave abusive situations and to avoid and remain out of situations in which they are vulnerable to violence. As Venis and Horton (2002) note, successful interventions are those that address the status of women economically, in societal attitudes, in interpersonal relationships, and in communities. Thus, for example, health care programs could be integrated with a broader community plan that includes social assistance, employment strategies, and child care programs.

Importantly, employee policy might attend to the fact that many nurses and other health care providers will themselves have experienced violence. So, for example, Employee Assistance Programs might be expanded to permit counselling by professionals with particular expertise in the area of violence, rather than the usual situation in which non-specialist counsellors are often assigned. Such policy would more effectively assist health care providers who experience abuse and would in turn help them to be more effective with patients.

At the level of government, the issues of violence and discrimination might be woven throughout various relevant policy areas. For example, despite the known intersections between violence and issues such as HIV/AIDS, substance use, and mental health, an examination of provincial health care policy in British Columbia found that there was little integration of the issue of violence in these areas (Morrow and Varcoe 2000). In a more recent example, cuts to social services, legal aid, and child care in British Columbia were anticipated by experts in family violence to have devastating effects on women who experience violence (particularly poor and racialized women), yet these policy changes were implemented without explicit attention to these effects (Varcoe, Morrow and Hankivsky 2003). Nurses and other health care providers can advocate for better policy integration using the ethical implications as an important rationale.

If we operate from a morality that values equity and justice, because gender-based violence is grounded in gender inequity, it is by definition an ethical issue. The health care response to violence against women continues to largely overlook violence, blame women, and fails to take into account the gender dynamics of violence. In addition to being an example of the dynamics of gender bias in health care, the health care response to violence offers a particularly clear example of how racism and classism operate in the provision of health care. Thus, the health care response has the potential to further harm those who experience violence through blame and inaction and through the creation of gender-based, class-based, and racialized barriers to access.

An ethical analysis based on feminist and post-colonial theory directs attention to inequity and injustice based on gender, race, and class that may underlie our current inadequacies of care. Thus, improvement in health care policy and practice must take into account the contextual features of violence against women. A consideration of the particulars of violence against women points to the need for ethical theory to attend to contextual features of health care in general. Whether in relation to issues as specific as HIV/AIDS or as general as home caregiving, theories, practices, and polices must be explicitly based on an understanding of the complexity of people's lives, their economic realities, and the range of forms of violence (such as racism) that they experience. Improvements in practice would be explicitly anti-racist and would take into account the attitudes and biases of health care providers so that practices are, at minimum, not harmful. Nurses have a significant role to play in widening the scope of ethical theory, practice, and policy so that women who experience violence are better served.

FOR REFLECTION

1. Given that every practitioner who encounters women necessarily deals with women who have experienced violence (probably about 25 percent of women have experienced physical or sexual assault at least once in their lifetime), to what extent have you recognized this fact? How have these women's experiences shaped your practice?

2. What experiences have you had in working with issues of race? If you have had none that readily come to mind, what does that say about the privileges you enjoy and your level of awareness about racism?

3. What is the most pernicious or pervasive form of "othering" that you encounter in your practice? How do you contend with these practices?

4. What are the most significant contextual features shaping the health and health care of clients in your care? In what ways do these features shape the "informed consent," "autonomy," "choice," or "access" of your clients?

5. For any scenario that comes to mind relative to the above questions, consider how you might explain that scenario as an ethical issue (e.g., using words like "justice," "fairness," "autonomy," "access," and so on). What might be the benefit of thinking in ethical terms about such issues?

ENDNOTES

1. Throughout this chapter, the terms "violence against women" and "gender-based violence" are used interchangeably and refer to a range of experiences perpetrated against women that includes emotional, physical, financial, and sexual abuse by intimate partners, sexual assault both by known and unknown assailants, and sexual harassment. **"Violence"** is defined as an abuse of power (British Columbia Institute on Family Violence, 1994). "Violence against women" is defined as "any act of gender-based violence that results in or is likely to result in physical, sexual, or mental harm or suffering to women, including threats of such acts, coercion, or arbitrary deprivation of liberty, whether occurring in private or public life" (United Nations General Assembly 1993, Resolution 48/104, December 20). In intimate relationships, violence may be

perpetrated against women by men in heterosexual relationships or by women in lesbian relationships. Although men may also be victims of violence, particularly when they are vulnerable because of age, race, ability, sexual orientation, and so on, such violence is not the focus of this chapter.

2. See Chapter 5 and Chapter 7 for descriptions of the forms of theory in contextual and nursing ethics.

3. The speaker identified a particular community, whose religion is predominantly Islam, by their pre-immigration country of origin. The identifier has been changed to protect the identity of the research site, community, and participants.

4. This excerpt is taken from an interview with a staff nurse conducted during a study of nursing practice in relation to violence against women (Varcoe 1997; 2001).

5. This study, titled "Project Violence Free," included four lesbians, two of whom had been battered by (former) male partners, two by female partners.

6. Although there is no biological basis for the notion of "race"—that is, race is a social construction, not a biological reality—in Canada, as elsewhere, people often perceive race as indeed biological. Race as a social construction is a powerful influence in structuring the lives of people. For discussions of racism as a social construction and its influence on health and health care, see Anderson and Kirkham (1998); Henry et al. (2000a); Krieger (1999); Rattansi (1995); and Shaha (1998).

7. This excerpt is also taken from an interview with a staff nurse conducted during a study of nursing practice in relation to violence against women (Varcoe 1997; 2001). I wish to note that the nurse cited in this excerpt was struggling with these ideas, as was I. The excerpt represents her thoughts at a particular moment in time and does so in a static way. She found this interview very useful and at a second interview drew attention to many of the dynamics outlined in this chapter. Undoubtedly she has continued to develop her ideas about violence, race, ethical practice, and so on.

8. Shaha (1998) defines "racism" as the execution of a deterministic theory (in which genetic or biological background is used as a basis for assumptions about individuals or groups who are seen as different from other individuals or groups) that is supported by the structure of a country and reinforced through daily practices.

9. In the study from which the examples were drawn, all but one of the health care providers who participated were Caucasian. This was reflective of the composition of the staff on the units studied and was in marked contrast to the ethnically diverse patient population that the units served. Although this imbalance is shifting, health care providers in Canada generally belong to various dominant groups because of their education, professional status, income, and facility in official languages.

10. Rather than the sense of minority in terms of sheer numbers, Valdivia (2002) is referring to minority in terms of share of power and resources.

11. Cultural safety involves the "recognition of the social, economic and political position of certain groups within society... and is concerned with fostering an understanding of the relationship between minority status and health status as a way of changing nurses' attitudes from those which continue to support current dominant practices and systems of health care to those which are more supportive of the health of minority groups" (Smye and Browne 2002, 46–47).

REFERENCES

Agnew, V. 1998. *In search of a safe place: Abused women and culturally sensitive services.* Toronto: University of Toronto Press.

Anderson, J. and Kirkham, S.R. 1998. Constructing nation: The gendering and racializing of the Canadian health care system. In V. Strong-Boag, S. Grace, A. Eisenberg and J. Anderson (Eds.), *Painting the maple: Essays on race, gender, and the construction of Canada* (pp. 242–261). Vancouver, BC: University of British Columbia Press.

Austin, W., Gallop, R., McCay, E., Peternelj-Taylor, C. and Bayer, M. 1999. Culturally competent care for psychiatric clients who have a history of sexual abuse. *Clinical Nursing Research, 8*(1), 5–25.

Babbitt, S.E. 1996. Personal integrity, politics, and moral imagination. In S.E. Babbitt (Ed.), *Impossible dreams: Rationality, integrity and moral imagination* (pp. 102–129). Boulder, CO: Westview.

Barnett, O.W. 2000. Why battered women do not leave. Part 1: External inhibiting factors within society. *Trauma, Violence, and Abuse, 1*(4), 343–372.

Bell, M. and Mosher, J.E. 1998. (Re)fashioning medicine's response to wife abuse. In S. Sherwin (Ed.), *The politics of women's health: Exploring agency and autonomy* (pp. 205–233). Philadelphia: Temple University Press.

Bourdieu, P. 2000. *Pascalian meditations.* Translator: R. Nice. Stanford, CA: Stanford University Press.

British Columbia Institute on Family Violence. 1994. *Family violence in British Columbia: A brief overview.* Vancouver, BC: British Columbia Institute on Family Violence.

Browne, A.J. and Fiske, J. 2001. First Nations women's encounters with mainstream health care services. *Western Journal of Nursing Research, 23*(2), 126–147.

Browne, A.J., Johnson, J.L., Bottorff, J.L., Grewal, S. and Hilton, B.A. 2002. Recognizing discrimination in nursing practice. *Canadian Nurse, 98*(5), 24–27.

Campbell, J., Rose, L., Kub, J. and Nedd, D. 1998. Voices of strength and resistance: A contextual and longitudinal analysis of women's responses to battering. *Journal of Interpersonal Violence, 13*(6), 743–762.

Canadian Centre for Justice Statistics. 1993. *Violence against women survey highlights and questionnaire package.* Ottawa: Statistics Canada.

Canales, M.K. 2000. Othering: Toward an understanding of difference. *Advances in Nursing Science, 22*(4), 16–31.

Cann, K., Withnell, S., Shakespeare, J., Doll, H. and Thomas, J. 2001. Domestic violence: A comparative survey of levels of detection, knowledge, and attitudes in healthcare workers. *Public Health, 115*(2), 89–95.

Centerwall, B.S. 1995. Race, socioeconomic status, and domestic homicide. *Journal of the American Medical Association, 273*(22), 1755–1758.

Chalk, R. and King, P.A. 1998. *Violence in families: Assessing prevention and treatment programs.* Washington, D.C.: National Academy Press.

Cochrane, D.A. 1987. Emergency nurses' attitudes toward the rape victim. *AARN Newsletter, 43*(7), 14–18.

Collins, P.H. 1990. *Black feminist thought: Knowledge, consciousness, and the politics of empowerment.* New York: Routledge.

Collins, P.H. 1993. Toward a new vision: Race, class and gender as categories of analysis and connection. *Race, Sex & Class, 1*(1), 23–45.

Corbally, M.A. 2001. Factors affecting nurses' attitudes towards the screening and care of battered women in Dublin A&E departments: A literature review. *Accident and Emergency Nursing, 9*(1), 27–37.

Crenshaw, K.W. 1994. Mapping the margins: Intersectionality, identity politics, and violence against women of color. In M.A. Fineman and R. Mykitiuk (Eds.), *The public nature of private violence* (pp. 93–118). New York: Routledge.

D'Avolio, D., Hawkins, J.W., Haggerty, L.A., Kelly, U., Barrett, R., Toscano, S.E.D., Dwyer, J., Higgins, L.P., Kearney, M., Pearce, C.W., Aber, C.S., Mahony, D. and Bell, M. 2001. Screening for abuse: Barriers and opportunities. *Health Care for Women International, 22*(4), 349–362.

Ellis, J.M. 1999. Barriers to effective screening for domestic violence by registered nurses in the emergency department. *Critical Care Nursing Quarterly, 22*(1), 27–41.

Erickson, M., Hill, T. and Siegel, R. 2001. Barriers to domestic violence screening in the pediatric setting. *Pediatrics, 108*, 98–103.

Ewing, W.A. 1987. Domestic violence and community health care ethics: Reflections on systemic intervention. *Family & Community Health, 10*(1), 54–62.

Fishwick, N.J. 1998. Assessment of women for partner abuse. *Journal of Obstetric, Gynecologic, & Neonatal Nursing, 27*, 661–670.

Garimella, R., Plichta, S.B., Houseman, C. and Garzon, L. 2000. Physician beliefs about victims of spouse abuse and about the physician role. *Journal of Women's Health and Gender-Based Medicine, 9*(4), 405–411.

Gerbert, B., Johnston, K., Caspers, N., Bleecker, T., Woods, A. and Rosenbaum, A. 1996. Experiences of battered women in health care settings: A qualitative study. *Women & Health, 24*(3), 1–17.

Groth, B., Chelmowski, M.K. and Batson, T. P. 2001. Domestic violence: Level of training, knowledge base and practice among Milwaukee physicians. *Western Journal of Medicine, 100*(1), 24–28, 36.

Grunfeld, A., Ritmiller, S., MacKay, K., Cowan, L. and Hotch, D. 1994. Detecting domestic violence against women in the emergency department: A nursing triage model. *Journal of Emergency Nursing, 20*, 271–274.

Gurr, J., Mailloux, L. and Kinnon, D. 1996. *Breaking the links between poverty and violence against women*. Ottawa: Health Canada.

Henry, F., Tator, C., Mattis, W. and Rees, T. 2000a. *The colour of democracy: Racism in Canadian society*. Toronto: Harcourt Brace.

Henry, F., Tator, C., Mattis, W. and Rees, T. 2000b. Racism and human-service delivery. In F. Henry, C. Tator, W. Mattis and T. Rees (Eds.), *The colour of democracy: Racism in Canadian society* (pp. 207–227). Toronto: Harcourt Brace.

Humphreys, J., Parker, B. and Campbell, J. 2001. Intimate partner violence against women. *Annual Review of Nursing Research, 19*, 275–306.

Krieger, N. 1999. Embodying inequality: A review of concepts, measures, and methods for studying health consequences of discrimination. *International Journal of Health Services, 29*(2), 295–352.

Lambert, L. and Firestone, J.M. 2000. Economic context and multiple abuse techniques. *Violence Against Women, 6*(1), 49–67.

Larkin, G.L., Moskop, J., Sanders, A. and Derse, A. 1994. The emergency physician and patient confidentiality: A review. *Annals of Emergency Medicine, 24*(6), 1161–1167.

Lazzaro, M.V. and McFarlane, J. 1991. Establishing a screening program for abused women. *Journal of Nursing Administration, 21*(10), 24–29.

Lee, R.K., Sanders Thompson, V.L. and Mechanic, M.B. 2002. Intimate partner violence and women of color: A call for innovations. *American Journal of Public Health, 92*(4), 530–535.

Limandri, B.J. and Sheridan, D.J. 1995. Prediction of interpersonal violence: An introduction. In J.C. Campbell (Ed.), *Assessing dangerousness: Violence by sexual offenders, batterers, and child abusers* (pp. 1–19). Thousand Oaks, CA: Sage.

Limandri, B.J. and Tilden, V.P. 1993. Domestic violence: Ethical issues in the health care system. *AWHONN's Clinical Issues in Perinatal and Women's Health Nursing, 4*(3), 493–502.

Loring, M.T. and Smith, R.W. 1994. Health care barriers and interventions for battered women. *Public Health Reports, 109*(3), 328–338.

Lugones, M.C. and Spelman, E.V. 1983. Have we got a theory for you! Feminist theory, cultural imperialism and the demand for "the woman's voice." *Women's Studies International Forum, 6*(6), 573–581.

McCauley, J., Yurk, R.A., Jenckes, M.W. and Ford, D.E. 1998. Inside "Pandora's box": Abused women's experiences with clinicians and health services. *Journal of General and Internal Medicine, 13*(8), 549–555.

McFarlane, J., Greenberg, L., Weltge, A. and Watson, M.G. 1995. Identification of abuse in emergency departments: Effectiveness of a two-question screening tool. *Journal of Emergency Nursing, 21*(5), 391–394.

McFarlane, J.M., Campbell, J.C., Wilt, S., Sachs, C.J., Ulrich, Y. and Xu, X. 1999. Stalking and intimate partner femicide. *Homicide Studies, 3*(4), 300–316.

McLeer, S.V. and Anwar, R.A.H. 1989. A study of battered women presenting in an emergency department. *American Journal of Public Health, 79*(1), 65–66.

McMurray, A. and Moore, K. 1994. Domestic violence: Are we listening? Do we see? *The Australian Journal of Advanced Nursing, 12*(1), 23–28.

Moore, M.L., Zaccaro, D. and Parsons, L.H. 1998. Attitudes and practices of registered nurses toward women who have experienced abuse/domestic violence. *Journal of Obstetric, Gynecologic & Neonatal Nursing, 27*(2), 175–182.

Morrow, M. and Varcoe, C. 2000. *Violence against women: Improving the health care response—A guide for health authorities, health care managers, providers and planners.* Victoria, BC: Ministry of Health.

Mosher, J.E. 1998. Caught in tangled webs of care: Women abused in intimate relationships. In C.T. Baines, P.M. Evans and S.M. Neysmith (Eds.), *Women's caring: Feminist perspectives on social welfare,* 2nd ed. (pp. 139–159). Toronto: Oxford University Press.

Nye, A. 2000. It's not philosophy. In U. Narayan and S. Harding (Eds.), *Decentering the center: Philosophy for a multicultural, postcolonial and feminist world* (pp. 101–109). Indianapolis, IN: *Hypatia,* Indiana University Press.

Pauly, B. and Varcoe, C. In review. Negotiating difference in everyday ethical practice. (Manuscript submitted to *Nursing Inquiry.*)

Polaschek, N.R. 1998. Cultural safety: A new concept in nursing people of different ethnicities. *Journal of Advanced Nursing, 27*, 452–457.

Ramsey, J., Richardson, J., Carter, Y.H., Davidson, L.L. and Feder, G. 2002. Should health professionals screen women for domestic violence? Systematic review. *British Medical Journal, 325*(7359), 314–318.

Ratner, P. 1995. *Societal responses as moderators of the health consequences of wife abuse.* Unpublished doctoral dissertation. University of Alberta, Edmonton.

Rattansi, A. 1995. Just framing: Ethnicities and racisms in a "postmodern" framework. In L. Nicholson and S. Seidman (Eds.), *Social postmodernisms: Beyond identity politics* (pp. 250–286). Cambridge: Cambridge University Press.

Richie, B.E. and Kanuha, V. 1993. Battered women of color in public health care systems: Racism, sexism and violence. In B. Bair and S.E. Cayleff (Eds.), *Wings of gauze: Women of color and the experience of health and illness* (pp. 288–299). Detroit, MI: Wayne State University.

Rodney, P., Varcoe, C., Storch, J.L., McPherson, G., Mahoney, K., Brown, H., Pauly, B., Hartrick, G. and Starzomski, R. 2002. Navigating toward a moral horizon: A multisite qualitative study of nurses' enactment of ethical practice. *Canadian Journal of Nursing Research, 34*(3), 75–102.

Rose, K. and Saunders, D.G. 1986. Nurses' and physicians' attitudes about women abuse: The effects of gender and professional role. *Health Care for Women International, 7*, 427–438.

Saunders, M.J. 1996. Feminist ethics and "privilege." *Resources for Feminist Research/Documentation pour la Researche Feministe, 25*(3/4), 18–25.

Shaha, M. 1998. Racism and its implications in ethical–moral reasoning in nursing practice: A tentative approach to a largely unexplored topic. *Nursing Ethics, 5*(2), 139–146.

Sherwin, S. 1992. Feminist and medical ethics: Two different approaches to contextual ethics. In H. Bequaret Holmes and L. Purdy (Eds.), *Feminist perspectives in medical ethics* (pp. 17–31). Indianapolis, IN: Indiana University.

Sherwin, S. (Ed.) 1998. *The politics of women's health: Exploring agency and autonomy.* Philadelphia: Temple University Press.

Shields, G., Baer, J., Leininger, K., Marlow, J. and Dekeyser, P. 1998. Interdisciplinary health care and victims of domestic violence. *Social Work in Health Care, 27*(2), 27–48.

Smye, V. and Browne, A.J. 2002. Cultural safety and the analysis of health policy affecting Aboriginal people. *Nurse Researcher, 9*(3), 42–56.

Sugg, T., Thompson, R.S., Thompson, D.C., Maiuro, R. and Rivara, F.P. 1999. Domestic violence and primary care. Attitudes, practices, and beliefs. *Archives of Family Medicine, 8*(4), 301–306.

Taylor, C.R. 1992. *Multiculturalism and "The politics of recognition."* Princeton: Princeton University Press.

Tilden, V.P. and Schmidt, T.A. 1994. Family abuse and neglect: A case-based ethics model. *Academic Emergency Medicine, 1*(6), 550–554.

Tilden, V.P. and Shepherd, P. 1987. Increasing the rate of identification of battered women in an emergency department: Use of a nursing protocol. *Research in Nursing and Health, 10*, 209–215.

Tjaden, P. and Thoennes, N. 1998. *Prevalence, incidence, and consequences of violence against women: Findings from the national violence against women survey.* Washington, D.C.: U.S. Department of Justice, Office of Justice Programs, National Institute of Justice.

United Nations General Assembly. 1993. Declaration on the elimination of violence against women. New York: United Nations.

Valdivia, A.N. 2002. bell hooks: Ethics from the margins. *Qualitative Inquiry, 8*(4), 429–447.

Varcoe, C. 1997. *Untying our hands: The social context of nursing in relation to violence against women.* Unpublished doctoral dissertation. University of British Columbia, Vancouver, BC.

Varcoe, C. 2001. Abuse obscured: An ethnographic account of emergency nursing in relation to violence against women. *Canadian Journal of Nursing Research, 32*(4), 95–115.

Varcoe, C. 2002. Inequality, violence and women's health. In B.S. Bolaria and H. Dickinson (Eds.), *Health, illness and health care in Canada,* 3rd ed. (pp. 211–230). Scarborough, ON: Nelson Thomson Learning.

Varcoe, C., Jaffer, F. and Kelln, P. 2002. *Protecting Women? Women's experiences of seeking protection from abuse by intimate partners.* Victoria, BC: University of Victoria.

Varcoe, C., Morrow, M. and Hankivsky, O. 2003. *No Lessons Learned? Developing a dialogue about the BC provincial cuts and the impact on women who experience violence.* Vancouver, BC: Research Advisory on the Provincial Cuts and Violence Against Women, BC Institute Against Family Violence.

Venis, S. and Horton, R. 2002. Violence against women: A global burden. *Lancet, 359*(9313), 1172.

Waalen, J., Goodwin, M.M., Spitz, A.M., Petersen, R. and Saltzman, L.E. 2000. Screening for intimate partner violence by health care providers. Barriers and interventions. *American Journal of Preventive Medicine, 19*(4), 230–237.

Walker, L.E.A. 1995. Racism and violence against women. In J. Adleman and G.M. Enguidanos (Eds.), *Racism in the lives of women: Testimony, theory and guides to antiracist practice* (pp. 238–249). New York: Harrington Park.

Warren, V.L. 1989. Feminist directions in medical ethics. *Hypatia, 4*(2), 73–87.

Warshaw, C. 1998. Domestic violence: Changing theory, changing practice. In J.F. Monagle and D.C. Thomasma (Eds.), *Health care ethics: Critical issues for the 21st century* (pp. 128–137). Gaithersburg, MD: Aspen.

Whaley, A.L. 1998. Racism in the provision of mental health services: A social-cognitive analysis. *American Journal of Orthopsychiatry, 68*(1), 47–57.

Wiebe, E. and Janssen, P. 2001. Universal screening for domestic violence in abortion. *Women's Health Issues, 11*, 436–441.

Wilkerson, A.L. 1998. "Her body her own worst enemy": The medicalization of violence against women. In S.G. French, W. Teays and L.M. Purdy (Eds.), *Violence against women: Philosophical perspectives*. Ithaca: Cornell University Press.

Williams, O.J. and Becker, R.L. 1994. Domestic partner abuse treatment programs and cultural competence: The results of a national survey. *Violence and Victims, 9*(3), 287–296.

Willson, P., Cesario, S., Fredland, N., Walsh, T., McFarlane, J., Gist, J., Malecha, A. and Schultz, P.N. 2001. Primary healthcare provider's lost opportunity to help abused women. *Journal of the American Academy of Nurse Practitioners, 13*(12), 565–570.

Woodtli, M.A. 2001. Nurses' attitudes toward survivors and perpetrators of domestic violence. *Journal of Holistic Nursing, 19*(4), 340–359.

Yeo, M. 1994. Interpretive bioethics. *Health and Canadian society: HCS, 2*(1), 85–108.

chapter twenty-one

Being an Ethical Practitioner: The Embodiment of Mind, Emotion, and Action

Gweneth Doane

... [S]ince ethics is a deeply personal, embodied process, being and becoming a moral agent requires the cultivation of mindful, critical awareness and attunement to emotion and bodily experience.

ETHICS AND NURSING

People indicate their theories or "truths" in three manners—by what they seek when they search for truth, by what they think they have found when they obtain it, and by what they do when they receive or impart its influence (Lansing 1908). In looking at the field of nursing ethics—at what we have sought, what we have imparted, and how we have imparted it—the positivist traditions are evident. Dominated by ethical theories and principles evolved in biomedicine (Fry 1989), ethics in nursing has traditionally focused on (1) the ethical dilemmas that typically arise from medical-technological advances (e.g., euthanasia), (2) learning and using supposedly neutral, culture-free principles rationally and logically to analyze the dilemmas, and (3) reaching a value-free "right" answer.

This rational approach to ethics is not unique to nursing, or even to health care. As Bauman (1993) describes, the broader field of philosophy and ethics has been dominated by a modernist approach to the search for truth. According to Bauman, early modern thinkers thought that rather than being a natural trait of human life, morality was something that needed to be created and injected into human conduct. As a result, the product of the search for moral truth was the development of an all-comprehensive unitary ethics—theories and codes of moral rules that people could be taught and expected to obey (Bauman 1993). Williams (1985) contends that this reductive enterprise of producing ethical theory and responding to moral challenges through normative regulation has been "unblinkingly" undertaken "if for no obvious reason except that it has been going on a long time" (76).

Many in the ethics field have critiqued this rationalist approach to moral truth and the ethical decision-making process it gives rise to (Bauman 1993; Damon 1999; Dewey 1891/1957; Elliot 1999; Flanagan 1996; Niebuhr 1963; Williams 1985). As Dewey (1891/1957) concluded, although these tools of analysis may help people to consciously consider their choices, the moral situation is an extremely complicated affair. A theory, principle, or rule cannot tell one how to act in any specific case (Dewey 1891/1957), and one danger of an overemphasis on rational principles is that they divorce people from their own identities and thereby risk destroying people's motivation to be moral (Walker 1999). Functional or procedural codes and the responsibilities they outline serve to blunt rather than reinforce personal responsibility—which, according to Bauman (1993), is "morality's last hold and hope" (35). As a collective, these ethicists have called for morality to "be let out of the stiff armor of the artificially constructed ethical codes" (Bauman 1993, 34). Emphasizing the re-personalizing of ethical decision-making, they have highlighted the importance of recognizing the passionate and complex reality of moral life.

This critique and call for re-personalization of ethics has also been occurring in nursing. Seeing the rationalist theories and principles as too abstract and distant from the complex human milieu in which nurses work, nurse ethicists have argued that they fall short when dealing with the relational and contextual nature of nursing care (Benner 1991). As a result, different suggestions for addressing this inadequacy have been made, including grounding ethical practice in nursing theory (Yeo 1989), developing a philosophy of ethics that evolves from nursing practice (Bishop and Scudder 1990), articulating a nursing ethic based on care (Fry 1989; Gadow 1990; Watson 1988), understanding human experience within relationships as the foundation for ethics (Bergum 1994; Pauly 2001), and developing a feminist ethics (Liaschenko 1993; Sherwin 1998). Similar to the broader field of ethics, what each of these suggestions has in common is the emphasis on the everyday nature of morality (that is, that every minute of nursing practice involves ethics) and a call for a more personal, humanly involved approach to ethics. (See also Chapter 7.)

In this chapter, I continue this call for a humanly involved ethics. I present a summary of the findings of one study that highlighted the significance of nurses' moral identity and the embodied nature of ethics and ethical practice. I will argue that since ethics is a deeply personal, embodied process, being and becoming a moral agent requires the cultivation of a mindful, critical awareness and attunement to emotion and bodily experience.

RE-PERSONALIZING ETHICS

The validity of the call for re-personalization of ethics has been confirmed by a number of theoretical and empirical studies. These studies have concluded that a person's moral identity and the concerns that stem from that identity are the best predictors of a person's commitment to moral action (Damon and Gregory 1997). It is one's moral identity that includes both the personal aspect—what a person considers to be the right decision or action—and the rationale—why she or he is compelled to follow through with a particular course of action (Damon 1999). As Bauman describes, "What we are learning, and learning the hard way, is that it is the personal morality that makes ethical negotiation and consensus possible, not the other way around" (34).

Damon (1999), along with others, has argued for the importance of bringing moral identity into the centre of morality and ethics. Research has shown that sustained moral commitment requires a uniting of self and morality: "People who define themselves in terms of their moral goals are likely to see moral problems in everyday events, and they are also likely to see themselves as necessarily implicated in these problems. From there, it is a small step to taking responsibility for the solution" (Colby and Damon 1992, 307). As Bauman (1993) explains, "When competing moral demands arise in the moment, it is the moral self which moves, feels, and acts in the context of that ambiguity, and no moral impulse can implement itself unless the moral actor feels compelled to 'stretch the effort to the limit'" (34).

NURSES' MORAL IDENTITY: FINDINGS FROM ONE STUDY

A study that sought to examine the meaning and enactment of ethics in nursing across a variety of clinical settings (Storch et al. 2000 [see Appendix A]) validated the significance of identity in nurses' ethical practice and offered important insight into nurses' experience of moral identity. A significant finding in the study was the way in which moral knowledge and ethical decision-making were channeled through the nurses' personal narrative and identity (Doane 2002). For example, in listening to the nurses discuss their ethical practice in focus groups, it was possible to actually hear them constructing their moral identities and to hear how that process shaped what was deemed "ethical" and how the nurses followed through with action.

Specifically, a socially mediated process of identity development was evident as the nurse participants recounted their experiences of navigating their way through everyday nursing practice (Doane 2002). Their identity as moral agents and their experience of ethics in everyday practice was **narratively, dialogically, relationally, and contextually derived** (Doane 2002). In addition, the bodily experience of ethics and ethical knowledge was highlighted.

Identity as Narrative

Similar to Woods' (1999) finding that nurses describe and respond to ethical issues narratively, narrative was central to how the nurses' moral identities were constructed and experienced. The nurses told personal stories of times when they had or had not seen themselves as acting ethically. In these stories their personal moral identity was woven together with the relevant others in the stories and with the context of the social organization that served as the narrative backdrop. At the same time, there seemed to be general or grand narratives that depicted what constituted an ethical nurse. And these grand narratives profoundly affected the personal narrative identities the nurses constructed. For example, the nurses lived within the grand narrative that said they were responsible for the well-being of their patients. But there was also the grand narrative of scarce resources in health care and another that depicted nurses as powerless against the systemic forces. The combination of these often conflicting grand narratives offered confusing and ambiguous direction to nurses as they attempted to practise ethically. For many of the nurses in the study, their individual narrative identity had become that of a nurse who was not practising ethically. As one nurse stated, "It's everything I can do, but it isn't enough." This inability to "do good" and "do enough," and the identity narrative it sparked, gave rise to profound moral distress. And as systemic forces in the current health care system made it more and more difficult for these nurses to act ethically and to identify themselves narratively as ethical practitioners, their moral distress grew.

Identity as Multiple and Dialogical

The nurses' moral identity was also constructed through inner dialogue. As McNamee (1996) points out, few of us would describe an ethical person as someone who exercises a particular set of morals in one situation and a vastly different one in another. We expect ethical individuals to be consistent in the values they use to make their decisions and shape their actions. Yet, the nurses in the study consistently spoke of the different parts and voices within them that offered differing views of what "should" be done in any given situation. For example, in deciding whether or not to perform cardiac resuscitation on an elderly man, one nurse described her inner dialogue in which one voice was saying that "doing good" would be to let him die peacefully while another voice was saying that he could be "the most active 102-year-old gentleman I have ever met (and he might want to be resuscitated)." As can be seen from this example, these differing views often led to inner tensions.

Given this multiple self, moral action was determined through a process of inner dialogue. As the nurses opened up to their different voices and entered into a dialogue, they could reach a consensus within themselves. However, a major deterrent to this inner dialogical process was the pace of practice. The nurses described that they most often did not have time to listen and to fully engage in an inner dialogue—to think things through to reach an inner consensus. Thus, they were often left feeling conflicted and dissatisfied with their response. This dissatisfaction with action inadvertently influenced their sense of moral agency and the identity they constructed of themselves narratively.

Identity as Relational and Contextual

As well as being narratively and dialogically derived, the nurses' identities appeared to emerge through layers of negotiation with self, with others, and within a context of social organization. Confronted with many different events and situations in their practice, the nurses selected and organized their experiences of those events into a set of workable meanings. These workable meanings shaped how they identified themselves within the situations and how their "professional identity" blended with their "personal identity." As one student nurse explained,

> When you get into the ward, there are constraints. You've got the pressures of the other nurses, your colleagues, administration, clients and clients' families. I found [that] myself and what I believe can get lost.

Ultimately it was in the mesh of the interdependence with the collective that the nurses came to identify themselves and their actions as ethical (or not). That is, their identity and view of themselves was shaped by the values of the larger collective and what that collective tacitly deemed to be "right action." And, conversely, their conception of how ethical the collective was arose through their personal view of what constituted "right" action.

Ethics as Embodied

> You know you're out of balance... when your heart is so heavy you can't carry it around the ward with you while you're trying to do your work.

This comment from a nursing student describing her experience of ethical practice offers one example of how ethics and moral identity are experienced as bodily processes, not merely as rational ones. Yet, following what they perceived to be proper ethical comportment, many of the nurses in the study attempted to separate and discount their subjective, embodied experience in order to engage in a more rational process of ethical analysis and decision-making. However, it seemed that often their attempts were in vain. Many of the nurses told stories of previous experiences that still had significance for them. Even though many of the experiences had occurred a number of years previously, they were still feeling distressed and unresolved about what had taken place and how they had responded. The grand narrative told them that their personal feelings were not relevant to their professional comportment. Further, the contextual forces allowed little time for inner dialogue and/or relational collegial support, which meant that the nurses were left living the experiences in a deeply embodied way. Consequently, these experiences continued to profoundly shape their identity as an ethical and/or unethical nurse.

ETHICAL NURSING PRACTICE: A PERSONAL, EMBODIED PROCESS

Elias (1978; 1982) contends that the tendency to divide the objective from the subjective—to divide reason from emotion—arose through the social relations of the Enlightment period. Enmeshed in the attitudes and beliefs of that era, people perceived such a division only because Descartes and other thinkers of the time conceived these attributes as separate. People experienced themselves in this way because they were enmeshed in the social controls and norms that perpetuated this way of being and thinking. Although these controls and norms were externally perpetuated, they became internalized in the body (Elias 1978; 1982). That is, the perceived division between reason and emotion was not "the source of experience; rather, one of its products" (Burkitt 1994, 18). As people took this division up bodily, it became an ingrained, unconscious, and supposedly "proper" way of being.

Recent work in the cognitive sciences, however, has clearly shown that the subjective and objective are not separate entities. Cognition and reason are now understood to be constituted by emergent processes that span and interconnect the brain, the body, and the environment and to ultimately emerge from the dynamic co-determination of self and other (Thompson 2001). Said another way, we now know that the mind is not located merely in the head but is embodied in the whole person, who is in turn embedded in his or her environment (Thompson 2001). As Wilshire (1982) points out, "To be a self is to be a human body that is mimetically involved with other such bodies" (266). The **embodied self** is a totality of life and action (Schrag 1997).

Complementing this developing knowledge in cognitive science, the field of self psychology has offered important insights into the synergy of identity, action, and social context. Elias (1978; 1982) has described how the embodied self (including one's identity and action) is linked to the changing experiences within the broader context of dynamic networks of social relations. According to Elias (1978; 1982), people become themselves—are configured—within a mesh of social relations.

Although the socially constructed nature of self and action has been discussed by many writers, Elias is particularly significant because he highlights that these socially prescribed dispositions are ingrained as bodily responses. According to Elias, people actually learn to discipline and control their own bodies in ways that are socially prescribed and that mirror the social habits of their group. These disciplines and controls form into dispositions toward certain behaviours and activities (e.g., ways of thinking, ways of knowing, ways of practising) (Burkitt 1994). The patterns of activity taken up are constantly reproduced by people in a non-reflective way. As these patterns are learned, they become ingrained in our bodily responses and flow through us unconsciously. As Dewey (1922; 1929) argues, we develop habits of conduct, including habits of seeing, hearing, touching, moving, speaking, and thinking, through enculturation and social sensibilities. These habits extend far beyond the behavioural level to the bodily/personal. People literally become their habits (Dewey 1922; 1929).

The internalization of social ways of being into bodily responses and identity is highly significant to ethical nursing practice. As part of the social collective, nurses automatically orient themselves with the dominant social norms. Subsequently, nurses' agential powers are shaped and molded through their social training and learning in the health care milieu. Since the division between reason and emotion continues to dominate the norms shaping ethical practice, sound ethical analysis and decision-making are most often linked with a rational/reasoned stance and process. The more this objective (rational/reasoned) ethical stance is perpetuated, and at, times demanded in the health care milieu, the more embodied it becomes. Nurses divorce themselves from their bodily sense and emotion and begin experiencing their own self as if it were composed of two objects—the mind and the body, reasons and emotions (Elias 1978/1982).

This embodied pattern of mind-body split results in the development of a pattern of identity and self-control in which constraints are placed on nurses' experience and expression of emotion. Although nurses' emotions are part of the automatic response of the body and therefore continue to be experienced, this embodied pattern of dividing the objective and subjective does not allow their emotions into the experience. For example, many nurses described "knowing in their heart" that the way a patient was being treated was not right, but they would tell themselves, "It is just me, and my personal feelings have no place in the decision." Even seemingly minor bodily sensations such as bodily tension were cues that nurses often ignored, yet this bodily knowledge had the capacity to inform the ethical situation. This discounting of emotion is problematic in two ways. First, Elias explains that dividing reason and emotion often leads to inner conflict and dissonance between what become two warring factions (the objective and the subjective). Certainly, this inner conflict was evidenced in the research study previously cited (Storch et al. 2000 [see Appendix A]). As the nurses took up the embodied stance of objective moral agent and acted from a reasoned perspective, they were often left feeling emotionally distressed. Although "reasonably" they had done what they "could and should," in their subjective, embodied experience they had not done enough. Of particular significance is that even attempts to avoid the emotional turmoil are ultimately fruitless. Since nurses are embodied beings, their ethical experiences continue to live on within them (bodily) even if they consciously and intentionally decide to "not take it on." Even nurses who compromise their ethical standards and walk away from their experience telling themselves rationally that they have to just let it go (e.g., it is the only way they can feel peaceful at the end of the day) are left with the emotional tensions bodily imprinted in them.

The second problem with discounting emotion (e.g., dividing the objective from the subjective) is that, as Nussbaum (2001) and Vetlesen (1994) have argued, it is through emotion that people actually experience the objects of moral judgments. Emotions are our value feelings—they mark what matters to us—"we experience emotion only in regard to that which matters" (Donaldson 1991, 2). Thompson (2001) explains that if it is feeling in the sense of bodily affect that makes one experience one's body as one's own, then it is emotion or value feeling that makes one experientially aware of one's personal self. "Thus emotions, as value feelings, make possible the evaluative experience of oneself and the world, and therefore are the very precondition of moral perception, of being able to 'see' a situation morally before deliberating rationally about it" (Thompson 2001, 24). Similarly, Vetlesen (1994) explains that "we experience the objects of moral judgments through emotion... emotions anchor *us* to particular moral circumstance, to the aspect of a situation that addresses *us* immediately, to the *here* and *now*.... [Emotion is required] to identify a situation as carrying moral significance in the first place" (4).

Consequently, bodily experience is of primary importance in moral sensibilities and moral reasoning (Jaeger 2001; see also Chapter 22). Discounting bodily knowing such as emotion has potentially deleterious effects on the well-being of nurses (Rodney 1997; Rodney and Starzomski 1993). Furthermore, as Jaeger argues, reducing moral decision-making and justification to reason or rational principles results in impoverished and inhumane morality.

Embodied Knowing

Sound ethical practice in nursing requires **embodied knowing.** As Gendlin (1992a) explains, your body is a site where many forms of "knowing" come together, are present simultaneously, and are weighed and interrelated as possible next moves. This understanding of how knowledge comes together in the body has highlighted the significance of embodied moral agency. Through our bodies, we have an implicit sense of a situation and the intricacy of it. The body not only acts as an orienting centre of perception and knowledge, but also orients our action. If we pay attention, we can physically sense our bodies' implication of the situation and the next steps we should take (Gendlin 1992a). A simple example is how our body implies hunger and urges us to eat. Similarly, in nursing, feeling "heavy in the heart" while going through the workday implies a re-looking at the "heart" of the matter (e.g., what is and what is not being placed at the centre of the ethical decision-making process or what needs to happen to ensure that the emotional/psychological well-being of a patient is being fully attended to and so forth).

Although we may not tune into or be aware of it, this implicit, intricate body-sense functions in every situation, and, according to Gendlin (1992b), we would be quite lost without it. Gendlin (1992a) offers the example of walking home at night:

You sense a group of men following you. You don't merely *perceive* them. You don't merely hear them there, in the space back of you. Your body-sense instantly includes also your hope that perhaps they aren't following you, also your alarm, and many past experiences—too many to separate out, and surely also the need to do something—walk faster, change your course, escape into a house, get ready to fight, run, shout (346).

In this way, our bodies are the site of ethical knowledge and decision-making, as well as the medium for knowledge development and ethical action. Body-sense includes more than we are consciously aware of and more than it would be possible to list (Gendlin 1992a). Gendlin contends that body-sense is not merely perception or feeling, but involves an intricate interaction of conscious and unconscious "knowing" that offers more than you can see, feel, or think. As such, embodied knowing offers a rich resource and foundation for ethical nursing practice.

The following story exemplifies the importance of embodied knowing. Hilary, a nurse of more than 20 years, came to talk with me one day about a family she was working with and the distress she was feeling with regard to what she "should" be doing in her work with the family. Hilary began her story by describing her long bike rides home each day, during which she sorted through her experience with the family, including her feelings and thoughts and the responses of others in the situation. It became evident to me as I listened to her descriptions that Hilary was in the process of evolving a new framework of ethical knowing and decision-making. Her bike rides home offered an opportunity for her to tune into her embodied knowing to inform her ethical decision-making and action. Ethics in Practice 21-1 provides verbatim pieces of my conversation with Hilary. (Minor changes have been made to the information Hilary provided about the family in order to ensure the confidentiality of both Hilary and the family she describes.)

Ethics in Practice 21-1	**One Nurse's Story**[1]

I'm working with a very high-risk family at the moment. Sarah, the mother who has just had her second baby... came to our program a year ago with her three-year-old son Aaron, and [was] pregnant at the time. Social services have had a long-standing involvement with the family. At the time she came to our program Aaron was still nursing and still in a very loving relationship with a supportive mother who couldn't always deal with her other relationships, so she was having trouble setting boundaries with her partner and violence erupted still. So when I met them I met her two or three times, then there was a violent episode, several family members were involved, the police were there and Aaron was taken off and he was acting up horribly and using horrible language, and obviously he had observed a lot of other things. So this family to me felt very high-risk and in crisis. So I did regular visits and we got to know each other over the next six months. Sarah's partner was not actually living with her and the children because of the violence, and I knew the Ministry was heavily involved, so in a way that took some of the pressure off—I didn't feel I needed to report everything I heard. But there were junctures where I worried for her because she was so upset. I worried for the three-year-old and I worried, "Was she really able to protect the new baby?" But I felt she was a very caring mother and I just decided to be there for her. But then the problem is this little voice says, "Well what is your responsibility here, can she protect this baby, should I be calling the ministry about this particular incident. Is this something I need to report?" And the baby is Down's syndrome. So there are lots of issues here. And there are pressures in the agency where I work. They are nervously applying rules to some situations and I find it really hard to be put in the role and have the expectation of always reporting on the families.

And yet being with her, you have a caring mother who with the right support actually could bring her family together.... [W]hen it came down to the wire, I was being asked to forfeit the relationship with my client in order to have my professional stance. What that enlightened in me was I just thought NO! The nursing relationship is a healthy relationship. [I]t is everything I know about myself as a nurse and my experience as a nurse that allows me to make the decisions and to have the relationship with the patient.... [A]nd it was just that melding of being a person to this client and being a nurse to this client, so it all came together. So I realized I could do both and it wasn't separate.

Hilary's narrative highlights how her embodied knowing supported her navigation through three fundamental tensions: nursing concerns and family needs, reason/rational and emotion/bodily sensing, and stance of certainty and stance of contingency. These tensions led Hilary to deep reflection about what it was that was guiding her work and how she ought to respond to the family and to the expectations of her agency. Hilary felt duty-bound, to both the family and her agency, to ensure the children were safe. Rationally, it seemed to make sense to consider removing the children from the home. Yet, through her experience with the family she *felt* that this was a loving mother with the capacity to care for her children. She found herself vacillating between following her rational duty to control risk and following the authority of her deeper embodied knowing, which told her that what was most needed by this family was relational connection and support.

Hilary also felt a strong tension between the habit of being certain and her growing conviction that the truth and "the right thing to do" were contingent. Given the volatile situation and the potential risk to the children, the habit of certainty and the need to act pressed in upon her. The objective risk-assessment score indicated that this was a very high-risk situation. Yet, she felt compelled to authentically support the mother—to be there for her.

This process of reflection became a deeply personal experience, bringing Hilary's feelings and values to the forefront and raising questions about subsequent action. The reflective process initially left her feeling confused and ambivalent. As Dewey (1922) explains, when routine habits (e.g., the habit of following an objective truth) are interfered with, uneasiness is generated and a protest set up. This protest may be both internally and externally experienced. Similar to Hart's (1995) analogy of the person who has just dismantled the family clock, Hilary found she could take it (the situation) apart but was unsure what to do when the parts were on the table in front of her. She was compelled by the different habits and desires that pulled her in conflicting directions.

Within Hilary's story, one can see "the artist" Dewey (1922) speaks of at work. As an artist of ethical nursing, Hilary tunes into her bodily experience—to her embodied knowing—and is able to weave thought, feeling, and action together to re-create her ethical practice. She *thoughtfully* reflects on her experience and the important aspects within it (e.g., family needs, agency regulations), sorts through her *emotions and bodily sense*, and through this process comes to "know" how to *respond*. Her embodied knowing *implies action*. In addition, by attending to her bodily experience and knowing, she was able to re-create herself and her practice as an ethical nurse. Hilary's artistry is evident in the way she lived and navigated her way through the tensions, recognized the power that each force wielded, and thoughtfully considered how to respond. She blended the expertise of her embodied knowledge with action that was thoughtfully felt to be "right" in particular moments. As Hilary spoke with me about her experience, she explained how this navigation process was not a straight-forward matter—how it was wrought with personal struggle.

Hilary's story depicts the deep challenges that lie within ethical nursing practice—the contradictions, fears, joys, and angst, the conflicting emotions that accompany irrevocable decisions, and the imposed pressures to ensure that one is "doing the right thing" when the only thing that can be guaranteed is the uncertainty of any situation (Flanagan 1996; see also Chapter 22). Her story highlights how opening up to embodied knowing allowed her to examine the habits of conduct and the taken-for-granted behaviours of her practice and enabled her to achieve a greater degree of clarity and power in relation to them. What stood out most for me as I listened to Hilary's story was the courage she lived in light of her vulnerability. Stepping out from behind the protective screen of rationalism and certainty, she courageously re-formed her ethical knowledge and practice in the moment to be as ethically responsive as possible to the concerns of everyone in the situation.

Developing the "Habit" of Embodied Knowing

Jaeger (2001) contends that revised epistemologies that re-introduce bodiliness are essential in developing a communicative, responsive ethics:

> To be in a situation with others involves not just ideas, values and principles, but also movements, touch, sound, and other minute, but perceivable physiological behaviours, including the paling or flushing of skin as well as changes in body temperature, muscular tensity and subtle facial expressions. Perception is not reducible to a cognitively driven function. Meaningful interactions with others are constituted in fully embodied ways (138).

Therefore, ethical nursing practice requires an intense vigilance and conscious engagement through which one reaches out and opens to the flux of human experience. As a deeply embodied process, ethical nursing practice involves a mindful, critical awareness and attunement to bodily experience that includes a questioning of what is contributing to and/or giving rise to that experience. This attunement provides a living and continuous access to ethical knowledge.

Gendlin (1992c) contends that to develop such awareness requires learning to "let it come"—to focus on and open up to our embodied knowing in the moment. This development of bodily sense begins with our everyday experience—in that place where one is feeling unease. It is important to clarify that bodily sense is more than emotion and feelings. Bodily sense is wider and at first may be unclear and murky. Although a feeling such as anger is felt bodily, as Gendlin (1992c) describes, if one waits a few moments one often finds that the anger is part of something wider—a larger felt sense. At the same time, bodily sense is less clear. One might experience a slight unease, a tightness, or a jumpy feeling (Gendlin 1992a).

In feeling this bodily sense, the nurses in the study previously cited often recounted that if they did become aware of this bodily sense they tended to rationalize it away by saying to themselves "it's just me" or "my personal feelings aren't relevant." They exemplified Gendlin's description of the learned tendency to disavow or ignore bodily sense. This ignoring was a dominant theme amongst the nurses in the study. However, as evidenced in Hilary's story, enlisting bodily sense not only offers insight into the salient aspects of an ethical situation, but can also provide a sense of strength and conviction from which to act. Developing the "habit" of listening and responding to bodily experiences such as the inner dissonance or confusion created by moral tensions is perhaps a beginning way for nurses to cultivate more fully informed, responsive, and empowered ethical practice. Examples of practical ways in which nurses can develop the habit of enlisting bodily sense are (1) tuning into to their bodily sensations at coffee or lunch breaks or when they stop to chart on a patient (e.g., are their shoulders tight, and, if so, what is the tension they are carrying?), or (2) asking questions related to themselves off and on throughout the day. For example, in addition to asking themselves "What should I *do* next?" as they go about their day, they consciously ask themselves "How am I feeling about how I am practising today? What is going on around me that is shaping these feelings?" And so forth.

Honouring Our Embodied Knowledge

As a nurse researcher and educator who has listened to countless stories of nurses' ethical practice and witnessed the moral distress that occurs when nurses divorce reason from emotion, I have come to believe that as a profession we have a moral imperative to foster embodied knowing. Recognizing and supporting the development of embodied knowing is not only vital to advancing ethical practice in nursing, it is essential to promoting the well-being of nurses. Although ethical theory and professional codes of conduct can support nurses' decision-making and action, we need to move beyond the habit of thinking of ethics as something we *follow* to seeing it as something we *are*. Until ethical knowledge is part of our "every muscle and sinew" (Burkitt 1994, 23) we will continue to live out habits of conduct that constrain our moral agency as nurses.

As Jaeger (2001) reminds us, the development of embodied knowing and moral sensitivity can either be cultivated or undermined. This means that the development of embodied knowing is a sociopolitical issue as much as a philosophical, conceptual, or academic one (Jaeger 2001). In closing, therefore, I extend an invitation not only to individual nurses but to the profession as a whole—an invitation to listen to the valuable knowledge living in our bodies, to pay attention to the embodied patterns we are living in our everyday practice, and, most importantly, to honour our embodied knowing of what is ethical.

FOR REFLECTION

1. Reflect upon an ethically challenging situation that arose in your professional practice and how you chose to respond.

   • What ethical knowledge did you access to inform your decision-making and action?

   • How did you enlist and/or discount your embodied knowing?

   • What habits of conduct constrained your embodied knowing and practice in that situation?

   • How did you identify yourself as a moral agent in that situation? For example, what was the narrative you constructed, and how are you depicted in that narrative?

   • What contextual forces shaped the situation, your action, and your experience?

2. How might you begin to develop a mindful, critical awareness and an attunement to bodily experience?

3. Who is a "moral exemplar" for you, and what is it about this person that invites your respect? How would this person be described (identified) narratively?

ENDNOTE

1. Hilary's experience has also been referred to in a previous discussion of ethics education in nursing. See Hartrick Doane, G. 2002. In the spirit of creativity: The learning and teaching of ethics in nursing. *Journal of Advanced Nursing, 39*(6), 521–528.

REFERENCES

Bauman, Z. 1993. *Postmodern ethics.* Oxford: Blackwell.

Benner, P. 1991. The role of experience, narrative, and community in skilled ethical comportment. *Advances in Nursing Science, 14*(2), 1–21.

Bergum, V. 1994. Knowledge for ethical care. *Nursing Ethics: An International Journal for Health Care Professionals, 1*(2), 72–79.

Bishop, A.H. and Scudder, J.R. 1990. *The practical, moral and personal sense of nursing: A phenomenological philosophy of practice.* Albany: State University of New York Press.

Burkitt, I. 1994. The shifting concept of the self. *History of the Human Sciences, 7*(2), 7–28.

Colby, A. and Damon, W. 1992. *Some do care: Contemporary lives of moral commitment.* New York: Free Press.

Damon, W. 1999. The moral development of children. *Scientific American, 28*(2), 72–79.

Damon, W. and Gregory, A. 1997. The youth charter: Towards the formation of adolescent moral identity. *Journal of Moral Education, 26*(2), 117–131.

Dewey, J. 1891/1957. *Outlines of a critical theory of ethics.* New York: Greenwood Press/Hilary House.

Dewey, J. 1922. *Human nature and conduct.* New York: Henry Holt.

Dewey, J. 1929. *The quest for certainty: A study of the relation of knowledge and action.* New York: Minton, Balch.

Donaldson, M. 1991. *Human minds: An exploration.* London: Penguin.

Elias, N.J. 1978. *The history of manners: The civilizing process.* Volume 1. Oxford: Blackwell.

Elias, N.J. 1982. *State formation and civilization: The civilizing process*. Volume 2. Oxford: Blackwell.

Elliott, C. 1999. *Bioethics, culture and identity. A philosophical disease*. New York: Routledge.

Flanagan, O. 1996. *Self expressions. Mind, morals and the meaning of life*. New York: Oxford University Press.

Fry, S. 1989. Toward a theory of nursing ethics. *Advances in Nursing Science, 11*(4), 9–22.

Gadow, S. 1990. Existential advocacy. In T. Pence and J. Cantral (Eds.), *Ethics in nursing: An anthology* (pp. 41–51). New York: National League for Nursing.

Gendlin, E.T. 1992a. The primacy of the body, not the primacy of perception. *Man and World, 25*(3-4), 341–353.

Gendlin, E.T. 1992b. Thinking beyond patterns: Body, language, and situations. In B. den Ouden and M. Moen (Eds.), *The presence of feeling in thought* (pp. 21–151). New York: Peter Lang.

Gendlin, E.T. 1992c. The wider role of bodily sense in thought and language. In M. Sheets-Johnstone (Ed.), *Giving the body its due* (pp. 192–207). Albany, NY: State University of New York Press.

Hart, T. 1998. Inspiration: Exploring the experience and its meaning. *Journal of Humanistic Psychology, 38*(3), 7–29.

Hartrick Doane, G. 2002. Am I still ethical? The socially mediated process of nurses' moral identity. *Nursing Ethics, 9*(6), 623–635.

Jaeger, S. 2001. Teaching health care ethics: The importance of moral sensitivity for moral reasoning. *Nursing Philosophy, 2*, 131–142.

Lansing, R.G. 1908. *The psychology of inspiration. An attempt to distinguish religious from scientific truth*. New York: Funk & Wagnall.

Liaschenko, J. 1993. Can justice coexist with the supremacy of personal values in nursing practice? *Western Journal of Nursing Research, 21*(1), 35–50.

McNamee, S. 1996. Therapy and identity construction in a postmodern world. In D. Grodin and T. Lindloff (Eds.), *Constructing the self in a mediated world* (pp. 141–155). Thousand Oaks, CA: Sage.

Niebuhr, H. R. 1963. *The responsible self*. New York: Harper & Row.

Nussbaum, M. 2001. *Upheavals of thought*. New York: Cambridge University Press.

Pauly, B. 2001. *Weaving a tapestry of nursing ethics: Philosophical grounding and future directions*. Unpublished manuscript. University of Victoria.

Rodney, P.A. 1997. *Towards connectedness and trust: Nurses' enactment of their moral agency within an organizational context*. Unpublished doctoral dissertation. University of British Columbia, Vancouver.

Rodney, P. and Starzomski, R. 1993. Constraints on the moral agency of nurses. *Canadian Nurse, 89*(9), 23–26.

Sherwin, S. 1998. A relational approach to autonomy in health care. In S. Sherwin (Co-ordinator), *The politics of women's health: Exploring agency and autonomy* (pp. 19–47). Philadelphia: Temple University Press.

Schrag, C.O. 1997. *The self after postmodernity*. New Haven: Yale University Press.

Thompson, E. 2001. Empathy and consciousness. In E. Thompson (Ed.), *Between ourselves. Second-person issues in the study of consciousness* (pp. 1–32). Charlottesville, VA: Imprint Academic.

Vetlesen, J. 1994. *Perception, empathy and judgment: An inquiry into the preconditions of moral performance*. University Park, PA: Pennsylvania State University Press.

Walker, L.J. 1999. The perceived personality of moral exemplars. *Journal of Moral Education, 28*(2), 145–163.

Watson, J. 1988. *Nursing: Human science and human care.* New York: National League for Nursing.

Wilshire, B. 1982. *Role playing and identity: The limits of theatre as metaphor*. Bloomington: Indiana University Press.

Williams, B. 1985. *Ethics and the limits of philosophy*. London: Fontana Books.

Woods, M. 1999. A nursing ethic: The moral voice of experienced nurses. *Nursing Ethics, 6*(5), 423–433.

Yeo, M. 1989. Integration of nursing theory and nursing ethics. *Advances in Nursing Science, 11*(3), 33–42.

chapter twenty-two

Emotions and Ethics

Per Nortvedt

Emotions play a role in moral sensitivity both because emotions contribute to the understanding of a situation's human significance... and also because emotional understanding motivates genuine personal human involvement in another person's situation.

It is essential to good nursing that patients are treated with **care** and **carefulness**[1] and that human needs are properly attended to. In this chapter, I will elucidate how emotions overall are central to moral reasoning and moral behaviour in nursing. I will show how moral sensitivity is highly essential to moral judgment and action in nursing and how this faculty in an important way is based on emotion. Further, I will elucidate how emotions play a significant role in moral judgments. Overall, it is my goal to show how emotions shape attitudes of care and human concern—attitudes that are extremely important in clinical nursing.

Let me start, however, with some words about what I will not argue. I do not wish to argue that emotion can take the important place that reason has in moral judgments and in motivating moral behaviour. Also, I will not address all aspects of emotion and ethics, but will concentrate on the positive contribution that emotions make to moral behaviour in nursing. I am well aware of the existence of negative emotions such as envy, partiality, insecurity, fear, and general emotional turmoil that impose important challenges for nurses. I will mention some of these challenges, but a more extensive discussion of these matters is beyond the scope of this chapter. I will mainly be focusing on what Lawrence Blum calls **altruistic emotions** (Blum 1980; 1994). Altruistic emotions such as compassion, sympathy, and concern are, in an important sense, moral emotions. These are emotions whose object is another person's good for his or her own sake and not for the good of others (Blum 1980).

First, I will have something to say about moral sensitivity in general. Then I will give an introduction to the general philosophical arguments and debates about the role of emotions in ethics generally, with allusions to nursing care specifically. This means that I will address both how theories of emotions have influenced ethical theory and systematical ethical thinking (**ethics**) and also how emotions are taken up by philosophers (and some psychologists) to play a part in our acting for the good of others in general (**morality**). This includes an elaboration on two important components of emotion: its cognitive and affective dimensions as well as the importance of these aspects of emotion to clinical nursing. I will, on the whole, integrate the general philosophical discussions with examples and intuitions central to clinical nursing. Second, I will provide a discussion of the role emotion plays in moral deliberations with regard to nursing practice. Third, I will illuminate the important role that emotions have in motivating good care and shaping attitudes of care and concern for the best of the patient. Finally, I will present some conclusions and a summary of the main points.

THE ROLE OF MORAL SENSITIVITY IN MORAL PERFORMANCE

To discuss the role of emotion in ethics generally and in nursing specifically necessitates some words on the role of moral sensitivity as a basis for moral judgment and action. This is partly because the role of moral sensitivity has been overlooked in many modern moral theories. It is also because if one takes moral sensitivity to be important for moral judgments, emotions play an essential part in this sensitivity.

In modern moral philosophy it is commonly or normally accepted that a conception of ethics, which mainly gives attention to reasoning and justification of actions, misses important aspects of morality in general (Blum 1994; Vetlesen 1994). Acting morally means to act for the right reasons and with the proper attitude guiding one's personal conduct. However, it is significant to note that acting morally presupposes **moral sensitivity**—that is, that the morally relevant features of the situation are properly recognized. In short, moral excellence is based on perceiving the salient features of the situation so that moral judgments can be sufficiently reliable and so that the action itself can display proper respect for the patient's dignity. Vetlesen (1994) calls this way of perceiving, judging, and acting with moral attitude the "moral performance." The notion of **moral performance** captures the fact that acting morally in a profound way bears on moral sensitivity, both in seeing and perceiving as well as in *how* one cares for the other person. This holistic approach of regarding the whole sequence of moral sensitivity, judgment, and action as essential dates back to Aristotle. In his *Nichomachean Ethics* (350 BCE/1985), Aristotle states that virtue is virtue of character. What is noteworthy is that he states that character is concerned with rational deliberation, feelings, and actions. About feelings, he famously states,

> But (having these feelings) at the right times, about the right things, towards the right people, for the right end, and in the right way, is the intermediate and best condition, and this is proper to virtue (44).

Yet what, more specifically, is moral sensitivity? One definition of moral sensitivity might be as follows: *Moral sensitivity is a capacity to be addressed by the morally significant aspects of a particular situation.* The words "to be addressed by" are important here. "To be addressed by," means, for instance, to be affected emotionally by the fact that a person is suffering. It means to be emotionally engaged and involved in another person's human condition.

Many people tend to think that arguing for the role of moral sensitivity only means to focus on the role of emotions. This is incorrect. We must have a diverse picture of what is involved in seeing a situation morally. Understanding the nature and importance of this capacity is very important. Moral sensitivity also involves a cognitive aspect of understanding a situation morally. For instance, in many cases what makes a nurse aware of certain aspects of value depends on his or her ability to judge a situation on the basis of his or her theoretical knowledge. What he or she takes as morally important in a situation also bears upon knowledge about moral theories and principles and how such knowledge is integrated into his or her total moral makeup. If we are conscious that autonomy and self-determination are significant moral rights, we tend to be aware of cases when these rights are jeopardized. If we are attentive to principles of justice, it is more likely that we are capable of distinguishing between various dilemmas of prioritizing in nursing and treating patients with respect for their common humanity.

Moral sensitivity therefore has a theoretical and cognitive foundation. Importantly, this affects how we ought to use our moral imagination in clinical understanding. Having learned that it is important to be attentive to the patient's human needs, a nurse might be more able to be sensitive to pain and suffering and to understand the situation of other persons. Nightingale's (1860) view of good nursing bears on this kind of moral sensitivity when she asks questions like the following:

> How is it for the patient to stay in bed the whole day, and never be able to look out the window? How is it for him to be awakened when he has just fallen asleep? How is it for the sick person when the doctor and the nurse at the round whisper over his head and he knows that they talk about him?

Rather laconically, Nightingale remarks here that such a strain might make the patient even more sick for a long period afterwards. For Nightingale, cognitive imagination of a patient's illness and suffering is central to nursing.

What we now see is that moral sensitivity—understood as an awareness of moral principles and an understanding of a patient's actual situation—is central to clinical nursing care. The ability of reflection plays a role in transcending a person's particular self-interest and makes him or her engage properly in another person's situation. Similarly, to be conscious about moral principles and simultaneously about the values that guide these principles is paradigmatically essential to perceiving what is morally important.

Further, clinical and moral experiences play a role in cultivating moral sensitivity. Experiences of cases when patients' rights to autonomy are not properly attended to often elevate our sense of responsibility in future situations in which we can see that a patient's right to self-determination and informed consent is threatened. For instance, if a nurse witnesses and reflects on the inappropriate restraint of a confused elderly patient, he or she would intervene in that situation and be more prepared to intervene more quickly for other patients. He or she would also be more prepared to engage in policy work and education about the use of restraints. To summarize, knowledge about and internalization of moral principles and the theories on which they are based serve as an important foundation for moral sensitivity. Moral experience and knowledge about moral principles focus and situate moral awareness and make us conscious of the importance of understanding a patient's experiences of illness.

Still, to portray this role of the intellect in moral sensitivity and judgment is only one part of the picture here. Aristotle (350 BCE/1987) was right when he claimed that moral perceptions as well as moral reasoning do not rely solely on cognition, but also on emotion. Canadian philosopher Charles Taylor cultivates this Aristotelian insight when he argues that without the proper emotional attunement, **moral perception** will not capture the human import of the situation, which is the true personal significance of human experiences (Taylor 1985).[2] Taylor states, "By 'import' I mean a way in which something can be relevant or of importance to the desires or purposes or aspirations or feelings of a subject; or otherwise put, a property of something whereby it is a matter of non-indifference to a subject" (Taylor 1985, 48).

This means that emotions are important for nurses in order for them to understand what pain and pleasure mean to the patient—the understanding is not a product of intellectual labour but is, instead, a reflection of nurses' own sentiments. In clinical situations, emotions are central for nurses to be properly aware of and understand a patient's experience of his or her illness. To feel compassion means to be touched by and to understand the human impact of a person's pain and suffering. It is not sufficient to know the right ethical theories and their principles. A principle does not tell us how a patient is suffering and what the human impact of this suffering is. Emotion is needed to recognize the true human significance of a person's pain and suffering.

Emotions play a role in moral sensitivity both because emotions contribute to the understanding of a situation's human significance (what the experience means to the individual) and also because emotional understanding motivates genuine personal human involvement in another person's situation. This kind of emotional involvement and understanding is apparent in many clinical situations in nursing—for instance, when a nurse's carefulness is mobilized in attending to an aching body, in dressing an infectious wound, or in comforting a mourning relative. All these situations call for care that is sensitive to the import of human experiences and for an ability to understand another person's feelings.

Hence, while knowledge, thinking, reflection, and cognitive imagination are important, they are not sufficient. *In order to reason about difficult moral cases, and also to perceive what is morally at stake in situations of caring for others, emotion is needed to engage nurses personally.* Emotion is also essential to fully understand what the experience of illness means to the patient. Thus, this chapter will further investigate the philosophical basis for claiming that emotions play an important role in moral sensitivity and for claiming that emotions are significant for proper moral reasoning and motivation. My arguments here will be based on examples from clinical nursing and historical texts in nursing which emphasize the role of emotion in moral and clinical understanding. I will begin with some words on Immanuel Kant and his influential views on the role of emotion in moral behaviour.

Kant's Position on Emotion and Moral Virtue

When Kant, in *Groundwork for the Metaphysics of Morals* (1964), downplays the role that emotion can have in morality, it is to a large extent because he means that reason alone can serve as a reliable instrument for judging the moral rightness or wrongness of a person's actions.[3] Also, he claims that a pure and reliable moral motive is available only when we are guided by reason alone. American philosopher Korsgaard formulates this Kantian insight as follows:

> It is not because we notice normative entities in the course of our experience, but because we are normative animals who can question our experience, that normative concepts exists (Korsgaard 1996, 47).

According to Kant, only reason endows the ability for reflection and offers the capacity to evaluate actions and attitudes from a moral perspective. Only reason can serve as a motive that, through reflection, guarantees an internal connection to the rightness of an action. This means that *only* reflection can guarantee that our moral judgment is right and hence that our moral conduct is right. Only reason protects an action from being based mainly on a person's subjective inclinations and preferences.

The reason Kant argues along these lines is partly because of his theories of moral psychology and his view on the role of moral experiences in moral judgment. Even though Kant modifies his views on emotions in his later works (*The Doctrine of Virtue* and *The Metaphysics of Morals)*, he grants the emotions merely a supporting—that is, a conditional—moral value. Emotions support human actions with properly tuned sensitivity and they motivate sympathetic understanding, but, according to Kant, only the insight and motivation offered by reason alone has unconditional moral worth.

Recently, in moral philosophy many scholars have argued that Kant overlooks the role that emotion can have in moral judgment and, moreover, that he ignores how emotions can in fact serve as reliable moral motives. Kant also (it is argued) gives too little room for the role of moral perception and how moral understanding is constituted not by reason alone, but also by emotion (Blum 1994; Nortvedt 1996; Oakly 1992; Vetlesen 1994). Importantly, the basic philosophical and psychological premise for granting emotions a more substantial role in moral perception and reasoning is the claim that emotions have not merely an affective part but also an important cognitive dimension. Hence, it follows that emotions are not merely self-centred passions in opposition to reason. Much emphasis in recent philosophical work on emotions has been invested in substantiating the cognitive role of emotions. It has been important to show how emotions play a significant and reliable role in moral reasoning and action (Bowden 1997; De Sousa 1987; Little 1995; Solomon 1983).

Emotions are significant for moral sensitivity, judgment, and action for three essential reasons. The use of the concept "emotion" may vary here. Many take this term to cover the different components of emotions. As Oakly (1992) and others (e.g., Ben-Ze'ev 2001; Blum 1980; Nussbaum 2001) argue, emotions are feelings or affects as well as cognitions and desires. First, morally speaking, one can argue that emotions involve cognition and contribute to moral understanding. Second, emotions are spontaneous affective responses which may be morally important as an ability to be affected by another person's distress. Third, emotions also function as desires or motives in promoting another person's good. In the following, I will show that emotion (both as a certain type of cognition but also as a pure sensory and affective impulse) plays a significant role in moral sensitivity in nursing.

In the last part of the chapter, I will discuss the role of emotions as moral motives, and I will discuss to what extent moral judgments can be based on emotion.

Emotions: The Cognitive Dimension

Let us first look at the cognitive component of emotion. Emotions are judgments about value, about what is dear to us, and about what has human import (Nussbaum 2001; Taylor 1985). Hence, while emotions refer to external states of affairs, they are judgments about states of affairs as *we see them,* and hence are subjective judgments (Solomon 1983). When Solomon says that emotions are subjective judgments, he means to underline the very personal nature of emotional judgments—how they are closely attached to our own state of mind and our relationships and attachments. This is not comparable to judging whether a car is blue or green. "Subjective" here combines a story (an assertion) about the actual event and the character of my judgment, of what the event means to *me.* When we feel shame, for instance, this says something about the situation. There is something in the situation that evokes shame. The feeling of shame also says something about our reaction to the situation (that we evaluate it as shameful). An emotion says something about the object in the situation through our reaction to what happens. It reveals "a property of non-indifference to the subject" (Taylor 1985, 48).

There is a general agreement both in philosophy (De Sousa 1987; Solomon 1983; Vetlesen 1994) and psychology (Lazarus 1992) that emotions as subjective and evaluative judgments play an essential part in moral agency. In her book on emotions, Nussbaum (2001) describes the way in which emotions can be defended as judgments about value. According to Nussbaum, emotions have an intentional object that is interpreted by the person who has the emotion (27.) Second, complex beliefs, evaluations, and affective attitudes concerning the object shape these intentions: "As in love, grief, or anger, emotions are concerned with value; they see their object as invested with value or importance" (30). Nussbaum further argues that emotions form a complex set of beliefs about an object. For instance, to feel compassion for a person who is in pain involves seeing the kind of serious effects that the pain has for the individual. It entails a judgment concerning the degree of suffering caused by the pain that is occasioned by the "awareness of another person's undeserved misfortune" (301). At the same time, **compassion** is itself a *pained* awareness of another person's situation. It is a painful emotion, an emotion that affectively reflects the painful experience of the other person. Compassion, then, involves judgments about the situational content and the degree of significance that the pain has to the person in the situation. Compassion is itself an emotion that reflects the ordeal and painfulness of human suffering (see also Chapter 21).

Interestingly, a way of emotionally apprehending another person's situation is evident also in historical texts of nursing ethics. For instance, Norwegian deaconesses, as well as the St. Joseph sisters in the Catholic tradition, emphasize the importance of understanding the patient's experience of his or her illness. A textbook on nursing ethics from the St. Joseph sisters in Norway, originating from the beginning of the last century says, for example,

> What is judiciousness? Judiciousness is the capability to enter into and understand the conditions of our fellow humans, their uniqueness and emotional world, and then immediately behave as love for one's next [the other] in the actual situation demands. Judiciousness acts through

people who dispose the art of reading the souls of others and with a certain consideration are able to explore their moods, secret wishes, their vulnerable and hardly overgrown places (Fischer 1902, 31).

Similarly, Norwegian deaconess Elisabeth Hagemann tells the student in pre-war Norway that

> To be a good nurse requires more than technical proficiency, namely an inner understanding of what is essential for the sick. And that is something which cannot be learned in a year or two, but a goal to reach, a goal to be achieved by the help of every sick person that is assigned to our responsibility (Hagemann 1930, 43).

These texts do not explicitly link empathic understanding to emotional capacities. However, it is likely that *to read the inner states of another person* is by no means a detached cognitive representation of a person's situation, deprived of any affective engagement in a person's state of affairs. It is, rather, likely that the kind of empathic understanding that traditional nursing envisioned (and envisions) includes a distinct emotional component.

To summarize, emotional judgments are judgments that reflect the significance of situations to the person having the emotion. Emotions tell something about the human significance of a person's pain and something about our own involvement—that is, that his or her pain is of concern to us. Compassion is a subjective judgment about another person's situation, his or her state of affairs, that reveals something essential about his or her human experience. Hence, emotions have an intentional object; they are a way of understanding the significance of a particular situation. They are not the only way of moral understanding, as I have argued earlier and as has been shown in other chapters of this book. But they are a combined way of understanding the human magnitude of experiences of illness and suffering with personal engagement and human involvement in a way that theory- and principle-based knowledge of ethics cannot do. This fact of personal involvement in emotional understanding makes it natural to turn to another essential part of emotional judgments—namely, the affective component of emotions.

Before elaborating on the affective component of emotions (in the next section), I would like to restate that emotional judgments are not neutral, as one's own emotional engagement reflects the significance of the situation. Emotions are "affective modes of awareness of situations," says Taylor (1985, 48), who further argues that "Experiencing a given emotion involves experiencing our situation as being of a certain kind or having a certain property. But this property cannot be neutral, cannot be something to which we are indifferent, or else we would not be moved" (48).

Thus far I have argued that philosophers now generally seem to agree that emotions are ways of apprehending important aspects of human situations and, in particular, those situations that have moral importance. What is more controversial is the role of emotions as feeling—in other words, the role of emotional affect in moral sensitivity and judgment. Emotions do not merely represent situations of human suffering by way of immediate cognitive interpretation. Emotions are affects as well: the immediate bodily distress and worry that strike us when seeing another person in pain. Imagine that you move a patient in bed and she suddenly cries out in pain. Her pain strikes you physically and mentally as your pained awareness of her situation. It is "like a nail in your stomach" (Nussbaum 2001, 49). This is what the feeling component of emotion is about. And this kind of pain immediately felt upon another person's suffering, I will argue, has moral importance, which is over-looked in many mainstream philosophical theories of emotions.

Emotions: The Affective Dimension

Ethics in Practice 22-1 provides a clinical example that illustrates the affective dimension of emotions.

Ethics in Practice 22-1	On the Ward This Evening

Suddenly on the ward this evening, the pleasant elderly lady you are caring for falls out of bed. Naturally you are immediately stricken with panic, you run to the bed, you try to get her up from the floor, and you call for help and check that she is all right. You are relieved when she talks and seems OK.

What has happened here? The incident of your patient falling mobilizes a gut reaction of fear. And this affective distress caused by apprehending the lady fall out of the bed awakens human concern for her in a motivationally most abrupt and strong sense. You see her fall, which gives you an immediate reason to rush to help her. Of course, this situation certainly involves multiple reflective acts as well. You evaluate her condition sponta-neously, taking account of all the experience and all the medical and nursing knowledge that you possess.

But reflection is still not first on the scene here. Your being moved by her fall is not a product of reflection, but a product of **sensibility.** By "sensibility" I mean the immediate, pre-reflective affective experience of being pained by another person's pain. This kind of pre-reflective sensibility is best outlined using German and French philosophical phenom-enology. According to German phenomenologist Husserl (1998), the actual experience, the original, actual event displays an original act of consciousness: "an original act, constitut-ing the object in a most original way" (26). Phenomenologists such as Husserl and the late French philosopher Levinas elucidate ethical and aesthetic impressions as affective intu-itions. These affective intuitions, in the passivity of sense-endowment, awaken the reflec-tive and theoretical attitude of consciousness (Nortvedt 2003).

This means that human consciousness is vulnerable in a very profound way. It is vul-nerable into the very core of its being when it is pained by another person's suffering. Levinas (1986; 1991) talks about this pre-reflective sensibility as a suffering for the per-son's suffering and as a passivity of consciousness—a passivity as a product not of reflec-tion but of sensibility (see also Nortvedt 2003).

This is morally significant because, when trying to answer the fundamental questions, "Why does the patient concern me?" and "Why am I relieved by the perception of her being all right, or why am I pained by her fall?", it is this very basic experience of her hurt that we have to turn our attention to. According to Nussbaum (2001), when we are stricken by a person's immediate and strong pain, the full recognition of a terrible event is the upheaval. As I cited earlier, Nussbaum tells us that "It is like putting a nail into your stomach" (45).

This pre-reflective and affective awareness is evident in many important instances of clinical nursing. For instance, when carefulness is motivated by tension in a patient's body, the carefulness is not at first a reflective act, but originates as a spontaneous response induced by the patient's bodily reaction. The arousal of feeling is a specific response, an affective movement that initiates the reflective act of consciousness. Reflective consciousness is awakened by sensibility (Nortvedt 2003).

Just imagine that you are going to turn a terminally ill patient in bed. You know you have to be cautious because he has metastases in his pelvis and bladder. But cautiousness also emerges from the contact you have with the patient's body, your feeling of the tensions, and you immediately respond to the patient's signs of pain. It is important to understand and be aware of this sensory/pre-reflective aspect of emotion. It is this affective dimension of emotion that provides an insight into the role that emotions play in moral responsibility. *This movement of being touched by another person's situation—the claim issued by the vulnerability of the other—awakens responsibility and heightens clinical sensitivity.*

Interestingly, recent thinkers on Levinas (e.g., Levine 1999; Scheffler-Manning 2001) find in the Levinasian idea of vulnerability for the other person a primordial ethical sense, which is located in a non-verbal language of bodily expressions. Indeed, Levine (1999) says that obligation first takes hold of us bodily—in the flesh. This obligation takes hold at a time—that is, at each and every moment (both synchronically and diachronically)—prior to thematizing consciousness, prior to reflective cognition, and therefore prior to the ego's construction of a worldly temporal order (Levine 1999, 279).

Norwegian philosopher Vetlesen (1994) takes this way of being emotionally receptive to another person's distress to be fundamental for moral responsibility and moral agency. He argues that if humans were not able to respond emotionally to another person's distress and hurt, moral agency would be deeply impaired. We do not care for other persons because some principles and moral theories tell us to. We care about others because we are relationally and emotionally attached to them. This does not mean that we care for all people or are attached to all. It does mean that the world and humanity concern us in a very profound way. We are emotionally involved.

In some theories about human empathy and its development in early childhood, this involvement is clearly illustrated. Hoffman (2000), an American psychologist and researcher on empathy for almost a generation, displays how essential afferent feedback responses created by mimicry substantiate the primordial empathic response in the first months of early childhood. The sensibility of the little child is finely attuned to the mother or father, and the child responds and reacts to the parents' expressed emotions. Early in childhood, we experience each other's feeling states, and we respond on the basis of our emotions. In **empathy**, which Hoffman defines as an affective response to the human condition of others and a cognitive way of understanding other people's experiences, this kinetic, sensory impulse is essential.

> The simple form of empathic distress is important, however, precisely because it shows that humans are built in such a way that they involuntarily and forcefully experience another's emotion—that their distress is often contingent not on their own but someone else's painful experience (5).

Theories of empathy illustrate this affective dimension of emotional sensitivity that is sensory, impulse based, and immediate. This impulse is what works when we feel the hurt of someone else as an aching in our own body. Researchers on empathy often describe this affective moral impulse as an **empathic distress response,** as the distress evoked by another person's distress. Moreover, they frequently underline the significance of this impulse in originating sympathy and natural moral duty (e.g., Hoffman 2000).

An investigation into this sensory and affective part of emotion elucidates a dimension of clinical and moral sensitivity that is immensely important in nursing care. For instance, what, really, is it to care for a patient in a careful way? Is it merely how you intentionally plan the care when you move the painful body? Is carefulness granted by the wisdom stemming from knowledge about pathological facts concerning the body and the person—for example, that she has pain, that her spine is badly affected by cancer? Yes, clinical sensitivity is such preparedness offered by knowledge. But to be careful in nursing the patient is more than this. Carefulness is also this immediate sensibility, hesitation, and passivity directly induced by the painful expressions of the patient: when she cries out in pain, when her body stiffens, when you are worried about the sweat on her forehead. Carefulness as an essential part of good care is also the non-intentional and spontaneous sympathy and concern expressed in bodily awareness.

The affective part of emotion (its component as a feeling, not only its cognitive component) is central to ethics in nursing. It is this feeling of concern for the other—because we are touched and moved by a person's situation—that contributes to shape the authenticity of care in interpersonal nursing. Emotion, including its way of affectively understanding the other person's situation, its way of "seeing and understanding with the heart" (as the Norwegian nurse philosopher Martinsen [1996] phrases it), plays an essential role in seeing and being aware of the moral significance of illness experiences and expressions of pain and suffering (to mention some phenomena central to nursing care).

In many ways, I have taken up the argument of British philosopher Hume (1984), who emphasizes how emotions generate sympathy for the other and motivate benevolent duty. I will soon elaborate on the role that emotions play in moral motivation. Suffice it to say here that emotions contribute significantly to moral performance, both in how they contribute to moral sensitivity and to our capability to be personally moved by the situation of the other, the patient. This does not mean, however, that emotions can explain all there is to moral judgments and that we from our pure sensitivity can tell what is morally right or wrong. *But emotions anchor us to essential, ethically relevant aspects of a situation so that our rational judgments can be fully informed.*

EMOTIONS AND MORAL JUDGMENTS

Now, let us look at the more direct role emotions can have in moral judgments. By moral judgment I mean reasoning about cases with conflicting interests of value. Reasoning about moral conflicts is closely attached to decision-making procedures that aim at determining the right action to take in particular cases. Sometimes such judgments are situational, with very little time for reasoning and discussion altogether. On other occasions, judgments might call for discussion and reflection among many members of a professional team. But the essential view here is that determining what is morally right and wrong in a situation most frequently is a cognitive and primary intellectual process of critically evaluating situational constraints, including all the information provided to us by our emotional sensitivities. Many theorists, Kant included, would grant emotions a role in moral sensitivity, but would argue that emotions can have no say in our judging about right and wrong. This view is nicely expressed by Vetlesen (1994):

> Emotions, as I have noted earlier, anchor us to the *particular* moral circumstance, to the singularity, *here and now,* that addresses us immediately. Yet emotions do not tell us, of themselves, as it were, what is morally right. But they provide us with the perceptual material we need to engage in order to judge what is morally right. Judgment does not let emotions have the final say in settling matters of right and wrong (339).

Therefore, emotions cannot provide us with the personal distance and critical rationality that are necessary for moral evaluation in many difficult cases in nursing care. Often this seems obviously true. For example, as a nurse you might feel deep compassion for a patient, but you still have to send him to another ward or give priority to the needs of other patients. To give an extreme example, old German nurses bluntly describe how, during pre-war times in Nazi Germany, they killed hundreds of children but showed them great care and compassion before the execution (Steppe 1993). Overall, this tells us that if ethics is not anchored in some basic principles and arguments that state the moral value of persons as ends in themselves, then much can go terribly wrong.

This also tells us that emotions most often need the support of reason to guarantee the moral rightness of an action. And it tells us that while reason can provide us with the critical distance that is important for reflection, a vital function emotions can have is to support reason with the information necessary for judgment. But is this all there is to be said about the role of emotion in moral judgments? I think not, because the role that emotions play in moral judgments also depends on what kind of moral situations we have to deal with as nurses. Many cases in nursing are situations of moral ambiguity in which it is very difficult to see what is the right thing to do and in which judgment relies on professional experience and personal sensitivity. In some situations, various alternatives might seem to be equally right, and it is then the emotional and careful attitude displayed by the nurse that leads to proper moral action. Also, in cases in which ethical situations are unstable and it is difficult to decide what to do, a nurse's emotional attitudes (not only his or her reason) in clinical actions might have a decisive role in making a morally right action.

Ethics in Practice 22-2 presents a situation that demonstrates how the ambiguity and anxiety of a stroke patient confronted with demands of physical activity are captured by a nurse's heightened sensitivity. It demonstrates how a nurse's moral conflict concerning the patient's right to autonomy versus the nurse's concern for the patient's well-being is very dependent upon the nurse's emotional sensitivities.

Ethics in Practice 22-2	A Student Nurse

A student nurse was set to care for a 50-year-old man who was hemiplegic due to a severe cerebral hemorrhage. The patient also suffered from severe aphasia and had difficulty with even differentiating between simple answers of "yes" and "no." Due to his paralysis (he had spastic pain in his left arm and leg), he had a tendency towards contractures in the left extremities. He had been staying in bed for several days, he was depressed, and he was anxious when confronted with demands of physical activity. When the [nursing] student attended to him that particular morning, she could feel this worry and insecurity. When she asked the patient if he wanted to get out of bed, he seemed uncertain; he hesitated and slightly nodded. However, the student noticed his ambiguity and was quite unsure about what to do, whereupon she addressed a nurse who knew the patient well. This nurse also had extensive experience in caring for such patients. She reacted promptly and told the student that the patient had to be mobilized or else his pain and contractures would intensify and that a further stay in bed would make him even more depressed and worried. Accordingly, she herself went to see the patient. She talked calmly to him about the importance of physical activity, and, very carefully and compassionately, she moved him to an upright position at the bedside. While doing this, she focused closely on his body language, looking for expressions of pain and discomfort and signs of spasms in his extremities. Soon the patient was seated in a chair and seemed comfortable.

The situation in Ethics in Practice 22-2 shows how proper sensitivity can be crucial in solving conflicts between possible alternative actions. In this situation, it was of crucial importance to determine to what extent patient autonomy was endangered and whether it would be right, from the perspective of benevolence, to persuade and mobilize the patient (partly against his immediate wish). The rationale for such a presumed action would be to prevent further pain and physical deterioration.

Inevitably, a conflict arose about how to act in accordance with the patient's best interests. What was his main worry? Was it the expected pain? Was that the reason for him to stay in bed? To what degree was the patient so depressed that he felt incapable of being mobilized? Did he really want to get up, but needed a "push?" Or was his agreeing to be helped out of bed only a way to satisfy the nurses? How was his ambiguity actually to be interpreted?

All these reflections were initiated by the student's sensitivity to the patient's initial reply. While she recognized patient autonomy to be a salient value, she noticed the patient's uncertainty and anxiety as well. In this case, there was no easy way to find out what to do. Still, a decision had to be taken. Situational sensitivity did not so much ease the tension between the choices of letting the patient stay in bed or helping him up as it revealed the relevant moral choices. In this case, knowledge about rights and moral principles as well as emotional sensitivity contributed to capture a potentially complex situation in its intricacy. It might seem plausible to say that without compassion the full significance of the patient's uncertainty and frustration would not have been captured. The salience of his actual needs might have remained unnoticed; different alternative actions (with regard to letting him stay in bed or mobilizing him) might not have been sufficiently recognized. Indeed, without emotional sensitivity, the student's and nurse's actions might not have been competent.

Importantly, it seems difficult to determine the moral rightness of the action taken in Ethics in Practice 22-2 without recognizing the emotional attitude and sensitivity with which it was performed. Had the nurse not been competent and sensitive in her mobilization of the patient, she certainly would have done him wrong. But emotional sensitivity was revealed not only in her attentiveness, but also in her performance—in how she calmed the patient and in how, by her touch, she reduced muscular tension and did what was good for the patient. Her sensitivity clearly contributed to the patient's well-being, even if he was reluctant to get out of bed in the first place.

Emotions contributed to moral judgment in two important respects here. First, they contributed to a competent awareness of the patient's human and clinical needs in all their diversity and ambivalent intricacy. Second, and even more important, while the right course of action was difficult to determine exactly in advance, the emotional attitude and sensitivity of the nurse were essential for performing with respect for the patient's dignity. The emotional attitude conveyed in nursing this patient determined the action's overall moral worth. In fact, had not the nurse clinician acted with the required professional and moral competence, the action would have missed its moral quality and rightness altogether. In short, the rightness or wrongness of the action also depended to a significant extent on how the emotional attitude of the nurse was displayed in the clinical performance.

There are other situations of clinical decision-making in which prognostic certainty is almost impossible and in which nurses, physicians, and other health care providers must rely partly on emotional cues when deciding upon further action. Research on care for premature infants, for instance (Brinchmann and Nortvedt 2000), shows that in marginal situations intuitive feelings of the child's vitality and to what extent there is any "sparkle of life" serve partly as a basis for deciding whether to continue or terminate medical treatment for the child. Emotions also play an important role here as a basis for the clinicians' intuitions about the child's expected chances for survival.

So, it seems that in important clinical situations in nursing—situations that are indeterminate from a moral point of view—emotional attitudes and sensitivity can determine whether actions are morally right. In heterogeneous (that is, complex) situations, reason alone does not have the last say in determining right actions. Emotions, too, play a distinctive role in judgments about rightness as well as in the successful performance of acts. In such cases, we might modify Vetlesen's (1994) view and argue that emotions alone do not have the final say in judgments about rightness, but neither does reason. *What we see is that reason and emotion inform each other in a dialectic that contributes to proper judgment and to sincere and respectful moral behaviour, particularly in situations of great ambiguity.*

There are also situations in which a nurse's emotional attitudes are even more important in contributing to the rightness of an action. These are often situations in which the question is not *what to do*, but *how to* care. These are situations, for instance, of comforting mourning relatives and of giving information with proper respect and human involvement. These are situations in which good care and human concern are the prominent dimensions of nursing and which often involve deep human trauma and drama but in which there are no conflicts between possible different ways of acting morally. These are instances when we as clinicians know what to do, when we know that the patient has a right to information—and the question is how to give it to them with proper care, how to minimize hurt. Finally, these are situations in which the emotional attitude and intentions in a nurse's behaviour are so important as to make it necessary to look more closely into the role of emotion in moral behaviour and motivation.

THE ROLE OF EMOTION IN MORAL ACTION AND MOTIVATION

Many philosophers, particularly those in the Kantian tradition (e.g., Baron 1995; Herman 1993), have persistently argued that emotion has merely a supporting moral value.

Emotion supplies action and perception with the proper compassionate attitude, thus creating the careful environment where human well-being can flourish. But in cases of personal conflict and conflicting inclinations, philosophers in the Kantian tradition argue that only reason can serve as a reliable moral motive to guarantee that the action is right. For instance, American philosopher Herman (1993), one of the prominent neo-Kantian philosophers in today's Anglo-American moral philosophy, argues along these lines: "There needs to be some internal connection between a moral motive and the rightness of an action, and the idea here is that the motive of duty makes 'doing what is right' the agent's object of concern in acting" (237).

Reason is a very important aspect of professional care, in particular when dealing with negative emotions. Nurses are not saints, and in many situations our emotions do not comply with what we would consider morally acceptable behaviour. We can be exhausted, the patient can be extremely demanding, or he can be guilty of actions that disgust us. Still, as nurses we have to act with impartial and good care, being sensitive even if it is contrary to our emotions. How, then, can we be compassionate when we do not feel compassionate? It is particularly in these situations (when our spontaneous emotions do not provide us with a sense of duty) that our ability to reason and be guided by moral principles is essential.

Kant presents particularly strong views on this issue of motivation in *Groundwork for the Metaphysics of Morals*. He argues that, with regard to motivation, we can easily see the strength of an ethics based on duty and principles. Because even if we do not feel compassionate, our moral principles can tell us to act in the best possible compassionate manner. But Kant appears to overstate the role of reason in the relationship between emotion and duty. Here, he seems to argue that an action done for the sake of duty or rightness alone—even if our emotional inclinations contradict such an action—has a greater moral value compared to actions performed when duty and personal inclination harmonize. This means that for a nurse to provide careful and compassionate nursing in a situation of great stress, and to a person for whom he or she has no respect, has a greater moral value than merciful care under more favourable circumstances and for a patient he or she likes. Crudely put, a nurse's actions that are contrary to his or her emotions, but which are undertaken for the sake of moral rightness, have greater moral value than actions in which emotions and duty are in harmony. This is so because to be morally motivated in the Kantian way is to be motivated for the sake of duty, for the sake of an action's rightness alone. Emotions are seen as irrelevant for determining the overall moral value of actions. As explained earlier, many philosophers have launched criticisms against this rather strict and narrow view on moral motivation, and even Kant himself modified his views in later works.

It may in many ways appear counterintuitive to say that an action's moral value is diminished when our emotions are in accordance with what duty would say. Many would agree with Aristotle (350 BCE/1987) that moral virtue and virtue of character are shown by a person who acts for the right reason and with the right emotions (a person who is compassionate because the situation tells him to be so and not because of a sense of duty). Virtue ethics in the Greek and Aristotelian tradition argue that emotions are not unreliable and insignificant as moral motives. Annas gives us a fascinating understanding of this in her book *The Morality of Happiness* (Annas 1993). According to Annas, emotion is not alien to virtue or something that diminishes an action's overall moral worth. On the contrary, emotion contributes to moral value. To act with the proper emotional intent, to feel right in doing right and without personal struggle in doing so, is morally praiseworthy. To act in accordance with virtue means that our feelings correspond with the aim of the action. This means that we should feel careful when being careful, should feel compassion in situations when it is needed, and so forth. According to the ethics of virtue passed down from antiquity, conflict and stress in the person signify lack of virtue, while attitudes in harmony with situational demands and a person's dispositions signify virtue. The virtuous person does not merely do what is right, he or she does the right thing with the right attitude—that is, he or she has the right feeling in doing what is required (Annas 1993).

The big question for Kantian moral psychology is how to show authentic emotions and authentic compassion out of a sense of duty when our personal moods and feelings are contrary to acting thusly. The role of duty and motivation in Kantian ethics is a highly debated issue that we cannot solve here. Suffice it to say that it is an important discussion for nursing because it captures many conflicts in daily nursing care—that is, when nurses have to act professionally and demonstrate caring, but do not feel so inclined.

There is another issue, however, which is similarly important and which we finally must address. This shows not how duty has to interplay with emotion, but how in certain circumstances being emotionally motivated might be more important than being motivated by duty in caring for persons. Influential moral philosophers such as Blum (1994), Williams (1981), and many others have persistently argued that the internalization of moral motives, including emotional motives, may under certain circumstances have true significance for the moral rightness of actions. The following hypothetical example from Blum (1980) illustrates this point: You visit your friend in hospital out of duty and not out of a personally felt sympathy for the friend. If when asked by the patient, "Why did you come?" you reply that it is because it is the duty of every true friend to visit one's friends at the hospital, the patient would certainly take it to be a strange answer. If you only visit your friend because it is what general duty demands and not out of some kind of emotional and intrinsic concern for your friend as a friend, you seem to have deeply misunderstood that friendship is about *acting for your friend for his own sake and not for the sake of impersonal duty*. As stated earlier, to do what is right because it is felt to be right, and to perform it with the proper emotional attitude, may in fact determine the moral worth of actions.

CAREFULNESS AND COMPASSION IN NURSING

As I have argued in this chapter, emotion and compassion are important in nursing care. *More precisely, emotional motivation is significant both because it makes us care for a person's well-being and also because emotion helps us care with the proper attitude.* In theories about virtue, it is important to understand how a person's emotional character has a bearing on right action. What we ought to do and how we should act are closely linked to the kind of person each of us is. To act carefully means that we each have to be a careful person. To act in a friendly and compassionate manner means that we should *be* friendly and compassionate people. Emotional attitudes must be deeply embedded in a person's character as a trait—as a stable disposition shaping his or her personality—for these to play an authentic ethical role in action.

In nursing, we see that the emotional tone and intention conveyed in action have a profound significance for respectful care, for how information is received, and for how friendliness in care is felt by the patient. In the Catholic tradition of nursing, it was claimed that "Those who care for the sick know... from [their] own experience the profound therapeutic effect a sole friendly word or serene gaze can contribute to the life of the sick person" (Fischer 1902, 57).

The tone, atmosphere, and attitude created by emotion shape carefulness in nursing, creating the necessary respect and attentiveness for individual needs to be addressed. An action, even if judged to be right according to the standards of moral principles, might be wrong if not performed with the right attitude and human concern for the person. In daily and "simple" situations of caring, respect for the patient and his or her relatives is shown in a nurse's simple compassionate attitudes and receptiveness. Sometimes, the moral rightness of what we do is dependent upon how we care and our emotional way of being in the situation. Martinsen (1996) illustrates this aspect of ethical nursing:

> We shape our interpersonal world and co-existence through our sensitive expressions. In such expression we address each other. In addressing the other there is an obligation to be listened to. What is important here is not the proposition, what is being said. But it is the expression, how it is being said. Our authentic being shows up in the expression. The expression continues and manifests in the voice, in its tone and in gesticulations. It is the tone of what is being said— expressed in the word spoken, in the wordless bodily speech that stretches into the norms— which creates sincerity, which shows us the welcoming of the other person. We can disagree in views and in cases. But in the tone of the voice we have no neutrality. It must either be received or neglected. In the tone, in the expression, the person himself is present (89).

Martinsen describes how attitudes are expressed in nonverbal sayings and how these expressions are normative—that is, how they influence and shape the interpersonal reality of human relationships. This moral reality of emotional expressions is crucial in nursing because how we care for the sick person is so important—in how carefulness is shown, in how the patient is informed and welcomed. In all these significant aspects of nursing care, emotion has a part in shaping the caring clinical attitude. We do not always speak of intriguing moral dilemmas and normative conflicts. But these are still the situations in nursing care that are the most prominent and in many cases the most important to the patient.

In this chapter, I have described aspects of emotions and the debate about emotions in moral psychology and moral philosophy. These are in no way new debates. In fact, their origin dates back to classical Greek philosophy—to Aristotle, Plato, and the Stoics (Annas 1993; Nussbaum 2001). Even if not all issues are settled in these debates (and perhaps will never be), there is much we can learn by understanding the role emotion plays in moral life generally and in nursing specifically. We can agree that emotions contribute significantly to moral sensitivity and to our understanding of moral situations and that they thereby have an impact on sincere moral judgments. We can agree that emotions are important for authentic and well-motivated caring behaviour. Thus, we can clearly see the role that emotions play in nursing in various respects. Because of the vulnerability of persons in the context of disease and illness, we see that emotions create the essential foundation in nursing for good care, clinical sensitivity, and respectful behaviour.

FOR REFLECTION

1. How can one argue that emotional judgments can be judgments about value?

2. Is it right that some moral situations or judgments can be based on emotion alone?

3. When reason and principles tell us what emotions to display, can these be sincere and authentic emotions?

4. In giving a significant role to the emotional affect in moral sensitivity, is the role of rational reflection downplayed or jeopardized?

ENDNOTES

1. I choose to use both the words "care" and "carefulness" because they have a slightly different meaning. Sometimes I will use only "carefulness" as this word expresses the emotional sensitivity involved in caring for others. Carefulness is a way to describe the emotional attitude which shapes and governs the caring action. Care, on the other hand, has a much broader meaning. Care not only explains the actual emotional involvement for another person's good, but also explains the principal intention of willingly acting for the good of others. Carefulness is a way in which care is realized in actual action. (See also Chapters 5 and 7 for a discussion of the ethics of care and feminist theory.)

2. Here, I use the term "moral perception" as a synonym for "moral sensitivity."

3. See Chapter 4 and Chapter 5 for a (brief) overview of Kantian thinking and critiques of Kant, who lived and wrote in the 18th century. See Kant (1949; 1964) for two examples of his extensive works.

REFERENCES

Annas, J. 1993. *The morality of happiness.* Oxford: Oxford University Press.

Aristotle. 350 BCE/1985. *Nicomachean ethics.* Translator: T. Erwin. Indianapolis, IN: Hackett.

Baron, M. 1995. *Kantian ethics almost without apology.* Ithaca: Cornell University Press.

Ben-Ze'ev, A. 2000. *The subtlety of emotion.* Cambridge, MA: MIT Press.

Blum, L. 1980. *Friendship, altruism and morality.* Cambridge, UK: Cambridge University Press.

Blum, L. 1994. *Moral perception and particularity.* Cambridge, UK: Cambridge University Press.

Bowden, P. 1997. *Caring.* New York: Routledge.

Brinchmann, B. and Nortvedt, P. 2000. Ethical decision making in neonatal units—the normative significance of vitality. In *Medicine, health care and philosophy* (pp. 25–34) Netherlands: Kluwer Academic.

De Sousa, R. 1988. *The rationality of emotions.* Cambridge, MA: MIT Press.

Fischer, P.M. 1902. *Sykepleien i sitt Etiske, Sœdelige krav.* Lærebok for sykepleiere, del 2. (*The ethical obligations of nursing,* Textbook for Nurses, Part 2) Handwritten manuscript, translated from German into Norwegian.

Hagemann, E. 1930. *Sykepleieskolens etikk (The Ethics of Nursing Education).* Oslo, Norway: Gyldendal.

Herman, B. 1993. *The practice of moral judgment.* Cambridge, UK: Cambridge University Press.

Hoffman, M.L. 2000. *Empathy and moral development—Implications for caring and justice.* Cambridge, UK: Cambridge University Press.

Hume, D. 1984. *A treatise of human nature.* London: Penguin.

Husserl, E. 1998. *Ideas pertaining to a pure phenomenology and to a phenomenological philosophy.* Volume II. Netherlands: Kluwer Academic.

Kant, I. 1949. *Fundamental principles of the metaphysics of morals.* New York: Liberal Arts.

Kant, I. 1964. *Groundwork for the metaphysics of morals.* Oslo: Harper & Row.

Korsgaard, C. 1996. *The sources of normativity.* Cambridge, MA: Harvard University Press.

Levinas, E. 1986. *Collected philosophical papers.* Boston: Kluwer Academic.

Levinas, E. 1991. *Otherwise than being or beyond essence.* 2nd edition. Boston: Kluwer Academic.

Levine, D.M. 1999. *The philosopher's gaze—Modernity in the shadows of enlightment.* Berkeley, CA: University of California Press.

Little, M. 1995. Seeing and caring: The role of affect in feminist moral epistemology. *Hypatia, 10,* 117–136.

Martinsen, K. 1996. *Phenomenology and care—Three dialogues.* Oslo, Norway: Tano.

Nightingale, F. 1860. *Notes on nursing.* London: Lippincott.

Nortvedt, P. 1996. *Sensitive judgment—Nursing, moral philosophy and an ethics of care.* Oslo, Norway: Tano.

Nortvedt, P. 2003. Subjectivity and vulnerability—Reflections on the foundation of ethical sensibility. *Nursing Philosophy, 4*(3).

Nussbaum, M.C. 2001. *The upheaval of thought.* Oxford: Oxford University Press.

Oakly, J. 1992. *Morality and the emotions.* London: Routledge.

Scheffler-Manning, R.J. 2001. *Beyond ethics to justice. Through Levinas and Derrida: The legacy of Levinas.* Quincy, IL: Franciscan.

Solomon, R. 1983. *The passions.* Notre Dame, IL: University of Notre Dame Press.

Steppe, H. 1993. *Krankenpfleger im nazionalsosialismus.* Hamburg, Germany: Mabuse Verlag.

Taylor, C. 1985. *Philosophical papers.* Volume 2. Cambridge, UK: Cambridge University Press.

Vetlesen, A.J. 1994. *Perception, empathy and judgment—An inquiry into the preconditions of moral performance.* University Park, PA: Pennsylvania State University Press.

Williams, B. 1981. *Moral luck.* Cambridge, UK: Cambridge University Press.

chapter twenty-three

Ethics for an Evolving Spirituality

Jane A. Simington

All nurses are taught the therapeutic use of self. All are educated in the skill of listening and responding with empathy. When we do so we touch the soul of another.

Some years ago, when I began teaching gerontology, a friend gifted me with a copy of a poem. It was signed "author unknown" but has since been titled "The Crabbed Old Woman." In this autobiographical poem, the author challenges her nurses to see beyond her physical image as a feeble old woman who is unable to perform the most basic tasks. She reminds them of the full life she has lived and the memories that she still cherishes. The author, whether aware of it or not, was not only describing her own inner pain but was also portraying the collective soul pain of many who are imprisoned within bodies that no longer respond to their commands. She was depicting the life of captives who are at the bid and call of those who provide for their physical needs. Communicating for each and every resident in long-term care, the author expressed her longing to be known, to feel a sense of worth and a sense of being valued. She described the soul pain she experienced because of her lack of feeling connected to those around her. No one knew who she really was, what her life story had been. No one knew what she had contributed to the world. No one knew of her talents and her abilities. No one knew what joys she had experienced during her lifetime. No one knew of the sorrows she had overcome and of the soul pain she still carried. No one knew what healing still needed to happen so that this one soul might feel the integrity that comes from being able to bless one's life and feel a true sense of peace with the One Who Gives Life.

The author of "The Crabbed Old Woman" was sharing her life review process and in so doing was delivering her message from a spiritual framework (Simington 2000). It appears that those around her were incapable of administering to the needs she was expressing, for they could not hear her desperate cries. Their eyes and ears were attentive to what was required in order to meet her physical care needs, for that, it appears, was the paradigm within which they operated. The worldview held by the staff regarding resident care was likely similar to the guiding philosophy and the ethic for practice held and continually reinforced by the organization in which they worked. Not only could the staff not hear her spiritual distress, but they likely saw little need to listen for such pain.

"The Crabbed Old Woman" is a catalyst for discussion about spirituality, spiritual distress, and spiritual care. The author begs us to ask ethical questions about our practice—about the norms, values, and principles that govern our professional conduct. Professional ethics are more than a written code. Ethics are the moral obligations that guide professional activities (Kornblau and Sterling 2000; Nisbett, Brown-Welty and O'Keefe 2002; Randall 2002). According to Wurzback (1999), development of the nurse-patient relationship is crucial to nursing practice. The crabbed old woman challenged the quality of this relationship. The author appealed for justice, autonomy, empowerment, care, and caring, and for recognition of her personhood. The poem is a vivid and bleak reminder of how we can lose sight of the human being and human wholeness. The poem helps us get in touch with the human story and the soul reality "housed" within the physical body. The poem calls us to adjust our perspective, to peek beyond the physical aspects of those around us, and to gaze in a direction where attitudes and actions are more holistic in nature.

As nurses, we have a professional responsibility to practise according to our code of ethics. According to this code, our primary responsibility is to promote patient well-being (Maier-Lorentz 2000). Promoting well-being means acknowledging, supporting, and advocating well-being in each of the human aspects—physical, emotional, mental, and spiritual—as well as paying attention to social and environmental influences on each of these aspects. Yet nurses sometimes work in environments in which the organizational values are incongruent with their own ethical values. This not only makes it extremely difficult for them to minister to the total needs of their patients but also forces them into a moral dilemma regarding this incongruence. Maier-Lorentz argues that to deal with these dilemmas we, as nurses, must be more willing to become leaders in creating environments where applying the ethical principles of doing good, having respect for people, and promoting their total well-being is not only tolerated but is the norm.

The author of "The Crabbed Old Woman" begs us to think about the ethical environment of the organization in which she received care and, in so doing, to reflect on the ethical environment of our own institutions. The author compels us to ask, "Where were the nurse advocates?" And it follows that we also ask, "Where are they in our work place?" As we begin our discussion of promoting an ethical environment in which the total well-being of our patients, including their spiritual well-being, is honoured and advocated, think about whether you identify a difference between an environment that promotes ethics and one that honours and values dignity, hope, and the other components that contribute to the spiritual makeup of a human being.

As we reflect on "The Crabbed Old Woman," we must ask whether working in a setting such as the one where this woman was cared for would cause us moral distress. Would we be morally sensitive and attuned to her cries of spiritual distress? And, if so, how would we muster the moral courage to move against the status quo and act as a moral agent on her behalf? If we were working in an environment similar to that described in the poem, how would we act as a responsible and accountable nurse to advocate for care in which the spiritual concerns of our patients could be more adequately addressed?

A CALL FOR ATTENTION TO SPIRITUAL CONCERNS

In the past five years, over 300 articles addressing the lack of attention to the spiritual concerns of people have been published in the scholarly journals of psychology, social work, nursing, medicine, physiotherapy, and occupational therapy. The authors remind us that the spiritual dimension of our humanness has a pervasive influence on thought, behaviour, and general health and well-being. And while care of the human spirit is primary to healing in virtually all other cultures past and present, Western society's practices of religion and models of helping have, in many ways, paid more attention to maintaining these systems than to addressing the needs of the human soul (Bernstein 1993; Carr 2003; Doran 1997). The resurgence of interest in spiritual concerns is based upon a growing recognition of this void—of the need for soul healing and of the differences between spirituality and religion (Baumann and Englert 2003, Boryshenko 1993; Cowan 1991; Levine 1996).

My purpose in writing this chapter is, first, to examine ethical decision-making in a framework that extends outside a Judeo-Christian philosophy, for people of numerous cultures and religions now reside in Canada and are recipients of health care services. Second, I want also to acknowledge that not only Christianity, but all major religions, hold as a basic belief the importance of love for self and for others and apply this principle as a guide for moral living (Johnson 1997; Scott 1999). Third, I wish to raise awareness of the rapid expansion of our Aboriginal population and to honour the many who are returning to traditional ways of expressing their spirituality (Bopp et al. 1985; Waxler-Morrison, Anderson and Richardson 1990). My fourth purpose is to acknowledge that many who seek health services do not belong to an organized religion and that many, as they move through a spiritual crisis, come to define their evolving spirituality in terms other than religion (Hague 1995; Malmo and Laidlaw 1999). Fifth, I wish to help expand present-day definitions of spirituality so that care providers might more courageously and effectively meet their ethical obligations in this regard. My final purpose in writing this chapter is to raise questions, so we might prepare answers that will support the new ethic of an evolving spirituality.

AN HISTORICAL PERSPECTIVE ON THE RELATIONSHIP BETWEEN RELIGION AND ETHICS

Cave drawings and preserved and rediscovered writings of the practices of ancient religions indicate that long before formalized health care, human beings saw little distinction between the sacred and the secular, between religion and spirituality, between healing and spirituality, and between curing and healing (Godwin 1981; Jung 1959). Strong links existed between religious and ethical practices. The discernment of right and wrong, good and evil (a task of ethics) was tied to each tradition's theology. Cottone and Tarvydas

(1985) conclude that "religion is ethics and ethics is religion" (154). Carl Jung (1959) reminded us that, even in our times, as soon as we get a safe distance from Western Europe and the cultures influenced by it, people still make little, if any, distinction between the sacred and the secular and between physical and spiritual realities. Every act of daily living is a sacred act. Every act of worship is a sacramental re-enactment of their oneness with the spiritual world. The actions of our ancestors (as well as those of some of the more indigenous and traditional peoples of today, including practices of folk medicine and other alternative forms of healing) may not be consistent with ethical guidelines set forth to guide Western health care practitioners. Yet, just as we do, shamans, healers, and temple priests and priestesses performed their rituals in attempts to please the gods, to seek healings, and to maintain the social structure (Meyers 1987). How do we view the relationship between healing and spirituality? How do we view practices of folk healing and other alternate methods of healing?

AN HISTORICAL PERSPECTIVE ON THE RELATIONSHIP BETWEEN RELIGION, ETHICS, AND POLITICS

Not only is ethics fused to religion, it is also deeply rooted and closely intertwined with culture and politics. Practices established during the Middle Ages and the decades of colonization that followed continue to influence Western methods of health care delivery. In order to capitalize on the growing awareness of the relationship between religion and power, and between power and financial gain, Christian Church authorities instigated means of establishing controls over the people and their belief systems. Since many of the priests were themselves unable to render healings, there was a need to separate in the minds and practices of the Earth Peoples their long-held connections between physical healing and spiritual healing and their beliefs surrounding what is sacred and holy. Teachings and practices related to healing became purposefully associated with spiritual healing. The responsibility for spiritual healing was placed solely on Jesus (McNutt 1995). Indigenous healers, able to provide spiritual healing and therefore affect a change in the physical body, were barred from performing their sacred rituals, under threat of torture and death (Freke and Gandy 2001a). As the Church gained control over the indigenous belief systems, spirituality became increasingly separated from religious practices. Care of the sick became associated not with spirituality and spiritual healing, but with the new religion. The focus gradually shifted from healing to care of the sick and therefore to illness care; such care was administered not by indigenous healers but by men and women associated with a religious order. As medicine advanced, the focus shifted even further from spiritual healing, drifting from care to cure (Freke and Gandy 2001a; 2001b; Mircea 1987).

For many centuries the Church held a powerful religious and political influence in all of the countries influenced by Western thought. Moral codes and ethical principles that direct our attitudes, belief systems, and health care practices bear this influence. Much literature acclaims the benefits Judeo-Christian philosophy has added to our social structure and worldview (Fowler 1999; Whitlock 1989). One theory of ethics is called the "rule of authority" (Cottone and Tarvydas 1998). This is based upon the Judeo-Christian assumption that God gave the commandments to Moses, and these commandments therefore dictate what actions "are not allowed" if one is to live as a moral being. Christians believe in the Divine authority of Jesus. His Sermon on the Mount (Jesus's teachings of "what to do" for moral living) is, therefore, a further example of the rule of authority (Bible, Matthew, 5:3). His philosophy purports kindness, compassion, and brotherly love. Jesus further emphasized that the greatest commandment is love—of God, self, and others (Bible, Luke, 10:27). A follower of Jesus must love his or her neighbour as oneself (Bible, Luke, 10:37). The golden rule flows from this teaching and remains a major foundation upon which professional codes of ethics are built and which continues to guide Western health care practitioners (Cottone and Tarvydas 1998). While there is variation in priorities of the bioethical principles within professional codes, they include nonmaleficence, to keep from harm and injustice; beneficence, to promote good; autonomy, to respect freedom of choice; veracity, to tell the truth; fidelity, to honour commitments; confidentiality, to hold in trust personal information; and justice, to insure fair treatment (Beauchamp and Childress 1995; Turkoski 2001).

It is valuable to recognize the good that has flowed to modern health care from the influences of the past, but it is also essential to scrutinize what we often take for granted, to expand our paradigm and peek outside the boundaries of our worldview. It is necessary, as we step into the new frontier, to raise an ethical eyebrow and to ask pertinent questions. Do the social, cultural, and religious trends that inform our ethical decision-making always flow from love and compassion, truth-telling, respect, and the sincere desire to do only good? Or are there numerous occasions when they flow from a need to control in order to maintain the status quo? Do they always contribute to justice and to equality, or do our value systems frequently perpetuate injustice and inequality? Do the social, cultural, and religious trends that inform our ethical decision-making support an individual's spiritual journey, or do they interfere with personal spiritual growth?

How would we, for example, respond to a patient who told us today that she would prefer to seek the services of a spiritual healer? Consider the situation in Ethics in Practice 23-1.

Ethics in Practice 23-1	Advocating in a Morally Sensitive Situation

Mary is a 38-year-old woman who is receiving home care nursing services. She has severe chronic fatigue syndrome and a suppressed immune syndrome disorder that the medical profession is unable to completely diagnose. Her life's quality is decreasing and she is told her prognosis is poor. Mary has been doing considerable reading about the relationship between body, mind, and spirit and believes her physical symptoms are a result of stored emotional and spiritual distress. She has decided to terminate her conventional treatments and seek the services of someone who is not clergy from an organized religion, but who is acclaimed as a spiritual healer.

As Mary's nurse, what would you need to do in order to increase your own moral sensitivity for her reasons for such a choice? The nurse in this situation had a difficult time accepting Mary's choice but agreed to read some of the information Mary asked her to. After reading the material and doing some of her own research, the nurse was in a better position to help Mary examine the pros and cons and make an informed choice. By help-ing Mary make an informed choice and then supporting her choice, the nurse showed respect for the freedom of another to choose what is best for him- or herself. Working as partners, to achieve the overall good, Mary and her nurse designed a therapeutic regime that included some of the treatments prescribed by the medical practitioners, as well as some of those suggested by the woman Mary chose to assist her in her spiritual healing.

Many of our judgments and professional choices flow from a paradigm created from our socio-cultural and religious backgrounds and professional education and training. Most of us who are currently delivering health care services have been educated within a medical model. This model is strongly influenced by scientism and almost completely evades the notion that human beings are much more than the sum of their parts. Little, if any, credence is given to the spiritual aspects of human beings. Most practitioners in our profession see their clients as physical beings that happen to have a soul, rather than as spiritual beings having a physical, human experience, as do people from other traditions and religious and spiritual backgrounds. In order to support our clients who are struggling with the spiritual questions in their lives, we must broaden our understanding of how oth-ers view the spiritual reality.

HEALING, WHOLENESS, AND WELLNESS

Many perceive the notion of wholeness to be New Age thought when, in fact, ancient teachers and writers, including Plato, had much to say on the topic. Plato reminded his stu-dents of the interrelatedness and interdependence of parts and of the effect of the parts on the whole. Since early times, religious teachings have been built around the assumption that human beings are body, mind, and spirit, and that they influence and are influenced by their social and natural environments. Psychoneuroimmunology supports the notions of the interrelatedness and interdependence of the parts to each other and their effect on the whole. As Deepak Chopra (1993), a leading neurobiologist, writes, every thought and every emotion produces a neuroenzyme that affects the physical body for the positive or the less than positive, depending on the quality of the thought or emotion being expressed. Jesus taught similarly. He asked whether it "is easier to say your sins are forgiven or take up your bed and walk" (Bible, Matthew, 9:5). Jesus was reminding his followers that what goes on at a soul level has an ultimate effect on the physical body. Psychoneuroimmunologists emphasize that 85 to 90 percent of physical symptoms have their roots in unresolved spiri-tual and emotional concerns.

Those entering our culture who bring with them Eastern religions and philosophies, those who have learned to recognize, as Einstein did, that all is energy (Einstein 1956/ 1984), those who use, for healing purposes, their understanding of how energy works within the human body (Harper 1994; Simington and Laing 1993; Stein 1997), as well as those who have returned to the more traditional ways of practising indigenous spirituality, also acknowledge the interrelationship between the body, mind, and spirit (Sams 1990). Each of these groups has developed an increased awareness of the effects of the condition of the parts on the whole. They acknowledge that what affects one aspect of our humanness has an eventual and pervasive effect on every other aspect of our being, on those around us, and on the universe. For those with this awareness, the goal of healing is not only to bring balance to and between the physical, emotional, and spiritual aspects of the individual but to ensure that the energies moving into the social and natural environments are also more balanced and therefore more whole in nature.

The philosophy that guides practitioners in these arenas is, in many ways, inconsistent with the prevalent philosophy of Western medicine and health care. While considerable rhetoric is devoted to promoting holistic care, there is evidence that many who provide health care services are unable to apply the knowledge of holism, thus demonstrating a lack of true understanding of the concept. For while there is mounting evidence to indicate that the spiritual dimension is integrally related to health, well-being, and quality of life (Barris 2000; McIntosh 1997; Raholm 2002; Ross 1994; Sperry 2001), care providers have difficulty fitting the concepts of spirituality into their models of holism (Gustafson 2003). This appears to be most evident when clients are moving through traumatic life experiences (Boehm et al. 1999; Correctional Services of Canada 1990; Davis 2002). Yet, when care that is truly holistic in nature is provided (when the needs of the human soul are addressed), recovery is more complete and often has surprisingly rapid results (Buckwalter 2003; Krebs 2001; Floriani 1999; Wallis 1996).

In *Nursing: The Finest Art,* M. Donahue (1985) emphasizes that nursing developed around a tradition of healing and wholeness. Similarly, in a recent article, Diana Gustafson (2003) asks, "If we talk about our patients as if they are biological units disconnected from their mind and spirit, then are we, as nurses, also simultaneously creating ourselves as biological units disconnected from our souls?" (9). Further, she asks, "Have we embodied knowledge or disembodied knowing?" (9). These are poignant and ethical questions, and they must be addressed before we can cross the threshold and enter the new frontier so that healing and wholeness may once again truly be a part of health care.

The provision of spiritual care has roots deep in nursing history. Florence Nightingale is generally credited as the founder of modern nursing. While Nightingale had a strong belief in God, she was not a member of a religious community. Her success during the Crimean War gained her a hero's status. Her effectiveness was instrumental in the development of modern nursing as a profession, separate from membership in a religious order (George 1995). Nightingale encouraged her followers to pay attention to the spiritual as well as the biological concerns of patients (Barnum 1996). Of 26 nursing theorists examined, Oldnall (1996) found that only twelve theorists followed Nightingale's lead in directing nurses to provide spiritual care. Oldnall reported that Roy, Neuman, and Watson most clearly and specifically incorporated the spiritual dimension as a core element in their nursing theory.

Those influenced by indigenous thought, by Albert Einstein, by holographic theory, and by Eastern teachings and practices, acknowledge that "All" (including human beings) are delicate systems of energy and energy transfer and that the energy moving through "All" is Divine (Myss 1996; O'Marchu 1999; Simington 2003). Those who subscribe to this worldview would clearly note the strong spiritual undertones in the writings of those nurse theorists who articulate this awareness. Rogers, Newman, Parse, and Watson communicate (either covertly or overtly) their understanding of the relationships between the concepts of energy and energy transfer and the link between energy and concepts of spirituality.

Three decades ago Hubert (1969) questioned whether nursing students recognized a spiritual need and understood their responsibility for providing spiritual care. There remains a need to ask these same questions (Greasley, Chiu and Gartland 2001; Heliker 1992). Research indicates that while patients believe nurses have a responsibility to address the spiritual concerns of those within their care, nurses do not consistently respond to these needs (Highfield 1992; Reed 1991). Many nurses are aware that their clients have spiritual needs and acknowledge that the provision of spiritual care is within the scope of nursing practice. They describe a lack of educational preparation (and therefore a lack of knowledge about the spiritual dimension), a confusion between religion and spirituality, and a hesitancy to introduce the "non-scientific" realm into a science-based nursing practice as the three major reasons for neglecting to address the spiritual aspects of their clients' care (Piles 1990; Price, Stevens and La Barre 1995). Yet, when their spiritual concerns are addressed by nurses, clients report a profound and sustained healing effect (Hood-Morris 1995).

To find reasons for this knowledge deficit, a team of nurse educators recently examined whether aspects of the spiritual dimension of care were being taught in Canadian Schools of Nursing and whether students' knowledge about the spiritual aspects of care was being evaluated by the Canadian Nursing Association through the preparation guides for RN exams. Their findings indicated that conceptual confusion exists and that the spiritual dimension is rarely defined or included in curriculum objectives. Testing in this area is sporadic and limited (Olson et al. 2003a; 2003b). Examining the data, one cannot help but ask if the confusion created in the separation of spirituality and religion, apparently introduced into health care during the Middle Ages, still permeates Western health care systems, nursing theory, and nursing education and practice. And, more specific to this chapter, are nurses acting as moral agents? Are we fulfilling professional responsibilities and accountabilities in relationship to patients when as a professional group we maintain that we provide holistic care in the face of evidence indicating that an important aspect of holistic care (the spiritual component) is only minimally, if at all, addressed? Can we, as a group, validly claim to be providing morally sensitive care—meaning that we are attuned to the physical, emotional, cultural, psychosocial, and spiritual needs of patients—when there is evidence indicating otherwise?

DEFINING RELIGION AND SPIRITUALITY AND EXAMINING THE DIFFERENCES

What Is Religion?

Until the end of the 1980s most scholars made little distinction between the concepts of "spirituality" and "religion" and most commonly used the intertwined concept synonymously with institutionalized religion. While this trend continues to some degree, by the early 1990s academics were struggling to express their awareness that there was a difference between the concepts of religion and spirituality. Those attempting to describe what is now referred to as spirituality coined the phrase "religiosity." This term is rarely used today, for, in attempting clarity, researchers now distinguish between the concepts of religion and spirituality. In examining the definitions, Emblem (1992) noted that most authors defined **religion** in terms of practices, in terms of dogmas and creeds and rites and rituals.

It is important for nurses to recognize the differences between these concepts. Throughout the ages, authors and poets, and more recently academics, have emphasized that inherent in the human experience is a gnawing desire for a connection to the Divine and to that which is sacred. Most of these authors indicate that while all people have a spiritual dimension to their life, there is considerable uniqueness in how this aspect of their life is expressed. Burkhardt and Nagai-Jacobson (2002) emphasized that, by being human, all people are spiritual regardless of whether or how they participate in religious observation. As Osterman and Rogers-Seidl (1991) argue, people can be very religious and have very low levels of spirituality; they can be very spiritual and have very low levels of religious practice; they can have low levels of spirituality as well as low levels of religious activity; still others may have high levels of spirituality as well as be highly active in religions practice.

Bowker (1997) noted that the word "religion" comes from the root phrase meaning "to bind together." It is important for health care practitioners to recognize that many people find significant health and social benefits in belonging to a faith community (Koening 1994; Simington 1997) and that a direct relationship between faith and health has been demonstrated (Coyle 2002; Dossey 1993). Less clear, however, is how "faith" has been defined. Do people define their "faith" in terms of their personal spiritual journey, or do they identify "faith" in terms of remaining "faithful" to a particular religious creed and dogmas?

It is also important for care providers to acknowledge that others, even those who describe themselves as highly spiritual, may have few connections with a religious group or organization. In this regard, it is necessary to question the ways in which health professionals indicate they provide spiritual care. For example, does the initial history taking and assessment conducted in health care settings seek information about a client's spiritual well-being? Does checking or leaving blank a person's religious affiliation provide adequate data about a person's spirituality or assess for any indications of spiritual distress? And, perhaps most importantly, how frequently does the provision of spiritual care to clients by health care professionals consist only of the completion of this assessment?

What Is Spirituality?

A literature review reveals that nurses write more prolifically on the concept of spirituality and its associated constructs than do any other professionals. Nursing authors adamantly remind their colleagues of their roots and of their commitment to healing and wholeness and beg their readership to recognize that people's spirituality has a significant influence on their health and well-being. The overlap noted in the use of the words "religion" and "spirituality" extends to the concept of "spiritual." "Spirit" and noun form "spirituality" are often interchanged and are also often interchanged with the adjuncts to the concept which have appeared in recent literature, including "spiritual dimension," "spiritual need," and "spiritual distress."

The concept "spiritual" comes from the Medieval Latin word *spiritualis,* pertaining to breath, wind, air, or spirit. It first appeared in written English in the 1303 writings of Robert Mannyng, who borrowed the word from the Old French form "spiritualis," which had its roots in the word "spirit" as used in the Book of Genesis and refers to "the breath," suggesting that spirit energy is essential for life (Banhart 1988). Eastern and Aboriginal cultures view the spiritual as having timeless, spaceless, and immortal qualities and an interconnectedness with all humans, the environment, and the universe (Bopp et al. 1985; Heliker 1992). The spiritual is often explained with symbols such as the medicine wheel and in the symbols that appear in art forms and in dreams and guided imagery (DeLaslo 1991; Nelson 1994).

Phrases used to describe and define **spiritual** in the health care literature include "an animating, creative and unifying force," "the current of life," "the core of the individual," and "that part which gives meaning and purpose" (Burkhardt and Nagai-Jacobson 1994; Keegan 1994). Spirituality is viewed as a harmonious interconnectedness to God, self, others, and nature (Burkhardt and Nagai-Jacobson 2002; Goddard 1995).

Spiritual Dimension

The phrase "spiritual dimension" was coined in the early 1980s, apparently in an attempt to communicate the importance of including the spiritual as an aspect of human wholeness. Authors have viewed the **spiritual dimension** as a unifying force within individuals, integrating and transcending all other dimensions, giving meaning to life and providing a common bond to other individuals and to a Divine power (Fryback and Reinert 1999; Tanyi 2002). In an attempt to capture the collective ideas presented in the literature, one group of researchers defined the spiritual dimension as "the animating current that forms the core of all human beings; the real person, the active, living and continually unfolding core of the individual; the part that does not die, that provides meaning and purpose in life, that transcends, permeates and influences all other dimensions: physical, psychological, and social. The spiritual dimension is expressed through relationship with God (however defined by the individual), self, others and nature" (Olson et al. in press).

Spiritual Well-Being, Spiritual Distress, and Spiritual Needs

Desiring to further communicate the relationship between the spiritual and other aspects of the human being, and in an effort to measure this aspect, researchers have formulated the construct spiritual well-being and set about designing instruments to measure this quality of humanness. **Spiritual well-being** has been defined as "a personal attribute having one vertical dimension connecting one's perception of a relationship to God and one horizontal dimension connecting one's perspective of life's meaning and purpose or satisfaction with one's existence" (Paloutzian and Ellison 1991). **Spiritual distress** is defined as "a disruption in the life principle which pervades a person's entire being and which integrates and transcends biopsychosocial nature (Kim, Mcfarland and Lane 1984). In other words, spirituality cannot be ignored in an assessment of needs.

Ruth Stoll (1989) defined **spiritual needs** as "any factor necessary to establish and/or maintain a person's dynamic personal relationship with God (as defined by that individual) and out of that relationship to experience forgiveness, love, hope, trust, and meaning and purpose in life." A decade later, subjects reported that the human spirit longs for connection to others, to the world around them, and to a Divine presence (Hungleman et al. 1985). Both Stoll and Hungleman et al. emphasized that spiritual distress can result from unfulfilled spiritual needs. While their results were reported in the late 1970s and early 1980s, and personal narratives have supported their findings (Simington 1996a), research indicates that their efforts have had limited effect upon practice (Olson et al. in press). Minimal literature describes how spiritual concerns manifest or what resources health care providers might use (that are spiritual versus religious in nature) to assist individuals who are struggling with soul's agony as they attempt to re-order their lives after a difficult life experience (Friedmann, Mouch and Racey 2002; Simington 1998; Simington and the Victorian Order of Nurses 1999).

Spirituality as Personal Experience

Theologians, poets, and contemporary writers tend to view spirituality more in terms of a **personal journey**. With the recognition of the narrative approach as a method of inquiry into bioethics (see Chapter 14 and Taylor 1996), stories of personal survival and transformation have become more valued for their contributions to knowledge. As in the days of the great philosophers, experience is once again being acknowledged as the greatest of teachers. Philosophers of various perspectives note that it is not during our "sunny days," but during our "dark nights" that we turn inward in an attempt to discover the true meaning of and purpose for our lives (Campbell 1989; Frankl 1979; Simington 2003; Vardey 1995). Jung described the "wounded healer." He noted that those who have faced personal darkness and survived have much to offer others in their search for answers to the numerous questions that pour forth from their agonizing soul (Moyers 1993). Research findings concur with Jung's descriptors. Student nurses who attained higher scores on a measure of spiritual well-being were found to have a greater desire to administer to the spiritual needs of older and dying persons (Simington 1996b). There is a saying among therapists that they can really only bring a client as far as they themselves have come!

In *Journey to the Sacred: Mending a Fractured Soul* (Simington 2003), I offer a personal journey into the darkness of spiritual despair and share my story of spiritual transformation. I present my discovery of the sacred in my experiences and in the experiences of those I have walked beside. From this lived experience and subsequent research, I now apply a 3-R model of spirituality. The first R of spirituality is the R of **remembering:** remembering who we really are remembering that we are a brilliant light of Divine energy. All religious and spiritual teachings guide their followers to look within for the light of this truth. The second R is **relating:** beginning to acknowledge the Divine energy in all other human beings. The example in Ethics in Practice 23-2 illustrates the spiritual concept of "relatedness" and its relationship to ethics.

Ethics in Practice 23-2	Facing a Moral Dilemma: Acting as a Moral Agent

Following a series of complications, a young mother lay unconscious following the birth of her sixth child. During the night shift of the third day postpartum, the nursing supervisor broke with hospital regulations in order to meet the emotional and spiritual needs of the anxious husband and family. On his behalf, a friend begged the nurses to allow the infant to be brought from the nursery three floors above so she could bond with her dying mother. Choosing to relate to this man as she "would want done to herself" in a similar situation, the nursing supervisor brought the infant and cradled her in her unconscious mother's arms. Here the infant remained for most of the shift. As the child was placed in her mother's arms, the fretful infant ceased crying while tears flowed from every other eye in the room—including from the eyes of the unconscious mother (Simmons 2003).

In this situation the nursing supervisor became an advocate for the entire family. Because of her role, she automatically assumed the role of moral agent. The situation forced her into a moral dilemma. She was required to choose between assisting in alleviating emotional and soul pain versus upholding hospital policy. The nursing supervisor conveyed moral sensitivity to the husband's concerns and displayed moral courage in acting on his behalf. In so doing she accomplished a greater good—acting according to the ethical principle of beneficence.

The third R in my model of spirituality is **recognizing** that Divine energy is within all that has been created. In my work of listening to soul pain, I recognize the relationship between healing and advancing spiritually. I notice that as people heal they become more spiritually aware. As they become more spiritually aware, they automatically begin to have an increased sense of self-love and love and respect for the dignity of others. I also note that as they become more spiritually aware they desire to connect in numerous and various ways with nature and the natural world. Many feel a need to relocate to the countryside, the mountains, or to be near a water source. Some place plants in their homes or begin to garden. Others feel drawn to spiritual practices that help them establish and maintain their connections to the Earth. Some investigate the use of energy-transfer healing modalities, such as therapeutic touch, for at some level they instinctively recognize (as Eastern philosophies teach) that the source of this energy is Divine and that the same energy that flows through each human being also flows through all that has been created.

Many nursing homes, palliative care units, and mental health programs have already begun to incorporate plants, the elements, and other aspects of nature into their environments. Others have begun to introduce healing touch, therapeutic touch, and other alternative and complementary forms of therapy. There is growing literature describing the positive outcomes of these approaches (Hartley 2001; Richardson 2003; Simington 1995).

The acknowledgment that Divine energy dwells in every aspect of creation frequently heralds the recognition of an individual's connection to the cosmos and the responsibility that comes with knowing that each aspect of creation is affected by every other aspect of creation. In *The Holographic Universe*, Michael Talbot (1991) presents evidence from an array of sources, each affirming we are a part of an ever-expanding and ever-evolving universe. In *Evolving Spirituality*, William Hague (1995) writes, "It is a paradox and mystery that when we find the transcendent written across the cosmos in all its awesomeness and glory we find it is immanent—within us—written on our hearts. It is an epiphany of oneness with the seamless whole of all that is" (290).

Recognizing the Quest for Knowing: The Spiritual Journey

Nurses work with people when they are moving through difficult life experiences. During such times life can seem overwhelming. While many professionals recognize that crises can initiate a need to reframe the view we hold of the world and of our place within it, most do not comprehend the intense agony of this spiritual quest. Nor do practitioners comprehend that it may take months or even years before soul issues are grappled with (Simington 1999). This has consequences for therapeutic caring, for, most often, any resources available to assist those who are moving through a difficult life experience are long removed before the soul pain (described by many as "the greatest suffering") is experienced.

Listening to someone who is struggling with beliefs can be a challenging experience, for it brings us face to face with our own untested beliefs. When we hold a belief, our very core is threatened when others lament that they can no longer accept such a belief. Our initial response is often one of defense. Our language and body movements can quickly convey our discomfort in having this belief challenged. We may become angry and communicate a strong disagreement with others' opinions. We may argue in an attempt to convince them of their inaccuracy. We may try to "fix" them and their situation by emphasizing their need to continue to hold the belief. We might, for example, attempt statements of false reassurances such as, "Just trust in God and it will all work out." Or we might try advice such as, "You should pray harder."

The threat of having our own beliefs challenged stirs, within us, a deep need to maintain the status quo. For if the status quo is disturbed we might be forced to re-examine our own beliefs and ways of doing things, and we know too well the turmoil this can create. Yet, it is only through disturbing the status quo that true spiritual growth happens and that a true ethical practice can evolve.

In addressing soul pain, we must be able to move beyond the boundaries of religion and culture, beyond the boundaries of our limiting filtering system. We must expand our paradigm, our consciousness. In the 14th century, Hildegard of Bingen (Uhlein 1983) had a vision of consciousness. She saw consciousness, rather than being in her, as residing outside of her. She envisioned that the consciousness that moves from us connects person to person and persons to all things and brings us in each moment fully in communion with the sacredness in each moment of creation. Visionaries, modern writers, and researchers support her vision and ask us to pay attention to our holistic nature and to our need to be connected to the sacred in our lives (O'Brian 1999; Salmon 2001). Our institutions are filled with people who have lost their connection to what is sacred and in so doing have lost connection to themselves, to others, and to the world around them.

While Western medicine's approach has clearly advanced the scientific model of research and practice, resulting in an ever-accelerating ability to diagnose and treat physical symptoms, it has been less than effective in its ability to relieve human suffering. The fixing of parts and the proclamation of cure, quite in isolation from any real and concrete attempt to provide integrated caring measures, augments the brokenness experienced by human beings. And the separation of curing from the sacredness of healing contributes, in numerous and various ways, to the ripping apart that is occurring in our social fabric.

Jung stated that the sacred does not easily reveal itself in oral language forms (DeLaslo 1961). Oral language is connected to left-brain activity, and the language of the soul is most easily interpreted by the right brain. The right brain communicates and interprets in right-brain fashion. Symbol and sound and light and energy vibrations in the forms of energy work, music, drumming, dance, song, laughter, art, beauty, imagery, and the elements are much more readily interpreted by the right brain than is verbal language.

Oral language is culturally bound and is perhaps also bound to one lifetime. Soul does not recognize such limitations. Its language is much broader, more expansive. The language of soul transcends time and space. Words can be easily misconstrued. Their meanings change over time and are interpreted according to the accompanying nonverbal reflections sent from the giver of the message. The interpretation of verbal language is also dependent upon the feeling state and perception of the receiver of the message. Symbolic language carries a deeper truth—truth not altered by mood or circumstance. Symbol is comprehended by the individual receiving the message and carries a meaning often instantly interpreted, and at a very deep level. The Age of Scientism, with its focus on what is observable and measurable, has encouraged left-brain development, resulting in generations of human beings who have all but lost touch with their right brain capabilities—that is, their creative capabilities—at the expense of the needs of the human soul.

THE AUTHOR'S INTEGRATED APPROACH TO SOUL WORK

In my work as a consultant, educator, and counsellor in mental health, I use music/art, visualization and guided imagery. I introduce energy work and ask those I work with to pay attention to their dream life. These techniques each have research support as therapeutic tools. I ask those I work with to draw, paint, or sculpt the pain deep within. I ask them to journal; to create story, poem, and song; to take up pottery, stained glass work; to sing; and to dance. "All are creative expressions. All release soul pain. All allow for soul healing and soul growth. I believe that creativity is the expression of the soul. When I see creativity flowering, even the desire to repaint a wall, or hang a picture, I see a measure of soul healing."[1]

I allow myself to be vulnerable and to risk on my own behalf. As stated above, allowing another to share his or her soul concerns can threaten our belief system. When we feel threatened by the concerns of another it is usually because we do not know enough about the notion they are struggling with. Our moral and professional task, therefore, is to increase our sensitivity and to keep learning and growing in spiritual knowledge just as we do in acquiring knowledge of a physical concern or condition. When we adopt this attitude we begin to recognize that those who are struggling to find answers to the major truths in their lives can be our greatest teachers.

And (I dare to ask!), "Where is God in all of this?" I want to acknowledge that their struggle with beliefs is a spiritual process, more to be welcomed than feared, for I believe it heralds advanced spiritual awareness and personal knowing. And I listen, and as I do I ask further questions. I use as my assessment guide questions which flow from the spiritual needs presented by Stoll (1989) and Hunglemann et al. (1985) (and described earlier). I want to know of and to validate feelings of anger, fear, hurt, and a lack of trust, right now, in the Creator and in the universal order. I listen for a lack of hope and for a longing for self-forgiveness and for forgiveness from others. I want to know of struggles with shattered beliefs. I want to hear the questions that surface as those I work with attempt to find answers to the "why" questions about the meaning of their experience. I welcome misgivings about what it is they are now to become. I encourage calculated risk taking, for I know it takes great courage to tiptoe over the threshold of the door of a new beginning. And on frequent occasions, I conduct a life review and assist in bringing integrity to a life filled with despair (Butler 1982; Simington 2000). Consider the situation in Ethics in Practice 23-3.

Ethics in Practice 23-3	Meeting Spiritual Needs: An Ethical Obligation

A number of years ago, while visiting quite regularly in a long-term care facility, I would frequently witness Walter, a resident unknown to me, repeating over and over "never any good, never any good, never any good" as he angrily slapped the arm rest of his wheelchair. On a number of occasions I chatted with the staff about what might be going on for Walter. Their remarks ranged from his being "agitated" to being "confused." Several weeks later I noticed that Walter was no longer in his usual place in the hallway and was informed he had died. Several days later a stranger entered the room of the friend I was visiting. She said the staff had told her I had frequently stopped to spend time with Walter. She was his only sister. She had not seen him for many years. She wanted to know if he had shared anything that would be valuable for her to keep as a treasured memory. After a lengthy conversation I told of his repetitive behaviours and words. She wept and said her father had been abusive. He had frequently punished Walter, telling him over and over he would "never be any good." Walter fulfilled the prophecy. It appeared his life had "never worked out" and had ended in despair. I never forgot Walter's story. It was one of the reasons I chose to study mental health and spiritual well-being. I now know that Walter was engaged in a process of life review. He was trying to determine what had gone wrong and if there was a way he could make amends before he met his Creator. Had I had the skill then, I would have spent the time listening to his spiritual struggle. I would have listened to his despair and assisted in seeking ways to help him resolve his soul concerns in order that he might have had a more peaceful closure to his life.

Sadly, there continue to be many individuals who, like Walter, end their lives in spiritual distress because, as nurses, we are not meeting our ethical obligations to assist others with their spiritual concerns. While you may argue that all nurses are not skilled to do a life review, all nurses are taught the therapeutic use of self. All are educated in the skill of listening and responding with empathy. When we do so we touch the soul of another. When we do not, we tighten the bonds that hold their agonized souls in captivity. We have an ethical responsibility to do the former.

No two people will define their spirituality in the same way. No two will take the same route on their journey, and no two will experience the same spirituality in their lives, nor should they (Hague 1995). "It would be a mistake to think we are all pursuing the same goal by identical routes" (Hague 297). Spirituality is quite simply a measure of our attempts to live fully. It is how we, in our own unique ways, make sense of the God questions in our lives, and it includes both a viewpoint or a perspective on life and a way of actually experiencing life. The more spiritually aware we become, the more we experience. The more we fully experience life, the more we transcend the mundane and experience our bigger self. The more we transcend our little self, the more we recognize the Divine in others. The more we recognize the Divine in others, the more we follow it through in our practices of care, responsibility, respect, and justice-making. "Spirituality, like religion at its best, is an intensely moral endeavour" (Hague 1995, 290). In my opinion, the greatest of ethical questions is, "Do my actions create pain and distress, or do my actions assist in moving myself and others in a direction of healing and wholeness?" As illness and curing are concepts relative to the physical aspects of our nature, healing and wholeness are concepts relative to the emotional and spiritual aspects of our nature. Movement in the direction of healing and wholeness is, therefore, movement in the direction of evolving spirituality. To advance along such a path and to allow those we work with to also move in that direction, we, as nurses, must come to more fully recognize our advocacy role. Advocacy is about love, compassion, and caring. These qualities are recognized in all the major religions as the greatest of spiritual gifts. To act ethically, to be a nurse advocate, is to do all we can to remove barriers that interfere with the ability of individuals, groups, and the collective to live their lives fully. To be true nurse advocates, we must "pay attention." We must examine the status quo. We must recognize the rules and regulations that strip power. We must be willing to step forth in courage, offering alterative solutions—solutions that empower ourselves, our profession, and those to whom we provide care and support. While our own spiritual journey, and those of the people we walk beside, may not be without pain, it is up to us to ensure that it is also not without joy.

FOR REFLECTION

1. Write a brief description of what spirituality means to you. To do this you might like to list all the words that would be necessary for you to have in your definition of spirituality.

2. Do you view spirituality and religion as the same concept? In what ways do you see them as the same; in what ways do you see these concepts as being different?

3. How do you view the relationship between religion, spirituality, ethics, and morality?

4. Have your definitions of religion and spirituality changed since reading this chapter?

5. Discuss a situation in which you believe a person's spirituality was dishonoured due to a violation of one or more of the ethical principles.

ENDNOTE

1. This quotation is taken from *Listening to Soul Pain* (J. Simington and the Victorian Order of Nurses 1999), a film that raises awareness of the effects of trauma on the human spirit and emphasizes that complete healing requires attention to the spiritual concerns that surface in the wake of the experience. This AMPIA award-winning film can be obtained on video by calling 1 (866) 473-6732 or by visiting: www.takingflight books.com

REFERENCES

Banhart, R. (Ed.). 1988. *The Banhart dictionary of etymology*. New York: Wilson.

Barnum, B.S. 1996. *Spirituality in nursing: From tradition to New Age*. New York: Springer.

Barris, T. 2000. The power of faith: Can spiritual beliefs contribute to mental and physical well-being? *FiftyPlus Magazine, 16*(5), 30–34.

Baumann, S. L. and Englert, R. 2003. A comparison of three views of spirituality in oncology nursing. *Nursing Science Quarterly, 16*(1), 52–59.

Beauchamp, T.L. and Childress, J.F. 1995. *Principles of bioethics*. 4th edition. New York: Oxford University Press.

Bernstein, A.E. 1993. *The formation of hell*. Los Angeles: UCLA Press.

Boehm, R., Golec, J., Krahn, R. and Smyth, D. 1999. *Lifelines: Culture, spirituality, and family violence*. Edmonton: University of Alberta Press.

Bopp, J., Bopp, M., Brown, L. and Lane, P. 1985. *The sacred tree*. Lethbridge, AB: Four Winds Press.

Boryshenko, J. 1993. *Fire in the soul: A new psychology of spiritual optimism.* New York: Warner.

Bowker, J. (Ed.). 1997. *The Oxford dictionary of world religions.* New York: Oxford University Press.

Buckwalter, G. 2003. Addressing the spiritual and religious needs of persons with profound memory loss. *Home Healthcare Nurse, 21*(1), 20–24.

Burkhardt, M.A. and Nagai-Jacobson, M.G. 1994. Reawakening spirit in clinical practice. *Journal of Holistic Nursing, 12*(1), 9–12.

Burkhardt, M.A. and Nagai- Jacobson, M.G. 2002. *Spirituality: Living our connectedness.* Albany, NY: Delmar/Thomson Learning.

Butler, R.N. 1982. *Aging and mental health: Positive psychosocial and biomedical approaches.* 3rd edition. Toronto: Mosby.

Campbell, C. 1989. *Meditation with John of the Cross.* Santa Fe, CA: Bear & Co.

Carr, T. 2003. The spirit of nursing: Ghost of our past or force for our future. In M. McIntyre and E. Thomlinson (Eds.), *Realities of Canadian nursing: Professional practice, and power issues* (pp. 470–491). New York: Lippincott, Williams & Wilkins.

Chopra, D. 1993. *Ageless body, timeless mind.* New York: Harmony.

Correctional Services of Canada. 1990. *Creating choices: The report of the task force of federally sentenced women.* Ottawa: Correctional Services of Canada.

Cottone, R. and Tarvydas, V. 1998. *Ethics and professional issues in counseling.* Upper Saddle River, NJ: Prentice Hall.

Cowan, T. 1991. *Fire in the head: Shamanism and Celtic spirituality.* San Francisco: Harper.

Coyle, J. 2002. Spirituality and health: Toward a framework for exploring the relationship between spirituality and health. *Journal of Advanced Nursing, 37*(6), 589–597.

Davis, B. 2002. Addressing spirituality in pediatric hospice and palliative care. *Journal of Palliative Care, 18*(1), 59–67.

De Laslo, V.S. (Ed.). 1991. *Jung, C. G. Psyche and symbol.* Translator: R.F.C. Hull. Princeton: Princeton University Press.

Donahue, M. 1985. *Nursing: The finest art.* Toronto: Mosby.

Doran, R. 1997. *Birth of a worldview.* London: Westview Press.

Dossey, L. 1993. *The healing power of prayer.* San Francisco: Harper.

Einstein, A. 1956/1984. *The world as I see it.* Translator: A. Harris. New York: Carol.

Emblem, J. 1992. Religion and spirituality defined according to current use in nursing literature. *Journal of Professional Nursing, 8*(1), 41–47.

Floriani, C.M. 1999. The spiritual side of pain. *American Journal of Nursing, 9*(5), 24–25.

Fowler, M. 1999. Ethics as a context for practice. In P.A. Solari-Twadell and M.A. McDermott (Eds.), *Parish Nursing: Promoting whole person health within faith communities* (pp.181–194). Thousand Oaks, CA: Sage.

Frankl, V.E. 1979. *The unheard cry for meaning: Psychotherapy and humanism.* New York: Touchstone.

Freke, T. and Gandy, P. 2001a. *The Jesus mysteries.* London: Thorsons.

Freke, T. and Gandy, P. 2001b. *Jesus and the lost goddess: Secret teachings of the original Christians.* New York: Three Rivers Press.

Friedmann, M., Mouch, J. and Racey, T. 2002. Nursing the spirit: Framework of systemic organization. *Journal of Advanced Nursing, 39*(4), 325–332.

Fryback, P.B. and Reinsert, B.R. 1999. Spirituality and people with potentially fatal diagnoses. *Nursing Forum, 34*(1), 13–22.

George, J. (Ed.). 1995. *Nursing theories: The base for professional nursing practice.* 4th edition. Norwalk, CT: Appleton & Lange.

Goddard, N.C. 1995. Spirituality as "Integrative energy": A philosophical analysis as requisite precursor to holistic nursing practice. *Journal of Advanced Nursing, 22*(5), 808–815.

Godwin, J. 1981. *Mystery religions in the ancient world.* London: Thames and Hudson.

Greasley, P., Chiu, L.F. and Gartland, M. 2001. The concept of spiritual care in mental health nursing. *Journal of Advanced Nursing, 33*(5), 629–637.

Gustafson, D.L. 2003. Embodied knowledge or disembodied knowing. *Canadian Nurse, 99*(2), 8–9.

Hague, W.J. 1995. *Evolving spirituality.* Edmonton: Department of Educational Psychology, University of Alberta.

Harper, T. 1994. *The Uncommon touch: An investigation of spiritual healing.* Toronto: McClelland and Stewart.

Hartley, N.A. 2001. On a personal note: A music therapist's reflections on working with those who are living with a terminal illness. *Journal of Palliative Care, 17*(3), 135–141.

Heliker, D. 1992. Re-evaluating the nursing diagnosis: Spiritual distress. *Nursing Forum, 27*(4), 15–20.

Highfield, M.F. 1992. Spiritual health of oncology patients: Nurse and patient perspectives. *Cancer Nursing, 15*(1), 1–8.

Hood-Morris, L.E. 1995. The concept of spirituality in the context of the discipline of nursing. Unpublished Masters Thesis. University of British Columbia, Vancouver, BC.

Hubert, M. 1969. Spiritual care for every patient. *Journal of Nursing Education, 2*, 9–11; 29–31.

Hungleman, J., Kenkel-Rosssi, E., Klassen, L. and Stollenwerk, R. 1985. Spiritual well-being in older adults: Harmonious interconnectedness. *Journal of Religion and Health, 24*, 147–153.

Johnson, P.G. 1997. *God and world religions: Basic beliefs and themes.* Shippenburg, PA: Ragged Edge Press.

Jung, C. 1959. *Psychology and religion: West and East.* Translator: R.F.C. Hull. Princeton: Princeton University Press.

Keegan, L. 1994. *The nurse as healer.* Albany, New York: Delmar.

Kim, M. J., McFarland, G. K. and Lane, A. M. 1984. *Pocket guide to nursing diagnosis.* Toronto: Mosby.

Koenig, H.G. 1994. Religion, coping, and depression. In H.G. Koenig (Ed.), *In aging and God: Spiritual pathways to mental health in midlife and later years* (pp. 219–243). New York: Haworth Pastoral Press.

Kornblau, B.L. and Sterling, S.P. 2000. *Ethics in rehabilitation: A clinical perspective.* Thorofare, NJ: Slack Incorporated.

Krebs, K. 2001. The spiritual aspects of caring—an integral part of health and healing. *Nursing Administration, 25*(3), 55–60.

Levine, C. 1996. Take time to care for the soul. *Edmonton Journal*, Jan. 13, B4.

Maier-Lorentz, M.M. 2000. Creating your own ethical environment. *Nursing Forum, 35*(3), 25–28.

Malmo, C. and Laidlaw, T. 1999. *Consciousness rising: Women's stories of connection and transformation.* Charlottetown, PEI: Gynergy Books.

McIntosh, P. 1997. Faith is powerful medicine: Scientific research supports what people have believed for centuries. *Readers Digest*, Nov/Dec.,155–158.

McNutt, F. 1995. *Healing*. Notre Dame, ID: Ave Maria Press.

Meyers, M.W. 1987. *The ancient mysteries sourcebook*. San Francisco: Harper.

Mircea, E. 1987. *The encyclopedia of religion*. New York: Macmillan.

Moyers, B. 1993. *"Wounded healers": Bill Moyers: Healing and the mind*. Prod. David Grubin. PBS Series. New York: Ambrose.

Myss, C. 1996. *Anatomy of the spirit*. New York: Harmony.

Nelson, A. 1994. *The learning wheel*. Tuscon, AZ: Zephyr Press.

Nisbett, N., Brown-Welty, S. and O'Keefe, C. 2002. A study of ethics education within therapeutic recreation curriculum. *Therapeutic Recreation Journal, 36*(3), 283–295.

O'Brian, M.E. 1999. Sacred covenants: Exploring spirituality in nursing. *AWHONN Lifelines, 3*(2), 69–72.

O'Murchu, D. 1999. *Quantum theology: Spiritual implications of the new physics*. New York: Crossroads.

Oldnall, A. 1996. A critical analysis of nursing: Meeting the spiritual needs of patients. *Journal of Advanced Nursing, 26*, 289–294.

Olson, J., Paul, P., Douglass, L., Clark, M., Simington, J. and Goddard, N. 2003a. *Addressing the spiritual dimension in Canadian undergraduate nursing education*. Canadian Journal of Nursing Research, 35(3), 94–107.

Olson, J.K., Paul, P., Douglass, L., Clark, B.M., Simington, J. and Goddard, N. 2003b. *Spiritual dimension in Canadian nursing education*. Unpublished research report. Faculty of Nursing, University of Alberta, Edmonton, Alberta.

Osterman Fieser, K. and Rogers-Seidl, F.F. 1991. Spiritual distress. In F.F. Rogers-Seidl (Ed.), *Geriatric nursing care plans* (pp. 83–87). St. Louis: Mosby Year Book.

Paloutzian, R.F. and Ellison, C.W. 1991. *Manual for the spiritual well-being scale*. Nyack, NY: Life Advance Inc.

Piles, C.L. 1990. Providing spiritual care. *Nurse Educator, 15*(1), 36–41.

Price, C.L., Stevens, H.O. and LaBarre, M.C. 1995. Spiritual care-giving in nursing practice. *Journal of Psychosocial Nursing, 33*(12), 5–9.

Randall, J. 2002. The shaping of moral identity and practice. *Nurse Education in Practice, 2*, 251–256.

Raholm, M. 2002. Weaving the fabric of spirituality as experienced by patients who have undergone a coronary bypass surgery. *Journal of Holistic Nursing, 20*(10), 31–47.

Reed, P. 1991. Spirituality and mental health in older adults: Extant knowledge for nursing. *Family and Community Health, 14*(2), 14–25.

Richardson, S. 2003. Complementary health and healing in nursing education. *Journal of Holistic Nursing, 21*(1), 20–36.

Ross, L. 1994. Spiritual aspects of nursing. *Journal of Advanced Nursing, 19*(30), 439–447.

Salmon, D. Music therapy as psychospiritual process in palliative care. *Journal of Palliative Care, 17*(3), 142–146.

Sams, J. 1990. *Sacred path*. New York: Harper Collins.

Scott, S. L. 1999. *Stories of my neighbour's faith*. Toronto: United Church Publishing House.

Simington, J. 1995. The power of expressive touch. *Humane Medicine, 11*(4), 162–165.

Simington, J. 1996a. The response of the human spirit to loss. *Living with Our Losses Bereavement Magazine, 1*(1), 9–11.

Simington, J. 1996b. Attitudes toward the old and death, and spiritual well-being. *Journal of Religion and Health, 35*(1), 21–32.

Simington, J. 1997. Parish nursing: Working with older adults in a faith community, *Resource Education for Continuing Care, 12*(5), 2–4.

Simington, J. 1998. Spiritual aspects of older adult care: Determining supplemental learning requirements of health professionals. *Resource Education for Continuing Care, 13*(1), 5–6.

Simington, J. 1999. *Facilitators guide: Listening to soul pain*. Edmonton: Victorian Order of Nurses, Edmonton Branch.

Simington, J. 2000. *Stitched together by memories: Legacy and life review,* Available online: http://humanehealthcare.com/vol12e/Stitched.html

Simington, J. 2003. *Journey to the sacred: Mending a fractured soul*. Edmonton: Taking Flight.

Simington, J. and Laing, G.P .1993. Effects of therapeutic touch on anxiety in the institutionalized elderly. *Clinical Nursing Research, 2*(4), 438–450.

Simington, J. and the Victorian Order of Nurses. 1999. *Listening to soul pain*. Edmonton: Souleado Productions. Videocasette.

Simmons, K. 2003. *Surrounded by miracles*. Edmonton: Simmons.

Sperry, L. 2001. Spirituality, liturgy and biology. *Human Development, 22*(4), 23–26.

Stein, D. 1997. *Essential reiki: A complete guide to an ancient healing art.* Freedom, CA: The Crossing Press.

Stoll, R.1989. The essence of spirituality. In V.B. Carson (Ed.), *Spiritual dimensions of nursing practice* (pp. 4–23). Philadelphia: W.B. Saunders.

Talbot, M. 1991. *The holographic universe*. New York, NY: Harper.

Tanyi, R.A. 2002. Toward clarification of the meaning of spirituality. *Journal of Advanced Nursing, 39*(5), 500–509.

Taylor, D. 1996. *The healing power of stories*. New York: Bantam.

Turkoski, B.B. 2001. Ethics in the absence of truth. *Home Healthcare Nurse, 19*(4), 218–223.

Uhlein, G. 1983. *Meditation with Hildegard of Bingen*. Santa Fe: Bear & Co.

Vardey, L. (Ed.). 1995. *God in all worlds: An anthology of contemporary spiritual writing*. Toronto: Vintage.

Wallis, C. 1996. Healing: A growing and surprising body of scientific evidence. *Time Magazine, 147*(26), 33–44.

Waxler-Morrison, N., Anderson, J. and Richardson, E. 1990. *Cross cultural caring: A handbook for health professionals*. Vancouver: University of British Columbia Press.

Whitlock, R.A. 1989. Ethical issues and the nurse. In V. Carson (Ed.), *Spiritual dimensions of nursing practice* (pp. 292–319). Philadelphia: W.B. Saunders.

Wurzbach, M.E. 1999. The moral metaphors of nursing. *Journal of Advanced Nursing, 30*(1), 94–99.

chapter twenty-four

Relational Ethics in Nursing

Vangie Bergum

With relational space as the location of enacting morality, we need to consider ethics in every situation, every encounter, and with every patient. If all relationships are the focus of understanding and examining moral life, then it is important to attend to the *quality* of relationships in all nursing practices, whether with patients and their families, with other nurses, with other health care professionals, or with administrators and politicians.

The focus of attention in this chapter is on relationship itself—that space where nurse and patient make connection. While much discussion in nursing ethics is enclosed around concepts of moral agency, moral sensitivity, moral distress, moral dilemmas, and even moral courage, the relational context of ethical practice has recently been given more attention. In this chapter, I work from the assumption that all relationships as experienced are moral, for in each relationship one is enacting the question of what is the "right thing to do" both for oneself and for others. With use of a clinical example, presented as a series of Ethics in Practice scenarios, I focus on a number of themes that have been identified as useful in increasing understanding and development of a relational ethic.

The clinical example is written in story form and is in six parts, beginning with "Once upon a time...." Story tends to engage the reader with the complexity of a particular situation as well as to shed light on other particular situations. The example is taken from personal experience, with permission granted by the woman (patient) and her family. Distinguishing details have been removed or changed to protect privacy. One could think that this story is fiction, and in one sense it is, as any recounting captures only a part of the totality of any person's experience. If the woman, the patient herself, had written the story, it would look quite different. If one of the many nurses who cared for the woman as patient had written the story, it would have a different emphasis and language. An important use of story is that readers are invited to engage with it from their own perspective and to be touched and challenged by those parts of the story that resonate with personal experience. In conjunction with the clinical example, throughout the chapter, I use the breath as a factor that can bridge physiological concerns with personal, psychological, and social concerns. The breath, and the ability to breathe, also bridges individual and community (ecological) issues. I end the chapter with a discussion of dialogue, the place where relational ethics is vividly enacted. Before the relational themes are explored with the use of the case example, I will discuss relational ethics in a general way.

RELATIONAL ETHICS

Relational ethics is an action ethic. Instead of making *judgments* "about the goodness or badness of human actions and character" (Morris 1978, 852), we *act* in ways that lead to goodness without being absolutely sure if we are right. John Caputo (1989) says, "We act not on the basis of unshakable grounds but in order to do what we can, taking what action as seems wise, and *not without misgivings*. We act, but we understand that we are not situated safely above the flux and that we do not have a view of the whole.... *We act because something has to be done*" (59, italics added). There is no clear high mountain vantage point from which to view the situation with complete objectivity. Nor is there clear certainty found in the valley of subjective experience. Rather, in relationships, one is "inescapably, dialogically, in the midst," and it is this relational space that gives moral meaning to our actions (Gaita 1991, 142). A relational ethic is, as Peacock (1999) suggests, referring to Leopold's ecological ethic, "an evolving thing, expanding in scope and effectiveness as our collectively shared experience grows—and always a bit tentative, even when it must guide us in life-and-death situations" (703).

When, as in this chapter, we view ethical action from the perspective of relationship, we move away from direct attention to epistemology (traditionally defined in terms of ethical theory and principles), virtues (behaviours such as telling the truth and being compassionate), or problems (such as euthanasia, stem cell research, or disparities of health and illness, wealth and poverty). Rather, we attend to the moral space created by one's relation to oneself and to the other. Relational space, as a moral space, is where one enacts responsiveness and responsibility not just for oneself *or* for the other, but within the space of being for and with both oneself *and* the other (Jopling 2000).

In relationship, where intersubjectivity is a goal, we do not assume that the other person is like ourselves, but, rather, through dialogue we may come to see the other as radically different—two separated people (self and other, you and I) (Taylor 1993). The opportunity of intersubjectivity is to experience encountering another as "absolutely foreign" without "blending of the self with the other" (Jopling 2000, 153) where, through dialogue, something new has the possibility of arising. Within the "logic of dialogue," we experience our human ability "to listen to one another, the capacity to attend to another" (Gadamer 1996, 166–167). Dialogue builds on the presupposition "that the other may not just have a right *but may actually be right*, may understand something better than we do" (Gadamer 1996, 82, italics added). Even the definition of just who is "other" alters power relationships themselves (Taylor 1993). Thus, realities such as disparities of health and illness, wealth and poverty are not experienced only as problems to be solved, but rather are experienced as questions to be asked (Burch 1986). Attention to "women, students, the mad, the ill, the poor, blacks, the suffering, the marginalized of every sort" leads to ethical questions precisely because it is often the marginalized people who challenge the meaning of relational commitments—to "be in the midst of (*inter-esse*)" of ethics—"not in a plan of universal revolution but by local action" (Caputo 1989, 59, 61). How do we understand and enact an ethic that does not further marginalize others? How do we individually act in relation to the sick and the poor and others who are marginalized? In our current society, there seems to be a need to genuinely embrace, cherish, and celebrate difference (Olthuis 2000).

With relational space as the location of enacting morality, we need to consider ethics in every situation, every encounter, and with every patient. If all relationships are the focus of understanding and examining moral life, then it is important to attend to the *quality* of relationships in all nursing practices, whether with patients and their families, with other nurses, with other health care professionals, or with administrators and politicians. Of course each nurse in daily practice is not in a personal relationship with administrators or politicians, yet the practice of relational ethics can be shown to affect all levels through the relationships nurses have on a daily basis.

In a world where people are increasingly isolated from each other and communities are divided against each other, it is not surprising that a relational approach to ethics has been gaining interest and credibility. With this renewed attention to the quality of relationships—not only the quality of nursing science or clinical competency—we focus on the kind of relationships that allow for the flourishing of good rather than evil, trust rather than fear, difference rather than sameness, healing rather than surviving, and so on. In this chapter, we are not exploring normative distinctions such as what is good and evil, yet we do know that in relationship some actions are better than others. "There are limits; we are aware when someone behaves in an unbecoming manner. But we cannot set out the limits beforehand" for, in relationships, "suitable responses are multiple not just one" (Keiser 1996, 82).

Attention to relationship does not take away from the need to distinguish between different ethical foci; practical ethics, professional ethics, medical ethics, and bioethics or health ethics. Nor does it erase the need to learn about ethical principles such as respect for autonomy, beneficence, preventing harm, truth-telling, distributive justice, and so on (see Chapters 4–7). Placing the focus of ethics at different levels of the health system—either at the micro level, the meso level, or the macro level—is also helpful to provide the language for ethics of the health care system. Attention to relationship, however, has a way of dismantling these distinctions and categories as what happens at the bedside is not cut off from the broader levels, but is part and parcel of the same system—the same lived universe. The moral community of nursing includes each of us as morally responsible for our actions in relation to the people we care for, educate, supervise, or work with in partnership (who themselves have moral responsibility). It is within each of us wherever we are, and knowing who we are, that gives language to ethics as relationship. Whether we are clinicians, educators, administrators, or researchers, the place we are is where we practise relational ethics. In each interaction a relational ethic can flourish.

In this chapter, a relational ethic for nursing will be described by exploring the relational themes of environment, embodiment, mutual respect, and engagement. While these themes are not final or even the most important themes of relational ethics (nor are they specific to nursing), a relational ethic is useful in considering ethical activities where nurses, specifically, are engaged. Here we consider that nursing ethics is only separate and distinct because of the nature of the work nurses are called to do. Another way to think about ethics is that nurses are called to consider relationships within our work. Instead of developing a separate ethic that is good for nursing, in this chapter we explore an ethic in which the *good* of nursing can show itself brilliantly and clearly by integrating both principles and context through enacting a relational ethic. The relational themes identified here are one way to articulate a relational ethic.

RELATIONAL THEMES

The themes that are discussed here are an outcome of a relational ethic research project that spanned a number of years and a number of projects at the University of Alberta (for more specific details of the project and the identified themes, see Bergum and Dossetor [in press]). One reason why relational ethics is so difficult to articulate is that the themes only come alive in the disorderly realities of practice rather in orderly requirements of theory. In practice, too, it is difficult to confine discussion of one theme to one particular section, for in real life the themes show themselves and disappear throughout the whole of experience.

The four themes (environment, embodiment, mutual respect, and engagement) explored here within the framework of current literature can be useful in giving language to a relational ethic for nursing. Of course we know that many areas in health care, and particularly in nursing, already practise a relational approach to ethics. Yet, there remains a need for a well-developed perspective that gives voice to the significance of ethical relationships and how to improve them. The concrete example is used to guide the discussion in which we attempt to reground both autonomy and community in an integrated relational whole. The discussion of the tangible experience of breathing—the breath—is a natural and ethical way to connect autonomy to community and vice versa. We begin with the theme of environment.

Environment

Within the relational approach, environment is not an object such that it is out there to be manipulated and managed. When we consider environment as only "out there," then the health care system is something beyond ourselves as nurses or even as citizens: "The healthcare system is causing the problem." Of course it is important to search for ways in which the health care system can be improved by having enough nurses available for patient care, more dollars to spend on supplies and equipment, and increased ability for nurses to safely speak out about issues of ethical and clinical concern. A good example of the need to explore the system as "out there" is seen in the latest review of the health care system by Roy Romanow (2000), *Building on Values: The Future of Health Care in Canada.* As valuable as this study may be to the future of health care in Canada, it is also necessary to understand the environment or the health care system *relationally*—where we see that each action we take affects the whole system.

In a relational view, an **environment,** such as the health care system, is "each of us"—a living system—that changes through daily action. We are the health care system; we are environment. Perhaps one reason that studies of the health care system seem to produce little lasting change is that we have been looking in the wrong place—"out there" instead of "in here." The clinical example presented in Ethics in Practice 24-1 to 24-6 is used to lead us into considering environment as a relational theme—an environment in which all of us are intimately engaged and therefore constantly changing.

Ethics in Practice 24-1	The Breath—Connecting the Individual and the Environment

Once upon a time, not so long ago and not so far away, on a quiet spring day on one of Canada's major highways, two vehicles crashed into each other. The drivers of the two vehicles were similar in some ways—driving alone that day, both in similar age with busy active lives, both severely injured with their smashed vehicles crushing bones and organs. Both individuals were released from their vehicles with the "jaws of life" and rushed off in screaming ambulances to the nearest emergency department (ER)—an ER just reduced in staff and resources by provincial cuts to health care. But each person, now a patient, needed more specialized care, and when both were stabilized with open airways and blood, they were again rushed off to a larger regional hospital. Here, they separated. One person, a woman, was taken by air ambulance to the next major hospital. Even here the specialists could not attend to the severity of this woman's injuries and she was moved within the first couple of hours to a large university centre where the intensive clinical expertise of nurses and doctors saved her life—reducing brain pressures, closing contusions, splinting and straightening bones and muscles, adding bone transplant materials to reconstruct heels and ankles, and, all the while, monitoring all life processes.

Each nurse who touched the injured people enacted the whole of the health care system. Imagine the scene where nurses rush to assist, starting with breath—perhaps even catching their own breath—in an attempt to maintain each person's breathing (breathing air we all share). The nurse, along with the doctor and others, as the breath is stabilized, works to stop the bleeding, calls out the name of each person when discovered, starts the intravenous (IV) to administer blood and drugs, aligns broken bones, and contacts the family if possible. The person who witnessed the accident, the ambulance attendant, the nurse, the doctor, and other members of the team are the health care system that attended to each person's needs—to keep each person alive. As each injured person is moved through the various locations to find the best possible care, the system responds through individual action, and each action affects the system itself. While we need to question whether cutbacks in health care resources affected the care of these patients, one needs to also question how each patient and each nurse acts from a place of being "inescapably in the midst" of the environment that each affects and is affected by.

With this kind of attention to environment we begin to see that while the persons in the accident become the primary focus, all those who care for them are involved and personally affected as well. The system is enacted through each individual connection to save each person's life—the nurses and doctors who rush to give attention (which takes away attention from others less in danger of dying), the families of the patients (who are stopped in their tracks when they hear the news), or the neighbours who take on the responsibility to tell the children (so that the police would not be the first to break the news). Even the citizen, who decides that health care dollars will be available to all citizens (both rich and poor) and that hospitals and resources will be available with various degrees of available expertise, is affected and involved. The undulating vibrations of the ambulance siren are felt far beyond the ears of anyone who hears it, or indeed the life of any one particular person. Looking at the environment in this relational way brings us back to individual acts.

When we consider environment and the health care system in this broad way (as an interdependent and complex entity) we agree with Kent Peacock's (1999) assertion that ethics cannot be just personal, social, or political, but needs to be ecological (see also Chapter 11). Such ecological consciousness is a hopeful sign says Gadamer (1996), for it includes not only the ability to manage by oneself (autonomy) but also the ability to manage along with other people (community). Such "housekeeping" (Gadamer 1996) encompasses not only individual activities but also includes the "house" that is held in common—the health care system, and even the planet as a whole. In such a living relation, one begins to see the fluidity between breath of the individual and breath of the universe, between stabilizing each patient's breathing and making sure that the air is pure and toxin free. The breath is in continuous communion, in both its micro and macro circumstances, which in its purist form would be "breathing in tune with the breathing of the entire living universe" (Irigaray 2002, 36).

The breath is the origin of autonomous existence of the living human being. That "first" breath (Bergum 1997) is necessary for material existence of the body (of nature) but is also necessary for the becoming of the person (of culture). The breath maintains a person's life, but to breathe for survival is not enough. The ultimate goal for the woman in Ethics in Practice 24-1 is to again breathe on her own, to take her own breath as a particular person, a person with a name, a history, a family, and a community. As the woman is secured in the reality of having breath maintained by artificial means (intubations, ventilators), the health care team begins the process of moving toward assisting her to again become autonomous and take charge of her own breath and her own life. We often speak of the elementary need to eat or to drink, but we do not often consider the need to breathe, which, says Luce Irigaray (2002), is our first and most radical need: "Breathing in a conscious and free manner is equivalent to taking charge of one's life, to accepting solitude through cutting the umbilical cord, to respecting and cultivating life, for oneself and for others" (74). For the woman in our example to come back to her own life (her individual and communal life) over the next weeks, she will begin to transform the vital breath in the service of survival to the more subtle breath in the service of the heart, of thought, and of speech. She will need to learn to breathe again—to take a "second" breath—in order to take charge of her own life, her life related to heart and soul. Even with this discussion, it is necessary to consider how autonomy can be fostered with those who will never be able to breathe without mechanical support.

For the moment, though, the woman's breath is breathed by and with others, through oxygen machines—not unlike the umbilical cord that once tied her to her mother. But like the breathing experienced in utero, it is breathing that is shared—not given away. The first ethical task with respect to autonomy is to share the breath—to breathe together. With the breath we begin to see how the individual is autonomous and also how individuals are connected to each other, how they respect and share life. "Community is then composed of autonomous individuals in conscious relation to one another" (Irigaray 2002, 102). Irigaray further reminds us that it is impossible to appropriate breath or air—one can only cultivate it, for oneself and for others (79).

Consider how Gadamer's notion of housekeeping speaks to the relation between the need to live well for oneself and to also live well together (1996). We are now, as a society, becoming more realistic in recognizing that these needs are the same—we can only live well autonomously if we live well together. If we do not attend to our shared "home," we will have no home at all. Think about the extensive resources used in the woman's care—the latex gloves, the IV and feeding tubes, the sheets and blankets, the detergents, the plastics (that need to be available and need to disposed of), and the landfills that take both the benign and toxic waste. The environment (the health care system) is part and parcel of the ecological system. Relational ethics highlights the connection between care of the woman and care of the earth.

Indeed, nurses have a great deal of power and responsibility in making waste disposal choices, and nurses are taking the lead. Susan Forsyth, for instance, a registered nurse and a representative of the California Nurses Association, embraces a nationwide (and hopefully worldwide) movement toward hospitals creating less hazardous waste (Gonzales 2000). The California Nurses Association supports Health Care Without Harm, a nationwide coalition of public health and environmental groups with the goal of reducing hazardous wastes from hospitals. Not only do nurses and other staff need to be educated about the impact of their choices for the waste that is produced during patient care, but we need to aware of the use of resources that are taken for granted. Take, for example, the use of latex gloves that are a necessary part of the care of the woman in our example. Boxes and boxes of latex gloves are used each day in our major hospitals as nurses and other staff don them whenever they touch a patient—for giving oral medications, for turning the patient, for lifting blankets to observe wounds and dressings, or to hand the patient a glass of water. While the use of gloves is based on clear scientific reason, to prevent transfer of infection (made clearly evident with the rapid transmission of Severe Acute Respiratory Syndrome), it is possible that the practice may become thoughtless in some situations as gloves are used and discarded with ease. A minor issue, one could say, but when we see ourselves in the midst of the environment then the interconnection between the use of gloves and landfills is no longer minor. Would it make any difference to nursing practice if we were more consciously mindful of the connection between the use of resources in daily practice and the needs of the living earth?

Exploring environment in this interactive, lived way brings our attention to the lived life of the woman in our example. Embodiment shows her lived life, shows that she is more than an object that needs emergent attention as she is navigated through the various hospitals and the care of many different nurses and doctors. The second theme of relationship that will be highlighted through discussion of the scenario is embodiment.

Embodiment

Each person, when brought into hospital by ambulance, is immediately treated, according to Gadow, as "pure object, without interiority... [with] no inherent authority over her body [which now] logically... belongs to the expert" (1994, 298). Of course we would not want the situation to be different. Yet, at the same time, even during these kinds of critical episodes, patients are still tied to their own lives and worlds—their life worlds. Though the woman is not able to go about her regular world—take her own breath, drive her own car, call to her own children—she is still bound to the world in which we are usually forgetful of our bodies. As the nurses and doctors focus on the woman as an object (body), they also know that in actual life there is "absolute inseparability of the living body and life itself" says (Gadamer 1996, 71). Gadamer then asks, "How can we successfully reconnect our instrumental reason, especially in light of the vast scale of its modern development, with the totality of our being-in-the world in a fruitful and productive way?" (72).

Embodiment calls for healing the split between mind and body—an integrative consciousness—so that scientific knowledge and human compassion are given equal weight and so that emotion and feeling are as important to human life as physical signs and symptoms. It is the family, in the particular instance of our clinical example, which assists the nurses and doctors (in their world of objectivity) to be mindful of the embodied reality of the woman. If the woman did not have a family that could readily be present, the nurses and other professionals would actively be more cognizant of the need to attend to the woman's lived life.

Ethics in Practice 24-2	The Breath—Connecting Mind and Body

It so happened that a woman, from her garden, heard the quaver of the sirens and stood to watch two racing ambulances flash by. Little did this mother, this grandmother, this great grandmother realize that from that moment her life would irreversibly change—from the quiet enjoyment of planting her garden to the fear of losing her adult child and only daughter. Soon she had a call informing her that her daughter was in the hospital. Now this mother felt the fear. After locating her grandchildren and ensuring their protection and safety, she and the woman's father went to see their daughter, now at the second hospital. There was little recognition of the daughter they loved—face and head swollen beyond belief, legs and pelvis mangled, breathing through a ventilator, surrounded by tubes and bags with little evidence of life. Nurses and doctors worked with serious concentration to do what was needed. These parents were told that their daughter would be moved by air to another larger hospital. The parents then made the necessary calls—to the woman's husband working in the Artic, to her brother on a business trip, to nieces and nephews, and to friends. Life changed for each person—now affected by this moment of terror that a precious life would be lost.

The focus of attention of doctors and nurses in this crisis of life and death is on the woman's body—the breath, the blood, the pressure on the brain, and the bones that protruded the skin—the body that is now treated as if it were a machine laid out by medical definition. Yet, the focus of attention of the woman's parents is on her lived body—the daughter and her life with them. The parents leave the details of the mechanical body to the professionals while they rally to keep the lived body alive—looking after her life as a mother, wife, sister, and aunt, even a worker—the whole of her life. While the nurses and doctors focus primarily on the body as an object, the family and friends make the necessary and ethical connection to her lived body, her human everyday life. Nurses support the reconnection of the body as object to the body as lived because they know that the lived body is as ethically important as the object body. While the woman is unconscious the nurses need careful attention to do for the woman what throughout her life she has, without thinking, done for herself. They work within the reality of the inseparability of the lived body and the object body.

The woman needs multiple surgeries carried out by different professional teams. Now the issue of consent becomes of particular concern. Who is this woman lying unconscious in the intensive care unit? Who is this woman entangled by tubes and machines? What treatment does she want? Of course, she does not even know she has been in an accident—she will not completely grasp this fact for days, indeed months. She cannot make decisions for herself. It is up to those close to her (her husband) to give consent for the various treatments. Her autonomy (self-knowledge and responsibility) is fostered by her connections to others—those who know her best. Again we see the lived reality of autonomy as a concept that is achieved through human connections. Self-knowledge and autonomy are "activity pursued with others and for others, and in a moral context in which the self's responsiveness to others, and its epistemic and moral responsibility for others, reaches an equilibrium with the self's concern for itself" (Jopling 2000, 152). Our relationships comprise who we are. The lived body is more important to the principle of autonomy than the object body as there is no autonomy for human beings in isolation from each other. Being alone and independent is primarily experienced because there are others to miss.

Issues of personal privacy also reflect embodied understanding. As her brother stands steadily by this woman's battered and unconscious body the day after the accident, he is always asked to leave the room when care is given by the nurses—care that might expose the woman's body in ways she would not, if able to make that decision for herself. In the same way as the nurses are respectful of patient needs, they recognize and encourage the presence of the family, who maintain vigilant attention to those aspects of the woman's life which the professionals have no knowledge of. They know that respectful attention to the lived body of the patient is vital to her healing.

Commitment to others is felt in the body. Do bodies hold knowledge that is not so easily articulated rationally and, therefore, a source of knowledge that is not easily understood? The mother remembers the physical connection to the daughter as she looks to find the face of the daughter she loves. But the nurse too must become bodily connected to the woman—to remember the lived body of the woman at the same time as she is engaged with the body as object (Gadow 1980). Not only is the patient embodied (connecting the lived body of the breath to the object body of the medical gaze), but so do nurses need to remember their own lived life—to take time to breathe for themselves. Gadamer (1996) asks another important question:

> What can intervention, our own actions, our dependency on the help of others, and our perhaps greater dependency on helping ourselves, contribute towards bringing the achievements of modern society, with all of its automated, bureaucratized and technological apparatus, back into the service of that fundamental rhythm which sustains the proper order of bodily life? (79)

There must be deep ethical commitment to *who* the woman is and not just *how* she breathes. The sharing of the breath reminds nurses that the woman is both embodied and autonomous yet connected to others through the embodiment of the nurse (Gadow 1989). Of course, when nurses feel (imagine) in their own bodies the bodily experience of the woman, they acknowledge their own vulnerability as they resonate with the other's pain (she could be me, my daughter, or my mother). Even when nurses imagine or "feel" the woman's pain, they need to remain vigilant to the reality that it is the woman's pain and not their own. It is a fine balance to allow sensitivity to another's pain (the embodied reality of the other person) while being true to the reality of one's own embodiment as separate and distinct (see also Chapter 21 and Chapter 22). This self-knowledge and self-respect is as important as respect for the other, which is the next relational theme to be discussed.

Mutual Respect

Mutual respect arises from the reality that we are fundamentally connected to one another. Our experience of our world and of ourselves is shaped by the attitude of others toward us and by our attitude towards others. Mutual respect is the challenge of daily life in health care, surely, but also in politics, in culture, and in gender relations. How can we truly respect one another, especially if we have differences of opinions, beliefs, or even activities? How can we truly respect someone who holds different knowledge, a different culture, and different values? In coming to mutual respect there is a need to be both respectful of others and also respectful of oneself (Dillon 1992). In fact we cannot respect others unless we first respect ourselves.

Ethics in Practice 24-3	The Breath—Connecting Self and Other

Time passed. Life unfolded. Nurses, neurologists, orthopedic specialists, physiotherapists, occupational therapists, rehabilitation psychologists, rehabilitation physicians, transfer teams, laboratory technicians, and so on enacted their special knowledge in the care of the woman. Each team member, working alone with the woman but in concert and collaboration with other team members, was directed toward the goal of restoring the woman to a full functioning life.

The woman's family, too, worked as a team to connect the woman to the life she had lived prior to the road accident. Her brother rushed to her bedside, flying across the country, renting a car to speed the trip, only to be left waiting impatiently at the border because of prolonged security checks. Then her husband arrived after hours in flight. Over the weeks, her mother, sister, and brothers-in-law, children, and finally friends were able to stay at her side as she gradually came back to her own world.

Each family member and each friend offered unique qualities and abilities, no less important than the professionals, just remarkably different. Each contact was necessary in the life of the woman. Each contact was also necessary for those who cared for her. In the first days after the accident the brother talked of the "technical wizard nurses and expert doctor carpenters" who acted out their roles as he stood by her bedside, singing and speaking healing words into her ear.

Mutual respect is probably the central theme of a relational ethic. It sounds so easy: "Of course, everyone deserves respect." Yet with the different teams (professional and family) looking after this woman, the question of respect needs foreground consideration. Different disciplines, different genders, different access to power, and different knowledge(s) are present in all health care relations and are embodied on any interdisciplinary team, including patients and their families. With the kind of care this woman received, the recognition of the varied skills and roles was paramount. Right from the very beginning there were different teams of specialists taking charge of her care—the nurses in the ER and intensive care unit (ICU), on the trauma general ward, on the rehabilitation (rehab) ward, and on various shifts; the surgeons for her pelvis, for her left leg, for her right foot, for the facial bone; neurologists for the pressure on her brain and the fracture of her spine; the rehab specialists such as occupational therapists, physiotherapists, and psychologists. Each had expertise that was unique yet overlapped with others.

Respect for difference (e.g., power, knowledge, beliefs and values, experience, attitudes) does not come easily. When professionals are grounded in their own perspective, it is sometimes hard to realize that others also have valuable perspectives—that in fact they may have it right. The word *mutual* directs attention to the interactive and reciprocal nature of respect. It seems easy to speak of respect—"I respect your wish for..."—yet harder to practise the attitude of "I respect you," especially if I think what you do is inappropriate. Too often the "other" is reduced to an object of study or integrated as one and the same as us in "our" world. Either way, it allows one to "avoid the problem of meeting with the stranger, with the other. We avoid letting ourselves be moved, questioned, modified, [and] enriched by the other" (Irigaray 2002, 125).

With the theme of **mutual respect,** we are asked to look for ways to achieve cohabitation or coexistence between people who are different but of equivalent worth and dignity. Teamwork is essential, with the patient and family taking on important roles on the team. Often the nurse is the co-ordinator of the team. In the clinical example, the nurse was the person who the woman's family was encouraged to call. The nurse has the tough, and often thorny, job of assisting all members to work in collaboration rather than in hierarchical pockets—a responsibility that cannot be the nurse's alone. If mutual respect is the central challenge of relational ethics, then teamwork is the prime opportunity for relational action. There is a need to learn ways to engage the other, the *you,* without reducing *you* to the same as *me,* or *me* to the same as *you.* From now on, the challenge is to know how to intertwine love of the same and love of the different while being faithful to oneself and the becoming of the other (Irigaray 2002). The relational theme of engagement focuses attention on being true to oneself and still attending to the other.

Engagement

Ethical action needs to start with an attempt to understand the other's situation, perspective, and vulnerability. This understanding requires a true movement toward the other as a person, a movement toward genuine engagement. When this is not possible, the lack of involvement of person-to-person needs to be recognized as the ethical issue it is. If we believe that the quality of relationship needs ethical attention, then lack of engagement could be understood as an ethical concern.

| Ethics in Practice 24-4 | **The Breath–Breathing Together** |

Again, time passed. The woman was now in the hospital where she began her journey. Now she breathed on her own—even using her breathing to both ease the pain and ease the anxiety. A feeding tube was inserted in her stomach in an attempt to give the necessary nutrition to heal the various fractures. Her neck brace was off, leaving her cheekbone as smooth and lovely as before the accident, the external pelvic brace was gone, and her scarred legs began to move through her own effort rather than only with the aide of the continuous rotating machine. Both family and professional teams surrounded her. But she was still losing weight, had a rash, felt discouraged, and said she was "so, so sick." Now she demanded drugs to kill the pain, shouted at nurses and doctors and husband. Everyone was worried.

Then came one nurse. Would she like to go to the college basketball game—where her teen son was a star? The social worker arranged the van, the doctors agreed, the nurses helped her dress, and family members came to escort her to the gym under the nurse's guidance and vigilance. As the van carried her through her own town, which she had not seen for months, the woman wept.

This event moved the woman to gain new vigour for life. It changed the course of her healing. Realistic and wise, the nurse reminded the woman that ups and downs are part of the healing life—meaning the "downs" would come again. Yet, the nurse also reminded her that she or someone else would assist her through difficult times whenever she needed.

Now the feeding tube and the urinary catheter were removed, and the woman wheeled her own chair.

In Ethics in Practice 24-4, the woman begins to be demanding. What can this mean when she has had such effective and skilled care? What more can she demand? The word "demand" means to ask urgently and firmly, leaving no chance for refusal, from the Latin *demandāre*, meaning to entrust (Morris 1978, 350), to give into someone's hand (1527). The woman seems to be asking for more now. She seems to realize that as a person she must now move to take charge of her own life, to more radically take "her own breath"—a second breath, a second birth assumed by oneself—willed by oneself and not by the demands of physiology (Irigaray 2002). But she still cannot do this alone, so she again entrusts herself to others, gives herself into other's hands *by her own request*. By her demands she asks for engagement. Because she cannot be fully vigilant in all parts of her life she entrusts herself to others—in order to bring herself into harmony with herself and her renewed life.

Relational **engagement** is located in the shared moment when people have found a way to look at something together. They "compose a mutually satisfactory interpretation of their situation... freely accepting or declining the interpretation that each other offers, until they reach a meaning that both affirm" (Gadow and Schroeder 1996, 131). This meaning is found in those moments when the nurse comes to see what the patient really needs—to connect to her son and to her community. The moment brings the woman to tears when she is driven through her own town. These tears acknowledge the reality of mortality and what she has lost (such as walking freely or looking after children) and what she has gained (re-connection to her world—love for husband and family and community support). There is power in the experience of people with different experiences (nurse and patient) coming to understand something together.

Yet how can nurses engage with patients and with one another? How can we stand close to someone else in order to understand someone else's experience and to recognize someone else's pain? Often there is concern about over-involvement between nurse and patient—standing too close, leading to abusive situations. Yet there is a need to be equally concerned about under-involvement and the disengagement that some say has led to a humanitarian crisis in which there is little connection between people—a crisis that harms patients and professionals alike. How can busy professionals have time for engagement with patients? How can nurses be asked to do more than they are already doing? Perhaps engagement is not something that can be required by any professional body (e.g., the Canadian Nurses Association in its Code of Ethics). Rather, engagement is something that each nurse and each professional has to consider individually. With this woman, it was just one nurse, one person, whose action seemed to change the course of care. Of course, this is not the only example that can be found, but it is a significant one.

The health care encounter brings into focus a particular kind of relation that connects strangers together in meaningful and even intimate ways. The nurse comes with specific competencies and a commitment to exploring what needs to be done for *this* person (respecting autonomy, values, confidentiality, and so forth) who comes for care. When a relationship is engaged, the patient comes with willingness to discuss health care needs in an environment where trust (entrusting) is an essential ingredient. According to Charles Taylor (1985), it is the self-interested focus of modern life and the primacy of technological or instrumental reasoning (with its search for control and domination of life and death) that fragments community life and leads to general malaise or indifference to the needs of others.

In a technical relationship, one nurse is interchangeable with another nurse and patients can be identified according to diseases or problems. As nurses find that they are expected to do more with insufficient time, and while they want to do good, they find that they cannot do so in the manner they believe is best for their patients (Rodney and Varcoe 2001). This reality can lead to a bigger problem, for when patients are treated as objects (diseases or problems) because of too many expectations, nurses become objects as well—faceless prac-titioners who mechanically carry out their professional duties. Is it possible that when we distance ourselves from others we all lose? Perhaps this is when nurses experience "burnout"—that feeling of exhaustion and overload that occurs when we take on (either by demand or choice) more than we can handle. Reasons for burnout can include the unrecog-nized separation of body and mind that leads to lack of embodiment, when we are not able to be fully present in the moment, when there is no time for care for the self, and where we become focused only on outcomes—the need to accomplish more. Engagement, attention to *this* moment, *this* nurse, *this* patient, *this* place may be one way for nurses to renew attention to the meaning found in their work. For patients it might offer opportunities to find meaning in their illness. Engagement may offer a way for each to make meaning out of tragic experi-ences—a meaning that can only be found by each person in his or her own way. Through the experience of responsiveness to the needs of both oneself and the other, the nurse discovers and responds to the moral commitment of relationship.

Bauman (1993) suggests that the moral impulse arises because one person elicits a response from another. Engagement with others allows one to discover abilities that one did not previously know one had: "The Other enables me to do more than I can do" (Lippitz 1993, 59). Such engaged relationships make it possible, not just necessary, to be moral: we gain ourselves, so to speak, and find out what we are capable of. Each of us does not lose the self through attention to the other. From this point of view, engagement does not ask for *selflessness* on the part of the nurse, but for both nurse and patient to be recognized as *whole beings* (both self-interested and other-focused) in what Dillon (1992) calls person-directed attention.

The notion of reciprocity, or mutuality, is sometimes hard to grasp for nurses and other health care professionals because a major impetus for becoming a professional is the desire to do good for others. Yet the moment we step out of mutuality, moral angst and depletion become a danger—we feel we give more than we receive. With engagement, nurses receive as well as give. Could increased attention to mutuality and engagement with each other lead to a new creativity in professional practice, decreased stress, increased self-confidence and satisfaction? A new creativity would require the "imaginative grasp of the relevant webs of interdependency" in which "concepts like sufficiency, wholeness, health, participation, diversity, possibility, creativity become the keywords, instead of privation, rationing, authority, centralization, rationalization, downsizing, inevitability, and management"(Peacock 1999, 705, 710). Here we begin to see the rippling effects of a relational ethic; the ethical space that begins between professional and patient needs to extend to organizational spaces as well. Perhaps this is why relational ethics cannot be understood as an ethic only for nursing, nor even health professionals, but an ethic for living life together in a finite and interdependent world.

One difficulty that is frequently raised about engagement between nurse and patient is the matter of time. There is just is not enough time in the health care environment for engagement. Even with the benefits of technology there is not enough time. Perhaps it is *because* of technology (and the technological attitude) that there is not enough time. Yet the image of patients lined up in emergency rooms gives reality to the fact that time and resources are limited. Approaches to time management or efforts to simplify activities may not be enough to deal with the reality of busier and more hectic lives. So while it is true that there is need for more time and resources available for nurses and other professional staff, this outward resource may not be the *only* consideration. Would engagement with patients and colleagues in more meaningful ways be helpful, or would it only make matters worse?

With attention to time, it might be useful to think of the measure of an engaged relationship to be inner rather than outer. Let us look at the notion of lived time—time in which we are fully present to the other person and the needs of the moment. Richard Niebuhr (1963) describes being present to another person as a *time-full* encounter. The time-full self is a "self that is always in the present to be sure, always in the moment, so that the very notion of the present is probably unthinkable apart from some explicit reference to a self, I and now belong together" (93). For the nurse in the clinical example to be present in *this* moment, she or he will need to hold past activities and future responsibilities at bay to be able to be in the moment with the woman. Or perhaps, as Niebuhr (1963) states, when one is in the present moment, past, present, and future "are dimensions of the active self's time-fullness" (99)—past and future are part of the present. By being truly present to another through engagement, we may make it possible to expand time—at least for that moment.

Anita Tarzian (1998) distinguishes between the Greek notion of non-linear time (*kairos*) and chronological time (*kronos)*. With non-linear time, we remain fully present in the moment, to the point of losing track of time or finding that time loses its demands. Tarzian says that when nurses say they *spend time* with patients, they may be focusing on the chronological sense of time. When nurses say that they are *being with* patients, there is a sense of time stopping so that it is time that cannot be "spent." "*Spending* refers to attaching monetary value to an experience and exchanging units of equal value. *Waiting upon* [being with], as a gift, cannot be spent or bought" (Tarzian 1998, 180, italics in original).

Nurses often realize that being with patients (*kairos*) at crucial moments will save chronological time (*kronos*) in the end. Being with patients is often actualized by dialogue. We will now turn to a discussion of dialogue as an activity that is needed in relational ethics.

RELATIONAL ETHICS THROUGH DIALOGUE

Genuine dialogue is the place where relational ethics is most easily realized—the place where the themes of relational environment, embodiment, mutuality, and engagement are enacted. Dialogue is not a one-sided interview for the purpose of diagnosis so that treatment can begin. Rather, **dialogue** is the beginning of treatment itself—a conversation that must be sustained throughout the whole process of recovery (Gadamer 1996). Placing emphasis on dialogue reminds us that healing does not lie within the jurisdiction of the nurse, doctor, or patient, but within nature itself. Dialogue, when recognized as an aspect of the treatment, expects something from nurses and doctors. It also expects patients to make their own contribution to sustaining this treatment. As we see in Ethics in Practice 24-5, as the woman recovers her breath, her second breath, she becomes more demanding. She begins to speak, to demand. She wants dialogue.

Ethics in Practice 24-5	The Breath—Breathing and Speaking Together

And so the days, weeks, and months passed, and the woman was moved to a rehab ward. Her arms were getting stronger, her legs still too fragile, it seemed, to imagine walking or even standing on them. Yet the woman did imagine. She wanted to have a picture taken when she was able to stand on her own. It was the picture she wanted to send to the specialists who had reconstructed her shattered bones. She wanted them to know how grateful she was that she had their special, unique ability to care for her. And one specialist, too, must have imagined the possibilities of her standing and walking again as she called her family, as well as her current physician, to find out how the woman was—concerned that she not stand too soon, that she lay on her stomach to avoid contractors of her hips from long periods in the wheelchair. The professionals wanted to know that the work of the team was a success for this woman. The talk continued between husband and family, between doctors, nurses, social workers, and rehab therapists. The conversation grew to include brothers and sisters, nieces and nephews, friends, and neighbours. While in hospital, the woman's contact with nurses offered the consistent (daily) opportunity for conversation.

If we recognize that dialogue is part of treatment rather than a preparation for treatment or for evaluating treatment, we realize the ethical responsibility to promote, maintain, or revive dialogue. In Ethics in Practice 24-5, dialogue is not merely a mode of communicating instructions or evaluating effectiveness. Rather, it is seen as necessary in order for nurse and patient to understand together.

Let us come back to breath. Proper attention to the breath, re-learning to breathe, is, as Irigaray (2002) points out, necessary for us to take charge of our own life, and with this attention we begin to see the relationship between breathing and speaking. As we allow ourselves to take the breath within our body, to expand our lungs, to let go of the air again, we feel the rhythm of our own life that makes it possible to be able to speak from an inner truth. McPherson (2000), paralyzed due to childhood polio, uses glossopharyngeal breathing in which he activates the muscles of the glossa and the pharynx. This "frog breathing" (McPherson 2000, 30) is a skill that he has mastered that allows him to be free of the respirator while awake. With this skill, he gasps for air by moving his jaw up and down, and as he releases the air he is able to speak. In McPherson's situation the connection between breath and speech is obvious. Irigaray (2002) suggests that it is patriarchal philosophies and religious traditions that have immobilized breathing by giving emphasis to words and speech ("have substituted words for life without carrying out the necessary links between the two" [Irigaray 2002, 51]). Irigaray goes on to suggest that one way to recover the links between words and life is to recover the breath, which would "allow reciprocally conserving, regenerating, and enriching life and speech" (51). Perhaps even for nurses there may be a need to take time to breathe, to help us to feel grounded in our own bodies so that activities and speech are strong and appropriate to the moment (see also Chapter 21).

Dialogue involves attention to both the body and the mind—to the experiences of the feeling body as well as the logic of rational thinking. Jopling (2000) identifies six characteristics of a dialogic encounter that are useful for this discussion:

1. Dialogue is open textured, not goal oriented. One does not know what will come of it. One does not know how each partner in the dialogue will be changed, how own self-understandings will be expanded. In genuine dialogue nothing is predetermined as there may be unexpected outcomes.

2. In dialogue there is mutual respect in order to encounter the other as other. It is otherness, rather than sameness or like-mindedness that is manifest. One cannot learn from the other if one consistently puts what is said into one's own terms in order to fit one's own point of view. In mutual respect one regards the other as a responsible partner within established norms of trustworthiness.

3. In dialogue one addresses the other with forthrightness and therefore responds with forthrightness. One is present to the other's company. "One of the most common events of everyday life is the act of addressing and responding to another person face to face, engaging the other in a way that is frank and unrehearsed in order to establish a commonly understood meaning. Language would be a rootless and impersonal system of signs if it were not anchored in the face-to-face confrontation" (156).

4. When dialogue is embodied with evocative components, one recognizes that feelings and emotion are not accompaniment to careful responses to questions. Rather, feelings (such as compassion, anger, sympathy, shame, desire) themselves constitute the response. Feelings give body to words—and bring back words to the body.

5. Dialogue signals mutual recognition by addressing the other as *you*. The pronoun "you" is personal and calls forth the personal in "me" as well.

6. Dialogue is found in the ethical moment—when one is present *with* and *for* someone, not merely thinking about them. Here the person is not an object of observation but is "called into conversation" with an actual other, bringing about an understanding of moral and social identity (152–157).

The ethical space is filled with dialogue, embodied dialogue, which includes silence as well as speech. "To be standing humanly... is to be not only at the brink of silence, but also in the depth of silence, awaiting the arrival of the poetic word that affirms the life of this life" (Aoki 1991, 45). Through dialogue, which could be in the actual words, in the silences, or in touch, the patient and nurse find their own way.

RELATIONAL ETHICS: UNDERSTANDING AND KNOWING OURSELVES AS WE ENGAGE WITH OTHERS

Throughout this chapter, we have explored relational ethics in nursing. We began with the proposition that all relationships, as experienced in daily life, are moral. With such a perspective, it is an ethical responsibility for nurses to consider the quality of their relationship with patients and with colleagues. The quality of relationship needs as much attention as the quality of nursing science and the quality of clinical competence. Throughout the chapter we used a clinical example to highlight relational themes: environment, embodiment, mutual respect, and engagement. The breath, one of the most important physical aspects of life, was used to evocatively provide another avenue for connecting to the relational themes: environment (the importance of the breath/air for survival of the individual and the world); embodiment (the breath as connecting the body as object to the body as lived); mutual respect (the need to breathe for oneself and to support the breath for others); and engagement (the need for breath to speak). In the final section of the chapter, we looked more closely at dialogue, a foundational action that explores the ethical space between people. As Ethics in Practice 24-6 illustrates, the bridge between the individual and community brings both together, to the enrichment of both.

Ethics in Practice 24-6	The Breath—Bridging Autonomy and Community

It was not long after the woman was settled in the fourth hospital that she received, at her home address, a bill from the third hospital where she spent less than two hours. The bill was for services rendered at a cost of more than U.S. $14,000. Neither the woman nor her family could have managed to pay this huge cost of just one short episode in this woman's care. In Canada, citizens are committed to financing a universal health care system in which all people get the care they need. The woman, through the concrete financial support of the health care system and the competent physical, emotional, and social support of professional staff and family, moved from bed to wheelchair, to crutches, and to canes in her desire to walk again. Unlike a fairy tale, this story does not end with a statement that the woman lived happily ever after. Nor does it tell the story of the other person in the accident whom the woman met again as they both worked at recovering their own lives. Rather this story shows the need for individual and community to support each other on the road to health. It cannot happen alone.

In this chapter, I have discussed how a relational ethic could assist professionals, especially nurses, to improve ethical care. As readers will recognize, relational ethics is not a panacea for easy ethical care; rather the focus on relationship may make ethical considerations even more complex. Yet individual nurses, who number in the hundreds in the months and years of this woman's care, each have opportunity to practise relational ethics. Each nurse has the opportunity to enact the health care environment, embodiment, mutual respect, and engagement through the daily care of people who experience illnesses, traumas, and even death. For the woman in our six-part clinical example, nurses were integral to her healing and growth, and, perhaps, their relationship with this woman may have also assisted nurses to come to know themselves better.

In the end, it seems that relational ethics is really about understanding and knowing ourselves as we engage with others. In nursing and in health care, the particular environment of health and illness is a profound and important means by which we confront ourselves in a community of other people within a focus on relationships. "Not only does dialogue open the self to itself by opening it to the other person; it is by means of reflective dialogue that persons are 'talked into' knowing who they are" (Jopling 2000, 157). Perhaps relational ethics for nursing reminds nurses as well as other caregivers to consider how important it is to continue to know more about ourselves, as nurses and as human beings. In that self-knowledge and openness, we can care for and know others.

FOR REFLECTION

1. Consider how relational ethics is already part of nursing practice using the relational themes of environment, embodiment, mutual respect, and engagement.

2. How, specifically, can nurses support a relational approach to ethics in working with other members of the health care team, including patients?

3. While ethical principles and virtues are already a part of ethical teaching and nursing, how might a focus of relational ethics be taught in nursing ethics?

4. How can we foster relational values in health care organizations so that nurses are better supported in enacting a relational ethic?

REFERENCES

Aoki, T. 1991. *Inspiriting curriculum and pedagogy: Talks to teachers*. Edmonton: Faculty of Education.

Bauman, Z. 1993. *Postmodern ethics*. Oxford: Blackwell.

Bergum, V. 1997. *A child on her mind: The experience of becoming a mother*. Westport, CT: Bergin & Garvey.

Bergum, V and Dossetor, J. In press. *Relational ethics. The full meaning of respect.* Hagerstown, Maryland: University Publishing Group.

Caputo, J.D. 1989. Disseminating originary ethics and the ethics of dissemination. In A.B. Dallery and C.E. Scott (Eds.), *The question of the other: Essays in contemporary continental philosophy* (pp. 55–62). Albany, NY: State University of New York Press.

Dillon, R.S. 1992. Respect and care: Toward moral integration. *Canadian Journal of Philosophy, 22*(1), 105–132.

Gadamer, H-G. 1996. *The enigma of health.* Stanford, CA: Stanford University Press.

Gadow, S. 1980. Existential advocacy: Philosophical foundation of nursing. In S. Spicker and S. Gadow (Eds.), *Nursing: Images and ideals: Opening dialogue with the humanities* (pp. 79–101). New York: Springer.

Gadow, S. 1989. Clinical subjectivity: Advocacy with silent patients. *Nursing Clinics of North America, 24*(2), 535–541.

Gadow, S. 1994. Whose body? Whose story? The question about narrative in women's health care. *Soundings: An International Journal, 77*(3–4), 295–307.

Gadow, S. and Schroeder, C. 1996. An advocacy approach to ethics and community health. In E.T. Anderson and J. McFarlane (Eds.), *Community as partner: Theory and practice in nursing*, 2nd ed. (pp. 123–137). Philadelphia: J.B. Lippincott.

Gaita, R. 1991. *Good and evil: An absolute conception.* London: Macmillan.

Gonzales, A. 2002. Hospitals adopting new methods of handling waste. *Sacramento Business Journal.* Available online: www.bizjournals.com/sacramento/stories/2000/03/06/focus2.html

Irigaray, L. 2002. *Between east and west. From singularity to community.* Translator: S. Pluhácek. New York: Columbia University Press.

Jopling, D.A. 2000. *Self-knowledge and the self.* New York: Routledge.

Keiser, R.M. 1996. *Roots of relational ethics: Responsibility in origin and maturity in H. Richard Niebuhr.* Atlanta, GA: Scholars Press.

Lippitz, W. 1990. Ethics as limits of pedagogical reflection. *Phenomenology and Pedagogy, 8*, 49–60.

McPherson, G. 2000. *With every breath I take. One person's extraordinary journey to a healthy life and how you can share it.* Edmonton: Gary McPherson.

Morris, W. (Ed.). 1978. *The American heritage dictionary of the ethics language.* Boston: Houghton Mifflin.

Niebuhr, H.R. 1963. *The responsible self: An essay in Christian moral philosophy.* New York: Harper and Row.

Olthuis, J.H. (Ed.). 2000. *Towards an ethic of community: Negotiations of difference in a pluralist society.* Waterloo, ON: Wilfrid Laurier University Press.

Peacock, K.A. 1999. Symbiosis and the ecological role of philosophy. *Dialogue, 38*, 699–717.

Robert, B. 1986. Confronting technophobia: A topology. *Phenomenology and Pedagogy, 4*(2), 3–21.

Rodney, P. and Varcoe, C. 2001. Towards ethical inquiry in the economic evaluations of nursing practice. *Canadian Journal of Nursing Research, 33*(1), 35–37.

Romanow, R.J. 2002. *Building on values. The future of health care in Canada—Final report.* Commission on the Future of Health Care in Canada. Ottawa: National Library of Canada. Available online: www.healthcarecommission.ca

Tarzian, A. 1998. *Breathing lessons: An exploration of caregiver experiences with dying patients who have air hunger.* Unpublished doctoral dissertation. University of Maryland, Baltimore, MD.

Taylor, C.A. 1993. Positioning subjects and objects: Agency, narration, relationality. *Hypatia, 8*(1), 55–79.

Taylor, C. 1985. *Philosophy and the human sciences.* Volume 2 of *Philosophical Papers.* New York: Cambridge University Press.

chapter twenty-five

Toward a Moral Horizon

Janet L. Storch,
Patricia Rodney, and
Rosalie Starzomski

Well, we have to have some hope. And so that's how I look at it.... I am in no way thinking that there's not more work to be done. There definitely is. But I have seen successes and so I think it is possible.... [W]e need to engage everybody... it has to be a level playing field. So... all people, physicians, nurses... and our health care team [have] to... have basically the same value and mission really, about what we're trying to do (Nurse research participant, Rodney et al. 2002, 91; see also Appendix A).

The challenges nurses face in attempting to enact the ethics of their practice are rooted in history and are unlikely to go away in the near future. As we conclude this book, the events surrounding SARS (Severe Acute Respiratory Syndrome) continue to evolve. These events have included a variety of occasions in which nurses spoke out about the unmistakable public safety concerns that were evident as SARS continued to spread. Specifically, nurses warned that the incidence of SARS was being underestimated and that some illness and deaths might have been prevented. They requested more resources to deal safely with the new cases, and, in Ontario, called for a comprehensive public inquiry into the handling of the SARS crisis. The government of Ontario eventually announced that an inquiry would be held into the management of the SARS outbreak. It was not the *public* inquiry nurses had hoped for, and they continued to press for a meaningful, transparent inquiry.

In the wake of this outbreak, we are left with some too-familiar questions. Why did it take so long for nurses to be heard as SARS continued to wreak havoc in the health care system? And why was the response only partial? Will the lessons of recent history—for example, the Sinclair Inquiry in Winnipeg (see Chapter 2 and Chapter 5)—ever be learned? How is it that nurses continue to be marginalized and devalued in health care when their role is all about the *care* in health care?

We do not purport that our text contains definitive answers to the multitude of questions arising from the management of the SARS outbreak or other major ethical questions. But we believe that within the preceding chapters readers should find deeper and newer ways to consider what it means to engage in safe, competent, ethical nursing practice. Throughout the text, the authors emphasize the ways that nurses can enact their role as advocates and influence change within the health care system. Such engagement involves understanding the background (the *moral landscape*), the environment (the *moral climate*), and the current and future challenges (the *moral horizon*) of nursing ethics.

WHAT WE HAVE OFFERED

In Section I: Moral Landscape, historical and philosophical analyses are provided in Chapters 2 and 3 as background to an understanding of nursing ethics and as tools in meeting and addressing future challenges. In the "theory quartet" (Chapters 4–7), an extensive overview of health ethics, organizational ethics, and nursing ethics is provided. This includes attention to theories, principles, contextual features, and models. The intent of this group of chapters is to ground nurses in ethical theory and application—to equip readers to become more "ethically fit" and to enable them to more capably assess newer ways of thinking about ethics. To conclude the analysis of our *moral landscape*, moral agency and its import for nursing practice is then explored in Chapter 8.

Section II: Moral Climate focuses on the current situation in which nurses and other health professionals seek to be ethical. Beginning with an analysis of health care funding and delivery in respect to health reforms, Chapter 9 stresses that these involve ethical choices that cannot be considered irrelevant to nursing ethics. In focusing on the *moral climate* of nursing practice, Chapter 10 emphasizes the power structures in health care that often interfere with appropriate ethical decisions and actions and authors call for the development of a moral community. Considering health care through an ecological lens, Chapter 11 provides new ways of understanding and recognizing possibilities for healing the health care system. Two situated examples are presented in Section II—one on home health care and ethics (Chapter 12) and the other on care at the end of life (Chapter 13). These serve as illustrations of the effects of our ethical choices in structuring the climate of health care. Concluding this section, a focus on narrative approaches in ethics (Chapter 14) offers ways to sharpen our moral sensitivity and to help others see the ethics in the everyday more clearly.

In Section III: Moral Horizons, a wider array of ethical concerns and challenges that we consider to be highly relevant to frontiers in nursing ethics are highlighted. Biotechnology (Chapter 15), globalization (Chapter 16), and research ethics (Chapter 17) are among these significant developments about which nurses will need to develop greater knowledge and ethical awareness. Three chapters challenge our thinking about the breadth of our ethical scope: the analyses of genetics and disability (Chapter 18); children and moral agency

(Chapter 19); and violence against women (Chapter 20) all demand that we consider the limitations of taken-for-granted current health care practices and enlarge our thinking about ethical practice in these areas. Concluding Section III are four chapters that call us to a heightened awareness of how we engage in ethical nursing practice. The authors discuss four approaches that can guide advances in nursing practice: focusing on embodiment of mind, emotion, and action (Chapter 21); allowing emotion its place in ethical awareness and judgment (Chapter 22); attending to the spirituality of those we care for (Chapter 23); and understanding what it means to be in relational ethical practice (Chapter 24). These chapters furnish thought-provoking material encouraging nurses to renew their commitment to using the full resources of their being—to be in relationship in practice.

WHAT REMAINS

As our work on this book has progressed, we have become mindful of the many other chapters we might have included. We might have included full chapters on ethics in the care of the elderly (discussed in Chapter 6), on the ethics of health promotion (discussed in Chapter 8), on the ethics of Aboriginal health care (discussed in Chapter 5 and Chapter 7), and on the ethics of interdisciplinary teamwork (touched on in Chapters 1, 8, 10, 24, and others); and greater attention might have been given to issues in developing codes of ethics (a discussion begun in Chapters 1 and 2). No doubt there are many other issues not yet in the realm of our own thinking. Such may well be the subject for inclusion in further editions of our book and in the writing that our colleagues in nursing and other disciplines are doing or may do.

ON THE HORIZON

As we close, we offer a cautionary note that deals with the status of nursing as a profession in the 21st century and the critical need for us, as nurses, to sharpen our political acumen. We began this final chapter with a concern about the continued marginalization of nurses' voices. The importance of achieving greater equity in whose voices are heard in health care planning and delivery cannot be overemphasized. The health of the community depends upon equity of access to input into health policy. How will nurses work to employ ethics in their political strategizing?

Two developments in nursing could lull nurses into thinking that their concerns will receive greater voice. Both of these developments relate to educational and practice *gains* for nurses. The first development is the legislative mandate in most provinces to raise the educational level required for entry into registered nursing practice across Canada. This move to require a baccalaureate degree for entry to practice is to begin in 2005. The second key development is the gradual implementation of advanced nursing practice, through legislation, to allow nurse practitioners a fuller scope of practice in primary health care. Both of these changes could be considered to raise the status of nursing. These types of legislative developments have been long-sought goals of the majority of Canadian nurses. On the other hand, acknowledged and documented in this text in many places are the brutal effects of past and current health care "reforms" on nurses, patients, families, communities, and other health care providers. For the most part, these reforms have not been kind to nurses and the important (largely invisible) work that nurses do. So, what does it mean that the need for increased nursing knowledge is being recognized by politicians in the form of a baccalaureate degree as entry to practice and that advanced nursing knowledge is being recognized as an important contribution to the health care system?

Nurses must continue to be clear about their first priority in health care—that is, the needs of the people for whom they provide care. Achieving a baccalaureate degree as entry to practice will not do our profession or the persons we care for much good if nurses' conditions of work continue to threaten competent and ethical practice (see Chapters 10–12), or, worse yet, if registered nurses are (inappropriately) replaced even more than they have already been replaced with less qualified staff. Similarly, having nurses show their strength and potential in advanced practice roles will not do our profession or the persons we care for much good if attention is diverted from the urgent needs of frontline nurses practising in hospitals, communities, and long-term care settings, or if nurses are used (inappropriately) to replace physicians. Clearly, achieving the baccalaureate as entry to practice and obtaining recognition of advanced nursing practice roles are potential solutions to the problems that plague health care *but only if individual nurses and the nursing profession as a whole have a meaningful say in their own destiny, and choose and act wisely.*

We are at a convergence of several realities. We know that nurses rate high in public trust[1]—indeed highest among those professions with inside knowledge of the health care system; there is data available (with more being collected) that describes the state of nursing in Canada; recognition is being given for the complexity of the professional nursing role; and it appears that governments are interested in making changes in how health care is delivered. This suggests that nurses are in a position to be heard, both by the public and by decision-makers (Haines 2002, 2). However, we must not be complacent. To ensure that our voices are heard, we must show vision and leadership, and at the same time, develop and use appropriate approaches to continue to influence change. Continuous critical reflection and political action are required to ensure that our messages are given prominence in the health care arena. And in this arena, we need to be very clear about *who we serve*—that is, persons who require care rather than governments and politicians.

This means that our future horizon ought to include a more purposeful linking of ethics with politics (see Chapters 5, 6, and 9). Effecting *the good* of individuals and of society through nursing practice should never be taken for granted. We must continue to examine our values and our ethics and how to further them in a democracy that is supposed to be founded on an egalitarian ideal and that is supposed to respect diversity. We need to be thoughtful and careful as we chart the course ahead in our current sociopolitical climate. In some small way, we hope our text can add to the potential for nurses to make ethical and political choices knowingly and wisely. We agree with the nurse whom we cited at the outset of this chapter. As a profession, we have achieved a great deal, yet a great deal more remains to be done. And we most definitely have hope for the future.

ENDNOTE

1. In an editorial written by Judith Haines in *Canadian Nurse* (2002), she described a Canadian Press/Leger marketing poll conducted in January 2002, in which it was reported that 96 percent of Canadians trust nurses—the second highest trust for any of the professions noted in the survey. Firefighters were ranked first at 98 percent; farmers third at 93 percent; doctors fourth at 92 percent, and police officers fifth at 88 percent. Haines concluded that because the status of the health care system is one of the key issues identified by the public as an area of concern, it suggests that nurses are well located to influence change

in the system and are positioned to be heard by the public and politicians (who, by the way, received a remarkably low [18 percent] trust rating in the marketing poll). In December 2002, when the poll was repeated with a sample of 1,529 Canadians, of the 20 professions, firefighters, nurses, and farmers were again ranked the most trusted professionals at 96 percent, 94 percent, and 91 percent, respectively. The top five included doctors (89 percent) and teachers (88 percent), with politicians (14 percent), car salespeople (20 percent), and publicists (38 percent) at the end of the list.

REFERENCES

Canadian Press. Feb. 16, 2003. Canadians really trust firefighters, nurses and farmers, poll suggests.

Haines, J. 2002. The convergence of trust and concern. *Canadian Nurse, 98*(4), 2.

Rodney, P., Varcoe, C., Storch, J.L., McPherson, G., Mahoney, K., Brown, H., Pauly, B., Hartrick Doane, G. and Starzomski, R. 2002. Navigating toward a moral horizon: A multi-site qualitative study of nurses' enactment of ethical practice. *Canadian Journal of Nursing Research, 34*(3), 75–102.

Appendix A

The Ethics of Practice: Context and Curricular Implications for Nursing

J. Storch, Principal Investigator
Co-Investigators: Gweneth Hartrick, Paddy Rodney,
Rosalie Starzomski, and Colleen Varcoe.
Graduate Students: Bernadette Pauly, Helen Brown, Gladys
McPherson, and Karen Mahoney

Project funded by Associated Medical Services, Inc.

BACKGROUND TO THE STUDY

Our project in the Ethics of Practice was stimulated by our questioning whether our teaching of nursing ethics was meaningful to our students. In considering how to revise our curriculum we believed we should seek answers from clinical practice. Thus, we designed a study to gain a better understanding about how nurses understand ethics and how they engage in ethical practice.

FOCUS OF THE STUDY

Because we recognized that understanding more about the meaning of ethics for nurses providing direct care would be a first step in a series of steps to revisit and revise our teaching of nursing ethics, we designed an exploratory study with a broad focus. Our initial research question to participants was "What does ethics mean to you in your practice?" Prompts included asking nurses to tell us about a time when they believed they were practising ethically, or times when they believed they were not practising ethically.

PARTICIPANTS AND DATA COLLECTION

Our qualitative data was collected through a series of focus groups across a wide variety of nursing units and community nursing services. Administrative and ethics approvals for the study were obtained from the University of Victoria and from the research ethics committee of a mid-sized metropolitan area. Administrative and ethics approvals were also obtained from each of the regions in a larger metropolitan area. Data collection took place between 1999 and 2001.

Unit managers, clinical resource nurses, or staff nurses in various units or services were contacted, and, if interested, a meeting time was established for us to meet with 2–7 nurses in a focus group. At the time of the meeting, the study was explained to the nurses and consent forms were provided and collected (leaving each nurse with a copy for future contact). Nineteen focus groups were conducted in and surrounding a large metropolitan area and in and around a mid-size metropolitan city. The focus groups included nurses working in maternity, long-term care, home care, community care, critical care, the operating room, emergency, rehabilitation, medical, surgical, and pediatric care. The nurses included staff nurses (12 focus groups), student nurses (4 focus groups), and nurses in advanced nursing practice (3 focus groups). Meetings were held on the unit or service, normally with two members of the research team—a faculty member facilitating the discussion and a graduate student taking responsibility for the logistics (e.g., room arrangements, notices to nurses, operating the tape recorder, obtaining consent, etc.) and taking field notes during the meeting.

DATA MANAGEMENT AND ANALYSIS

Following each focus group the tape was submitted to a secretary for transcription. A copy was then checked by the graduate student (RA) prior to being copied and distributed to the whole team. We followed a constructivist mode of inquiry using field notes and transcriptions with frequent team meetings to discuss and compare our thematic findings and to develop suggestions for analysis of specific themes. Our data analysis was concurrent with our data collection over the first year of the project (2000), and into the second year of our work we were able to construct thematic clusters with a visual map to suggest linkages.

FINDINGS

We learned from our participants about how ethical decisions actually unfolded and were acted upon, what they experienced when they were unable (or were able) to follow through on their decisions, what they believed the consequences were, and the effects of their practice environments on their decision-making. Further detail about the design, the analysis, and the outcomes is available in four publications based upon this project.

Publications

Rodney, P., Varcoe, C., Storch, J.L., McPherson, G., Mahoney, K., Brown, H., Pauly, B., Hartrick, G. and Starzomski, R. 2002. Navigating towards a moral horizon: A multisite qualitative study of ethical practice in nursing. *Canadian Journal of Nursing Research, 34*(3), 75–102.

Storch, J.L., Rodney, P., Pauly, B., Brown, H. and Starzomksi, R. 2002. Listening to nurses' moral voices: Building a quality health care environment. *Canadian Journal of Nursing Leadership, 15*(4), 7–16.

Hartrick Doane, G. 2002. Am I still ethical? The socially mediated process of nurses' moral identity. *Nursing Ethics, 9*(6), 623–635.

Hartrick Doane, G., Pauly, B., MacPherson, G. and Brown, H. In press. Exploring the heart of ethical nursing practice: Implications for nursing education. *Nursing Ethics.*

Varcoe, C., Rodney, P., Hartrick Doane, G., Pauly, B., Storch, J., Brown, H., McPherson, G., Mahoney, K. and Starzomski, R. In press. Ethical practice in nursing: Working the in-betweens. *Journal of Advanced Nursing.*

CURRENT AND FUTURE RESEARCH PROGRAM IN NURSING ETHICS

Based upon our findings, we considered it a moral imperative that we pursue a study of ethics in practice. This involves participatory action projects on two nursing units to demonstrate how attention to ethics can matter to practice and practice settings. That three-year study, funded by the Social Sciences and Humanities Research Council, is in process.

Another current study, funded by Associated Medical Services Inc., focuses on the curricular implications for nursing educators. In effect, our first inquiry included an exploration regarding what students have experienced in their practice and how this was or was not addressed through the integration of ethical content in their current curriculum. Our current focus is to attempt to address the shortcomings of previous teaching and demonstrate how new approaches to teaching ethics can make a difference.

Appendix B

Ethical Decision-Making Models

A. AN ETHICAL DECISION-MAKING FRAMEWORK FOR INDIVIDUALS

Michael McDonald, PhD
W. Maurice Young Centre for Applied Ethics
University of British Columbia 2003

1. Collect Information and Identify the Problem(s)

a) Identify what you know and *what you don't know.* Be prepared to add to/update your information throughout the decision-making process.

b) Gather as much information as possible on the patient's physical, psychological, social, cultural, and spiritual status, including changes over time. Seek input from the patient, family, friends, and other health care team members.

c) Investigate the patient's assessment of his or her own quality of life and wishes about the treatment/care decision(s) at hand. This includes determining the patient's competency. If the patient is not competent, look for an advance directive. Identify a proxy decision-maker for patients who are not competent and seek evidence of the patient's prior expressed wishes. Regardless of the patient's competence (capacity), involve the patient as much as possible in all decisions affecting him or her.

d) Include a family assessment: their roles, relationships, and relevant 'stories.'

e) Identify the health care team members involved and circumstances affecting them.

f) Summarize the situation briefly but with all the relevant facts and circumstances. Try to get a sense of the patient's overall illness trajectory.

g) What decisions have to be made? By whom?

2. Specify Feasible Alternatives for Treatment and Care

a) Use your clinical expertise to identify a wide range and scope of alternatives.

b) Identify *how* various alternatives might be implemented (e.g., time trials).

3. Use Your Ethics Resources to Evaluate Alternatives

a) Principles/concepts

- *AUTONOMY:* What does the patient want? How well has the patient been informed and/or supported? What explicit or implicit promises have been made to the patient?
- *NONMALEFICENCE:* Will this harm the patient? Others?
- *BENEFICENCE:* Will this benefit the patient? Others?
- *JUSTICE:* Consider the interests of all those (including the patient) who have to be taken into account. Are biases about the patient or family affecting your decision making? Treat like situations alike.
- *FIDELITY:* Are you fostering trust in patient/family/team relationships?
- *CARE*: Will the patient and family be supported as they deal with loss, grief, and/or uncertainty? What about any moral distress of team members? What principles of palliative care can be incorporated into the alternatives?
- *RELATIONAL AUTONOMY:* What relationships and social structures are affecting the various individuals involved in the situation? How can these relationships and social structures become more supportive of the patient, family members, and health care providers?

b) Standards

Examine professional norms, standards and codes, legal precedents, hospital policy.

c) Personal judgments and experiences

Consider yours, your colleagues' and other members of the health care team.

d) Organized procedures for ethical consultation

Consider a formal case conference(s), an ethics committee meeting, or an ethics consultant.

4. Propose and Test Possible Resolutions

a) Select the best alternative(s), all things considered.

b) Perform a sensitivity analysis. Consider your choice(s) critically: Which factors would have to change to get you to alter your decision(s)?

c) Think about the effects of your choice(s) upon others' choices: Are you making it easier for others (health care providers, patients and their families, etc.) to act ethically?

d) Is this what a compassionate health care professional would do in a caring environment?

e) Formulate your choice(s) as a general maxim for all similar situations. Think of situations where it does *not* apply. Consider situations where it does apply.

f) Are you and the other decision-makers still comfortable with your choice(s)? *If you do not have consensus, revisit the process.* Remember that you are not aiming at "the" perfect choice, but the best possible choice.

5. Make Your Choice.

Live with it.

Learn from it.

This framework is to be used as a guide rather than a "recipe." *Ethical decision-making is a process, best done in a caring and compassionate environment.* It will take time and may require more than one meeting with patient, family, and team members. The goal is to arrive at a decision that best reflects *what the patient would want* if he or she were fully informed and well supported.

Developed by: Dr. Michael McDonald (1993–present), W. Maurice Young Centre for Applied Ethics

Adapted by: Dr. P. Rodney & Dr. R. Starzomski (2003), University of Victoria School of Nursing & W. Maurice Young Centre for Applied Ethics

Versions of this framework are posted on the Centre for Applied Ethics web page: http://www.ethics.ubc.ca

B. STORCH MODEL FOR ETHICAL DECISION-MAKING FOR POLICY & PRACTICE*

Janet Storch, RN, PhD
Professor, University of Victoria School of Nursing 2003

1. Information & Identification
- Concern
- People/Population
- Ethical Components

2. Clarification & Evaluation

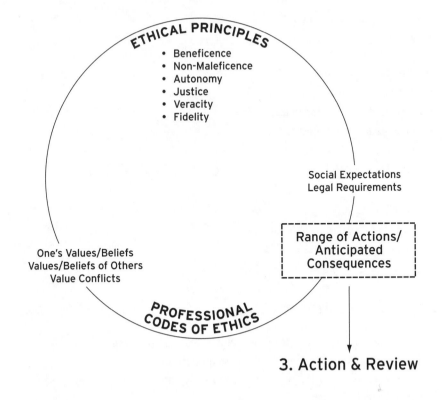

ETHICAL PRINCIPLES
- Beneficence
- Non-Maleficence
- Autonomy
- Justice
- Veracity
- Fidelity

Social Expectations
Legal Requirements

One's Values/Beliefs
Values/Beliefs of Others
Value Conflicts

Range of Actions/
Anticipated
Consequences

PROFESSIONAL
CODES OF ETHICS

3. Action & Review

*Reprinted from *Canadian Nursing Faces the Future*, 2nd edition, Alice J. Baumgart and Jenniece Larsen, eds., page 267, copyright 1992, with permission from Elsevier.

C. AN ETHICAL FRAMEWORK FOR MAKING ALLOCATION DECISIONS

Michael McDonald, PhD
W. Maurice Young Centre for Applied Ethics
University of British Columbia 2003

Step 1: Consultation Process

- Will it yield useful information?
- Do all the relevant parties have a fair say?
- competent representation for those who need help in presenting their interests?
- Does it avoid expert imperialism and conflicts of interest?

Step 2: Identify Distributional Issues

- What is being distributed?
- By which decision-makers?
- To what persons?
- From which persons?
- For what reasons?
- Are any of the above ethically suspect?
- Make the necessary corrections.

Step 3: Look Up, Down, Around

For impacts on:
- Population health
- Particular populations and patients
- Existing and future claims
- Systemic capacity and sustainability

Step 4: Four Ethical Tests

- Fiduciary test: best interests of present and future populations
- Fair dealing test: respecting the rights of all parties
- Good stewardship: using public resources efficiently for intended purposes
- Public processes: open and accountable

Step 5: Make Your Choice

- From the remaining options
- Live with the choice.
- Learn from it.
- Good CQI (continuous quality improvement)
- Good consultation and feedback

Appendix C

Code of Ethics for Registered Nurses*

Contents

*Reprinted with permission from the Canadian Nurses Association.

© Canadian Nurses Association 50 Driveway Ottawa ON K2P 1E2
Tel: (613) 237-2133 or 1-800-361-8404 Fax: (613) 237-3520
E-mail: pubs@cna-aiic.ca Web site: www.cna-aiic.ca August 2002 ISBN 1-55119-890-8

Preamble

This code of ethics for registered nurses is a statement of the ethical commitments[1] of nurses to those they serve. It has been developed by nurses for nurses and sets forth the ethical standards by which nurses are to conduct their nursing practice.[2]

Purpose of the Code

The code of ethics for registered nurses sets out the ethical behaviour expected of registered nurses in Canada. It gives guidance for decision-making concerning ethical matters, serves as a means for self-evaluation and self-reflection regarding ethical nursing practice and provides a basis for feedback and peer review. The code delineates what registered nurses must know about their ethical responsibilities, informs other health care professionals and members of the public about the ethical commitments of nurses and upholds the responsibilities of being a self-regulating profession. This code serves as an ethical basis from which to advocate for quality practice environments with the potential to impact the delivery of safe, competent and ethical nursing care.

While codes of ethics can serve to guide practice, it takes more than knowledge of general rules to ensure ethical practice. Sensitivity and receptivity to ethical questions must be part of nurses' basic education and should evolve as nurses develop their professional practice. Nursing practice involves attention to ethics at various levels: the individual person, the health care agency or program, the community, society and internationally.

Elements of the Code

The elements of this document include:

- A preamble highlighting changes influencing nursing practice;
- A description of the nature of ethics in nursing;
- A definition of values and the importance of relationships for ethical practice;
- A description of the eight values of the code;
- Explanatory responsibility statements based upon each value;
- Glossary;

---

1. In this document the terms moral and ethical are used interchangeably based upon consultation with nurse-ethicists and philosophers, while acknowledging that not everyone shares this usage.

2. In this document, nursing practice refers to all nurses' professional activities, inclusive of nursing education, administration, research and clinical or public health practice.

- Specific applications of the code (Appendix A);
- The code of ethics history (Appendix B); and
- Ethics reading resources.

Context of the Code

The Canadian Nurses Association's (CNA's) code of ethics reflects changes in social values and conditions that affect the health care system and create both new challenges and opportunities for the ethical practice of nursing. Examples of such challenges and opportunities are briefly below.

- Nurses have become more autonomous in their practice as a function of the development of nursing knowledge and research and changing patterns of care. For example, day surgeries and shortened lengths of stays have lead to nurses caring for people with complex care needs across acute, continuing, community and home care settings. With less direct supervision, greater individual accountability for safe, competent and ethical care is needed.
- Nurses have greater opportunities to provide benefit to people and communities through integrated team work. Effective team work requires clear and respectful communication which is essential to providing quality care. This goal has been difficult to achieve due to fiscal and systemic constraints.
- Traditionally nurses have been leaders in health promotion and primary health care, often in remote areas, and now increasingly in the community. These roles have become more important in the evolving climate of health care reform. Further, the emergence of communicable diseases, once thought conquered, and new infectious diseases have created serious public health challenges and reinforces the reality of the global community.
- The biological/genetic revolution, as well as other emerging technologies, raise profound changes in the human capacity to control disease and human reproduction as well as to govern access to health information. Comparable philosophical development in considering the ethics of these advances is, as yet, limited. The public needs knowledge and ethical guidance to make well-informed choices about the appropriate use of many of these advances.
- The adoption of a business approach to health care reform involves values of efficiency guided by outcome measures and often a re-orientation of priorities. Many have concerns that the values inherent in an industrial and/or for-profit approach could replace fundamental values underlying health care in Canada, such as provision for the care of vulnerable persons (eg. elderly), enhancing quality of life and solidarity in community. This might reflect a shift in public values.

The Nature of Ethics in Nursing

The ability of nurses to engage in ethical practice in everyday work and to deal with ethical situations, problems and concerns can be the result of decisions made at a variety of levels – individual, organizational, regional, provincial, national and international. Differing responsibilities, capabilities and ways of working toward change also exist at these various levels. For all contexts and levels of decision-making, the code offers guidance for providing care that is congruent with ethical practice and for actively influencing and participating in policy development, review and revision.

The complex issues in nursing practice have both legal and ethical dimensions. An ideal system of law would be compatible with ethics, in that adherence to the law should never require the violation of ethics. There may be situations in which nurses need to take collective action to change a law that is incompatible with ethics. Still, the domains of law and ethics remain distinct, and the code addresses ethical responsibilities only.

Ethical Situations

In their practice, nurses constantly face situations involving ethics. These can be described in several ways. Description allows nurses to name their source of discomfort, a first step in addressing these ethical situations.

Everyday ethics: the way nurses approach their practice and reflect on their ethical commitment to the people[3] they serve. It involves the nurses' attention to common ethical events such as protecting a person's physical privacy.

Ethical violations: neglecting fundamental nursing obligations in a situation where the nurse knows that the action or lack of action is not appropriate.

Ethical dilemmas: situations arising when equally compelling ethical reasons both for and against a particular course of action are recognized and a decision must be made, for example, caring for a young teenager who is refusing treatment.

Ethical distress: situations in which nurses cannot fulfill their ethical obligations and commitments (i.e., their moral agency), or they fail to pursue what they believe to be the right course of action, or fail to live up to their own expectation of ethical practice, for one or more of the following reasons: error in judgment, insufficient personal resolve, or other circumstances truly beyond their control (Webster and Baylis 2000). They may feel guilt, concern, or distaste as a result.

Moral residue: "...that which each of us carries with us from those times in our lives when in the face of ethical distress we have seriously compromised ourselves or allowed ourselves to be compromised" (Webster and Baylis 2000, p. 218). Moral residue may, for example, be an outcome for some nurses who are required to implement behaviour modification strategies in the treatment of mentally ill persons (Mitchell 2001).

Ethical uncertainty: arises when one is unsure what ethical principles or values to apply or even what the moral problem is (Jameton 1984).

Nurses may experience ethical situations differently. Regardless of this, the code provides guidelines for reflection and guides to action and is intended to assist nurses through these experiences. Naming situations can be a turning point from which nurses can begin to address difficult situations, for example, dealing with ethical distress and moral residue can often lead to "defining moments" in one's career (e.g., if the nurse determines that this specific situation shall not occur again), thus allowing for positive outcomes to emerge from a difficult experience.

---

3. In this document the terms 'people they serve', 'person' or 'individual' refers to the patient, the client, the individual, family, group or community for whom care and/or health promotion assistance is provided.

Ethical Decision-Making

The Code of Ethics for Registered Nurses is structured around eight primary values that are central to ethical nursing practice:

- Safe, competent and ethical care
- Health and well-being
- Choice
- Dignity
- Confidentiality
- Justice
- Accountability
- Quality practice environments

With each value, specific responsibility statements are provided. Ethical reflection, which begins with a review of one's own ethics, and judgment are required to determine how a particular value or responsibility applies in a particular nursing context. There is room within the profession for disagreement among nurses about the relative weight of different ethical values and principles. More than one proposed intervention may be ethical and reflective of good practice. Discussion and questioning are extremely helpful in the resolution of ethical issues. As appropriate, persons in care, colleagues in nursing and other disciplines, professional nurses' associations, colleges, ethics committees and other experts should be included in discussions about ethical problems. In addition legislation, standards of practice, policies and guidelines of professional nurses' associations, colleges and nurses' unions may also assist in problem-solving. Further, models for ethical decision-making, such as those described in CNA's *Everyday Ethics*, can assist nurses in thinking through ethical problems.

Values

A value is a belief or attitude about the importance of a goal, an object, a principle or a behaviour. People may hold conflicting values and often may not be aware of their own values. Values refer to ideals that are desirable in themselves and not simply as a means to get something else. The values articulated in this code are grounded in the professional nursing relationship with individuals and indicate what nurses care about in that relationship. For example, to identify health and well-being as a value is to say that nurses care for and about the health and well-being of the people they serve. This relationship presupposes a certain measure of trust on the part of the person served. Care and trust complement one another in professional nursing relationships. Both hinge on the values identified in the code. By upholding these values in practice, nurses earn and maintain the trust of those in their care. For each of the values, the scope of responsibilities identified extends beyond individuals to include families, communities and society.

It should be noted that nurses' responsibilities to enact the values of the code cannot be separated from the responsibilities for other health care providers, health care agencies and policy makers at regional, provincial, national and international levels to foster health care delivery environments supporting ethical practice. While the code cannot enforce responsibilities outside of nursing, it can provide a powerful political instrument for nurses when they are concerned about being able to practice ethically.

Nursing Values Defined

Safe, Competent and Ethical Care

Nurses value the ability to provide safe, competent and ethical care that allows them to fulfill their ethical and professional obligations to the people they serve.

Health and Well-Being

Nurses value health promotion and well-being and assisting persons to achieve their optimum level of health in situations of normal health, illness, injury, disability, or at the end of life.

Choice

Nurses respect and promote the autonomy of persons and help them to express their health needs and values and also to obtain desired information and services so they can make informed decisions.

Dignity

Nurses recognize and respect the inherent worth of each person and advocate for respectful treatment of all persons.

Confidentiality

Nurses safeguard information learned in the context of a professional relationship, and ensure it is shared outside the health care team only with the person's informed consent, or as may be legally required, or where the failure to disclose would cause significant harm.

Justice

Nurses uphold principles of equity and fairness to assist persons in receiving a share of health services and resources proportionate to their needs and in promoting social justice.

Accountability

Nurses are answerable for their practice, and they act in a manner consistent with their professional responsibilities and standards of practice.

Quality Practice Environments

Nurses value and advocate for practice environments that have the organizational structures and resources necessary to ensure safety, support and respect for all persons in the work setting.

Nursing Values and Responsibility Statements

Safe, Competent and Ethical Care

Nurses value the ability to provide safe, competent and ethical care that allows them to fulfill their ethical and professional obligations to the people they serve.

1. Nurses must strive for the highest quality of care achievable.

2. Nurses must recognize that they have the ability to engage in determining and expressing their own moral choices. Their moral choices may be influenced by external factors (e.g. institutional values and constraints).

3. Nurses should be sufficiently clear and reflective about their personal values to recognize potential value conflicts.

4. Nurses must maintain an acceptable level of health and well-being in order to provide a competent level of service/care for the people they serve.

5. Nurses must base their practice on relevant research findings and acquire new skills and knowledge in their area of practice throughout their career.

6. Nurses must practice within their own level of competence. When aspects of care are beyond their level of competence, they must seek additional information or knowledge, seek help from their supervisor or a competent practitioner and/or request a different work assignment. In the meantime, nurses must provide care until another nurse is available to do so.

7. Nurses seeking professional employment must accurately state their area(s) of competence. They should seek reasonable assurance that employment conditions will permit care consistent with the values and responsibilities of the code.

8. Nurses must admit mistakes and take all necessary actions to prevent or minimize harm arising from an adverse event.

9. Nurses must strive to prevent and minimize adverse events[4] in collaboration with colleagues on the health care team. When adverse events occur, nurses should utilize opportunities to improve the system and prevent harm.

10. All nurses must contribute to safe and supportive work environments.

11. Nurse leaders have a particular obligation to strive for safe practice environments that support ethical practice.

12. Nurses should advocate for ongoing research designed to identify best nursing practices and for the collection and interpretation of nursing care data at a national level.

Health and Well-Being

Nurses value health promotion and well-being and assisting persons to achieve their optimum level of health in situations of normal health, illness, injury, disability or at the end of life.

1. Nurses must provide care directed first and foremost toward the health and well-being of the person, family or community in their care.

2. Nurses must recognize that health is more than the absence of disease or infirmity and must work in partnership with people to achieve their goals of maximum health and well-being.

3. Nurses should provide care addressing the well-being of the person in the context of that person's relationships with their family and community.

---

4. Adverse events include physician and interdisciplinary team error.

4. Nurses must foster comfort and well-being when persons are terminally ill and dying to alleviate suffering and support a dignified and peaceful death.

5. Nurses should provide the best care that circumstances permit even when the need arises in an emergency outside an employment situation.

6. Nurses should respect and value the knowledge, skills and perspectives of the persons in their care and must recognize, value and respect these while planning for and implementing care.

7. In providing care, nurses should also respect and value the knowledge and perspectives of other health providers. They should actively collaborate and where possible seek appropriate consultations and referrals to other health team members in order to maximum health benefits to people.

8. Nurses should recognize the need to address organizational, social, economic and political factors influencing health. They should participate with their colleagues, professional associations, colleges and other groups to present nursing views in ways that are consistent with their professional role, responsibilities and capabilities and which are in the interests of the public.

9. Nurses should recognize the need for a full continuum of accessible health services, including health promotion and disease prevention initiatives, as well as diagnostic, restorative, rehabilitative and palliative care services.

10. Nurses should seek ways to improve access to health care that enhances, not replaces, care by utilizing new research based technologies, such as telehealth (eg. telephone assessment and support).

11. Nurses should continue to contribute to and support procedurally and ethically rigorous research and other activities that foster the ongoing development of nursing knowledge.

12. Nurses who conduct or assist in the conduct of research must observe the nursing profession's guidelines, as well as other guidelines, for ethical research.[5]

Choice

Nurses respect and promote the autonomy of persons and help them to express their health needs and values and also to obtain desired information and services so that they can make informed decisions.

1. Nurses must be committed to building trusting relations as the foundation of meaningful communication, recognizing that building this relationship takes effort. Such relationships are critical to ensure that a person's choice is understood, expressed and advocated.

2. Nurses should provide the desired information and support required so people are enabled to act on their own behalf in meeting their health and health care needs to the greatest extent possible.

3. Nurses should be active in assisting persons to obtain the best current knowledge about their health condition.

4. Nurses must respect the wishes of those who refuse, or are not ready, to receive information about their health condition. They should be sensitive to the timing of information given and how the information is presented.

5. Please see CNA's Ethical Research Guidelines for Registered Nurses, 3rd ed. (2002) for full details.

5. Nurses must ensure that nursing care is provided with the person's informed consent. Nurses must also recognize that persons have the right to refuse or withdraw consent for care or treatment at any time.

6. Nurses must respect the informed choices of those with decisional capacity to be independent, to choose lifestyles not conducive to good health and to direct their own care as they see fit. However, nurses are not obligated to comply with a person's wishes when this is contrary to the law.

7. Nurses must continue to provide opportunities for people to make choices and maintain their capacity to make decisions, even when illness or other factors reduce the person's capacity for self-determination. Nurses should seek assent of the person when consent is not possible.

8. If nursing care is requested that is contrary to the nurse's personal values, the nurse must provide appropriate care until alternative care arrangements are in place to meet the person's desires.

9. Nurses must be sensitive to their position of relative power in professional relationships with persons. Nurses must also identify and minimize (and discuss with the health team) sources of coercion.

10. Nurses must respect a person's advance directives about present and future health care choices that have been given or written by a person prior to loss of decisional capacity.

11. When a person lacks decisional capacity, nurses must obtain consent for nursing care from a substitute decision-maker, subject to the laws in their jurisdiction. When prior wishes for treatment and care of an incompetent person are not known or are unclear, nurses' decisions must be made based on what the person would have wanted as far as is known, or failing that, decisions must be made in the best interest of the person in consultation with the family and other health care providers.

12. Nurses should respect a person's method of decision-making, recognizing that different cultures place different weight on individualism and often choose to defer to family and community values in decision-making (ANA, 2001). However, nurses should also advocate for the individual if that person's well-being is compromised by family, community or other health professionals.

Dignity

Nurses recognize and respect the inherent worth of each person and advocate for respectful treatment of all persons.

1. Nurses must relate to all persons receiving care as persons worthy of respect and endeavour in all their actions to preserve and demonstrate respect for the dignity and rights of each individual.

2. Nurses must be sensitive to an individual's needs, values and choices. Nurses should take into account the biological, psychological, social, cultural and spiritual needs of persons in health care.

3. Nurses must recognize the vulnerability of persons and must not exploit their vulnerabilities for the nurse's own interest or in a way that might compromise the therapeutic relationship. Nurses must maintain professional boundaries to ensure their professional

relationships are for the benefit of the person they serve. For example, they must avoid sexual intimacy with patients, avoid exploiting the trust and dependency of persons in their care and must not use their professional relationships for personal or financial gain.

4. Nurses must respect the physical privacy of persons when care is given, by providing care in a discreet manner and by minimizing unwanted intrusions.

5. Nurses must intervene if others fail to respect the dignity of persons in care.

6. Nurses must advocate for appropriate use of interventions in order to minimize unnecessary and unwanted procedures that may increase suffering.

7. Nurses must seek out and honour persons' wishes regarding how they want to live the remainder of their life. Decision-making about life-sustaining treatment is guided by these considerations.

8. Nurses should advocate for health and social conditions that allow persons to live and die with dignity.

9. Nurses must avoid engaging in any form of punishment, unusual treatment or action that is inhuman or degrading towards the persons in their care and must avoid complicity in such behaviours.

Confidentiality

Nurses safeguard information learned in the context of a professional relationship and ensure it is shared outside the health care team only with the person's informed consent, or as may be legally required, or where the failure to disclose would cause significant harm.

1. Nurses must respect the right of each person to informational privacy, that is, the individual's control over the use, access, disclosure and collection of their information.

2. Nurses must advocate for persons requesting access to their health record subject to legal requirements.

3. Nurses must protect the confidentiality of all information gained in the context of the professional relationship, and practice within relevant laws governing privacy and confidentiality of personal health information.

4. Nurses must intervene if other participants in the health care delivery system fail to maintain their duty of confidentiality.

5. Nurses must disclose a person's health information only as authorized by that person, unless there is substantial risk of serious harm to the person or to other persons or a legal obligation to disclose. Where disclosure is warranted, information provided must be limited to the minimum amount of information necessary to accomplish the purpose for which it has been disclosed. Further the number of people informed must be restricted to the minimum necessary.

6. Nurses should inform the persons in their care that their health information will be shared with the health care team for the purposes of providing care. In some circumstances nurses are legally required to disclose confidential information without consent. When this occurs nurses should attempt to inform individuals about what information will be disclosed, to whom and for what reason(s).

7. When nurses are required to disclose health information about persons, with or without the person's informed consent, they must do so in ways that do not stigmatize individuals, families or communities. They must provide information in a way that minimizes identification as much as possible.

8. Nurses must advocate for and respect policies and safeguards to protect and preserve the person's privacy.

Justice

Nurses uphold principles of equity and fairness to assist persons in receiving a share of health services and resources proportionate to their needs and promoting social justice.

1. Nurses must not discriminate in the provision of nursing care based on a person's race, ethnicity, culture, spiritual beliefs, social or marital status, sex, sexual orientation, age, health status, lifestyle, mental or physical disability and/or ability to pay.

2. Nurses must strive to make fair decisions about the allocation of resources under their control based upon the individual needs of persons in their care.

3. Nurses should put forward, and advocate for, the interests of all persons in their care. This includes helping individuals and groups gain access to appropriate health care that is of their choosing.

4. Nurses should promote appropriate and ethical care at the organizational/agency and community levels by participating in the development, implementation and ongoing review of policies and procedures designed to provide the best care for persons with the best use of available resources given current knowledge and research.

5. Nurses should advocate for health policies and decision-making procedures that are consistent with current knowledge and practice.

6. Nurses should advocate for fairness and inclusiveness in health resource allocation, including policies and programs addressing determinants of health, along with research based technology and palliative approaches to health care.

7. Nurses should be aware of broader health concerns such as environmental pollution, violations of human rights, world hunger, homelessness, violence, etc. and are encouraged to the extent possible in their personal circumstances to work individually as citizens or collectively for policies and procedures to bring about social change, keeping in mind the needs of future generations (ANA, 2001).

Accountability

Nurses are answerable for their practice, and they act in a manner consistent with their professional responsibilities and standards of practice.

1. Nurses must respect and practice according to the values and responsibilities in this *Code of Ethics for Registered Nurses* and in keeping with the professional standards, laws and regulations supporting ethical practice. They should use opportunities to help nursing colleagues be aware of this code and other professional standards.

2. Nurses have the responsibility to conduct themselves with honesty and to protect their own integrity in all of their professional interactions.

3. Nurses, in clinical, administrative, research or educational practice, have professional responsibilities and accountabilities toward safeguarding the quality of nursing care persons receive. These responsibilities vary, but all must be oriented to the expected outcome of safe, competent and ethical nursing practice.

4. Nurses should share their knowledge and provide mentorship and guidance for the professional development of nursing students and other colleagues/health care team members.

5. Nurse educators, to the extent possible, must ensure that students will possess the required knowledge, skills and competencies in order to graduate from nursing programs (ANA, 2001).

6. Nurse administrators/managers, to the extent possible, must ensure that only those nurses possessing the required knowledge, skills and competencies work in their practice areas.

7. Nurses should provide timely and accurate feedback to other nurses and colleagues in other disciplines and students about their practice, so as to support and recognize safe and competent practice, contribute to ongoing learning and improve care.

8. If nurses determine that they do not have the necessary physical, mental or emotional well-being to provide safe and competent care to persons, they may withdraw from the provision of care or decline to engage in care. However, they must first give reasonable notice to the employer, or if self-employed to their patients, and take reasonable action to ensure that appropriate action has been taken to replace them (RNABC, 2001).

9. Nurses planning to participate in job action or who practice in environments where job action occurs, must take steps (see Appendix A) to safeguard the health and safety of people during the course of the job action.

10. Nurses must give primary consideration to the welfare of the people they serve and to any possibility of harm in future care situations when they are pondering taking action with regard to suspected unethical conduct or incompetent or unsafe care. When nurses have reasonable grounds for concern about the behaviour of colleagues or about the safety of conditions in the care setting, they must carefully review the situation and take steps, individually or in partnership with others, to resolve the problem (see Appendix A).

11. Nurses should advocate for discussion of ethical issues among health team members, patients and families.

12. Nurses should advocate for changes to policy, legislation or regulations in concert with other colleagues and their professional associations or colleges, when there is agreement that these directives are unethical.

Quality Practice Environments

Nurses value and advocate for quality practice environments that have the organizational structures and resources necessary to ensure safety, support and respect for all persons in the work setting.

1. Nurses must advocate, to the extent possible within the circumstances, for sufficient human and material resources to provide safe and competent care.

2. Nurses individually or in partnership with others, must take preventive as well as corrective action to protect persons from incompetent, unethical or unsafe care.

3. If working short staffed, nurses must set priorities reflecting the allocation of resources. In such cases, nurses must endeavour to keep patients, families and employers informed about potential and actual changes to usual routines (CRNM, 2000).

4. Nurses must support a climate of trust that sponsors openness, encourages questioning the status quo and supports those who speak out publicly in good faith (e.g. whistle blowing). It is expected that nurses who engage in responsible reporting of incompetent, unsafe or unethical care or circumstances will be supported by their professional association.

5. Nurses must advocate for work environments in which nurses and other health workers are treated with respect and support when they raise questions or intervene to address unsafe or incompetent practice.

6. Nurses must seek constructive and collaborative approaches to resolve differences impacting upon care amongst members of the health care team and commit to compromise and conflict resolution.

7. Nurses are justified in using reasonable means to protect against violence when, following an informed assessment, they anticipate acts of violence toward themselves, others or property. In times when violence cannot be prevented or anticipated nurses are justified in taking self-protective action.

8. Nurse managers/administrators must strive to provide adequate staff to meet the requirements for nursing care as part of their fundamental responsibility to promote practice environments where fitness to practice and safe care can be maintained (AARN, 2001). With their staff, they should work towards the development of a moral community.[6]

9. As part of a moral community, nurses acknowledge their responsibility in contributing to quality practice settings that are positive, healthy working environments.

10. Nurses should collaborate with nursing colleagues and other members of the health team to advocate for health care environments conducive to ethical practice and to the health and well-being of clients and others in the setting. They do this in ways that are consistent with their professional role and responsibilities.

Glossary

Accountability: the state of being answerable to someone for something one has done (Burkhardt & Nathaniel, 2002).

Advance Directives: a person's written wishes about life-sustaining treatment meant to assist with decisions about withholding or withdrawing treatment (Storch, Rodney & Starzomski, 2002). Also called living wills or anticipatory health plans.

Assent: the agreement by a child or incapacitated person to a therapeutic procedure or involvement in research following the receipt of good information. Assent from the individual affected is encouraged in addition to informed consent from the guardian or parent.

---

6. A moral community is one where there is coherence between what the agency publicly professes to be their goal and what employees, persons in care, and others witness and participate in (Webster & Baylis, 2000). A moral community for nurses would include, for example, a community in which the development of effective teams was fostered, ethics education opportunities were available and provision was made for ethics rounds and/or an ethics committee.

Autonomy: self-determination; an individual's right to make choices about one's own course of action (AARN, 1996).

Belief: a conviction that something is true (AARN, 1996).

Confidentiality: means the duty to preserve a person's privacy.

Consent: see informed consent.

Ethical: a formal process for making logical and consistent decisions based upon ethical values.

Ethical Commitment: ethical obligations health providers have to those they serve.

Ethical/Moral Uncertainty: arises when one is unsure what ethical principles or values to apply or even what the ethical problem is (Jameton, 1984).

Fair: equalizing people's opportunities to participate in and enjoy life, given their circumstances and capacities (Caplan, Light & Daniels, 1999).

Health Care Team: a number of health care providers from different disciplines working in collaboration to provide care for individuals, families or the community.

Informational Privacy: is the right of persons to control the use, access, disclosure and collection of their information.

Informed Consent: a legal doctrine based on respect for the principle of autonomy of an individual's right to information required to make decisions.

Justice: a principle focusing on fair treatment of individuals and groups within society. Justice is a broader concept than fairness, one example of its application is the just allocation of resources at a societal level.

Moral Agent/Agency: The concept of moral agency reflects a notion of individuals engaging in self-determining or self-expressive ethical choice. Moral agency designates nurses enacting their professional responsibility and accountability through relationships in particular contexts. A moral agent is the individual involved in fulfilling moral agency (Rodney & Starzomski, 1993).

Moral Community: is a community in which there is coherence between what a healthcare organization publicly professes to be, i.e. a helping, healing, caring environment that embraces values intrinsic to the practice of healthcare, and what employees, patients and others both witness and participate in (Webster & Baylis, 2000).

Moral Residue: "… that which each of us carries from those times in our lives when in the face of ethical distress we have seriously compromised ourselves or allowed ourselves to be compromised" (Webster and Baylis, 2000, p. 218).

Nurse: Refers to registered nurse.

Physical Privacy: refers to withdrawing or being protected from public view, particularly applicable to protecting persons from exposure while providing body care.

Social Justice: involves attention to those who are most vulnerable in society, e.g. those who have been excluded or forgotten due to handicap, limited education or failing health.

Appendix A   Suggestions for Application of the Code in Selected Circumstances

Steps to address incompetent, unsafe and unethical care

- Gather the facts about the situation and ascertain the risks and undertake to resolve the problem;
- Review relevant legislation and policies, guidelines and procedures for reporting incidents or suspected incompetent or unethical care and report, as required, any legally reportable offence;
- Seek relevant information directly from the colleague whose behaviour or practice has raised concerns, when this is feasible;
- Consult, as appropriate, with colleagues, other members of the team, professional nurses' associations, colleges or others able to assist in resolving the problem;
- Undertake to resolve the problem as directly as possible consistent with the good of all parties;
- Advise the appropriate parties regarding unresolved concerns and, when feasible, inform the colleague in question of the reasons for your action;
- Refuse to participate in efforts to deceive or mislead persons about the cause of alleged harm or injury resulting from unethical or incompetent conduct.

Nurse managers/administrators, professional associations and client safety

- Nurse managers/administrators seek to ensure that available resources and competencies of personnel are used efficiently;
- Nurse managers/administrators intervene to minimize the present danger and to prevent future harm when persons' safety is threatened due to inadequate resources or for some other reason;
- Professional nurses' associations support individual nurses and groups of nurses in promoting fairness and inclusiveness in health resource allocation. They do so in ways that are consistent with their role and functions.

Considerations in student-teacher-client relationships

- Student-teacher and student-client encounters are essential elements of nursing education and are conducted in accordance with ethical nursing practices;
- Persons are informed of the student status of the care giver and consent for care is obtained in compliance with accepted standards;
- Students of nursing are treated with respect and honesty by nurses and are given appropriate guidance for the development of nursing competencies;
- Students are acquainted with and comply with the provisions of the code.

Considerations in taking job action

- Job action by nurses is often directed toward securing conditions of employment that enable safe and ethical care of current and future patients. However, action directed toward such improvements could work to the detriment of patients in the short term.
- Individual nurses and groups of nurses safeguard patients in planning and implementing any job action.
- Individuals and groups of nurses participating in job action, or affected by job action, share the ethical commitment to person's safety. Their particular responsibilities may lead them to express this commitment in different but equally appropriate ways.
- Persons whose safety requires ongoing or emergency nursing care are entitled to have those needs satisfied throughout any job action.
- Members of the public are entitled to information about the steps taken to ensure the safety of persons during any job action.

Appendix B   A Code of Ethics History

1954   CNA adopts the ICN Code as its first Code of Ethics

1980   CNA moves to adopt its own code entitled, *CNA Code of Ethics: An Ethical Basis for Nursing in Canada*

1985   CNA adopts new code called, *Code of Ethics for Nursing*

1991   *Code of Ethics* for Nursing revised

1997   *Code of Ethics for Registered Nurses* adopted as updated code for CNA

2002   *Code of Ethics for Registered Nurses* revised

The Canadian Nurses Association prepares position papers, ethics-issue specific practice papers, an ethical dilemma column in the *Canadian Nurse* journal, an ethics listserv, booklets and other ethics related resources. In addition, CNA works with other health professional associations and colleges to develop interprofessional statements (e.g. about no resuscitation policies, resolving conflict) related to issues or concerns of an ethical nature.

References

Alberta Association of Registered Nurses. (1996). *Ethical decision-making for registered nurses in Alberta: Guidelines and recommendations.* Edmonton: Author.

Alberta Association of Registered Nurses. (2001). *Working extra hours: Guidelines for registered nurses on fitness to practice and the provision of safe, competent, ethical nursing care.* Edmonton: Author.

American Nurses Association. (2001). *American Nurses Association code of ethics.* Washington: Author.

Burkhardt, M. A. & Nathaniel, A.K. (1998). *Ethics & issues in contemporary nursing.* Toronto: Delmar Publishers.

Canadian Nurses Association. (2002). *Ethical research guidelines for registered nurses* (3rd ed.). Ottawa: Author.

Caplan, R. L., Light, D. W. & Daniels, N. (1999). Benchmarks of fairness: A moral framework for assessing equity. *International Journal of Health Services, 29*(4): 853-869.

College of Registered Nurses of Manitoba. (2002). *Working short staffed.* Winnipeg: Author.

Jameton, A. (1984). *Nursing Practice: The ethical issues.* Englewood Cliffs, N.J.: Prentice Hall.

Mitchell, G. J. (2001). Policy, procedure, and routine: Matters of moral influence. *Nursing Science Quarterly, 14*(2): 109-114.

Registered Nurses Association of British Columbia. (2001). *Nursing Practice guidelines: Duty to provide care.* Vancouver: Author.

Rodney, P. & Starzomski, R. (1993). Constraints on moral agency of nurses. *Canadian Nurse, 89*(9), 23-26.

Storch, J., Rodney, P. & Starzomski, R. (2002). Ethics in health care in Canada. In B.S. Bolaria & H. Dickinson (Eds.), *Health, illness and health care in Canada* (3rd edition, pp. 409-444). Scarborough, ON: Nelson Thomas Learning.

Webster, G. & Baylis, F. (2000). Moral residue. In S. B. Rubin & L. Zoloth (Eds.), *Margin of error: The ethics of mistakes in the practice of medicine* (pp. 217-232). Hagerstown, MD: University Publishing Group.

Ethics Reading Resources

CNA Resources

Canadian Dental Association, Canadian Medical Association, Canadian Pharmacists Association, Canadian Health Care Association, Canadian Nurses Association, Consumer Association of Canada. (2000). *Principles for privacy protection of personal health information in Canada.* Ottawa: Authors.

Canadian Healthcare Association, Canadian Medical Association, Canadian Nurses Association, Catholic Health Association of Canada (with Canadian Bar Association). (1995). *Joint statement on resuscitative interventions.* Ottawa: Authors.

Canadian Home Care Association, Canadian Healthcare Association, Canadian Long Term Care Association, Canadian Nurses Association, Canadian Public Health Association, Home Support Canada. (1994). *Joint statement on advance directives.* Ottawa: Authors.

Canadian Healthcare Association, Canadian Medical Association, Canadian Nurses Association, Catholic Health Association of Canada. (1999). *Joint statement on preventing and resolving ethical conflicts involving health care providers and persons receiving care.* Ottawa: Authors.

Canadian Nurses Association. (1992). *The role of the nurse in the use of health care technology.* Ottawa: Author.

Canadian Nurses Association. (1994). *A question of respect: Nurses and end-of-life treatment dilemmas.* Ottawa: Author.

Canadian Nurses Association. (1998, May). Advance directives: The nurse's role. *Ethics in Practice.*

Canadian Nurses Association. (1998, June). Ethical issues related to appropriate staff mixes. *Ethics in Practice.*

Canadian Nurses Association. (1998). *Everyday ethics: Putting the code into practice.* Ottawa: Author.

Canadian Nurses Association. (1999, November). I see and am silent / I see and speak out: The ethical dilemma of whistleblowing. *Ethics in Practice.*

Canadian Nurses Association. (2000, September). Working with limited resources: Nurses' moral constraints. *Ethics in Practice.*

Canadian Nurses Association. (2001). *Nursing professional regulatory framework.* Ottawa: Author.

Canadian Nurses Association. (2001). *Privacy of personal health information.* Ottawa: Author.

Canadian Nurses Association. (2001). *Quality professional practice environments for registered nurses.* Ottawa: Author.

Canadian Nurses Association. (2001). *The role of the nurse in telepractice.* Ottawa: Author.

Canadian Nurses Association. (2001, May). Futility presents many challenges for nurses. *Ethics in Practice.*

Canadian Nurse—Ethical Dilemma Columns

Ellerton, M. L. (2000). When parents and children disagree about care. *Canadian Nurse, 96*(7), 35–36.

Ellerton, M. L. (2002). Client restraints: More than a safety issue. *Canadian Nurse, 98*(2), 32–33.

McAlpine, H. (2001). Refusal to care. *Canadian Nurse, 97*(6), 33–34.

Moorhouse, A. (2001). When CPR is not an option. *Canadian Nurse, 97*(1), 37–38.

Storch, J. (2000). Exposure to body fluids. *Canadian Nurse, 96*(6), 35–36.

Storch, J. (2002). When a client considers surrogacy. *Canadian Nurse, 98*(5), 32–33.

Infirmière canadienne—Articles on ethics

Saint-Arnaud, J. Technologies biomédicales et enjeux éthiques en soins infirmiers : La fin justifie-t-elle les moyens?, *infirmière canadienne,* 3 (4), 2002, p. 4-8.

Saint-Arnaud, J. Technologies biomédicales et enjeux éthiques en soins infirmiers : La vie, oui… mais à quel prix?, *infirmière canadienne,* 3 (3), 2002, p. 4-8.

Pelletier, C. Recherche sur la maltraitance infantile : Les incontournables de l'éthique, *infirmière canadienne,* 2 (6), 2001, p. 4-8.

Saint-Arnaud, J. Les théories éthiques et l'éthique des soins, *infirmière canadienne,* 2 (2), 2001, p. 8-10.

Saint-Arnaud, J. Pourquoi une chronique en éthique des soins?, *infirmière canadienne,* 1 (3), 2000, p. 10-11.

Provincial and Territorial Resources

Alberta Association of Registered Nurses. (1997). *Professional boundaries: A discussion paper on expectations for nurse-client relationships.* Edmonton: Author.

College of Nurses of Ontario. (1999). *Ethical framework for nurses in Ontario.* Toronto: Author.

College of Registered Nurses of Manitoba. (2002). *Professional boundaries for therapeutic relationships.* Winnipeg: Author.

Registered Nurses Association of British Columbia. (2000). *Advocacy and the registered nurse.* Vancouver: Author.

Registered Nurses Association of Nova Scotia. (1996). *Violence in the workplace: A resource guide.* Halifax: Author.

Registered Nurses Association of Nova Scotia. (2000). *Guidelines for telenursing practice.* Halifax: Author.

Other Resources

Nurses may consult with members of the health team, ethics committees, practice consultants at associations and colleges, religious leaders etc.

Austin, W. (2001). Nursing ethics in an era of globalization. *Advances in Nursing Science,* 24(2), 1–18.

Canadian Nurses Protective Society. (1993, September). Confidentiality of health information: Your client's right. *Info Law, 1*(2).

Canadian Nurses Protective Society. (1994, December). Consent to treatment: The role of the nurse. *Info Law, 3*(2).

Corley, M.C. and Goren, S. (1998). The dark side of nursing: Impact of stigmatizing responses on patients. *Scholarly Inquiry for Nursing Practice,* 12(2), 99–122.

International Council of Nurses. (1999). *Guidelines on coping with violence in the workplace.* Geneva: Author.

International Council of Nurses. (2000). *The ICN code of ethics for nurses.* Geneva: Author.

Johnstone, M. J. (1999). *Bioethics: A nursing perspective.* Toronto: Harcourt Saunders.

Peter, E. & Morgan, K. (2001). Explorations of a trust approach for nursing ethics. *Nursing Inquiry,* 8(1), 3-10.

Varcoe, C. and Rodney, P. (2002). Constrained agency: The social structure of nurses' work. In B. S. Bolaria and H. Dickinson (Eds.), *Health, Illness and health care in Canada,* (3rd ed., pp.102–128). Scarborough, ON: Nelson Thomas Learning.

Waters, W. F. (2001). Globalization, socioeconomic restructuring and community health. *Journal of Community Health,* 26(2), 79-92.

Webster, G. & Baylis, F. (2000). Moral residue. In S. B. Rubin & L. Zoloth (Eds.), *Margin of error: The ethics of mistakes in the practice of medicine* (pp. 217–232). Hagerstown, MD: University Publishing Group.

White, G. (2001). The code of ethics for nurses: Responding to new challenges in a new century. *American Journal of Nursing,* 101(10), 73, 75.

Yeo, M. & Moorhouse, A. (Eds.). (1996). *Concepts and cases in nursing ethics.* (2nd ed.). Peterborough, ON: Broadview Press.

Websites for International Documents on Human Rights

Numerous documents can be found on websites. For example, the *Universal Declaration on Human Rights, Article 25; International Convenant on Economic, Social and Cultural Rights, Article 12; International Convention on Elimination of all Forms of Racial Discrimination; Convention on Elimination of all Forms of Discrimination Against Women; Convention on the Rights of the Child; Convention on Torture and Other Cruel, Inhuman or Degrading Treatment or Punishment; UN Resolution 46/119 Protection of Persons with Mental Illness and Improvement of Mental Health Care; World Health Organization Constitution.*

http://www.un.org/rights

http://www.who.int/archives/who50/en/human.htm

http://www.unesco.org/ibc/index.html

Appendix D

Ethical Research Guidelines for Registered Nurses*

Contents

*Reprinted with permission from the Canadian Nurses Association.

© Canadian Nurses Association 50 Driveway Ottawa ON K2P 1E2
Tel: (613) 237-2133 or 1-800-361-8404 Fax: (613) 237-3520
E-mail: pubs@cna-aiic.ca Web site: www.cna-aiic.ca September 2002 ISBN 1-55119-894-0

These guidelines apply to all nurses. They speak to:

- Staff nurses caring for people who may be research subjects, or staff nurses who may be collecting information for the research team;
- Nurses who are engaged as research assistants on projects involving humans;
- Nurses who are engaged as research or clinical research coordinators (sometimes called research program directors) in health research;
- Nurses (i.e., principal or co-investigators) engaged in health research;
- Nurses who are members or chairs of research ethics boards or research review committees;
- Nursing administrators/managers who may be responsible for making provision for research ethics boards and for monitoring their activities; and
- Nursing educators who oversee the research of their students and/or teach research ethics.

Preamble

Canadian nurses value research that can lead to improved health for all. They are involved in caring for individuals and communities who are research subjects in health research,[1] or they are directly involved in the research process itself. This research may involve randomized controlled clinical trials or other experimental designs, other types of quantitative research and qualitative research including participatory action research. In all research involving human subjects, care must be taken to ensure the research design is procedurally and ethically rigorous. All those who agree to become human subjects must be informed about the purposes and methods of research, as well as the risks and benefits associated with participation. Further, they must freely volunteer to be involved. The research methodology must limit as much as possible exposure to risk and harm and make provisions for foreseen or inadvertent harms occurring as a result of the research. To that end, ethical guidelines for registered nurses in research involving human subjects are important for **all** nurses.

The intent of this document is to link ethical guidance for nurses involved in research with humans to the ethical guidance offered by the Code of Ethics for Registered Nurses (CNA, 2002). This code gives guidance for decision-making concerning ethical matters, serves as a means for self-evaluation and reflection regarding ethical practice and provides a basis for peer review initiatives (CNA, 2002). Much of the guidance for ethical nursing practice provided in the code can be applied to relationships with research subjects. However, the field of research ethics is changing rapidly and has become significantly more complex over the past years. Numerous national and international

---

1. Health research, for purpose of this document, includes research involving all health disciplines, medical, nursing and others.

guidelines now exist for both general and specific research. Thus, there is a need to provide nurses with an overview of research ethics, an update on resources available and references for consultation.

Introduction

The relationship of researcher and research subject must be characterized by trust. The public's trust in research is considered critical to the government's continuation of research funding and to the willingness of the public to volunteer for research. In order to maintain public trust, good ethics and procedurally rigorous research are requirements of good research (McDonald, 2000).

In Canada, several recent initiatives have been taken to promote greater attention to ethics in research involving humans and the protection of human subjects. In 1998, the three main federal granting agencies, the Social Sciences and Humanities Research Council (SSHRC), the Natural Sciences and Engineering Research Council (NSERC) and the Medical Research Council (MRC), released the *Tri-Council Policy Statement on the Ethical Conduct of Research Involving Humans* (TCPS, 1998). The TCPS was developed to protect human subjects in all types of research. In the previous year, Health Canada adopted the *Good Clinical Practice: Consolidated Guidelines* (*GCP*) to provide more specific guidelines for researchers and research coordinators involved in conducting clinical trial research (GCP, 1997). The *GCP* is based upon international agreements to harmonize technical requirements for registration of pharmaceuticals for human use. In June 2001, the *TCPS* was specified by Health Canada as the guideline for human subject research in Canada, with the *GCP* specified as the guideline for all clinical trial research involving human subjects. At the same time, Health Canada also provided additional regulations for clinical trials.[2] This latter set of regulations is important for all clinical trial research. When uncertainty exists in the interpretation or application of any of these guidelines, or when there appear to be conflicts among them, nurses should seek professional ethics advice or consult a Research Ethics Board (REB).

An important element of these official guidelines is that any research study involving human subjects must first be reviewed and approved by a research ethics committee before the research can proceed. Research ethics committees are formally called Research Ethics Boards (REBs)[3] in Canada and Institutional Review Boards (IRBs) in the United States. The composition and operating procedures for these boards are outlined in the TCPS guidelines.[4] Many of these REBs include nurses: some are chaired by nurses. The need to protect the persons who volunteer as subjects in health care research has increased. This has led to added responsibilities for all nurses. Nurses engaged in direct care also

---

2. On 7 June 2001 the Regulations Amending the Food and Drug Regulations (1024 – Clinical Trials) were published in the Canada Gazette, Part II, (2001-06-20).

3. The term Research Ethics Board was adopted in the Tri Council Policy as the Canadian designation of the committee with the mandate to conduct an ethical review of research proposals (and approve or disapprove the proposed research) involving human subjects. In health agencies across Canada, the actual title of this committee may vary, but in this document, the term Research Ethics Board refers to all the variously named committees designed to provide an ethics review of proposed research.

4. The TCPS (Tri-Council Policy Statement: Ethical conduct for research involving human subjects), Section 1.B.

need to know about the existence of these various guideline documents, about the need to protect human subjects and about the resource of an REB. Nurses engaged in research need to know and understand national guidelines and research ethics boards. In this document *Ethical Research Guidelines for Registered Nurses*, reference will be made to these other national guidelines and to other resources.

The values of CNA's *Code of Ethics for Registered Nurses* (2002) serve as an organizing framework for *Ethical Research Guidelines for Registered Nurses*. This capitalizes on the strength of the code, allows for consistency and coherence between the two ethics documents and allows for ease in location of specific guidelines. The eight primary values in the code, considered central to the practice of nursing, are the following:

- Safe, Competent and Ethical Care
- Health and Well-being
- Choice
- Dignity
- Confidentiality
- Justice
- Accountability
- Quality Practice Environments

These values are also primary values for nurses engaged in research with human subjects.

Registered Nurses and Research

Nurses are in a good position to know persons in their care well. Thus, they are able to recognize people who may be experiencing harmful or potentially harmful effects from the research study in which they are involved or are considering. Every nurse who interacts with people requiring care needs to appreciate the importance of the nurse's role in safeguarding individuals during research.

Nurses involvement in human subject research could include:

1. nurses acting as principal investigators or co-investigators on nursing or other health-related research studies (see Appendix A);
2. nurses serving as clinical research coordinator (or research program director) or as research assistant in medical, nursing or other health related research studies;
3. nurses in practice settings or working in academic settings where research studies are underway;
4. nurses chairing or serving on a research ethics board, or a local agency's research review committee or administrative review committee;
5. nurses serving in an administrative capacity with responsibility to provide for an REB that is appropriately composed and attentive to ethics guidelines; and
6. nurses sharing administrative responsibility for the ethical conduct of research with other managers or administering areas in which research is in progress.

From the perspective of the protection of human research subjects, all registered nurses are held to meet their provincial or territorial standards of practice, many of which speak to ethical conduct in patient or client care, like the *Code of Ethics for Registered Nurses* (CNA, 2002). While these standards, guidelines and codes are general in nature, they appropriately serve as the basis for the research specific guidelines in this document.

Nursing Values and Research

Nurses recognize and support the importance of research and its benefits. They are also aware of the risks and harms that research may pose. This section builds upon CNA's code of ethics and utilizes value statements with basic descriptors as they relate to research involving humans. In each area, one or more short case studies are provided to illustrate the value and complexity of ethical considerations in research with human subjects.

Safe, Competent and Ethical Research and Practice

Nurses value the ability to provide safe and competent nursing practice and to engage in nursing research to fulfill their ethical and professional obligations to the persons they serve.

1. Nurses engaged in research must comply with the *Code of Ethics for Registered Nurses* (2002) and conduct themselves with honesty and integrity in all their interactions with research subjects and research colleagues.

2. Nurses involved in research or in practice must be sensitive to the need to protect the integrity of the research design so the value of the research can be realized.

3. Nurses involved as principal investigators, clinical research coordinators or research assistants must base their research on relevant knowledge of research methods and continue to acquire new skills and knowledge to develop and maintain their level of competence in research.

4. Nurses involved in research, particularly as principal investigators or co-investigators, have an ethical duty to analyze their data with integrity, to disseminate both positive and negative findings of their research and to be fair in representing team responsibilities and authorship.

5. Nurses must be aware of conflict of interests and declare conflicts of interest to research ethics boards and research colleagues (see *TCPS* 1998, section 4).

Case Example	A STAFF NURSE WHO IS A MEMBER OF THE RESEARCH ETHICS BOARD EXPERIENCING A CONFLICT OF INTEREST

A senior staff nurse in a community hospital is an active promoter of nursing research in the hospital. She has done a great deal to facilitate and coach a small group of interested nurses to complete a research proposal and submit it for funding. The senior staff nurse also serves as a member of the research ethics board (REB). At the meeting where the nurses' research proposal is being reviewed, the

REB has difficulty reviewing the proposal, because of lack of familiarity with nursing research. The senior staff nurse educates the REB about nursing research methodologies. In this case, she cannot advocate for acceptance of this proposal, because she recognizes her conflict of interest due to her involvement in the research proposal. She raises this with the REB. The REB requests that she provide more information about the study and then asks her to leave the room while they discuss the acceptance or rejection of the proposal.

Health and Well-Being

In all research studies, care needs must never be sacrificed for research needs. All nurses must safeguard the person's physical and mental integrity, whether the person is involved in a research study or not.

1. Nurses engaged in nursing practice must hold people's optimum health and well-being as first and foremost in their interactions with all those they serve.

2. The priority accorded the person's well-being can often create conflict for research nurses, particularly research investigators, between their care-giver role and their research role. As a general rule, nurses should not be both care-giver and researcher unless there are good reasons to do so. In such cases, the REB needs to be convinced that a dual role[5] is justified and that ethical problems encountered in the dual role can be overcome.

3. If nurses providing direct care become involved in recruiting research subjects or in collecting data for the study, they must be mindful that their first duty is the health and well being of the persons for whom they are caring.

4. Nurses must recognize that most research imposes some level of risk for the research subject, thus it is important that the effects of involvement in the research project be carefully monitored. Nurses must be alert to risk, harm or the imposition of serious burden for persons for whom they are caring.

5. Nurses should value procedurally and ethically rigorous research that incorporates into the research design ways to minimize risk (eg. physical, psychological, financial) and protect persons from unnecessary burden.

6. Nurses should support research that has the potential to enhance the health and well-being of people.

7. Nurses should recognize the importance of bringing a nursing perspective to health research and engage with other health professionals in interdisciplinary health research promoting health and well being.

8. Nurses should recognize that health status is influenced by a variety of factors. Nurses have an important role in advocating for research that promotes greater emphasis on disease prevention and health promotion.

---

5. A dual role means a relationship in which a researcher also serves as caregiver or educator for the subjects involved in the research.

| Case Example | A STAFF NURSE ALERT TO POTENTIAL RISK/HARM FOR RESEARCH SUBJECT |

A staff nurse notices that one of the persons for whom she is caring is becoming extremely anxious over a 3–4 day period. He is having difficulty sleeping and has begun to worry about what seem to be minor issues in his life. His appetite has diminished and he is fidgety. The only change in the person's treatment plan is that during that same time period he was enrolled in a clinical drug trial—he began his course of medication five days ago. She is concerned that research might be jeopardizing the person's well-being. She decides to speak to the research coordinator to determine if the person's anxiety might be caused by the study drug.

| Case Example | A NURSE CLINICAL RESEARCH COORDINATOR EVALUATES BURDEN |

A nurse who is working as a clinical research coordinator is involved in a clinical trial in which a number of elderly men are required to travel to the clinic on a weekly basis for blood tests and other measurements. The nurse becomes concerned about the difficulties that these subjects experience in coming in for weekly monitoring since the visits are solely for research purposes. He discusses his concerns with the investigators, asking if they might be able to alter the monitoring plan by either scheduling clinic visits less often than weekly, or arranging for nurses to visit these subjects in their homes to conduct the monitoring (Fry and Veatch, 2000).

Choice

Nurses promote and respect the autonomy of persons involved in research and do their part in facilitating an informed choice (see *TCPS*, Section 2, Free and Informed Consent).

1. Nurses caring for people involved in research should do their part in ensuring that consent is free and informed. The investigator, or the individual designated by the investigator, should fully inform the subject of all pertinent aspects of the study including the type and level of commitment required and potential benefits and risks.

2. Nurses should help subjects and potential subjects to raise questions and receive appropriate information about the research, their level of participation, its potential benefits and its risks (see Appendix A).

3. If nurses see evidence of a deficit in the subject's understanding of the research project, they must contact the research coordinator or investigator.

4. Nurses must support and advocate the individual's right to decline to participate in research, or to withdraw from a study, and ensure to the extent possible that no discriminatory care arises from that person's choice.

5. Nurses caring for persons must be alert to any signs that these individuals feel pressured or coerced into participating in a research study. If they suspect that these individuals feel pressured or coerced, nurses must advise the investigator and/or the agency's REB.

6. Nurses, who are directly involved in research involving human subjects must ensure the person's consent is informed and voluntary, be clear in explaining the research and ensure there is adequate time for questions. In addition, nurse researchers must ensure that they do not apply coercion or manipulation in obtaining consent.

7. Nurses serving as research investigators, clinical research coordinators or research assistants must be particularly mindful of the power imbalances and the ways in which people may feel coerced or influenced to consent to involvement in a study. For example, people may feel obliged to agree to participate in a study because of a sense of loyalty to a physician, a nurse or other care provider who is the researcher. Further, people may participate, because they believe that the quality of the care they will receive depends upon their participation. In addition, people may be coerced if they believe that their participation is the only means by which they may have access to expensive or innovative treatments. Finally, paying individuals to be involved in a research project can also be a form of coercion.

8. In some cases, cultural sensitivity may require that researchers seek permission from community leaders, councils or families before they can approach potential research subjects. Often the community or family may also be involved in the informed consent process. Nurses involved in such research must be respectful of the norms of the culture while seeking ways to be assured of the individual's consent or assent (eg. translation and interpreter services).

9. Nurses must respect adults who are unable to provide consent due to lack of decisional capacity and ensure they are protected. Each province may have laws or guidelines regarding a substitute decision-maker's ability to consent on behalf of a person. In most cases, a substitute decision-maker can only consent to involve an incapacitated or incompetent person in a research study if that study involves minimal risk. Even when a substitute decision-maker consents, nurses should seek the assent of the individual research subject.

10. Nurses must also be aware of provincial legislation and guidelines when children are recruited as research subjects. Nurses should first seek the child's consent. In cases where parents or guardians have given authorization to the child's participation, nurses should also seek the assent of the child (NCEHR, 1994).

Benefits and Risks of Research

Benefits may include:

- access to potentially helpful interventions;
- contact/access to a clinical research coordinator who may facilitate continuity of care and provide support;
- modest material or financial gain (e.g. a stipend for being a research subject);

- satisfaction in having contributed to a worthwhile project, which can lead to increased self-esteem;
- a sense of purpose, an opportunity to help others;
- an opportunity to ventilate anger or to express feelings; or/and
- an opportunity for increased insight or self-knowledge.

Risks to avoid or minimize may include:

- the potential for physiological harms;
- psychological harm such as increased anxiety, guilt, fear, false hope, self doubt, loss of privacy or re-traumatization;
- social harm such as stigma by being included in a research study on alcohol abuse, HIV-AIDS, anorexia, bipolar disorder, etc.; or/and
- economic harm such as costs of being involved in the study (child care, travel time, days off work), threats of job loss and/or loss of life insurance if participation in the study becomes known.

(Talbot, 1995; Norwood, 2000)

| Case Example | A NURSE CLINICAL RESEARCH COORDINATOR CONFIRMING CONSENT |

A nurse serving as a clinical research coordinator on a medical research study (a clinical drug trial) is required to confirm the consents of individuals who volunteered to be part of the clinical trial. The person considering becoming a research subject has already been given printed information from her physician-investigator, along with a discussion of the study in the physician's office the previous week. As the nurse research coordinator proceeds to review the information with the individual prior to asking for a signed consent, the person tells the nurse that she would prefer not to be part of the clinical trial. She states she felt duty bound to help her physician with his study. The nurse research coordinator considers the research guidelines on 'choice' and decides this client has not chosen to participate freely. The nurse coordinator postpones confirming the consent until she can speak to the physician. She re-assures the person that quality of her care will not be jeopardized by her decision to decline to participate. The nurse clinical research coordinator then speaks with the physician-investigator, asking that he reassure the person that her care will not be jeopardized.

Dignity

Nurses involved in studying or caring for people involved as human subjects in research must ensure their dignity is respected.

1. Nurses demonstrate equal respect for persons who choose to become research subjects and for those who choose not to participate.

2. Nurses, whether directly involved in research or providing care, are often involved in recruiting persons to be research subjects. In recruitment, nurses must carefully consider when a person should be approached for involvement in a study. Even when the person matches the criteria the researchers are seeking, nurses must consider first the well being of the person in making an approach or in suggesting to researchers that such an approach/request might be made. At the same time, nurses should be sensitive to the desire of individuals to be given opportunities to be involved in research.

3. Nurses providing care must intervene if researchers fail to respect the dignity of people who are involved as research or potential research subjects. Nurses may, for example, seek to obtain more information from the researchers and alert them to concerns about the study, contact the REB to gain more information and express their concerns or approach their supervisor to register their concern. Nurses should advocate for subjects or potential subjects:

   - if nurses suspect the researchers have used coercive tactics in gaining subject consent;
   - if they believe information provided about the research project is inadequate or dishonest;
   - if the researchers fail to minimize harm to the subject's well-being;
   - if the researchers do not provide opportunities for the subject to withdraw from the study; or/and
   - if the study is not discontinued when there is good evidence that one treatment is superior to another.

4. Nurses should respect the process by which communities determine whether and under what conditions research can be conducted (e.g. First Nations communities).

Case Example	PUBLIC HEALTH NURSES ANTICIPATING RISKS IN RECRUITMENT

Public health nurses were asked by a team of investigators to assist them in developing a research proposal for a study on parents' responses to sudden infant death syndrome (SIDS). The nurses were concerned that the investigators did not understand the trauma some of the parents might experience in being studied. Keeping in mind the need to ensure that the dignity of the people in their care must be respected, both in approaching them for involvement in such a study and in protecting them from research risks, the nurses discussed their concerns with the investigators. They urged the researchers to be sensitive to the psychological risks involved for these parents. They also asked the researchers to build the provision for counselling assistance into their study in the event that some parents' grief or guilt might surface.

Confidentiality

Nurses observe practices that protect the anonymity of each human subject in research whenever possible. When that is not possible, they protect the confidentiality of each research subject's personal and health information. They should also intervene if others fail to protect this information (see *TCPS*, Section 3, Privacy and Confidentiality).

1. Nurses caring for persons involved in research must be attentive to the subject's privacy and exercise caution in use, access, collection and disclosure of information. They should be aware of relevant provincial legislation about the confidentiality of health and research information.

2. Nurse research investigators, clinical research coordinators and research assistants must find ways to manage information to fulfill their obligation of not divulging identifying information learned in the research. Strategies typically include disguising the subject's identity by the use of pseudonyms and distorting non-relevant information, reporting data as a group response rather than by individual response, separating identifying information such as name or chart number from study data, securing pledges of confidentiality from research personnel and limiting access to the data through careful storage of data (Talbot, 1995; Norwood, 2000).

3. Nurse research investigators must be sensitive to the subject's need to have his/her identity protected. It may be necessary to secure optional places for data collection (i.e. interviews, focus groups, etc.) so that no one knows that the particular subject is part of a study.

4. Nurses must be aware and should inform the research subject if the release of some research data may be required e.g., by statute or common law, sponsors or the REB for monitoring purposes.

5. Nurse researchers, clinical research coordinators and research assistants must inform human subjects about the limits to confidentiality prior and during data collection. For example, revelation of child abuse by the abuser (who is a research subject) would create an obligation on the nurses to report this to child welfare authorities. These are often difficult situations to anticipate at the onset of the study, but nurses must be sensitive to the flow of information being given, particularly in qualitative research and inform the subject when protection of confidentiality would no longer be possible and disclosure of information would be required.

6. In all cases where research data must be released, nurses should release only the minimum amount of data required and restrict the number of people to whom data is released.

7. In research with communities, nurses must protect subjects from unnecessary exposure, particularly if the information has the potential to stigmatize the community.

Case Example	A NURSE INVESTIGATOR DEALING WITH RELEASE OF PERSONAL RESEARCH INFORMATION

A nurse investigator is studying the experience of adult children who are caring for their elderly parents. In his qualitative research study, he is listening to middle aged individuals sharing the rewards and trials of being thrust into the role of care-giver. One of his subjects becomes very emotional and blurts out that on several occasions she has struck her mother as a result of frustration in dealing with her mother who is suffering from dementia. The investigator knows that, in this particular province, legislation exists that requires mandatory reporting of such information, yet he has promised the subjects that their information will be kept in confidence. He feels caught between breaking a promise to the subject and knowing that this mother is at risk of harm if he does not report it.

He considers these competing obligations, and seeks guidance from his professional colleagues and his professional regulatory body to find ways to report the matter in a way that is sensitive to the dynamics of the relationship.

Justice

Nurses must promote unbiased selection of research projects and research subjects so that methodologically rigorous and ethically sound research has the potential to benefit all. Nurses must work to influence research and research agendas to promote principles of equity and fairness (see *TCPS*, Section 5, Inclusion in Research and Section 6, Research Involving Aboriginal People).

1. Nurses must seek to ensure that all persons have access to opportunities, subject to availability, to be involved as research subjects.
2. Nurses must safeguard against an unfair burden being placed upon one group over another, for example, the over-use of institutionalized elderly, populations of prisoners, students, employees or military personnel who may be used as research subjects because of their easy accessibility (Talbot, 1995).
3. Nurses should be sensitive to subjects' potential sense of abandonment following a study and should anticipate and advocate for the services and treatments subjects may continue to require once the research is over.
4. Nurses should promote participatory research where research subjects can work in partnership with researchers in design, implementation and dissemination of research.
5. Nurses should promote research reflective of diversity in society, i.e., race, ethnicity, culture, spiritual beliefs, social or marital status, sex, sexual orientation, age, health status, lifestyle, physical and mental attributes.
6. Nurses involved in international research must ensure that their proposed study is reviewed by the appropriate REB and relevant research review bodies in the country where the research will be conducted.
7. Nurses involved in international research should, to the extent possible, ensure that the research responds to the health needs of the population being studied, since only then can it offer potentially relevant benefits to the population (NBAC, 2001).
8. Nurses must raise concerns if claims for use of equipment for research purposes take preference over people's need for diagnosis and treatment.

Case Example	A NURSE INVESTIGATOR CONSIDERS INCLUDING HER EMPLOYEES AS RESEARCH SUBJECTS

A nurse investigator wishes to conduct a study involving some of the employees with whom she works. She is a

nurse manager completing her master's program in nursing, and her research focuses on improving the environment for nursing practice. She wishes to observe and interview staff nurses, some of whom report to her in her managerial role. She wonders about the conflict of interests that might arise because of her roles, as administrator and research investigator. She considers various ethical codes and guidelines and determines that asking her staff to be subjects in her research could put them in a compromising position. She also notes that their inclusion might lead to questions about the validity of her findings. Although she will lose a significant group of nurses and her data collection will be more challenging if she does not include her own staff, she decides to exclude them.

Accountability

Nurses involved in research directly (as investigators, coordinators or assistants) conduct their research in a procedurally rigorous manner consistent with ethical guidelines for research provided by their professional organizations, federal government agencies and international bodies. They seek to keep abreast of emerging ethical issues in research and participate in promoting strategies that protect people who serve as human subjects.

1. Nurses engaged in research must conduct the research within their own level of competence. Even if others assume that nurses know and should be able to perform certain research interventions required in the study, nurses must advise researchers and clinical staff if they do not feel they have the level of competence needed to perform these tasks. If placed in such a position, they should seek information and help from investigators and other knowledgeable researchers.

2. Nurses who are research investigators must accurately represent their qualifications for research. They are responsible for the research design, supervision of research personnel, the standard and process of informed consent, the monitoring of the project, confidentiality of the research data, the dissemination of findings and fostering the transfer of research knowledge into practice and policy.

3. Nurses must observe Canadian guidelines (e.g. the Tri-Council Policy Statement, Good Clinical Practice Guidelines) and good practices in all research.

4. When nurses agree to serve on an REB, they must ensure they acquire adequate information and preparation for this ethical responsibility, including knowledge of applicable national and international regulations and guidelines.

5. Nurses, individually or in partnership, must take preventive as well as corrective action to protect persons from unsafe, incompetent or unethical research practices. If nurses suspect a breach of research ethics, they have an obligation to report their concern. They should review ethical guidelines for research, speak to knowledgeable colleagues, undertake to resolve the problem directly if it is feasible or report it to the principal investigator or the chair of the REB. Nurses caring for persons who are research subjects should take these initial steps outlined and discuss their concerns with their supervisor or with the REB.

6. Nurses responsible for administering REBs must monitor research within their agency to ensure that standard operating procedures are being followed according to protocol and that research is conducted according to ethical guidelines.

7. Nurses engaged in research and nurse educators should seek to ensure their students learn about research design, research ethics and the need for ethics approval. They should also help students be aware of their level of competence in conducting research.

8. Nurse educators must ensure that graduate students conducting research are well supervised and attentive to research ethics at all times. This is particularly critical when students are engaged in research in countries where few ethical research guidelines exist. If graduate student supervision is not possible in such cases, the research should not be approved.

Case Example	A NURSE RESEARCH ASSISTANT IS CONCERNED ABOUT HER COMPETENCE

A registered nurse with less than one year of experience in clinical practice agrees to work as a research assistant on a medical research study with a very busy principal investigator. At the interview for the position, the research investigator explains the role the research assistant is required to take in the study. The registered nurse is comfortable with the description and is certain she has the qualifications to do the job described. However, after the study begins, she finds she is frequently placed in the very uncomfortable position of being expected to conduct assessments she is not yet competent to do, and there is no one to help her learn these new procedures. She carefully considers her ethical dilemma. She worries about harming the research subjects by making a mistake and/or invalidating the project, thereby wasting everyone's time and research resources. Yet, she enjoys this type of nursing, and she needs the job to support her family. She decides to meet with the principal investigator to tell him that she needs training to do the tasks he is asking her to do, and if training cannot be provided, she will have to resign. This would be a costly proposition for her, but she believes it is the right thing to do.

Quality Research Environments

Nurses advocate for research environments enabling nursing and other types of research to be conducted in such a way that protects human subjects and is procedurally and ethically rigorous.

1. Nurses advocate for a research environment that fosters:
   - voluntary and non-coercive consent;
   - non-pressured recruitment of research subjects, e.g., they are not working for rewards based on the number of subjects they recruit;
   - safe disclosure of ethical concerns in research;
   - freedom to raise questions about research agendas, clinical studies and research infrastructure;

- collegial and mutually supportive relationships between researchers and clinical staff are; and
- protection of research data, e.g., storage.

2. Nurses involved in research should share their knowledge about processes in research design and implementation with other nurses and the health care team. They should provide mentorship and guidance for student nurses who are developing knowledge and skills in research as well as for staff and practising nurses.

3. Nurses seeking employment as clinical research coordinators or research assistants must accurately state their level of competence and seek reasonable assurance that employment conditions will permit research consistent with the values and responsibilities articulated in these guidelines and in the *Code of Ethics for Registered Nurses* (2002).

Case Example	A NURSE CLINICAL RESEARCH COORDINATOR SEEKING TO PROTECT PRIVACY

A nurse who works as a clinical research coordinator on a nursing research project is involved in obtaining the subjects' consent for the research study. This study entails interviews that will include some highly personal information about the subjects' mental health over their lifetime. The subjects are being recruited from a group of outpatients in a mental health clinic. Even as the nurse coordinator tries to obtain consent, she realizes the area in which the research team will be interviewing is not private. It is a highly visible area and conversations can be easily heard. She is troubled about obtaining consent in such a setting and even more concerned about the inevitable lack of privacy that would prevail during the interviews planned for the study. She decides to bring this matter to the attention of the nurse investigator, and she assists the investigator in locating a more appropriate interview space.

Glossary

Accountability: to be answerable to oneself and others for one's own actions (ANA, 2001)

Anonymity: means client information is de-identified and non-linkable, i.e., no one knows who is the participant in the research study, and there is no way to link responses to individual subjects (Norwood, 2000)

Assent: the agreement by a child or incapacitated person to a therapeutic procedure or involvement in research following the receipt of good information; assent from the individual affected is encouraged in addition to informed consent/authorization from the guardian or parent

CIHR: Canadian Institutes for Health Research, which funds health research in Canada

Clinical research coordinator: a person responsible for all aspects of managing a clinical research study, is accountable to the principal investigator

Clinical study nurse: a nurse responsible for data collection and other aspects of the research study (see research assistant)

Clinical trial/study: an experiment involving a test of the effectiveness of a clinical treatment, generally involving a large and heterogeneous sample of subjects (Polit, Beck & Hungler, 2001)

Confidentiality: protection of subjects in a study such that their individual identities will not be linked to the information they provide and will never be publicly divulged (Polit, Beck & Hungler, 2001)

Dual role: a relationship in which a researcher also serves as care-giver or educator for the subjects involved in the research

Good Clinical Practice: Consolidated Guideline (*GCP*): a document that includes the standard for the design, conduct, performance, monitoring, auditing, recording, analyses and reporting clinical trials, following the guide provides assurance that the data and reported results are credible and accurate and that the rights, integrity and confidentiality of trial subjects are protected (GCP, 1997)

Health research: research undertaken by all health disciplines – medical, nursing and other disciplines involved in studying health and illness

Human subjects: patients or people who have agreed to be participants in human research

Informed consent: a legal doctrine based on respect for the principle of autonomy of an individual's right to information required to make decisions

Institutional Review Board (IRB): United States equivalent of the Canadian Research Ethics Board (REB)

MRC: stood for Medical Research Council, a health research funding body that existed until April 2000 when it was transformed into the Canadian Institutes for Health (CIHR)

Minimal risk: anticipated risks not greater than those encountered by the person in his or her every day life (*TCPS*, 1998)

Monitoring: the act of overseeing the progress of research and ensuring it is conducted, recorded and reported in accordance with the research protocol and in keeping with rigorous research design

NCEHR: the National Council on Ethics in Human Research, an independent national organization designed to advance the protection and well-being of human subjects in research and to foster high ethical standards for the conduct of research involving humans by assisting REBs through educational offerings and site visits

NSERC: the Natural Sciences and Engineering Research Council of Canada, funds bio-medical and psychological research

Nurse: Refers to registered nurse

PRE: the Panel on Research Ethics, a tri-council panel mandated to review and update the *TCPS*

Principal investigator (Co-principal investigator): a person who is the lead researcher and has primary responsibility for overseeing the project

Privacy: the right of an individual to control the use, collection, access and disclosure of information; physical privacy refers to withdrawing or being protected from public view

Program Director: a person responsible for managing all aspects of the research study and accountable to the principal investigator (see clinical research coordinator, term often reserved for clinical research)

Qualitative research: a blanket definition for all forms of social inquiry relying primarily on qualitative data, aims at understanding the meaning of human action and its data are generally in the form of words (Schwandt, 2001)

Quantitative research: a term used to refer to any type of design (e.g. experimental or survey) or procedure (e.g. statistical) that relies mainly on the use of numeric data (Schwandt, 2001)

Research assistant: a person who serves as assistant to the principal investigator and research coordinator in a study

Research Ethics Board (REB): the Canadian designation for the committee that is designed to conduct ethical review of research proposals and approve or disapprove the research proceeding

Serious Adverse Events (SAE): any untoward medical occurrence that at any dose of a drug results in death, is life-threatening, requires hospitalization, results in significant disability or is a congenital anomaly/birth defect

SSHRC: the Social Science and Humanities Research Council, a granting body that funds social sciences and health research

Tri-Council Policy Statement (TCPS): a document designated as the guideline for all research involving human subjects in Canada

Appendix A

A Summary of Ethical Obligations in Research According to Role
WHAT STAFF NURSES NEED TO KNOW

1. Some persons in their care may be involved in research studies.
2. They have a duty to ensure that all persons they care for receive high quality care, whether they choose to be research subjects or not.
3. People have made an informed and voluntary choice to participate in a research project and that, if the research subject seems unclear about the purposes of various interventions, nurses should remind them about the research and contact the investigator or coordinator to assess the person's willingness to continue in the study.
4. The agency in which they work should have, or have access to, a Research Ethics Board (REB) or a similar committee designated to review research proposals against the standard of research ethics guidelines.
5. They have a duty to question the effects of the research on persons in their care and to raise any concerns. They may, for example, want to speak to a member of the research team or the REB Chair.

6. They have a right to information about the expectations of research investigators in terms of data collection, patient monitoring, etc. since these may impose an added burden on nursing resources for which they are not staffed. If these requirements are found to be unworkable due to the level of knowledge needed, excessive workload or conflicting values that could compromise the care of those they serve, nurses should register their concerns with their supervisors and/or the investigators.

WHAT RESEARCH COORDINATORS, RESEARCH ASSISTANTS, CO-INVESTIGATORS AND PRINCIPAL INVESTIGATORS NEED TO KNOW

1. They have a responsibility to choose research studies that are relevant and timely for health care and nursing.

2. There are common research ethics guidelines, such as the Tri-Council Policy, Good Clinical Practices Guidelines and Regulations from Health Canada, governing research with human subjects.

3. They must receive ethics approval from an REB before commencing research that involves human subjects.

4. They must ensure a high standard of consent by the research subject, including continuing consent, with attention to both the information given and the subjects' comprehension of that information (see *TCPS* Section 2 – Free and Informed Consent).

5. They are responsible for preventing known harms and minimizing harmful effects of the research and must be sensitive to person's physiological, psychological and social reactions as well as response to interventions. They have a responsibility to identify, report and manage serious adverse side effects, always keeping the well-being of the person/subject foremost in their thinking and actions.

6. Their role in protecting privacy and confidentiality of personal information and research subject information is significant (see *TCPS* Section 3 – Privacy and Confidentiality).

7. They need to be mindful of the research subject at the close of the study and attempt to link subjects to other resources, similar to those provided through the study, if that is important for the person's well-being.

ADDITIONAL RESPONSIBILITIES FOR PRINCIPAL INVESTIGATORS

1. They carry ultimate responsibility to create a methodologically rigorous research design that minimizes risks to human subjects and conforms to research ethics guidelines.

2. Their selection of subjects for their study must be sensitive to inclusiveness of the population, for example, the ability of the subject to be involved in the approach taken in the study. For example, a qualitative research project in which subjects are required to describe their inner world of feelings may be difficult for those who have not known the sharing of basic emotions and feelings with others (Crigger, Holcomb & Weiss, 2001).

3. They must ensure that research staff are fully trained and that such training is documented. They are fully responsible for overseeing all aspects of the research study. They must also ensure their research staff understands the significance of the study, of

sound data collection, of careful analysis and of handling research data. They should never place a research staff member in a position beyond his/her competency.

4. They should ensure they, or a knowledgeable co-investigator, are available to respond to the research subject should that person wish to speak with them.

5. They must remain sensitive to the type of data being collected and allow sufficient time for their researchers or themselves to build relationships with subjects prior to some types of data collection, for example, mentally ill persons who may need time to develop trust and acquaint themselves with the researcher.

6. In dealing with research data, they must exercise care in reporting findings, for example, in qualitative research, they must strive to protect the privacy of the research subject in their reporting. Confidentiality must be maintained when dealing with all research data.

7. They report all findings, even those where there may be, for example, discrepancies between theory and practice or where they may experience negative reaction from their colleagues.

8. If they oversee the research of students, they must ensure the student's research conforms to ethical standards. They must communicate the importance of research integrity verbally and in their actions.

WHAT NURSES SERVING ON RESEARCH ETHICS BOARDS AND NURSES IN ADMINISTRATION MAKING PROVISION FOR RESEARCH ETHICS BOARDS NEED TO KNOW

1. There are a series of ethical guidelines governing research involving human subjects such as the *Tri-Council Policy Statement*, 1998; *Good Clinical Practice Guidelines*, 1997; and Health Canada Regulations, 2001, by which REBs are to assess the research proposals they review.

2. The composition of REBs is set according to the *TCPS*, and meetings of this committee are to be face to face. There are also a series of stipulations about the processes the REBs are to employ (see *TCPS* Section 1, Ethics Review).

3. There are national agencies designed to promote high ethical standards of research ethics that offer workshops and additional guidance. They can be consulted if there is difficulty in performing the reviews.

4. They must assess whether the clinical environment can safely accommodate a research project and whether research funds can adequately reimburse the unit or agency for human and material resources used in the project.

5. Human research subject protection and well-being remain the foremost concern.

Appendix B

A Brief History of CNA's Ethical Guidelines for Nurses Involved in Research

In 1980 a discussion paper entitled Guidelines for Ethics in Nursing Research was prepared during CNA's Code of Ethics Project. This paper served as the background for preparation of the first CNA guidelines for research.

1983 Ethical Guidelines for Nursing Research Involving Human Subjects

This document defined nursing research and established three key areas of guidance; the scientific merit of the research, the relationship of mutual trust between subject and researcher manifested in attention to informed consent, confidentiality, protection of client well-being, and the setting where the research is done.

1994 Ethical Guidelines for Nurses in Research Involving Human Participants

A revision to the 1983 guidelines. The foci of these guidelines were to provide nurses in all domains of practice with guidelines relevant to the complex realities of research. Based upon relevant value statements from CNA's 1991 *Code of Ethics for Nursing*, it encompassed nursing research and research related to other disciplines. It provided case examples and used the word participants rather than subjects to characterize the relationship of researcher and research volunteer.

2002 Ethical Research Guidelines for Registered Nurses

This document is designed to provide nurses with guidance in research involving humans. It is developed to complement the CNA 2002 *Code of Ethics for Registered Nurses* (which provides guidelines for research relative to each of the eight values of the code) and to alert nurses to current national guidelines for research ethics as well as to complement those guidelines. In addition, it makes explicit reference to the range of roles nurses take in human subject research, from staff nurses and student nurses caring for a person on a research protocol to nurses who serve as research assistants, clinical research coordinators, principal investigators and on REBs.

REFERENCES

American Nurses Association. (2001). *American Nurses Association code of ethics.* Washington: Author.

Canadian Nurses Association. (2002). *Code of ethics for registered nurses.* Ottawa: Author.

College of Nurses of Ontario. (1999). *The ethical framework for nurses in Ontario.* Toronto: Author.

Fry, S. T. & Veatch, R. M. (2000). *Case studies in nursing ethics* (2nd ed.). Toronto: Jones & Bartlett Publishers.

Health Canada. (1997). Good clinical practice: Consolidated guideline. Therapeutic products directorate guidelines: ICH harmonised tripartite guideline. *International conference on harmonisation of technical requirements for the registration of pharmaceuticals for human use.* Ottawa: Ministry of Public Works and Government Services Canada. [Available through Health Canada Publications, Brooke Claxton Building, A.L.#0913A, Tunney's Pasture, Ottawa ON K1A 0K9]

Health Canada. (2001). Regulations amending the food and drug regulations (1024 – *Clinical Trials*). *Canada Gazette,* Part II, 135(13).

McDonald, M. (2000). *The governance of health research in Canada.* Ottawa: Law Commission of Canada.

Medical Research Council of Canada, Natural Sciences and Engineering Research Council of Canada & Social Science and Humanities Council of Canada. (1998). *Tri-Council Policy Statement: Ethical Conduct for Research Involving Humans.* Ottawa: Authors.

National Bioethics Advisory Council. (2001). *Ethical and policy issues in international research: Clinical trials in developing countries.* Bethesda, MD: Author.

National Council on Ethics in Human Research. (1994). *Research involving children.* Ottawa: Author.

National Council on Ethics in Human Research. (1999). *Research involving aboriginal individuals and communities: Genetics as a focus.* Proceedings of a Workshop of the NCEHR Consent Committee.

Norwood, S. L. (2000). *Research strategies.* New Jersey: Prentice Hall.

Schwandt, T. (2001). *Dictionary of qualitative inquiry* (2nd ed.). Thousand Oak: Sage.

Talbot, L. A. (1995). *Principles and practice of nursing research.* Toronto: Mosby.

READING RESOURCES

Beauchamp, T. & Childress, J. (2001). *Principles of biomedical ethics* (4th ed.). New York: Oxford University Press.

Canadian Association of Universities of Northern Studies. (1997). *Ethical principles for the conduct of research in the north.* Ottawa: Author.

Crigger, N. J., Holcomb, L., & Weiss, J. (2001). Applying ethical guidelines in nursing research on people with mental illness. *Nursing Ethics, 8*(5), 459-468.

Grinyer, A. (2001). Ethical dilemmas in nonclinical health research from a UK perspective. *Nursing Ethics, 8*(2), 123-132.

International Council of Nursing. (1996). *Ethical guidelines for nursing research.* Geneva: Author.

National Council on Ethics in Human Research. (1996). *Informed choice in research.* Ottawa: Author.

Polit, D. F., Beck, C. T., & Hungler, B. P. (2001). *Essentials of nursing research: Methods, appraisal and utilization* (5th ed.). New York: Lippincott.

Silva, M. (1995). *Ethical guidelines in the conduct, dissemination, and implementation of nursing research.* Washington, D.C.: American Nurses Association.

Strumpf, N. & Gamroth, L. (1989). Ethics and research in teaching nursing homes. In M. Mezey, J. Lynaugh & M. Cartier (Eds.), *Nursing homes and nursing care: Lessons from the teaching nursing home.* New York: Springer Publishing.

Yeo, M. & Moorhouse, A. (Eds.). (1996). *Concepts and cases in nursing ethics* (2nd ed.). Peterborough, Ontario: Broadview Press.

Websites

Canadian Institutes of Health Research (CIHR)   **www.cihr.ca**

Canadian Health Services Research Foundation (CHSRF)   **www.chsrf.ca**

Health Canada (HC)   **www.hc-sc.gc.ca**

Inter-Agency Panel on Research Ethics (IPRE)   **www.nserc.ca/programs/ethics/english/index.htm**

National Council on Ethics in Human Research (NCEHR)   **www.ncehr.org**

Solicitor General of Canada   **www.sgc.gc.ca/index_e.asp** (research on inmates)

Canadian Nurses Association 50 Driveway Ottawa ON K2P 1E2   Tel: (613) 237-2133 or 1-800-361-8404   Fax: (613) 237-3520   E-mail: pubs@cna-aiic.ca   Web site: **www.cna-aiic.ca**   ISBN 1-55119-894-0

Index